Atlas of
Echocardiography

Second Edition

Editor-in-Chief

Scott D. Solomon, MD

Director, Noninvasive Cardiac Laboratory
Cardiovascular Division
Brigham and Women's Hospital
Associate Professor of Medicine
Harvard Medical School
Boston, Massachusetts

Series Editor

Eugene Braunwald, MD, MD (Hon), ScD (Hon)

Distinguished Hersey Professor of Medicine
Harvard Medical School
Chairman, TIMI Study Group
Brigham and Women's Hospital
Boston, Massachusetts

With 51 contributors
Developed by Current Medicine Group, LLC
Philadelphia

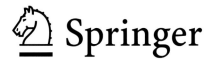

CURRENT MEDICINE GROUP LLC, PART OF SPRINGER SCIENCE+BUSINESS MEDIA LLC

400 Market Street, Suite 700 • Philadelphia, PA 19106

Developmental Editor	Elizabeth Fetterman
Editorial Assistant	Juleen Deaner
Design and Layout	Daniel Britt
Illustrators	Dan Britt, Kim Broadbent, Bernard E. Bulwer, Theresa Englehart, Heather Hoch, Wiesława Langenfeld, Jacqueline Leonard, Maureen Looney, and Andrea Penko
Production Coordinator	Carolyn Naylor
Indexer	Holly Lukens

Library of Congress Cataloging-in-Publication Data

Atlas of echocardiography. -- 2nd ed. / editor-in-chief, Scott D. Solomon ; with 51 contributors.
    p. ; cm.
  Rev. ed. of: Atlas of echocardiography / editors, Mani A. Vannan ... [et al.]. c2005.
  Includes bibliographical references and index.
  ISBN 978-1-57340-323-8 (alk. paper)
  1. Echocardiography--Atlases. I. Solomon, Scott D. II. Title.
  [DNLM: 1. Echocardiography--Atlases. WG 17 A88158 2008]

RC683.5.U5A86 2008
616.1'207543--dc22

ISBN 978-1-57340-323-8

www.springer.com

For more information, please call 1 (800) 777-4643
or email us at orders-ny@springer.com

www.currentmedicinegroup.com

10 9 8 7 6 5 4 3 2 1

Printed in China by Hong Kong Graphics and Printing LTD.

This book was printed on acid-free paper

Preface

If a picture is worth a thousand words, then there are few images in all of medicine that are as compelling or as captivating as those of the beating human heart. Despite a plethora of new cardiac imaging techniques, echocardiography remains the bread and butter imaging modality for cardiologists worldwide. Indeed, no other modality offers as comprehensive a look at all aspects of cardiac function and morphology, as echocardiography can be used to assess both systolic and diastolic function, cardiac size and structure, and valvular morphology and function. Moreover, echocardiography can be performed in hospitals or clinics in any country, in intensive care units or in the operating room, and it can be performed with increasingly powerful yet portable machinery, including devices that are now able to fit in the palm of the hand.

Echocardiography is, by definition, a visual discipline; hence, learning echocardiography also needs to be visual. The second edition of the *Atlas of Echocardiography* is as comprehensive as any textbook, but it is arranged in atlas form with figures and captions. The figures consist of echocardiographic images, tables, and diagrams designed to cover all aspects of echocardiography. In addition to the basics of echocardiography (including the underlying physical principles), the atlas covers some of the newer areas in the field, including contrast echocardiography, strain imaging, assessment of diastolic function, assessment of cardiac dyssynchrony, transesophageal echocardiography, echocardiography in the operating department, handheld echocardiography, and three-dimensional echocardiography.

The CD version of the atlas contains all of the figures and captions in the text, as well as many examples of moving images to complement the still images in the text. Ultimately, this book should appeal to all students of echocardiography: sonographers, fellows, cardiologists in practice, or other physicians who use echocardiography to care for their patients.

Scott D. Solomon, MD
Director, Noninvasive Cardiology
Cardiovascular Division
Brigham and Women's Hospital
Harvard Medical School
Boston, Massachusetts

Contributors

Theodore P. Abraham,
MD, FACC, FASE
Associate Professor of Medicine
Associate Director, Clinical
  Echocardiography Laboratory
Division of Cardiology
Johns Hopkins University
Baltimore, Maryland

Brijesh Anantharam,
MBBS, MRCP (UK)
Research Fellow
Department of Cardiovascular Medicine
Northwick Park Hospital
Harrow, Middlesex, United Kingdom

Gerard P. Aurigemma, MD
Professor of Medicine and Radiology
Director
Non-invasive Cardiology and Fellowship
  Training Program
Division of Cardiovascular Medicine
Department of Medicine
University of Massachusetts Medical School
Worcester, Massachusetts

Jeroen J. Bax, MD, PhD
Professor of Medicine
Department of Cardiology
Leiden University Medical Center
Leiden, The Netherlands

Gabe B. Bleeker, MD, PhD
Department of Cardiology
Leiden University Medical Center
Leiden, The Netherlands

Bernard E. Bulwer, MD, MSc
Cardiovascular Division
Harvard Medical School
Brigham and Women's Hospital
Boston, Massachusetts

Meryl S. Cohen, MD
Associate Professor of Medicine
Director of Echocardiography
Children's Hospital of Philadelphia
Philadelphia, Pennsylvania

Veronica Lea J. Dimaano, MD
Senior Research Fellow
Division of Cardiology
Johns Hopkins University
Baltimore, Maryland

Hisham Dokainish, MD, FACC, FASE
Associate Professor of Medicine
Director of Echocardiography
Department of Medicine/Cardiology
Baylor College of Medicine
Houston, Texas

Maurice Enriquez-Sarano, MD
Professor of Medicine
Mayo Clinic Medical Center
Rochester, Minnesota

Raul E. Espinoza, MD
Mayo Clinic
Rochester, Minnesota

Rodney H. Falk,
MD, FRCP, FACC, FAHA
Harvard Vanguard Medical Associates
Associate Clinical Professor of Medicine
Harvard Medical School
Director, Brigham and Women's Hospital
Cardiac Amyloidosis Program
Boston, Massachusetts

Elyse Foster, MD
Araxe Vilensky Endowed Chair in Cardiology
Director
UCSF Adult Echocardiography Laboratory
Professor of Medicine
University of California
San Francisco, California

Rosario V. Freeman, MD, MS
Assistant Professor
Department of Internal Medicine/Cardiology
University of Washington
Seattle, Washington

Linda D. Gillam, MD
Professor of Clinical Medicine
Columbia University College of Physicians
  and Surgeons
Medical Director Cardiac Valve Program
  (Non-Invasive)
Columbia University Medical Center
Past President
American Society of Echocardiography
New York, New York

Carolyn Y. Ho, MD
Medical Director, Cardiovascular
  Genetics Center
Cardiovascular Division
Brigham and Women's Hospital
Boston, Massachusetts

Judy Hung, MD
Cardiac Ultrasound Laboratory
Massachusetts General Hospital
Boston, Massachusetts

Ron Jacob, MD
Fellow
Department of Cardiovascular Medicine
Cleveland Clinic Foundation
Cleveland, Ohio

Jorge R. Kizer, MD, MSc
Associate Professor of Medicine and
  Public Health
Weill Medical College of Cornell University
New York-Presbyterian/Weill Cornell
  Medical Center
New York, New York

Suma H. Konety, MD, MS
Clinical Instructor
Division of Cardiology
University of California, San Francisco
San Francisco, California

Kaitlyn My-Tu Lam, MBBS, FRACP
Research Fellow in Medicine
Department of Medicine
Harvard Medical School
Massachusetts General Hospital
Boston, Massachusetts

Roberto M. Lang, MD, FACC
Professor of Medicine
Director
Noninvasive Cardiac Imaging Laboratories
University of Chicago Medical Center
Chicago, Illinois

Robert A. Levine, MD
Professor of Medicine
Harvard Medical School
Cardiac Ultrasound Laboratory
Massachusetts General Hospital
Boston, Massachusetts
Program Coordinator
Foundation Leducq Transatlantic Network of
  Excellence in Mitral Valve Disease
Paris, France

Fay Y. Lin, MD
Fellow
Division of Cardiology
Weill Medical College of Cornell University
New York-Presbyterian/Weill Cornell
  Medical Center
New York, New York

Judy R. Mangion,
MD, FACC, FASE, FAHA
Associate Director
Non Invasive Cardiac Laboratory
Division of Cardiovascular Medicine
Brigham and Women's Hospital
Boston, Massachusetts

Sunil V. Mankad, MD
Assistant Professor of Medicine
Consultant
Cardiovascular Diseases
Mayo Clinic College of Medicine
Rochester, Minnesota

Barry J. Maron, MD
Director
Hypertrophic Cardiomyopathy Center
Minneapolis Heart Institute Foundation
Minneapolis, Minnesota

David McCarty, MB, BCh, MRCP (UK)
Research Fellow in Medicine
Department of Medicine
Harvard Medical School
Massachusetts General Hospital
Boston, Massachusetts

Hector I. Michelena, MD
Assistant Professor of Medicine
Consultant
Cardiovascular Diseases
Mayo Clinic College of Medicine
Rochester, Minnesota

Victor Mor-Avi, PhD, FASE
Research Associate
Professor
Director of Cardiac Imaging Research
Department of Medicine
Section of Cardiology
University of Chicago
Chicago, Illinois

Rita Novello
Cardiovascular Technologist
Adult Congenital Heart Disease Program
Hospital of the University of Pennsylvania
Philadelphia, Pennsylvania

Jae K. Oh, MD
Professor of Medicine
Co-Director
Echo Lab
Director
Pericardial Diseases Clinic
Mayo Clinic
Rochester, Minnesota

Catherine M. Otto, MD
J. Ward Kennedy-Hamilton Endowed
  Professor of Cardiology
Director, Cardiology Fellowship Programs
University of Washington School of Medicine
Seattle, Washington

Robert F. Padera, MD, PhD
Assistant Professor of Pathology
Harvard Medical School
Associate Pathologist
Brigham and Women's Hospital
Boston, Massachusetts

Patricia A. Pellikka, MD
Professor of Medicine
Mayo Clinic College of Medicine
Co-Director
Echocardiography Laboratory
Rochester, Minnesota

Michael H. Picard, MD
Associate Professor
Department of Medicine
Harvard Medical School
Director of Echocardiography
Department of Medicine
Massachusetts General Hospital
Boston, Massachusetts

Theodore Plappert
Manager
Center for Quantitative Echocardiography
Department of Cardiology
Hospital of the University of Pennsylvania
Philadelphia, Pennsylvania

Jose Rivero, MD
Brigham and Women's Hospital
Boston, Massachusetts

Roxy Senior,
  MD, DM, FRCP, FESC, FACC
Consultant Cardiologist
Director of Cardiac Research
Department of Cardiovascular Medicine
Northwick Park Hospital
Middlesex, Harrow, United Kingdom
Honorary Professor
Middlesex University
Honorary Senior Lecturer
Imperial College
London, United Kingdom

Amil M. Shah, MD
Brigham and Women's Hospital
Boston, Massachusetts

Stanton K. Shernan, MD, FAHA, FASE
Associate Professor of Anesthesia
Director of Cardiac Anesthesia
Department of Anesthesiology, Perioperative
and Pain Medicine
Brigham and Women's Hospital
Harvard Medical School
Boston, Massachusetts

Scott D. Solomon, MD
Director, Noninvasive Cardiac Laboratory
Cardiovascular Division
Brigham and Women's Hospital
Associate Professor of Medicine
Harvard Medical School
Boston, Massachusetts

Kirk T. Spencer, MD
Associate Professor of Medicine
University of Chicago Medical Center
Chicago, Illinois

Martin St. John Sutton, MD
Cardiovascular Medicine Division
Department of Medicine
Hospital of the University of Pennsylvania
Philadelphia, Pennsylvania

Lissa Sugeng, MD
Assistant Professor of Medicine
University of Chicago Medical Center
Chicago, Illinois

James Thomas, MD
Director, Cardiovascular Imaging
Cleveland Clinic Foundation
Cleveland, Ohio

Dennis A. Tighe, MD, FACC, FACP
Professor of Medicine
University of Massachusetts Medical School
Associate Director
Non-invasive Cardiology
University of Massachusetts Memorial
  Medical Center
Worcester, Massachusetts

Justina C. Wu, MD, PhD, FACC
Assistant Professor
Department of Medicine
Harvard University Medical School
Associate Director
Non-invasive Laboratory
Division of Cardiology
Brigham and Women's Hospital
Boston, Massachusetts

Kibar Yared, MD, FRCPC
Research Fellow in Medicine
Department of Medicine
Harvard Medical School
Massachusetts General Hospital
Boston, Massachusetts

Cheuk-Man Yu, MD
Prince of Wales Hospital
Shatin, NT, Hong Kong

William A. Zoghbi,
  MD, FASE, FAHA, FACC
Professor of Medicine
Weill Cornell Medical College
Director
Cardiovascular Imaging Institute
William L. Winters Chair in CV Imaging
Department of Cardiology
The Methodist Hospital
Houston, Texas

Contents

1

Basic Principles of Echocardiography and Tomographic Anatomy

Bernard E. Bulwer, Jose Rivero, and Scott D. Solomon

Echocardiography relies on the use of ultrasound—high-frequency sound waves—to interrogate bodily tissues. Ultrasound waves penetrate through and are reflected by tissues before returning to the transducer, where they are then converted into images. Modern ultrasound equipment uses three principal modalities. They include M-mode imaging, B-mode (or two-dimensional imaging), and Doppler imaging. This chapter will introduce the basic physical principles of ultrasound and tomographic anatomy in cardiac imaging with ultrasound.

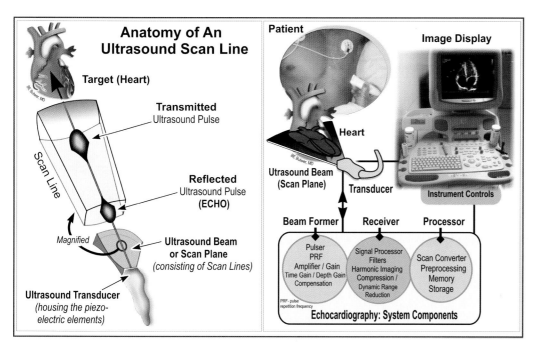

Figure 1-1. Ultrasound waves used in medical ultrasound imaging are generated by the piezoelectric elements housed within the transducer (*left panel*). In order to generate an ultrasound image, the ultrasound pulse must make a round trip between the piezoelectric elements (housed inside the transducer) and the region of interest (imaged structure). The ultrasound waves that are emitted travel along scan lines and interact with tissue structures. Ultrasound waves or echoes are differentially reflected from cardiac structures and returned to transducer where they are then converted to electrical impulses and subsequently converted to images by system components (*eg*, signal processor and scan convert-

ers) housed within the ultrasound equipment. Two-dimensional images representing cardiac cross-sectional anatomy are composed of several scan lines (*see* Fig. 1-3).

The principal method used in order to produce ultrasound images is referred to as B-mode or "brightness mode" imaging (*right panel*). Echocardiographic images are processed and displayed as pixels, or picture elements, of varied shades of gray (black-to-white). Each pixel has its own anatomical "address" and echoreflectivity and is mapped accordingly.

The major components of a modern ultrasound scanner include the following: 1) Transducer. The transducer is the interface between the patient and the beamformer. Electrical energy is converted here into ultrasound and returning ultrasound (echoes) into electrical energy. 2) Beamformer. The beamformer has several components with various functions, including the pulser and the amplifier. 3) Receiver/ signal processor. Returning echoes from the imaged tissue must be processed and filtered. 4) Processor/ scan converter. The scan converter converts echo-cardiographic data into echocardiographic images that can be displayed, stored, or further processed. 5) Display monitors. These are cathode-ray tubes or liquid crystal display (LCD) screens that display the image. PRF—pulse repetition frequency.

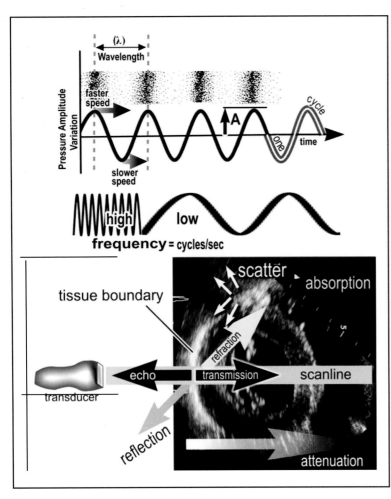

Figure 1-2. Ultrasound waves are high-frequency sound waves, which have a general range of over a million cycles per second. In contrast, sound that is audible to humans fall within the 20 to 20,000 Hz range. The oscillatory nature

of sound waves is caused by the compression and rarefaction of particles. The properties of ultrasound (as is the case in all waves) include 1) frequency (f): the number of cycles occurring per second; 2) wavelength (λ): the length of the wave—one cycle; and 3) velocity (c): propagation speed or velocity. These properties are related by the equation $c = f\lambda$ (*top panel*).

Amplitude represents the "height" or power of the wave. The intensity represents the power in watts divided by the area in square centimeters. Ultrasound waves are subject to attenuation—the decrease in amplitude relative to the distance traveled as sound waves weaken as they travel through a medium.

Ultrasound waves are primarily reflected from the boundaries between tissues of different acoustic impedance (*bottom panel*). This type of reflection is referred to as a "specular" reflection. Although part of the ultrasound is reflected as the echo, a percentage is transmitted (transmission) through the reflector. Ultrasound waves can interact with tissue in the following ways: 1) Refraction is a change in the direction of a non perpendicular incident ultrasound beam without a change in frequency. This results in the bending of a portion of the incident ultrasound waves away from the main beam axis. 2) Scattering is a combination of reflection and refraction of incident ultrasound waves within tissues, which diverts them in multiple directions. Interaction with tissues and tissue boundaries produces a pattern of echoes that are characteristic of the tissues imaged, which gives them their signature appearance. Hyperechoic structures produce greater amplitude of reflections and appear white. Hypoechoic tissues produce echoes with smaller amplitudes and appear as various shades of gray. Anechoic or echolucent structures appear echo-free because they completely absorb all the incident ultrasound waves. 3) Attenuation refers to the loss of amplitude or beam intensity with distance traveled within the imaged tissue due to absorption and scattering. 4) Absorption is the transmission of ultrasound waves with complete loss of acoustic energy and with no reflected echoes. A fraction of the acoustic energy is lost as heat.

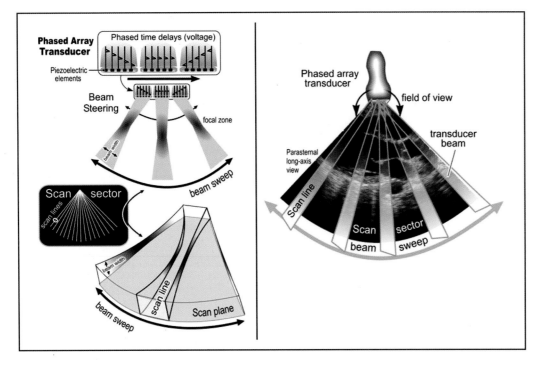

Figure 1-3. Modern ultrasound equipment have phased array transducers, which electronically generate and steer the ultrasound beams generated in sequence. Each beam results in the generation of a scan line. A defined sequence of scan lines is swept through the angle of view in order to generate a composite called the scan sector. A scan sector still frame from a phased array transducer typically consists of 96 to 512 scan lines.

Ultrasound beams for standard B-mode imaging are generated in "pulses." The frequency of these pulses is called the pulse repetition frequency.

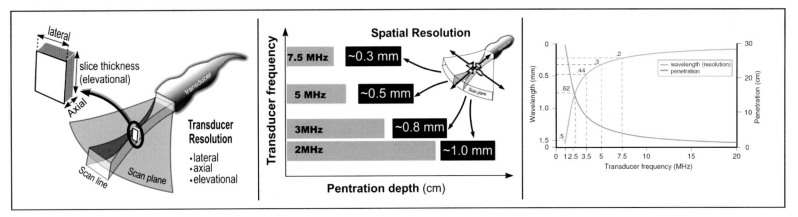

Figure 1-4. The resolution of ultrasound images (*ie*, the ability of the ultrasound beam to detect and display anatomical details within the structures imaged) is dependent on many factors, including the characteristics of the transducer combined with the physical principles of ultrasound. Each ultrasound beam emitted has a defined slice thickness (*left panel*). The components of overall resolution include axial, lateral, elevational (slice thickness), temporal, and contrast resolution. Axial resolution, which is also called depth, longitudinal, linear, or range resolution, refers to the ability to resolve or detail echoes that are reflected from two contiguous structures oriented along the axis of the scan line. It is influenced by transducer frequency and wavelength (pulse length) and is equivalent to one-half spatial pulse length. Increased transducer frequency results in increased axial resolution, although this is a trade-off of penetration, which decreases with increasing transducer frequency. Lateral resolution refers to the ability to resolve or detail echoes from two side-by-side structures oriented perpendicularly to the scan line axis and is influenced by the beam width and imaging depth. Spatial resolution refers to the ability to resolve detail in an ultrasound image (averaging 1 mm) and is dependent on both axial and lateral resolution. It is heavily influenced by transducer frequency (*middle panel*). Slice thickness (elevational) resolution refers to the ability to resolve details situated "out of plane" of the ultrasound beam or scan plane. Temporal resolution refers to the ability to precisely "capture" still frames of moving structures as they move from instant to instant "accuracy in time," averaging 50 m/sec. The greater the pulse repetition frequency (*ie*, the more pulses emitted from the transducer per second), the greater the ability of the transducer to accurately "capture" a still frame of a moving structure. Contrast resolution refers to the ability to discern differential reflectivity between different tissues (*eg*, endocardial border) and the myocardium, and is influenced by pre and postprocessing. (*Right panel from* Otto et al. [1]; with permission.)

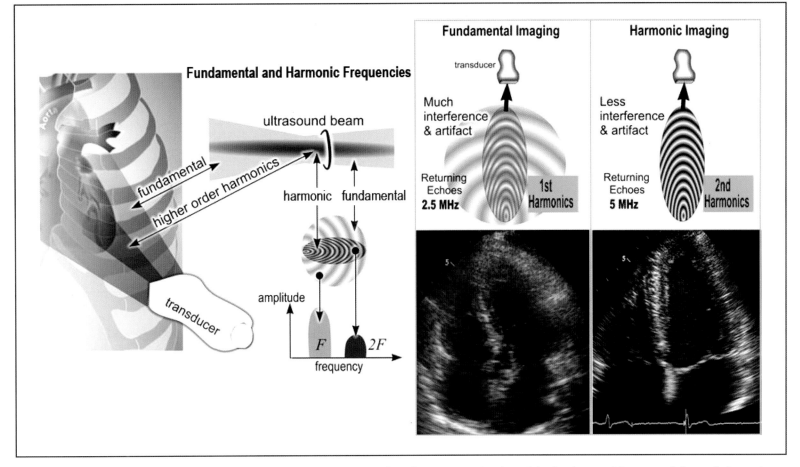

Figure 1-5. Harmonic imaging is an important development that has greatly improved ultrasound image quality. Harmonic images rely on the fact that tissues may reverberate at frequencies that are multiples of the original ultrasound beam. Harmonic images are created from returning echoes that have frequencies twice that of the fundamental frequency (*left panel*). Second harmonics (*right panel, right side*) undergo less distortion than first harmonics (*right panel, left side*) and result in increased signal-to-noise ratio. Image quality and endocardial definition are considerably better with harmonic imaging.

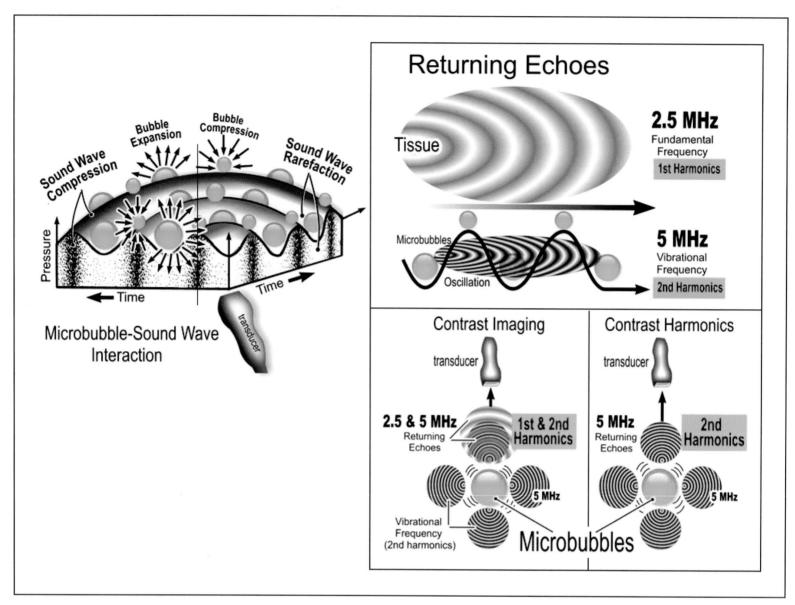

Figure 1-6. Contrast echocardiography has been an important advancement in echocardiography. It has clinical use in the assessment of both cardiac structure and function. Encapsulated microspheres or microbubbles measuring ~3 to 6 μm in diameter can pass through capillaries. Microbubbles contain a "shell or gas" comprised of one or a combination of air, lipid, polymer, perfluorocarbon, insoluble gas (*eg*, perflutren lipid microsphere). These improve their echoreflectivity. Microbubbles may have resonant frequencies ranging from 2 to 10 MHz.

Encapsulation enables gas to stay within blood vessels, and to not be lost to diffusion. Microbubbles create increased echogenicity during interaction with ultrasound waves. **Left panel,** At the low-pressure (rarefaction) regions of the incident ultrasound wave, microbubbles expand (may expand 2- to 10-fold). At the crest of the ultrasound waves—the regions of peak pressures—the microbubbles are compressed. This creates bubble oscillations, which produce new echoes. These echoes contain harmonic frequencies of the incident ultrasound that improve their echoreflectivity, and hence image analysis. The differential acoustic impedance of microspheres is lower than that of blood, which leads to increased linear backscattering and reflectivity at the microsphere-blood interface. The microspheres produce echoes in response. **Right panels above and below,** Contrast harmonic imaging with generation of microbubble harmonics.

Causes of Ultrasound Artifacts

Faulty equipment

Instrument malfunction

Interference from other equipment (eg, electrocautery during surgery); malfunctioning transducer

Improper instrument settings

Too much time gain compensation (gain)

No harmonic imaging (fundamental frequency only)

Suboptimal imaging technique: inadequate transducer frequency, sector width, depth, dynamic range, and power output

Improper technique or patient characteristics

Sonographer inexperience

Suboptimal imaging due to patient movement, breathing, obesity, COPD, post-chest surgery

Suboptimal imaging technique: inadequate transducer frequency, sector width, depth, dynamic range, and power output

Acoustic or sonographic artifacts

Attenuation artifacts: shadowing and enhancement

Propagation artifacts: Poor spatial resolution, section/slice thickness, speckling, reverberation, comet-tail or "ring down," mirror image, range ambiguity, and slide lobe artifacts

Figure 1-7. All imaging modalities are subject to artifacts, which can have adverse effects on the interpretation of studies. Artifacts are false images that can be caused by faulty equipment, improper technique, or by acoustic phenomenon or interference. Understanding artifacts and their mechanisms is important in echocardiography because they commonly occur. Their recognition is crucial to proper interpretation because they can cause unnecessary alarm and unwarranted clinical studies. COPD—chronic obstructive pulmonary disease.

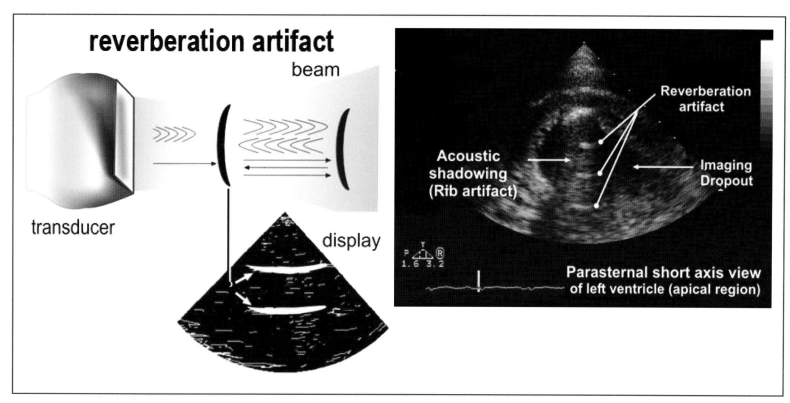

Figure 1-8. Reverberation artifacts are caused by internal reverberations, or back-and-forth echoes within the imaged tissue itself, which result in equipment miscalculation of the "return trip" time of the emitted pulses. Reverberation artifacts occur at greater depths than the true image, but at distances that are multiples of the true image. **Left panel**, The ultrasound is both reflected from and transmitted through a structure (ie, an area of calcification) before reflecting off a second structure. The reflected echo is re-reflected in the direction of the original beam returning to the deeper structure and is then reflected back to the transducer. An artifact is generated at a distance that is a multiple of the original reflecting structure. **Right panel**, The image resulting from the inflow conduit of an LV assist device positioned in the LV apex. With reverberation artifacts, the artifacts are equally spaced, located parallel to the sound beam axis, and are seen at depths deeper than the true reflector. Acoustic shadowing or dropout artifacts appear as hypoechoic or anechoic regions below structures with high attenuation (eg, calcified structures).

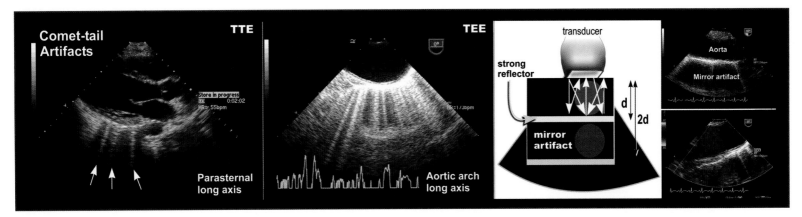

Figure 1-9. Left panel, Comet tail or "ring down" artifacts (*arrows*) on the parasternal long-axis view (PLAX). These appear as hyperechoic, comet tailed, and linear in appearance and are located parallel to the ultrasound beam axis. They arise from merger of closely spaced reverberations (*middle panel*). Mirror image artifacts are commonly seen when imaging the thoracic aorta on transesophageal echocardiography (TEE). This is a long-axis view of the descending thoracic aorta long-axis view (*right panel*). TTE—transthoracic echocardiography.

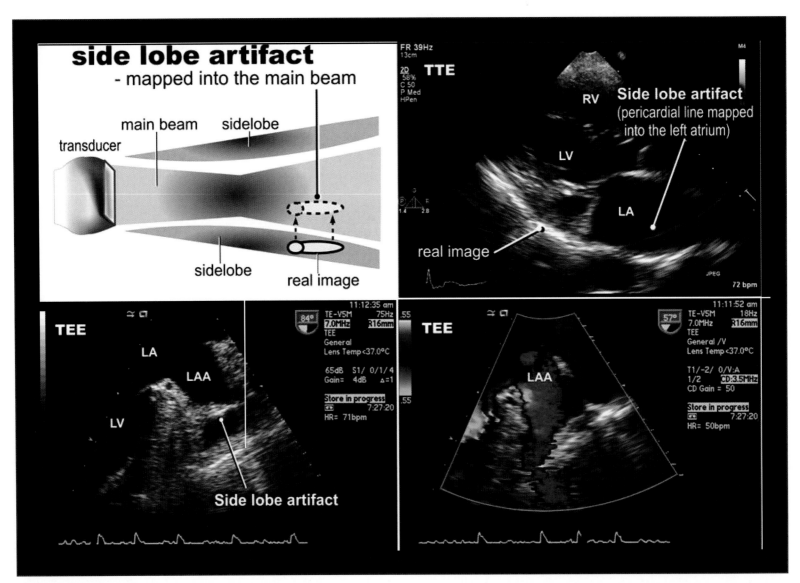

Figure 1-10. Upper left, Side lobes degrade lateral resolution. Artifacts appear side by side at the same depth. Grating lobe artifacts follow a similar principle in their manifestation, but they arise from the structural arrangement of multiple transducer elements within the transducer. **Upper right**, This side-lobe artifact, arising from the pericardium in this parasternal long-axis view, gives the impression of a linear echodensity in the left atrium (LA). **Lower left**, The hyperechoic linear echodensity seen in this left atrial appendage (LAA) on transesophageal echocardiography (TEE) does not share the same echoreflectivity pattern as thrombus or the pectinate muscles, which would appear isoechoic with the LAA wall. Neither does it exhibit the characteristics of the "warfarin ridge" that appear as linear shadowing within the LAA lumen, which moves synchronously with the fold of tissue separating the LAA from the left upper pulmonary vein. It is actually a side lobe artifact that is mapped into the LAA lumen. **Lower right**, Color flow Doppler "angiogram" shows no evidence of a physical presence within the LAA lumen. TTE—transthoracic echocardiography.

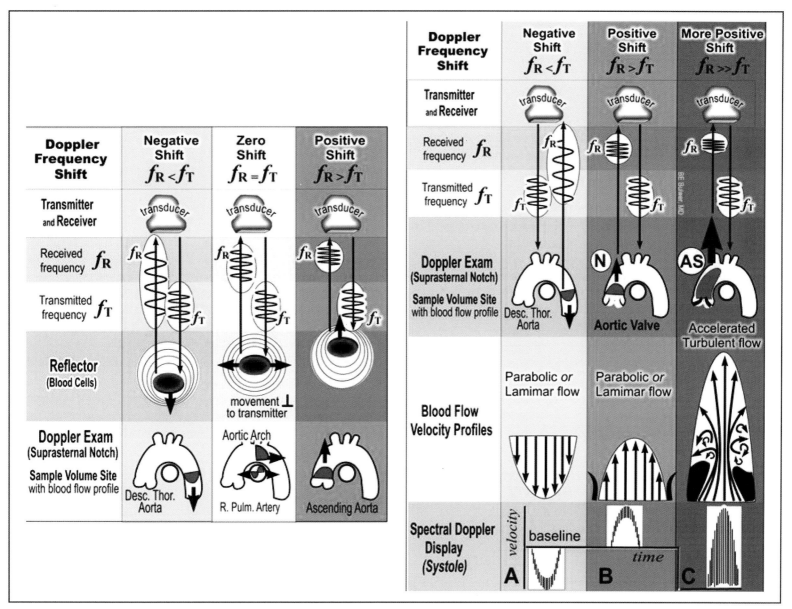

Figure 1-11. **Left panel**, The Doppler principle as applied to normal blood flow dynamics within the thoracic aorta. The Doppler frequency shift, sometimes referred to as Doppler frequency, is a shift in the frequency of the returning echoes compared with the frequency of emitted ultrasound waves. The Doppler frequency is itself a wave with its own frequency. Echoes reflected from blood flowing away from the transducer are at lower frequencies compared with those emitted from the transducer (*left panel, blue column*). Echoes reflected from blood flowing towards the transducer are at higher frequencies compared with those emitted from the transducer (*left panel, red column*). Echoes reflected from blood flowing perpendicular to the transducer show no changes in frequency compared with those emitted from the transducer (*left panel, white column*). **Right panel**, Doppler assessment of blood flow hemodynamics. Normal laminar flow exhibits a range of frequencies that are detectable by spectral Doppler, which is so named for its ability to exhibit the spectrum of frequencies. Note the narrow range or band of frequencies (*right panel, blue and red columns*) and their relationship to the baseline, which creates a "window" between the Doppler display and the baseline. **Right panel, deep red column**, During turbulent flow, there is a wider range of blood flow velocities seen on the spectral Doppler display (spectral broadening) with a "filled-in" window. **Right panel, blue column**, Flow away from transducer. **Right panel, red column**, Flow towards transducer.

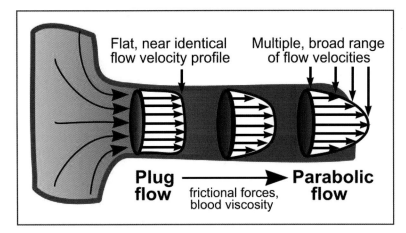

Figure 1-12. Understanding blood flow hemodynamics is crucial to understanding Doppler echocardiography. Several factors influence blood flow through vessels, including blood viscosity, vessel size, shape, wall characteristics, flow rate, and phase of the cardiac cycle. There is also a differential pattern of flow across the cross-section of a single blood vessel.

Laminar flow is streamlined flow where concentric "layers" of blood glide smoothly along the length of blood vessels. This is the normal pattern of blood flow throughout most of the cardiovascular system. Laminar flow can be seen in fast- or slow-moving blood. The two basic profiles of laminar flow are plug flow and parabolic flow. Fast laminar flow shows the highest velocities (Vmax) and is typically found at the axial center of tubular blood vessels, occurring during systole. This type of flow is called plug flow. The "plug" profile during systole occurs because almost all of the blood is flowing at the same velocity. Plug flow is also seen at the vascular inlets. During diastole, the loss of pump and the impact of frictional forces and blood viscosity exert a drag on blood near vessel walls, which leads to a more parabolic profile. Slow laminar flow with a parabolic profile can be seen within veins.

Turbulent flow is disorganized flow, exhibiting wide ranges and directions of velocities, and is typically seen with valvular stenosis, septal defect shunts, and prosthetic heart valves. Unlike laminar flow, turbulent flow results in significant energy losses in the form of heat, vortex formation, and turbulent friction (*see* Fig 1-11 *right panel* and Fig. 1-20).

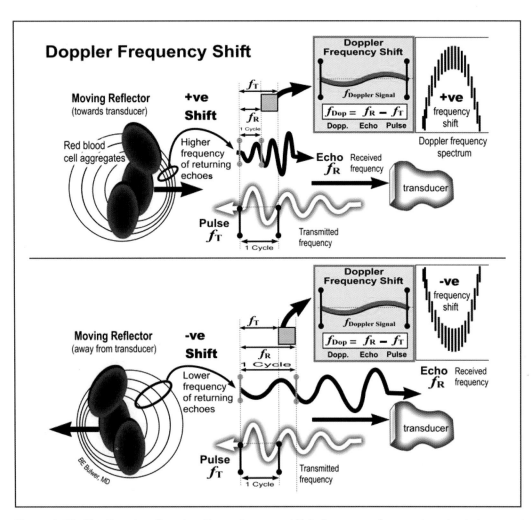

Figure 1-13. The Doppler effect describes a change or shift in frequency of sound emitted from a source moving relative to that of the observer. Doppler echocardiography uses this principle to determine the velocity of blood flowing within the heart or the velocity of myocardial motion. When ultrasound waves of a particular frequency are reflected from moving structures, such as red blood cells, the returning sound waves are at a slightly higher (*ie*, if the particles are moving towards the transducer) or lower (*ie*, if they are moving away from the transducer) frequency than the emitted sound waves. The ultrasound equipment calculates the difference in frequency of the transmitted and received ultrasound waves. From this difference (the Doppler shift), the ultrasound equipment can calculate the velocity of the blood flow using the Doppler equation: (*see* Fig. 1-14)

$$f_{Dop} = f_R - f_T = 2f\cos\theta\, v/c$$

A negative frequency shift is indicative of blood flow away from the transducer; a positive frequency shift is indicative of flow towards the transducer. +VE—positive; -VE—negative.

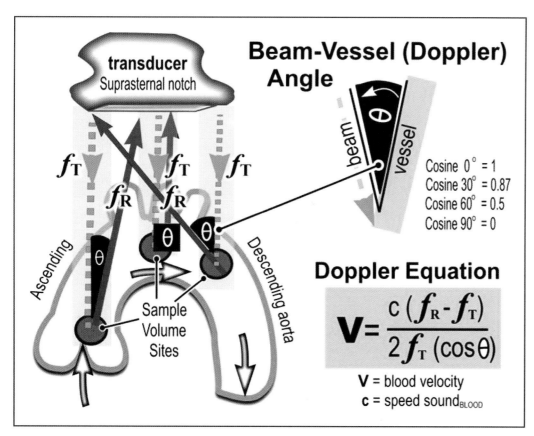

Figure 1-14. The Doppler equation is used to convert Doppler frequency shifts into blood flow velocities. However, the accuracy of the Doppler frequency shift is directly influenced by the beam-vessel alignment or the Doppler angle. The smaller the Doppler angle (θ), the more accurate the measurement. Although the actual angle can be used in the equation to correct Doppler beams that are not exactly parallel to the interrogated flow (most ultrasound equipment has the capability to do this), the further this angle is from 0 degrees, the less accurate the measurement will be. C—speed sound$_{blood}$; V—velocity; fR—frequency of the received or returning echoes; fT—frequency of the transmitted ultrasound pulses

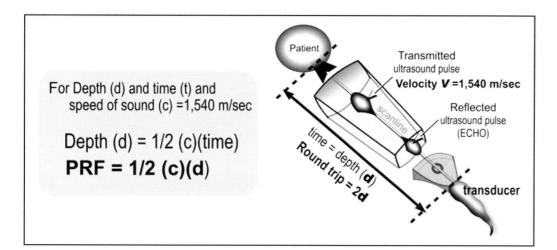

Figure 1-15. In order to construct an ultrasound image (*eg*, a scan sector), the ultrasound pulse must make a round trip between the transducer and the target. In pulsed Doppler studies, the transducer must "listen" for the Doppler signal following transmission. A new ultrasound pulse cannot be transmitted before the previous pulse has returned. The pulse repetition frequency (PRF) is the number of pulses transmitted each second. The further the imaging depth, the slower the PRF must be to allow for the round trip. D—depth.

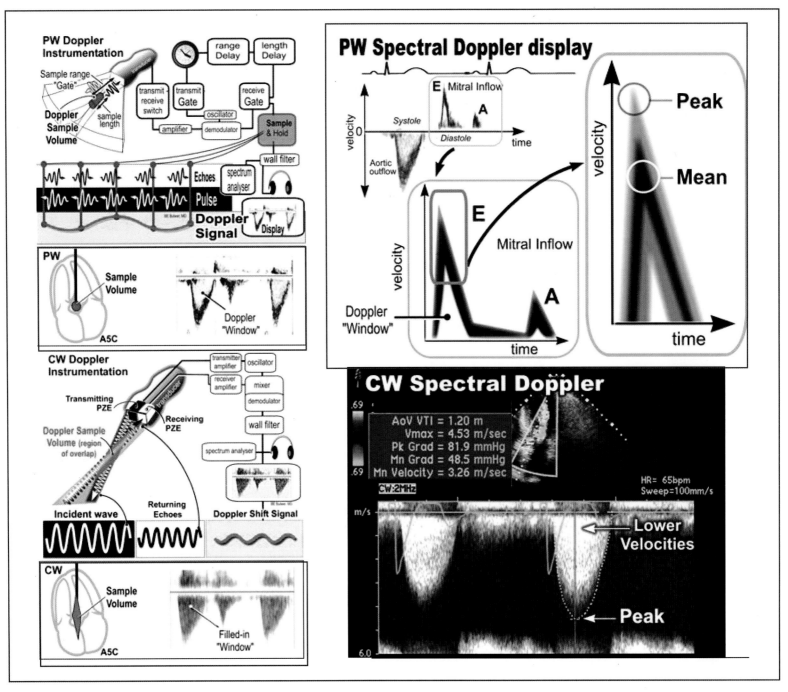

Figure 1-16. In pulsed-wave Doppler (*upper left panel*) the ultrasound signal is emitted repeatedly from the transducer and the return signal is "listened for" by the transducer. Sending out Doppler in pulses allows the equipment to interrogate velocities at particular depths by gating, or only "listening" at a certain time after the pulse is emitted. By focusing on a particular scan line, a region of interest (sample volume) can be defined by both the "depth" using time gating and the lateral location. Because pulsed Doppler is sent out and received in "pulses," the Doppler velocities are essentially being "sampled" at the pulse repetition frequency and are therefore subject to sampling issues, which can limit the velocity of the blood flow that can be interrogated. All spectral Doppler signals (*upper right panel*) show time on the X-axis and velocity on the Y-axis. When the pulsed-wave Doppler signal appears hollow (Doppler "window"), it is indicative of laminar flow where the majority of red blood cells are traveling within a narrow range of velocities.

With continuous wave (CW) Doppler (*lower left panel*) the Doppler signal is emitted continuously (similar to a continuous tone) and continuously listened for. For this reason, CW Doppler can be used to identify peak velocities, but cannot localize velocities to particular depths. Note the filled in appearance of the CW spectral Doppler display in the (*lower right panel*). This reflects the wide spectrum of velocities detected within the much larger sample volume.

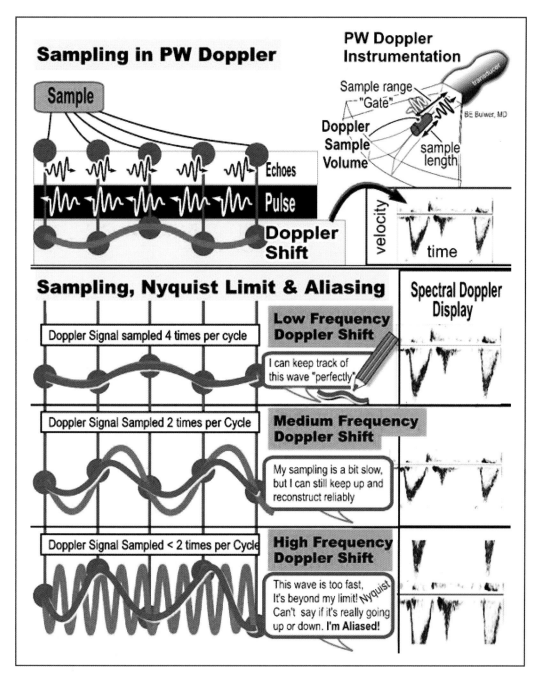

Figure 1-17. According to sample theory, the returning Doppler frequency shift—a wave—must be sampled at least twice per cycle in order to accurately reconstruct it. The Doppler shift (*ie*, the difference between the emitted and received Doppler signals) represents the velocity of blood flow and is the waveform that must be sampled. The sampling frequency is essentially the pulse repetition frequency (PRF). The point at which the sampling frequency cannot accurately sample the waveform is the Nyquist limit. This limit is reached when the Doppler shift frequency is half that of the PRF. When the interrogated velocities, and hence the Doppler shift, is too high based on the current PRF, the equipment cannot accurately define the waveform and thus cannot determine the velocity accurately.

On the pulsed wave (PW) Doppler display, aliasing appears as a wraparound, with the highest frequencies misplaced on the opposite side of the velocity scale. Aliasing may be overcome by either adjusting the baseline up or down as appropriate, or increasing the PRF, although the maximum PRF is determined by depth because the signal requires time in order to return to the transducer before the next pulse is emitted.

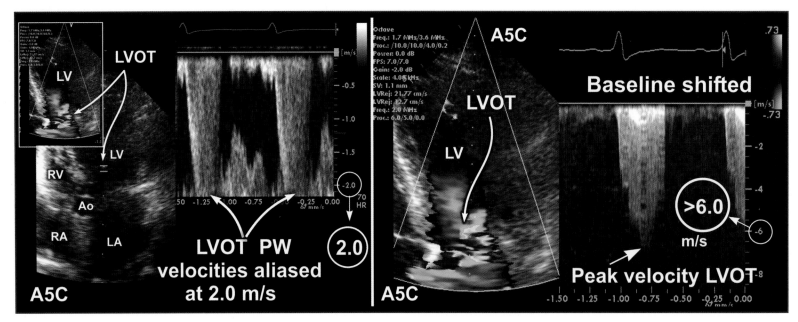

Figure 1-18. Left panel, Apical five-chamber view in a patient with dynamic LV outflow tract (LVOT) obstruction showing accelerated flow on color flow Doppler (*inset*). Pulsed wave (PW) Doppler showed aliased velocities with baseline set just above 2 m/s. **Right panel**, Nyquist limit and aliasing; baseline adjustment. The same patient with baseline set at 6.0 m/s and switch to continuous wave Doppler mode, the entire spectral display and peak velocities are now unambiguously displayed.

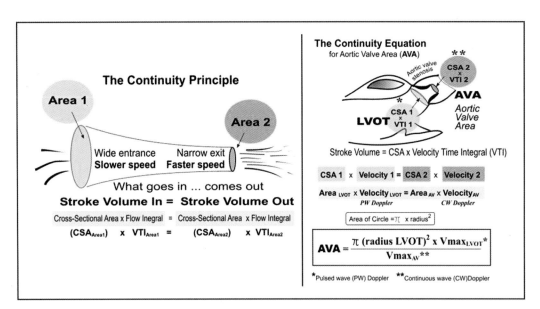

Figure 1-19. The law of conservation of mass states that the flow in one part of the heart has to be equivalent to the flow in another part; *ie*, flow rate in = flow rate out (*left panel*). Doppler ultrasonography harnesses this principle in order to calculate valve area (*eg*, in aortic stenosis). Blood flow velocities increase at sites where blood vessel diameter narrows. The differential flow velocities are detected by Doppler and used to calculate the valve areas. The continuity equation suggests that the area at a particular location multiplied by either the velocity of flow or the time integral of flow—velocity time integral (VTI) represents the area under the curve of the Doppler flow profile—will be similar in two locations assuming no shunt is present. For example, in order to calculate the valve area in a patient with suspected aortic stenosis (*right panel*), the cross sectional area (CSA) at the level of the LV outflow tract is calculated (in actuality, the diameter is measured and the area is calculated), and multiplied with the velocity or VTI obtained at the same location using pulsed wave (PW) Doppler. This product should equal the product of the velocity or VTI across the valve itself, which is estimated using continuous wave (CW) Doppler to find the highest velocity and the aortic valve area (AVA), which is then calculated. LVOT—LV outflow tract.

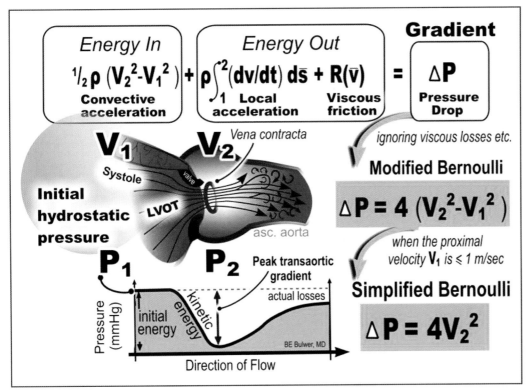

Figure 1-20. The Bernoulli principle serves as the basis of calculating pressure gradients ("driving pressure") across a narrowed orifice. The Bernoulli principle broadly states that as the velocity of a moving fluid increases, the pressure within the fluid decreases. It assumes the conservation of energy, though in reality some energy is lost through heat, turbulent friction, and vortex formation. Doppler-derived velocities are inserted into the modified or simplified version of the Bernoulli equation in order to calculate pressure gradients across cardiac chambers and valves. As a blood vessel or orifice narrows or becomes stenosed, the velocity of blood downstream from the stenosis must increase. Blood proximal to the stenosis (location 1) will therefore accelerate as it flows downstream from the stenosis (location 2) (law of conservation of energy).

The modified Bernoulli equation requires knowing velocities both proximal and distal to a stenosis. In the majority of cases in physiologic conditions, we can ignore the proximal velocities. This is not true, however, when velocities proximal to the stenosis are elevated. For example, if we were to use the Bernoulli equation in order to assess the gradient across a stenotic aortic valve, physiologic velocities proximal to the valve would be relatively low compared with the velocities distal to the valve. However, if that same patient had outflow tract obstruction due to hypertrophic cardiomyopathy or a sub aortic membrane, the proximal velocities would have to be considered. LVOT—LV outflow tract.

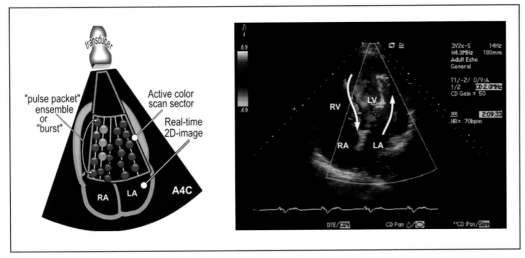

Figure 1-21. One of the advances in cardiac ultrasound has been the development of color flow Doppler (CFD) imaging. It has dramatically improved the assessment of cardiovascular hemodynamics, and complements the cross-sectional and spectral Doppler examination. CFD is a pulse wave (PW)–based modality that, unlike PW, uses multiple gates (ie, multiple sample volumes) simultaneously instead of a single gate and provides spatial display of real-time color-coded velocities superimposed upon real-time two-dimensional (2D) imaging. CFD thus provides information on flow velocity and direction. CFD imaging is subject to the same physical principles as PW Doppler and is thus subject to aliasing when velocities are high enough that the Doppler shift is greater than half the pulse repetition frequency.

Left panel, Schema of apical four-chamber (A4C) view showing CFD sector scan superimposed upon real-time two-dimensional grayscale image. The active color scan sector employs multiple gates (trains or ensemble) that are color-coded velocities. **Right panel**, A4C view showing color Doppler superimposed on B-mode two-dimensional imaging. Flow direction during early systole reveals blue flow along the LV outflow tract. Red flow indicating flow momentum from left atrium into LV is also visualized.

CFD provides an intuitive assessment of cardiovascular hemodynamics because it permits an "angiographic" view of the flow, and is therefore more intuitive than spectral Doppler. It allows for rapid qualitative assessment of abnormal flow patterns. It is an important guide to PW and continuous wave Doppler position and alignment. LA—left atrium; RV—right atrium.

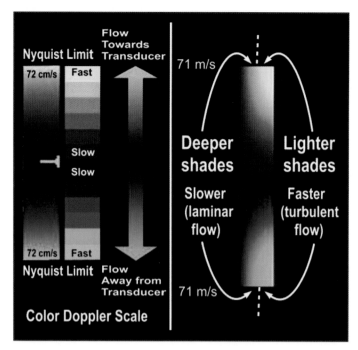

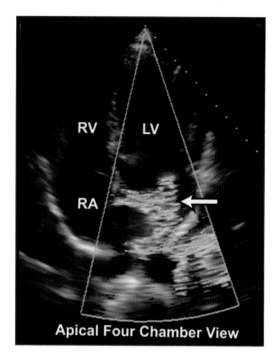

Figure 1-22. Images obtained by color flow Doppler (CFD) frames must be interpreted with reference to the velocity scales displayed on the image. These reference maps or scales provide information on average flow velocities based on three characteristics of color: 1) hue, 2) luminance, and 3) saturation. Two major modes of display are velocity mode and variance mode.

Left panel, Conventional velocity mode: flow towards transducer is coded (by convention) in shades of red. Flow away from transducer is color-coded in shades of blue ("BART": blue away, red towards). Black color on the sale indicates no flow. Lighter shades of BART indicate faster flow.

Right panel, Variance mode maps provide information in addition to velocity and direction. They can help distinguish laminar from turbulent flow. In laminar flow, the average velocities are not much different from the peak velocities. They are close together (ie, they exhibit minimal variance). When blood flow is turbulent, there are much greater differences between the average and peak velocities, namely greater variance. Deeper shades indicate slower laminar flow, while lighter shades may represent faster, turbulent flow.

Figure 1-23. The mosaic color pattern shown in this image reflects high-velocity turbulent flow (*arrow*) in a patient with severe mitral regurgitation. Note the mosaic pattern of bright hues indicative of aliasing due to turbulence and high-velocity flow.

Comparison of Doppler Modes

	Continuous wave Doppler	Pulsed wave Doppler	Color flow Doppler
Sample volume	Large (with spectral broadening)	Small (with spectral window due to narrow range of velocities); sample volume adjustable (best 2–5 mm)	Large with multigating; adjustable active color window in color scan sector
Detection of peak/ maximal velocities	Detects highest velocities along scan line; peak velocity measurements	Peak velocity measurements, but aliasing occurs at high velocities	Mean velocity measurements; aliasing occurs as it is a PW-based modality
Aliasing	No aliasing	Aliasing (Nyquist limit)	A PW Doppler-based technique; aliasing
Sensitivity	Best sensitivity	Good sensitivity	Good sensitivity (jet size very sensitive to gain settings)
Depth resolution/ range ambiguity	Range ambiguity	Range resolution; detects location of flow	Range resolution; real time 2D anatomy of flow
Spectrum analyzed	Wide (spectral broadening)	Narrow; spectral broadening seen with turbulent flow and large sample volumes	Wide color-encoded Doppler shifts on conventional *BART scale and color hues, saturation, and luminance

Blue away, red towards.

Figure 1-24. Comparison: continuous wave, pulsed wave, and color flow Doppler.

The Normal Echocardiographic Examination and Tomographic Anatomy

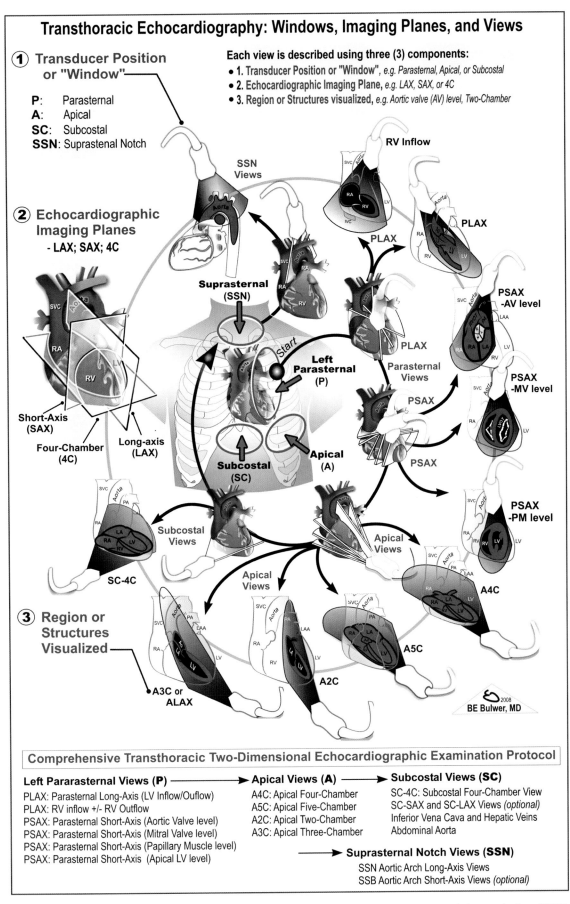

Transthoracic Echocardiography: Windows, Imaging Planes, and Views

(1) Transducer Position or "Window"

P: Parasternal
A: Apical
SC: Subcostal
SSN: Suprastenal Notch

Each view is described using three (3) components:
- 1. Transducer Position or "Window", *e.g. Parasternal, Apical, or Subcostal*
- 2. Echocardiographic Imaging Plane, *e.g. LAX, SAX, or 4C*
- 3. Region or Structures visualized, *e.g. Aortic valve (AV) level, Two-Chamber*

(2) Echocardiographic Imaging Planes
- LAX; SAX; 4C

Short-Axis (SAX)

Four-Chamber (4C)

Long-axis (LAX)

(3) Region or Structures Visualized

Comprehensive Transthoracic Two-Dimensional Echocardiographic Examination Protocol

Left Pararasternal Views (P)
PLAX: Parasternal Long-Axis (LV Inflow/Ouflow)
PLAX: RV inflow +/- RV Outflow
PSAX: Parasternal Short-Axis (Aortic Valve level)
PSAX: Parasternal Short-Axis (Mitral Valve level)
PSAX: Parasternal Short-Axis (Papillary Muscle level)
PSAX: Parasternal Short-Axis (Apical LV level)

Apical Views (A)
A4C: Apical Four-Chamber
A5C: Apical Five-Chamber
A2C: Apical Two-Chamber
A3C: Apical Three-Chamber

Subcostal Views (SC)
SC-4C: Subcostal Four-Chamber View
SC-SAX and SC-LAX Views *(optional)*
Inferior Vena Cava and Hepatic Veins
Abdominal Aorta

Suprasternal Notch Views (SSN)
SSN Aortic Arch Long-Axis Views
SSB Aortic Arch Short-Axis Views *(optional)*

Figure 1-25. Transthoracic two-dimensional echocardiography: imaging planes, transducer positions, and standard views. A2C—apical two-chamber view; A3C—apical three-chamber view; A4C—apical four-chamber view; A5C—apical five-chamber view; PLAX—parasternal long-axis view; PSAX— parasternal short-axis view; PSAX-AV—parasternal short-axis view-aortic valve level; PSAX-MV—parasternal short-axis view-mitral valve level; PSAX-PM—parasternal short-axis view papillary muscle level; SC-4C—subcostal view (four-chamber).

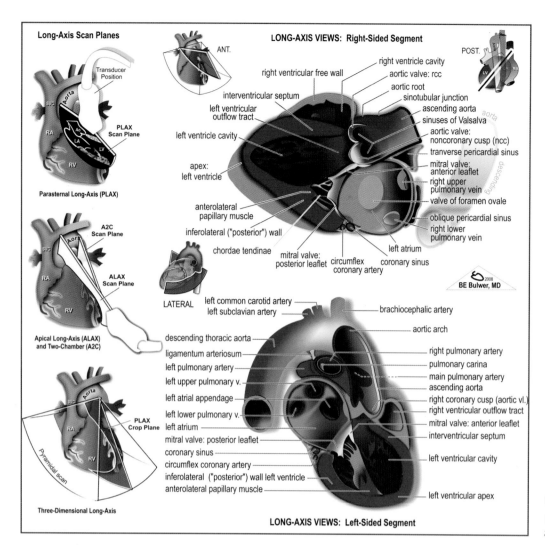

Figure 1-26. Echocardiographic long-axis scan planes and corresponding anatomy. RA—right atrium; SVC—superior vena cavity.

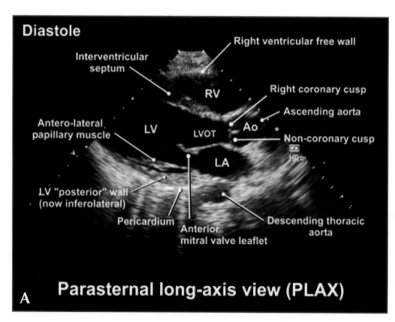

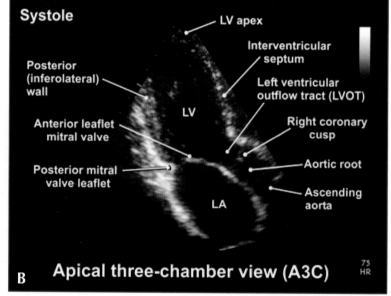

Figure 1-27. Two-dimensional long-axis views showing structures visualized on the parasternal long-axis (PLAX) view (**A**) and apical long-axis (ALAX) view, also called the apical three-chamber (A3C) view (**B**). Ao—aorta; LA—left atrium.

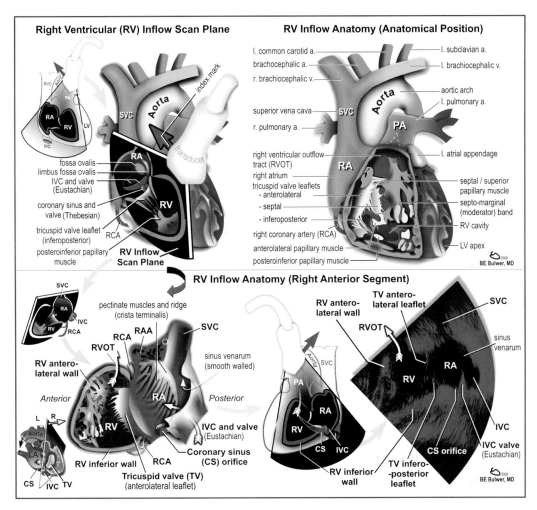

Figure 1-28. Echocardiographic parasternal RV inflow scan plane and corresponding anatomy. IVC—inferior vena cava; LLPV—left lower pulmonary vein; LUPV—left upper pulmonary vein; RA—right atrium; RAA—right atrial appendage; RVOT—RV outflow tract; SVC—superior vena cava.

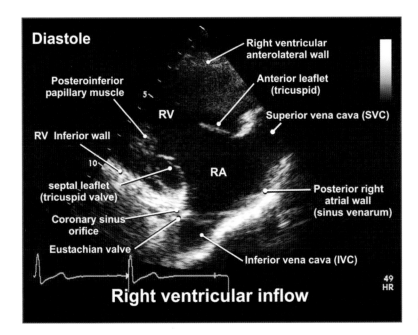

Figure 1-29. Two-dimensional long-axis view showing structures visualized on the RV inflow view. RA—right atrium.

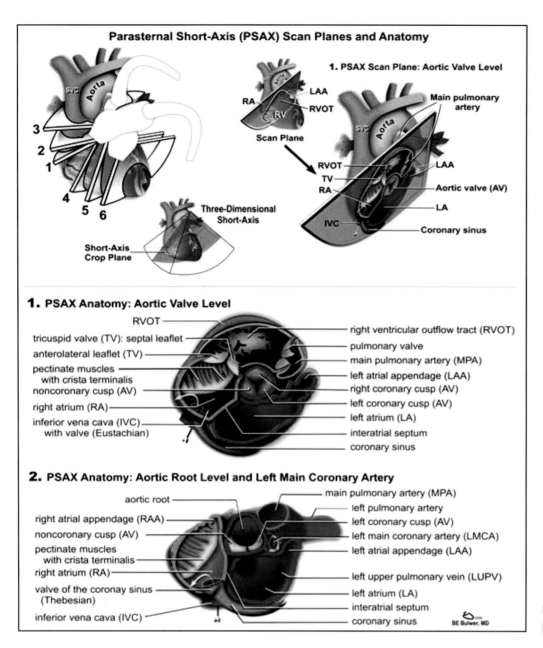

Figure 1-30. Echocardiographic short-axis scan planes and corresponding anatomy.

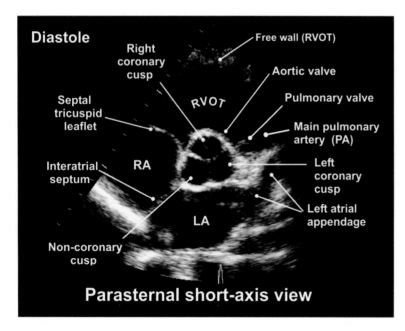

Figure 1-31. Two-dimensional parasternal short-view showing the structures visualized at the level of the aortic valve. RA—right atrium; RVOT—RV outflow tract.

Parasternal Short-Axis (PSAX) Scan Planes and Anatomy

3. High PSAX Scan Plane and Right Ventricular (RV) Outflow: Pulmonary Artery Level

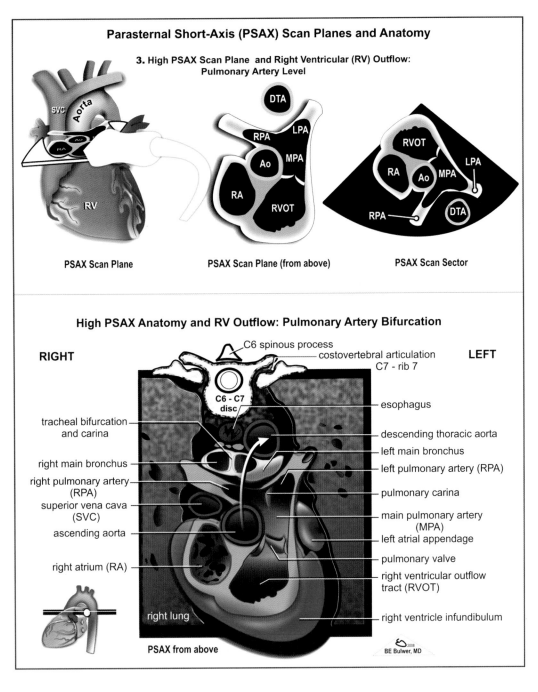

PSAX Scan Plane

PSAX Scan Plane (from above)

PSAX Scan Sector

High PSAX Anatomy and RV Outflow: Pulmonary Artery Bifurcation

RIGHT

LEFT

C6 spinous process

costovertebral articulation
C7 - rib 7

C6 - C7
disc

esophagus

tracheal bifurcation
and carina

descending thoracic aorta

left main bronchus

right main bronchus

left pulmonary artery (RPA)

right pulmonary artery
(RPA)

pulmonary carina

superior vena cava
(SVC)

main pulmonary artery
(MPA)

ascending aorta

left atrial appendage

pulmonary valve

right atrium (RA)

right ventricular outflow
tract (RVOT)

right lung

right ventricle infundibulum

PSAX from above

BE Bulwer, MD

Figure 1-32. Views of the high parasternal short-axis scan plane at the level of the pulmonary arteries and corresponding anatomy. Ao—aorta; DTA—descending thoracic aorta; PA—pulmonary artery.

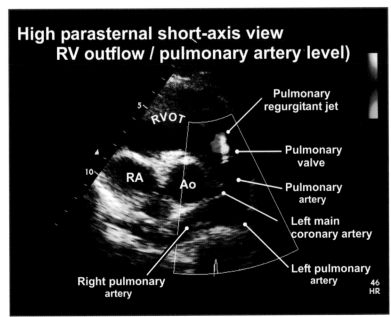

Figure 1-33. Two-dimensional echocardiographic frame showing the structures visualized on high parasternal short-axis view at the level of the main pulmonary artery (PA) and bifurcation into the right and left pulmonary arteries. Ao—aorta; RA—right atrium; RVOT—RV outflow tract.

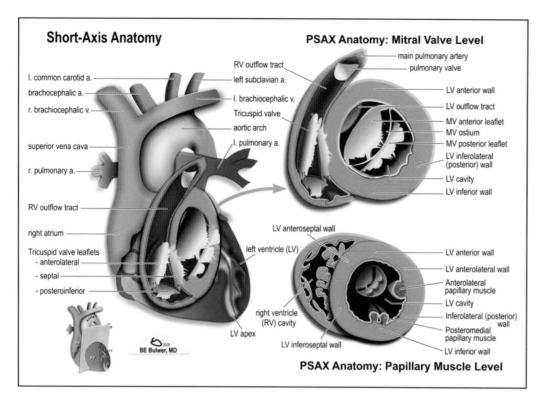

Figure 1-34. Anatomical structures corresponding to the parasternal short-axis (PSAX) scan planes at the level mitral valve (MV) and papillary muscle.

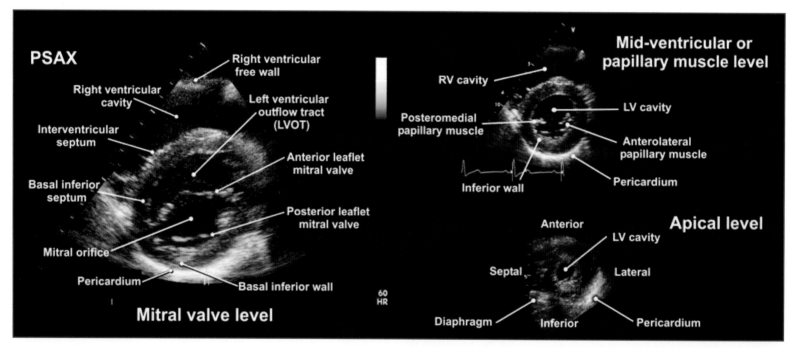

Figure 1-35. Two-dimensional short-axis frames showing structures visualized on the parasternal short-axis (PSAX) views at the mitral valve level (*left panel*), mid ventricular or papillary muscle level (*right panel*), and apical level (*right panel*).

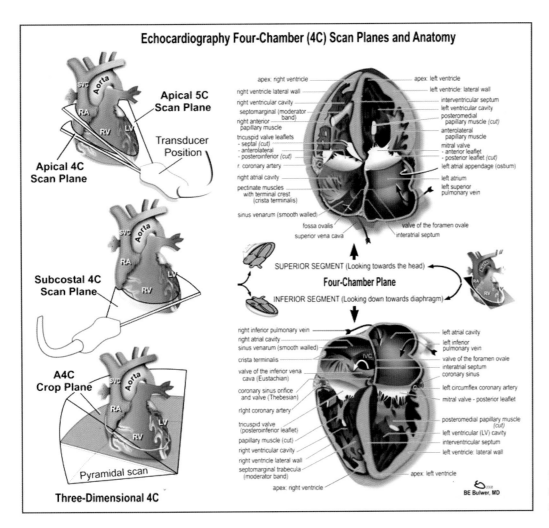

Figure 1-36. Echocardiographic four-chamber scan planes and corresponding anatomy. RA—right atrium; SVC—superior vena cavity.

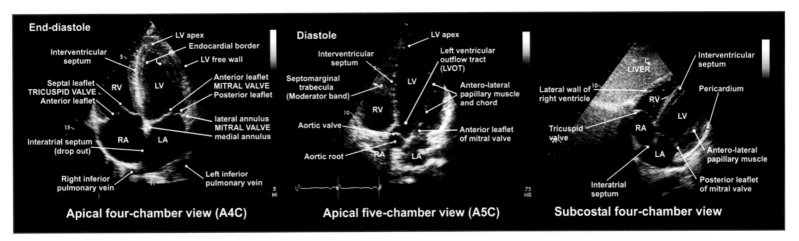

Figure 1-37. Two-dimensional four-chamber frames showing the structures visualized on the apical four-chamber (A4C) (*left panel*), apical five-chamber (A5C), (*middle panel*), and subcostal four-chamber views (*right panel*). LA—left atrium; RA—right atrium.

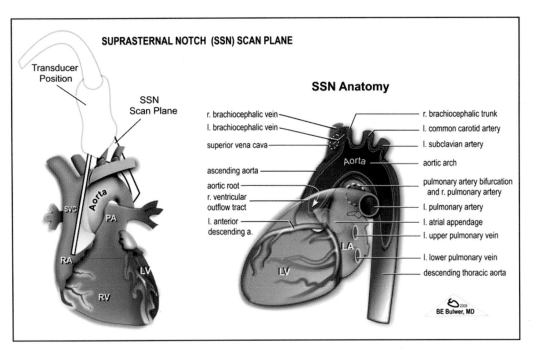

Figure 1-38. Echocardiographic suprasternal notch scan plane and corresponding anatomy. LA—left atrium; PA—pulmonary artery; RA—right atrium; SVC—superior vena cavity.

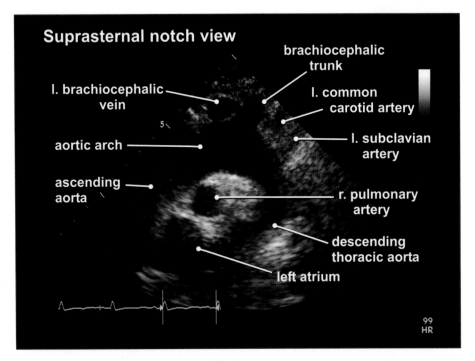

Figure 1-39. Two-dimensional frame showing structures visualized on the suprasternal notch view.

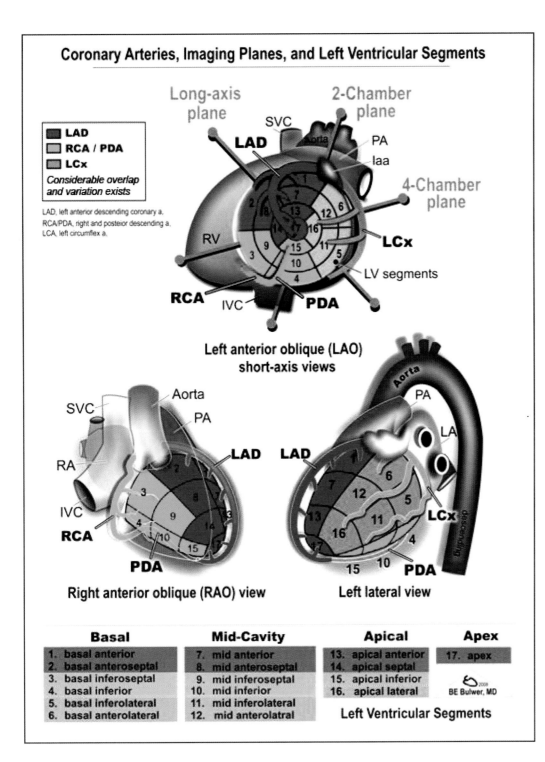

Coronary Arteries, Imaging Planes, and Left Ventricular Segments

LAD
RCA / PDA
LCx
Considerable overlap and variation exists

LAD, left anterior descending coronary a.
RCA/PDA, right and posterior descending a.
LCA, left circumflex a.

Long-axis plane
2-Chamber plane
SVC
LAD
Aorta
PA
laa
4-Chamber plane
RV
LCx
RCA
IVC
PDA
LV segments

Left anterior oblique (LAO) short-axis views

Aorta
SVC
PA
RA
LAD
LAD
PA
LA
IVC
LCx
RCA
PDA
PDA

Right anterior oblique (RAO) view

Left lateral view

Basal	Mid-Cavity	Apical	Apex
1. basal anterior	7. mid anterior	13. apical anterior	17. apex
2. basal anteroseptal	8. mid anteroseptal	14. apical septal	
3. basal inferoseptal	9. mid inferoseptal	15. apical inferior	
4. basal inferior	10. mid inferior	16. apical lateral	
5. basal inferolateral	11. mid inferolateral		
6. basal anterolateral	12. mid anterolatral		

Left Ventricular Segments

BE Bulwer, MD

Figure 1-40. Panoramic schema of coronary artery territories and LV segments using nomenclature recommended by the American Heart Association Writing Group on Myocardial Segmentation and Registration for Cardiac Imaging [2]. IVC—inferior vena cavity; LA—left atrium; laa—left atrial appendage; LAD—left anterior descending artery; PA—pulmonary artery; LAO—left anterior oblique; LCx—left circumflex; RAO—right anterior oblique; RCA/PDA—right coronary/posterior descending; SVC—superior vena cavity.

References

1. Otto C, ed: Principles of echocardiography imaging acquisition and Doppler analysis. In *Textbook of Clinical Echocardiography*, edn 3. Philadelphia: WB Saunders; 2004.

2. Cerqueira MD, Weissman NJ, Dilsizian V, *et al.*: Standardized myocardial segmentation and nomenclature for tomographic imaging of the heart: a statement for healthcare professionals from the Cardiac Imaging Committee of the Council on Clinical Cardiology of the American Heart Association. *Circulation* 2002, 105:539–542.

Recommended Reading

Bushberg JT, Siebert JA, Leidholdt EM Jr, Boone JM: *The Essential Physics of Medical Imaging*, edn 2. Philadelphia: Lippincott Williams & Wilkins; 2002:469–553.

Cape EG, Yoganathan AP: Principles and instrumentation for Doppler. In *Marcus Cardiac Imaging*, edn 2. Philadelphia: WB Saunders; 1996:273–291.

Feigenbaum H: *Echocardiography*, edn 4. Malvern, PA: Lea and Febiger; 1986.

Gardin JM, Adams DB, Douglas PS, *et al.*: Recommendations for a standardized report for adult transthoracic echocardiography: a report from the American Society of Echocardiography's Nomenclature and Standards Committee and Task Force for a Standardized Echocardiography Report. *J Am Soc Echocardiogr* 2002, 15:275–290.

Geiser EA: Echocardiography: physics and instrumentation. In *Marcus Cardiac Imaging*, edn. 2. Edited by Skorton DJ, Schelbert HR, Wolf GL, Brundage BH. Philadelphia: WB Saunders; 1996:273–291.

Hatle L, Angelsen B: *Doppler Ultrasound in Cardiology: Physical Principles and Clinical Applications*, edn. 2. Philadelphia: Lea & Febiger; 1985.

Henry WL, DeMaria A, Gramiak R, *et al.*: Report of the American Society of Echocardiography Committee on nomenclature and standards in two-dimensional echocardiography. *Circulation* 1980, 62:212–217.

Hung J, Lang R, Flachskampf F, *et al.*: 3D echocardiography: a review of the current status and future directions. *J Am Soc Echocardiogr* 2007, 20:213–233.

Kremkau FW: *Diagnostic Ultrasound: Principles and Instruments*, edn 6. Philadelphia: WB Saunders; 2002.

McAlpine WA: *Heart and Coronary Arteries: an Anatomical Atlas for Clinical Diagnosis, Radiological Investigation, and Surgical Treatment*. Berlin, Heidelberg, New York: Springer-Verlag; 1975.

Medical diagnostic ultrasound instrumentation and clinical interpretation: report of the ultrasonography task force. *JAMA* 1991, 265:1155–1159.

O'Rourke MF, Nichols WW: *McDonald's Blood Flow in Arteries*, edn 5. New York: Oxford University Press; 2005.

Quinones MA, Douglas PS, Foster E, *et al.*: ACC/AHA clinical competence statement on echocardiography: a report of the American College of Cardiology/American Heart Association/American College of Physicians - American Society of Internal Medicine Task Force on Clinical Competence. *J Am Coll Cardiol* 2003, 41:687–708.

Quinones MA, Otto CM, Stoddard M, *et al.*: Recommendations for quantification of Doppler echocardiography: a report from the Doppler Quantification Task Force of the Nomenclature and Standards Committee of the American Society of Echocardiography. *J Am Soc Echocardiogr* 2002, 15:167–184.

Seghal CM: Principles of ultrasonic imaging and Doppler ultrasound. In Textbook *of Echocardiography and Doppler in Adults and Children*. Edited by St. John Sutton MG, Oldershaw PJ, Kotler MN. Oxford, UK: Blackwell Science; 1996:3–30.

2 M-Mode Echocardiography

Judy R. Mangion

M-mode echocardiography provides superior temporal resolution. Subtle changes can be better appreciated with M-mode as opposed to two-dimensional or three-dimensional methods. These changes can include precise measurements of cardiac chambers (provided that they are obtained on-axis), valvular vegetations, early closure or early opening of the valve structures with respect to timing in the cardiac cycle, identification of prosthetic valves and their function, assessment of paradoxical interventricular septal motion and dyssynchrony of the LV, as well as fluttering of valve leaflets, which is seen in association with valvular regurgitation. The exaggerated motion of cardiac structure, as well as restricted motions of various cardiac structures, is also readily appreciated with M-mode echocardiography.

An M-mode echocardiogram provides one-dimensional information regarding a particular cardiac structure as it relates to time and distance. Time is displayed on the horizontal axis, and depth or distance is displayed on the vertical axis. The strength of the reflected echo is represented as the brightness of the structures appearing on the image display. The limitations of M-mode echocardiography involve having to draw conclusions in one dimension about a three-dimensional structure. Furthermore, measurements are dependent on the identification of clearly defined borders, which may not be obtainable in technically challenging patients. With respect to M-mode–derived ejection fractions, calculations may not be accurate when regional wall motion abnormalities are present.

M-mode echocardiography was described more than 50 years ago by Edler and Hertz; however, new concepts and technologies have allowed for M-mode techniques to expand. For example, color M-mode echocardiography evolved in the 1990s in order to provide rapid evaluation of time-related events (*eg*, diastolic mitral regurgitation), and it has also been used to provide less load-dependent information regarding diastolic function. Color M-mode techniques have also been used in assessing myocardial deformation or strain, in which a curved M-mode is traced along an area of interest on the myocardium, and information is displayed in both parametric and graphical format. This allows for a sensitive evaluation of normal and abnormal patterns of ventricular contractility.

This chapter provides case examples of normal M-mode examinations, as well as providing a diverse spectrum of abnormal M-mode examinations that illustrate classic cardiac anomalies. Each figure legend will provide a "clinical pearl," highlighting important concepts to understand in either technically obtaining or interpreting each image.

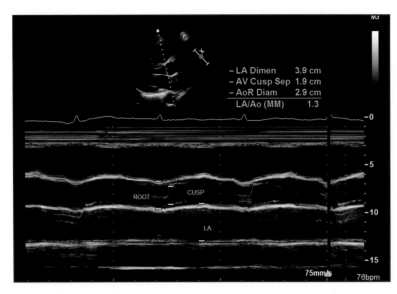

Figure 2-1. Normal M-mode examination of the aortic root, aortic valve cusps, and left atrium (LA). Measurements are obtained in the parasternal long-axis imaging plane. Note the holosystolic opening of the aortic valve cusps. M-mode measurements are made leading edge to leading edge. This differs from two-dimensional measurements. The M-mode cursor is placed perpendicular to the aortic valve leaflets. CUSP—aortic leaflet separation; ROOT—aortic root.

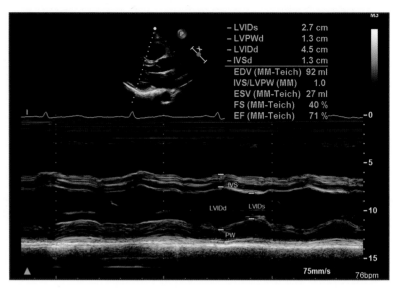

Figure 2-2. Normal M-mode examination of the LV obtained from the parasternal long-axis imaging plane. LV dimensions are made at end diastole and end systole, whereas septal and posterior wall thicknesses are usually only measured at end diastole. The M-mode cursor is placed perpendicular to the long axis of the LV at the level of the mitral valve chordae. EF—ejection fraction; ESV—end systolic volume; FS—fractional shortening; IVS—interventricular septum; EDV—end-diastolic volume; LVIDd—LV internal dimension in diastole; LVIDs—LV internal dimension in systole; PW—posterior wall.

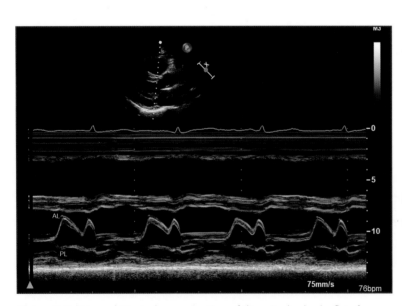

Figure 2-3. Normal M-mode examination of the mitral valve leaflets from the parasternal long-axis imaging plane. The M-mode cursor is placed perpendicular to the long axis of the LV at the level of the tips of the mitral leaflets. AL—anterior leaflet; PL—posterior leaflet.

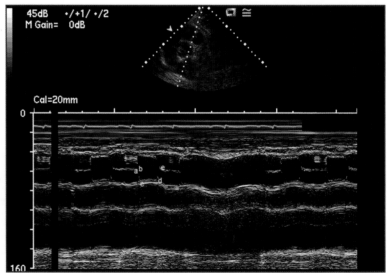

Figure 2-4. Normal M-mode examination of the pulmonic valve obtained from the parasternal short-axis view. This recording may also be obtained from the parasternal RV outflow view, as well as the main pulmonary artery and bifurcation view. Note the holosystolic opening of the cusps, which is similar to the aortic valve. Often, M-mode of the pulmonic valve only transects the right-posterior leaflet. In this example, both the anterior and right-posterior leaflets are transected. The M-mode letter designations for the pulmonic valve are as follows: a—atrial contraction; b—onset of ventricular systole; c—ventricular ejection; d—during ventricular ejection; e—end of ventricular ejection.

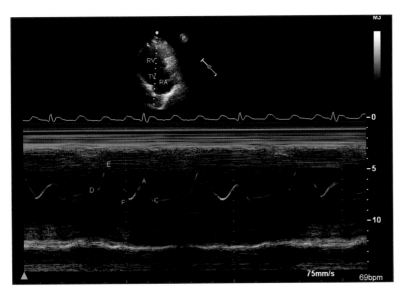

Figure 2-5. Normal M-mode examination of the tricuspid valve obtained from RV inflow view. Normally, only the anterior leaflet of the tricuspid valve (TV) is transected. A—leaflet reopening with atrial contraction; C—leaflet closure following ventricular systole; D—onset of diastole; E—maximal opening of the leaflet, E-F slope—closing motion of the leaflet; F—most posterior position of the leaflet; RA—right atrium.

M-Mode Examination of the Aortic Valve

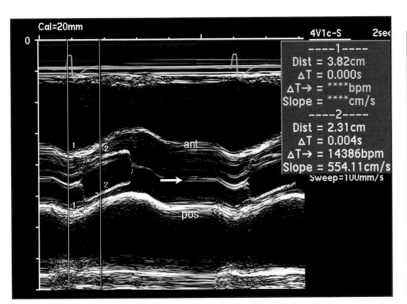

Figure 2-6. M-mode examination of a bicuspid aortic valve, obtained from the parasternal long-axis view. Note that the closing of the valve is asymmetric (*arrow*). This may be an important clue in establishing the diagnosis of bicuspid aortic valve, if present. In some situations, bicuspid aortic valves may open symmetrically. ant—anterior; pos—posterior.

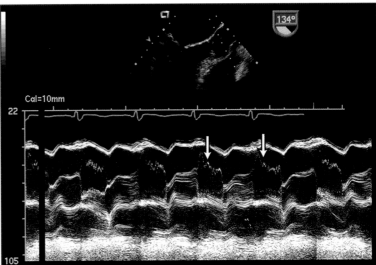

Figure 2-7. M-mode examination of the aortic valve demonstrating early systolic closure of the leaflets (*arrows*) due to a fixed subaortic membrane. The membrane decreases the pressure differential between the systemic circulation and LV, which causes the aortic valve to close early. The image was obtained from longitudinal view of the aortic valve with transesophageal probe.

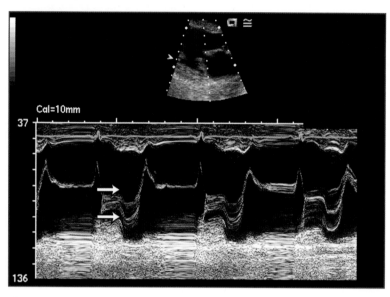

Figure 2-8. M-mode examination of the mitral valve demonstrating classic late systolic bileaflet mitral valve prolapse (*arrows*) obtained from the parasternal long-axis view. Prolapse can be missed or overdiagnosed with M-mode echocardiography alone because of dependence on the ultrasound beam. Therefore, the diagnosis needs to be confirmed by two-dimensional methods, demonstrating systolic prolapse of greater than 2 mm beyond the plane of the mitral annulus and into the left atrium.

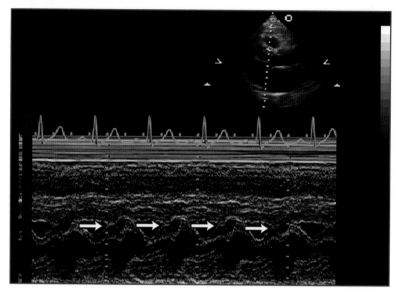

Figure 2-9. M-mode examination of the mitral valve, parasternal long-axis view, demonstrating systolic anterior motion of the mitral valve (*arrows*), which causes dynamic LV outflow tract obstruction. This is often observed in the setting of hypertrophic obstructive cardiomyopathy; however, it can also occur in the absence of hypertrophic cardiomyopathy. In the setting of hypertrophic obstructive cardiomyopathy, the anterior cusp of the mitral valve comes into forceful contact with the protruding interventricular septum as the LV chamber decreases in systole. The M-mode recording provides information pertaining to the timing of systolic anterior motion of the mitral valve.

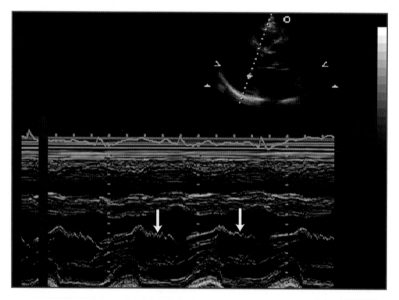

Figure 2-10. M-mode examination of the mitral valve, parasternal long-axis view, demonstrating high-frequency diastolic fluttering of the anterior mitral leaflet (*arrows*) due to severe aortic insufficiency. This is the equivalent of the Austin Flint murmur.

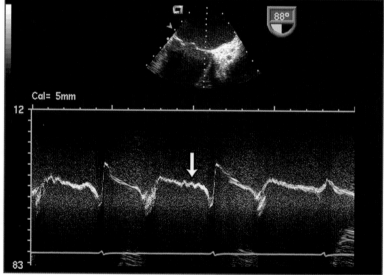

Figure 2-11. M-mode examination of the mitral valve, midesophageal two-chamber view, demonstrating high-frequency diastolic fluttering of the anterior leaflet of the mitral valve leaflet (*arrow*) due to severe aortic insufficiency impinging on the leaflet.

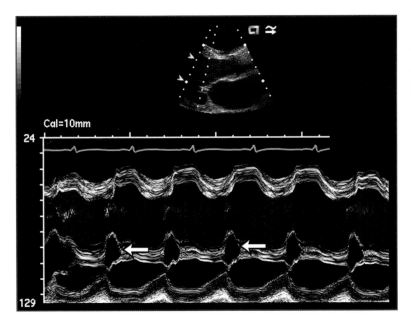

Figure 2-12. M-mode examination of the mitral valve, parasternal long-axis view, demonstrating early diastolic closure of the mitral valve (*arrows*) due to severe acute aortic insufficiency. The sudden increase in diastolic volume overload causes increased resistance by the ventricle to diastolic filling causing the early diastolic closure of the mitral valve.

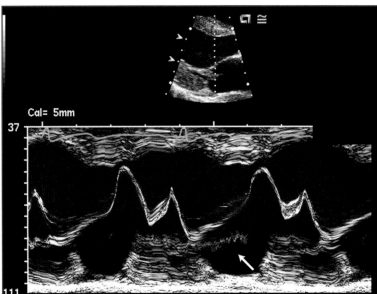

Figure 2-13. M-mode examination of the mitral valve demonstrating a large mobile mass with independent motion on the atrial surface of posterior leaflet in a patient with suspected endocarditis (*arrow*). M-mode echocardiography can sometimes identify vegetations that can be missed with two-dimensional echocardiography because of its higher frame rates.

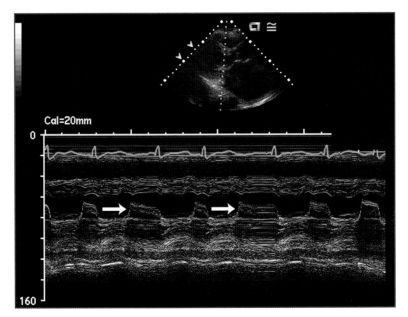

Figure 2-14. M-mode examination of the mitral valve affected by rheumatic valvular heart disease. There is reduced opening of the mitral leaflets during diastole (*arrows*) due to fusion of the commissures.

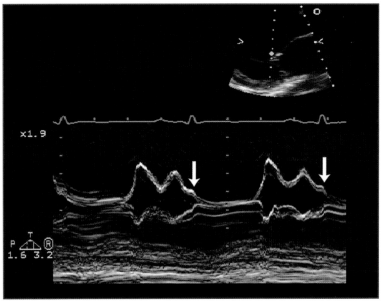

Figure 2-15. M-mode examination of the mitral valve demonstrating a "b-notch" on the anterior mitral valve leaflet (*arrows*) in a patient with dilated cardiomyopathy. Although the b-notch is not always present, it is indicative of an elevated LV end-diastolic pressure when identified.

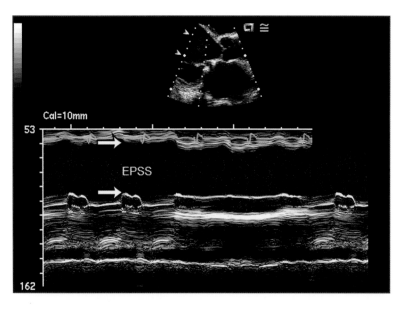

Figure 2-16. M-mode examination of the mitral valve demonstrating an enlarged E point septal separation (EPSS) (*arrows*) in a patient with dilated cardiomyopathy due to a reduced stroke volume with poor systolic function. A normal EPSS should generally be less than 1 cm. EPSS on M-mode can provide a useful marker of overall LV systolic function.

M-Mode Examination of the Left Ventricle

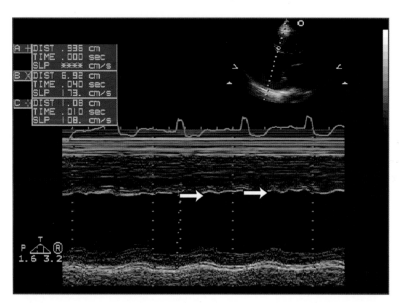

Figure 2-17. M-mode examination of the LV, parasternal long-axis view, in a patient with left bundle branch block. Note the paradoxical septal motion, or delayed contraction, of the interventricular septum in systole (*arrows*).

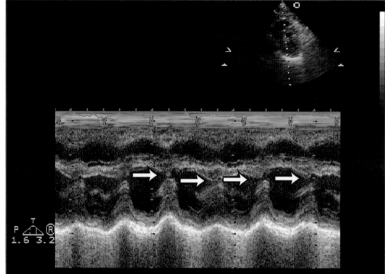

Figure 2-18. M-mode examination of the LV, parasternal long-axis view, demonstrating exaggerated respiratory variation of the position of the interventricular septum, the so-called septal bounce (*arrows*). This is a nonspecific finding in suspected constrictive pericarditis; if clinical suspicion of cardiac constriction is high, it should warrant additional directed comprehensive two-dimensional and Doppler evaluation.

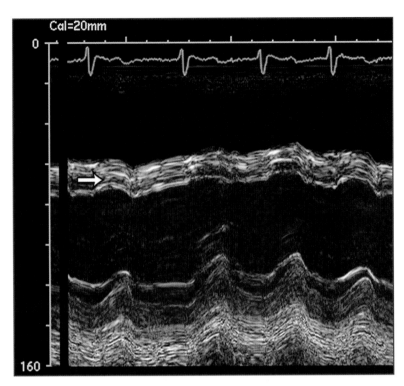

Figure 2-19. M-mode examination of the LV, parasternal long-axis view, in a patient with severe cor pulmonale, demonstrating both systolic and diastolic flattening of the interventricular septum, the so-called d-shaped septum (*arrow*). Systolic flattening of the septum represents pressure overload of the RV from pulmonary hypertension, whereas diastolic flattening of the septum represents volume overload of the RV, which in this example was secondary to severe wide open tricuspid insufficiency.

M-Mode Examination of the Pulmonic and Tricuspid Valves and Inferior Vena Cava

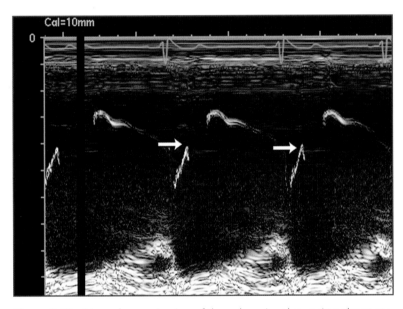

Figure 2-20. M-mode examination of the pulmonic valve, main pulmonary artery view, demonstrating early systolic closure of the pulmonic valve, so-called flying w (*arrows*) associated with severe pulmonary hypertension due to the elevated filling pressure of the RV. There is often an absent a-wave (atrial wave) of the M-mode tracing.

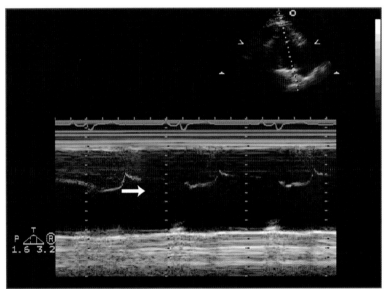

Figure 2-21. M-mode examination of the tricuspid valve, RV inflow view in Ebstein's anomaly. Ebstein's anomaly is a congenital deformity characterized by downward displacement of either part or all of the tricuspid valve into the RV cavity. Note the decreased diastolic opening of the anterior leaflet due to deformation (*arrow*) as compared with the normal M-Mode of tricuspid valve (*see* Fig. 2-5).

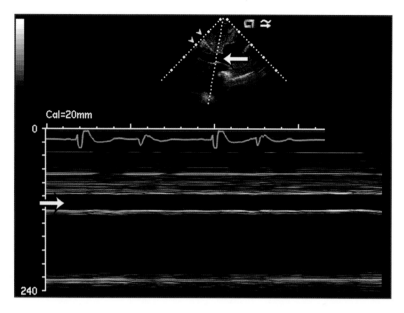

Figure 2-22. M-mode examination of the inferior vena cava, subcostal view, in the presence of markedly elevated right atrial pressure, such as tamponade, constriction, or cor pulmonale. Note the markedly dilated (> 2 cm) and plethoric (no inspiratory collapse) inferior vena cava (*arrows*). The M-mode cursor is placed at the junction of the inferior vena cava and the right atrium. The estimated right atrial pressure in this scenario is at least 20 mm Hg.

M-Mode Examination of Prosthetic Valves

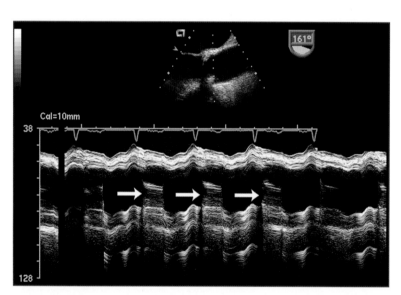

Figure 2-23. M-mode examination of a normally functioning St. Jude's bileaflet mechanical aortic valve prosthesis, longitudinal view, obtained with transesophageal echocardiography. In order to demonstrate correct motion of both prosthetic valve leaflets in systole (*arrows*), M-mode echocardiography continues to be an important part of the evaluation of prosthetic valve function.

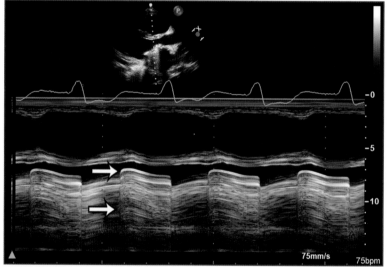

Figure 2-24. M-mode examination of a normally functioning St. Jude's bileaflet mechanical mitral valve prosthesis, parasternal long-axis view. M-mode echocardiography continues to be an important part of the evaluation of prosthetic valve function because of its ability to demonstrate correct motion of both prosthetic valve leaflets in diastole (*arrows*).

Color M-Mode Echocardiography

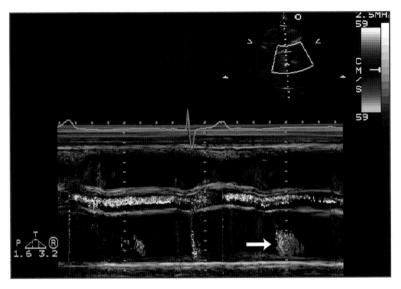

Figure 2-25. Color M-mode examination of the aortic root and left atrium, parasternal long-axis view, in a patient with mild diastolic mitral regurgitation (*arrow*), which is attributable to heart block. This demonstrates that M-mode echocardiography is an ideal modality for confirming the timing of events with respect to the cardiac cycle.

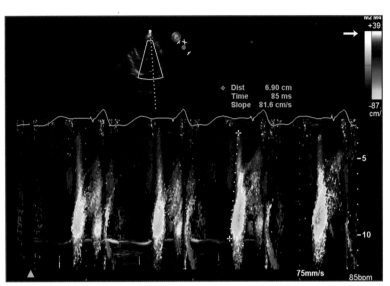

Figure 2-26. Color M-mode examination of the LV, apical four-chamber view, demonstrating normal propagation velocity of blood flow in the left ventricle of 81.6 cm/s during diastole, which is indicative of normal diastolic filling pattern. Normal propagation velocities are measured by the initial slope of the E wave on color M-mode and are always greater than 45 cm/s. Note that the Nyquist color scale is moved up to 39.4 cm/s (*arrow*), allowing color Doppler flow to be visualized all the way from the base of the mitral annulus to the LV apex.

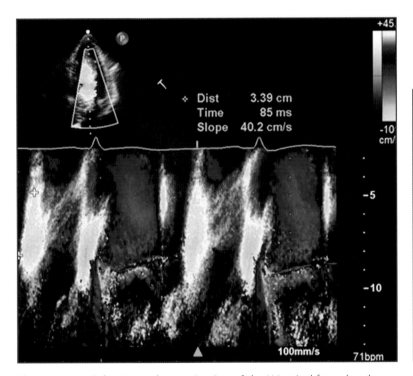

Figure 2-27. Color M-mode examination of the LV, apical four-chamber view, demonstrating a diastolic filling pattern consistent with impaired LV relaxation. In this case, the propagation velocity measures 40.2 cm/s and it is mildly reduced. Color M-mode is a useful tool in the assessment of diastolic function of the LV, and it is thought to be less flow dependent than pulsed wave Doppler.

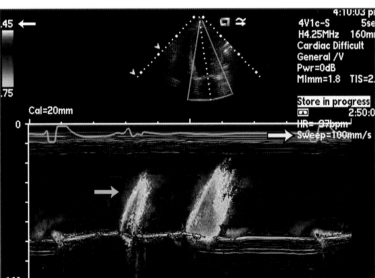

Figure 2-28. Color M-mode examination of the LV, apical four-chamber view, demonstrating a diastolic filling pattern consistent with markedly delayed propagation or restrictive physiology. In this example, the propagation velocity (Vp) measured significantly less than 45 cm/s (*blue arrow*). Note that the accuracy of the measurement of the Vp of early diastolic filling on color M-mode is improved by increasing the sweep speed to 100 mm/s (*yellow arrow*). The Nyquist scale of color Doppler propagation has been reduced to 45 cm/s (*white arrow*).

Strain Imaging of the Myocardium (Parametric M-Mode Echocardiography)

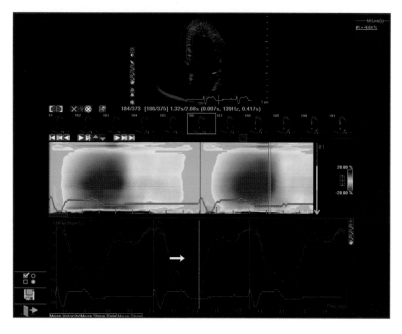

Figure 2-29. Parametric curved M-mode examination of the LV, apical four-chamber view, demonstrating normal strain pattern of the LV. Strain imaging represents load independent, cutting edge technology for measuring regional myocardial deformation of the ventricular myocardium, and it is measured in percentages in order to reflect the relative shortening of the myocyte during systole. In this example, a curved M-mode line is traced along the interventricular septum from apex to base. The orange wide band in systole represents shortening, whereas the yellow wide band in diastole represents lengthening. The four red curves below the parametric image represent four separate strain measurements from apex to base, with the apex (top curve) showing the least amount of strain or deformation during systole (*arrow*).

Suggested Reading

Foster E, ed: *Echo SAP*. American College of Cardiology Foundation. 2006

Sahn DJ, DeMaria A, Kisslo, J, Weyman A: Recommendations regarding quantitation in M-mode echocardiography: results of a survey of echocardiographic measurements. *Circulation* 1978, 58:1072.

Solomon SD, ed: *Essential Echocardiography*. Totowa, NJ: Humana Press; 2007.

Weyman, A, ed: *Principles and Practice of Echocardiography*, edn 2. Philadelphia: Lea & Febiger; 1994.

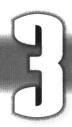

Cardiac Hemodynamics

Rosario V. Freeman and Catherine M. Otto

Doppler echocardiography is useful in assessing hemodynamic status and valvular function. The Doppler equation (*see* Fig. 3-1) describes the principle that sound reflected from a moving object returns with a different frequency than that of transmitted frequencies. Analysis of the Doppler frequency shift between transmitted and reflected ultrasound signals from moving structures (most commonly red blood cells) allows for the evaluation of flow direction and velocities (higher velocities create larger Doppler shifts). A nonparallel intercept angel "θ" between the ultrasound beam and blood flow underestimates velocity. At an angle of 20°, error in velocity estimation is only 6%, but at 60°, error increases to 50%. There are three basic Doppler modalities. The first two are pulsed wave Doppler (PWD) and continuous wave Doppler (CWD), which are nonscanned modalities in which velocity is plotted against time. Color flow Doppler (CFD) is a scanned modality where velocities are coded onto a color map and superimposed onto a two-dimensional image. Standard Doppler controls include power output, receiver gain, velocity range, baseline shift, and filters, which eliminate low-frequency Doppler shifts. If filters are set low and Doppler interrogation is focused on the myocardium (lower velocities), tissue motion can also be measured [1,2].

With PWD, the transducer alternates between sending and receiving signals and samples blood velocities at a specified depth along the ultrasound beam. There is a limited measurable maximum velocity with PWD, termed the "Nyquist limit," beyond which the signal aliases and peak velocity cannot be measured. Therefore, PWD is useful for localizing lower velocities at specified depths; this is most commonly used for the evaluation of normal valves and intracardiac flow. High-pulse repetition frequency is a modification of PWD, where velocities are taken from multiple samples proximal to the depth of interest. By measuring proximal velocities, higher velocities can be recorded, avoiding aliasing. With CWD, the transducer has two piezoelectric crystals, one that continuously transmits and one that continuously receives signals. There is no aliasing with CWD; however, specific velocities cannot be localized in space (*ie*, range ambiguity) because the signal is received continuously along the entire length of the ultrasound beam. CWD is useful for evaluating transvalvular flow where velocities are much higher, such as stenotic or regurgitant valves. Pres-

sure gradients can be calculated from CWD peak velocities using the Bernoulli equation.

Frequency shifts toward the transducer are shown above the zero baseline and shifts away from the transducer below the baseline in both PWD and CWD. The highest recorded signal is the peak velocity, with mean velocities averaged over the duration of flow (in milliseconds). Velocities are plotted against time on the baseline axis. The velocity time integral (VTI) is the integral of blood flow velocity over time, measured in distance (in meters). When interrogating blood flow, a flat-flow profile with equal velocities across the cross-sectional area (CSA) is optimal as a single velocity measurement would represent average flow velocity. However, parabolic flow with higher center velocities is often present due to blood viscosity, vessel wall effects (*see* Fig. 3-2), and entrainment of the anterograde jet. The shape, timing, and density of spectral Doppler images provide valuable qualitative evaluation of blood flow, and increased jet density suggests increased flow volume. Rapid equalization of transvalvular pressure gradients between two cardiac chambers leads to steeper jet slopes (*see* Fig. 3-3).

CFD is a form of PWD where velocities are sampled along multiple cursor lines in a sector. Averaged velocities are converted into color scale and are then superimposed onto two-dimensional images, allowing imaging of real time directional and spatial blood flow. By convention, flow away from the transducer is coded blue, and flow towards the transducer is coded red. Similar to PWD, CFD imaging is limited with a nonparallel intercept angle and is subject to signal aliasing at higher velocities. Because velocities are averaged across the scan plane, temporal resolution is less optimal than with PWD or CWD, but it can be improved by decreasing scan line number, pulses per scan line, or color sector size (generally with incremental adverse impact on spatial resolution).

Noninvasive echocardiographic evaluation of cardiac hemodynamics is centered on several principles. These include the principle of flow quantitation (stroke volume [SV] calculation), the principle of continuity of flow (continuity equation), and the pressure/velocity relationship (Bernoulli equation). When combined with qualitative measures, inferences on cardiac hemodynamics (including quantitation of stenosis and regurgitation severity), cardiac SV and output, ventricular systolic and diastolic function, and intracardiac pressure calculation can be obtained [1].

Quantitation and Continuity of Flow

The SV per cardiac cycle, traversing a cardiac orifice, is the product of the CSA at that point and the velocity time integral (VTI_{FLOW}) [3–5] (see Fig. 3-4 and 3-5). The CSA can be calculated by measuring the diameter at the point of interest (assuming a circular orifice). Accuracy in the diameter measurement is crucial because any error is squared in CSA calculation. Measurements of CSA and VTI_{FLOW} should be obtained at the same anatomical position. A flat-flow profile with equal velocity across the interrogated CSA is assumed. The intercept angle between the ultrasound beam and blood flow must be parallel so that maximum velocity and VTI_{FLOW} are measured. Cardiac output can be calculated by multiplying SV by heart rate. Anterograde SV through an orifice is the sum of both forward and retrograde (regurgitant) flow. SV calculations across an orifice with significant regurgitation will lead to incorrect cardiac output measurements. Accuracy and reproducibility of Doppler-derived measures of SV and cardiac output are comparable with other methods, including Fick thermodilution, contrast angiographic ventriculography, and radionucleotide ventriculography [2].

The principle of continuity of flow describes the concept that the SV passing just proximal to an orifice (SV_{pre}) is the same as the SV passing through the orifice ($SV_{orifice}$) (see Fig. 3-6). If the CSA and VTI_{pre} just proximal to the orifice and the $VTI_{orifice}$ at the orifice are known, orifice area can be calculated using the quantitation of flow principle ("continuity equation"). The most common application of the continuity equation is for an aortic valve area (AVA) measurement for stenosis with LV outflow tract (LVOT) area and VTI at the LVOT and aortic valve used for continuity calculation. Because the shape and timing of the VTI curves are similar in the LVOT and at the aortic valve, the peak velocity ratio is proportional to the VTI ratio and can be substituted (see Fig. 3-7). The correlation between Doppler-derived AVA and invasive measurements in the cardiac catheterization laboratory ranges from 0.83 to 0.96 [2,6,7]. Assuming the absence of significant mitral regurgitation, the continuity equation can also be used to calculate mitral valve area (MVA) (see Fig. 3-8 and 3-16) in mitral stenosis.

Pressure-Velocity Relationship (Bernoulli Equation)

With increased obstruction to blood flow, velocities increase and are correlated with increased pressure gradients across the orifice. The pressure-velocity relationship is described by the Bernoulli equation, where ρ represents the mass density of blood (1.06×10^3 kg/m³).

$$P_2 - P_1 = 1/2\rho(V_2^2 - V_1^2) + \text{viscous friction} + \text{local acceleration}$$

The following assumptions can be made: 1) effects of viscous friction between blood cells and the vessel wall are minimal; 2) local acceleration of individual blood cells is minimal; 3) the proximal velocity (V_1) is significantly smaller than the distal velocity (V_2). The proximal velocity (V_1) is usually ignored, and the equation can be simplified to: $P_2 - P_1 = 4V_2^2$ (see Fig. 3-9).

If V_1 is greater than 1 m/s or is comparable with V_2 in magnitude, it should be included in calculations. Doppler-derived pressure gradients correlate well with direct invasive measurement [2].

Evaluation of intracardiac and intrapulmonary pressures is a common application of the pressure-velocity relationship and the simplified Bernoulli equation. In the estimation of pulmonary arterial pressures, the gradient between the RV and the right atrium is calculated using the systolic blood velocity from the tricuspid regurgitant jet and the end-diastolic velocity from the pulmonic regurgint jet [8,9] (see Fig. 3-10 and 3-11). Right atrial pressure estimates are added

to the pressure gradients for pulmonary artery pressures (see Fig. 3-12 and 3-13). Estimates of left atrial and LV end-diastolic pressure (LVEDP) are made using velocities obtained from mitral and aortic regurgitant jets, respectively, assuming absence of significant aortic stenosis for the LVEDP calculation (see Fig. 3-14).

Peak and mean transvalvular pressure gradients are estimated from transvalvular velocities. In the evaluation of aortic stenosis, peak transvalvular velocities should be obtained from several views to ensure that the maximal velocity is recorded. Doppler-derived transvalvular pressure gradients are maximum instantaneous gradients as opposed to the "peak aortic pressure to the peak left LV pressure" gradients reported from the catheterization laboratory, resulting in a small discrepancy between the two methods (see Fig. 3-15). In addition to the continuity equation, MVA can be calculated from the empirically derived equation: MVA = 220/pressure half time (PHT), where PHT (or $T_{1/2}$) is the time duration for the peak early mitral inflow pressure gradient to drop by half. Because of the quadratic pressure-velocity relationship described in the Bernoulli equation, where the pressure change equals $4V_{max}^2$, PHT is also the time duration for early mitral inflow velocity to decrease by $V_{max}/2^{1/2}$ (see Fig. 3-16). Doppler-derived methods for MVA have been validated against invasive measurements in the catheterization laboratory [2,10,11].

Doppler Evaluation of Valvular Regurgitation

Echocardiography is the method of choice for the noninvasive evaluation of valvular regurgitation. In asymptomatic patients with significant regurgitation, timing of surgical intervention is predicated on adverse hemodynamic effects of regurgitation on receiving chamber size and function. Color Doppler mapping allows visualization and assessment of the regurgitant jet flow disturbance, jet size, direction, and jet eccentricity

(see Fig. 3-17). Measurement of the narrowest jet width (vena contracta) at or just distal to the regurgitant orifice correlates with regurgitation severity and is a simple measure, even with eccentric jets [12–14] (see Fig. 3-18). For atrioventricular valve regurgitation, PWD evaluation of the peak early inflow velocity (E wave) and the shape of the regurgitant CWD envelope jet provides additional data on regurgitation severity. Other markers of regurgitation severity include flow reversal of the Doppler signal in adjacent upstream vascular structures, which is typically seen when regurgitation severity is moderate or more severe [15–17] (*see* Fig. 3-19, 3-20, 3-21, and 3-22). Relative density of the regurgitant compared with anterograde CWD signal and the acuity of the regurgitant Doppler signal slope correlate with severity as well. For example, with severe aortic regurgitation, the Doppler signal is more intense and diastolic pressure equilibrium between the aorta and LV is established earlier with a steeper slope (expressed as a PHT) calculated in the same manner as described previously.

Quantitative evaluation of regurgitation severity uses continuity of flow (flow convergence) and quantitation of flow. The proximal isovelocity surface area (PISA) calculation assumes regurgitant flow accelerates in a laminar fashion towards a regurgitant orifice, forming concentric "hemispheres" of isovelocity [18,19] (*see* Fig. 3-23 and 3-24). The effective regurgitant orifice area (EROA) can be calculated based on the principle of continuity of flow once hemisphere surface area, blood velocity at that hemisphere ("aliasing velocity"), and orifice regurgitant velocity are measured. Calculation of EROA by PISA is more accurate when the regurgitant orifice is circular, and the jet is not eccentric. The aliasing velocity must be measured when flow convergence forms a well-defined hemisphere, as any error will be squared in the final calculation. The PISA calculation measures the EROA at the maximal instantaneous flow. If regurgitation is not holosystolic, such as in mitral valve prolapse, maximal

instantaneous flow rate will overestimate total regurgitation severity and EROA. Similarly, the vena contracta measurement may overestimate regurgitation severity if flow is not holosystolic. A simplified EROA calculation can be performed by setting color Doppler aliasing velocity at 40 cm/s (assuming a mitral regurgitant peak velocity of 5 m/s) and measuring the distance between the aliasing velocity to the valve orifice, where EROA = $r^2/4$ [20]. Regurgitant volume is the retrograde SV per heart beat. Using the principle of flow quantitation, regurgitant volume equals EROA $\times$ VTI_{FLOW}, and regurgitant fraction is the relative fraction of regurgitant flow to total transvalvular flow. Another method of assessing regurgitation severity is to compare anterograde volume across the regurgitant valve (including anterograde and regurgitant flow) with flow across a competent valve (difference = regurgitant volume), allowing calculation of regurgitant fraction and effective orifice area [14,21] (*see* Fig. 3-25). A clinical example of mitral regurgitation severity assessment is provided (*see* Fig. 3-26). Gradation of mitral and aortic regurgitation by the American Society of Echocardiography is now incorporated in the newly published American Heart Association/American College of Cardiology guidelines on valvular heart disease, which support use of these quantitative measures to grade regurgitation severity [22] (*see* Fig. 3-27). Quantitative measures are superior to qualitative assessment because CFD measures of regurgitant jet size and flow disturbance are subject to transducer frequency and instrument settings.

Doppler Assessment of Ventricular Function

Evaluation of LV systolic pressure generation provides a surrogate measure of systolic function. Using the simplified Bernoulli equation, LV rate of change in pressure over time (dP/dt) can be calculated by measuring the transmitral pressure gradient at two points on the velocity curve and time duration between these points. With impaired systolic function, there is a delay in LV systolic pressure generation, and the slope of intracardiac pressure over time increases [23,24] (*see* Fig. 3-28).

PWD echocardiography aids in the assessment of ventricular diastolic function. Diastolic indices include evaluation of LV inflow velocities with early filling E wave and atrial contribution to filling (A wave) at the mitral leaflet tips for peak velocities/deceleration time and at the mitral annulus for A wave duration. Other indices include

isovolumic relaxation time and left atrial inflow velocities with peak pulmonary vein A wave velocity and duration. Loading conditions (ie, heart rate, volume overload, and mitral regurgitation) affect left atrial inflow and outflow measurements. Mitral inflow evaluation repeated during Valsava maneuver (transient preload decrease) may unmask underlying diastolic dysfunction. Many of these indices can also aid in evaluation for pericardial disease. Tissue Doppler interrogation at the septum and lateral wall 1 cm below the mitral annulus allows measurement of early (E′) and atrial (A′) contribution to myocardial diastolic motion and is less sensitive to loading conditions. The ratio of transmitral E to myocardial E′ allows evaluation of LV filling pressures [25] (*see* Fig. 3-29 and 3-30).

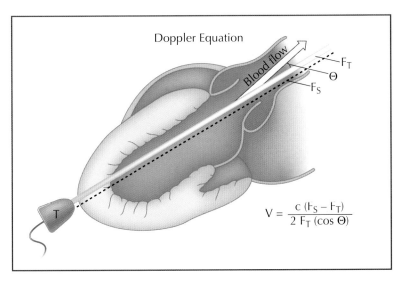

Figure 3-1. The Doppler equation calculating the velocity of blood flow (*V*) is shown. The difference in frequency between the transducer frequency (F_T) and the backscattered frequency (F_S) represents the frequency shift. The speed of sound in blood is represented by c, and the angle of incidence between the ultrasound beam and the flow of interest is "θ." A nonparallel intercept angle (θ) between the ultrasound beam and blood flow will underestimate velocity. For example, the error in velocity estimation at an angle of 20° is only 6%, but at 60°, error increases to 50%. (*From* Otto [2]; with permission.)

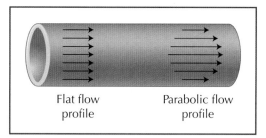

Flat flow profile   Parabolic flow profile

Figure 3-2. Blood flow through a vessel. Parabolic flow profile occurs with higher central blood velocities and progressively slower velocities, which are closer to the vessel wall because of entrainment of the anterograde jet and viscosity effects between blood cells and vessel walls. A flat profile is more optimal because a single velocity measurement represents average blood velocity across the cross-sectional area. In echocardiography, an assumption of flat-flow profiles is reasonable at great vessel inlets and across normal valves. Measured blood velocities are more accurate in larger vessels because of less viscosity effects on blood flow and a flatter flow profile. Flow acceleration and stream tapering, as seen in the LV outflow tract, also result in a flatter spatial flow profile.

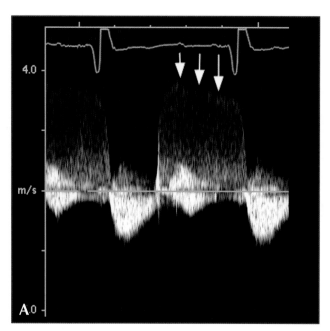

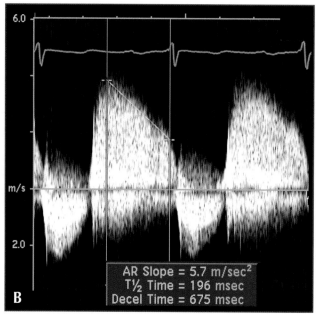

AR Slope = 5.7 m/sec²
T½ Time = 196 msec
Decel Time = 675 msec

Figure 3-3. Aortic regurgitation (AR) is seen during diastole. The AR Doppler signal represents diastolic equilibrium between the aorta and the LV. With significant AR, a faster rate of velocity decrease is associated with a steeper Doppler slope. The pressure half time (PHT) or $T_{1/2}$ is equal to the time from peak AR velocity to decrease to $V_{max}/\sqrt{2}$. A PHT of less than 200 ms is consistent with acute or severe AR. Increased density of the continuous wave Doppler signal relative to anterograde flow is another indicator of regurgitation severity. **A**, A continuous wave Doppler signal with mild AR. The slope of the regurgitant Doppler signal is less steep with a weak signal relative to anterograde flow. **B**, A patient with severe AR showing a steep slope with a dense Doppler signal. The PHT of 196 ms is consistent with severe AR.

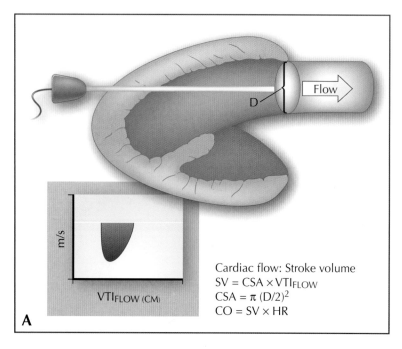

Cardiac flow: Stroke volume
$SV = CSA \times VTI_{FLOW}$
$CSA = \pi\,(D/2)^2$
$CO = SV \times HR$

Figure 3-4. Quantitation of flow. Stroke volume (SV) through a vessel or orifice is the velocity integral traversing that structure (VTI_{FLOW} [m]) multiplied by the cross-sectional area (CSA). Assuming a circular orifice, CSA can be calculated by measuring the orifice diameter (D). Calculation of SV and cardiac output (CO) at the aortic valve annulus in the LV outflow tract (LVOT) is demonstrated (**A**). SV measurements are generally most accurate at the aortic valve annulus because of relative ease in aligning a parallel Doppler ultrasound beam, and less variability in annular diameter change throughout the cardiac cycle. CO is calculated by multiplying SV and heart rate (HR). The VTI_{FLOW} is taken at the LVOT (*ie*, blood flow directed away from the transducer).

Continued on the next page

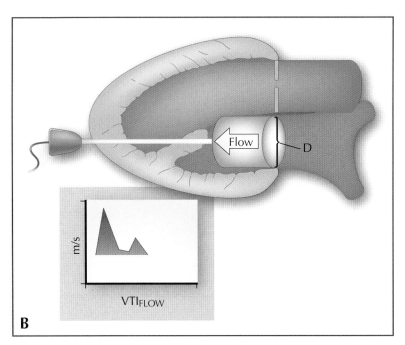

B

Figure 3-4. *(Continued)* SV and CO can also be calculated at other sites, such as the mitral (**B**) or pulmonic valves, with assumption of a circular orifice for calculation of CSA. However, the CO calculation reflects total transvalvular flow (anterograde and regurgitant volume), and will overestimate anterograde flow if there is significant valvular regurgitation at the point of interrogation. D—mitral annulus diameter.

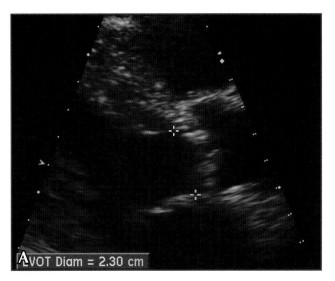

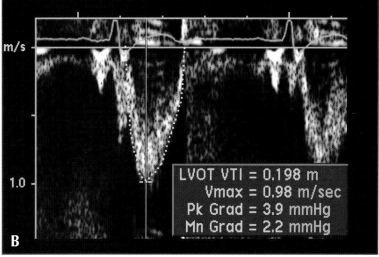

Figure 3-5. Cardiac output (CO) calculation in a patient with severe aortic stenosis and no aortic regurgitation. **A**, The diameter measurement of the aortic valve annulus from a parasternal long-axis view during midsystole is shown. **B**, The velocity time integral (VTI_{FLOW} [m]) in the LV outflow tract (LVOT) with the sample volume at the same position that the diameter measurement was taken is shown. The sample volume was obtained with the transducer anteriorly angulated in the apical four-chamber view. Unit conversion of distance to volume is 1 cm^3 = 1 mL. Cardiac output in this case is 6.5 L/min, which is normal.

$SV = CSA_{LVOT} \times VTI_{LVOT}$
$CSA_{LVOT} = \pi(D_{LVOT}/2)^2 = 3.1(2.3/2)^2 = 4.1\ cm^2$
$SV = 4.1\ cm^2 \times 20\ cm = 82\ cm^3$ or 82 mL
$CO = SV \times HR$
$CO = 82\ mL \times 79\ bpm = 6478\ mL/min$ or 6.5 L/min

CSA—cross-sectional area; HR—heart rate; SV—stroke volume.

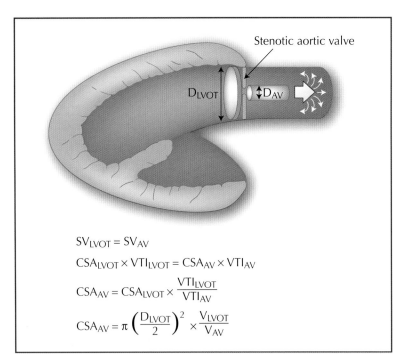

Stenotic aortic valve

D_{LVOT} $\updownarrow D_{AV}$

$SV_{LVOT} = SV_{AV}$

$CSA_{LVOT} \times VTI_{LVOT} = CSA_{AV} \times VTI_{AV}$

$CSA_{AV} = CSA_{LVOT} \times \dfrac{VTI_{LVOT}}{VTI_{AV}}$

$CSA_{AV} = \pi \left(\dfrac{D_{LVOT}}{2}\right)^2 \times \dfrac{V_{LVOT}}{V_{AV}}$

Figure 3-6. Continuity of flow: blood volume (stroke volume [SV]) passing just proximal to a stenotic orifice is the same as the SV passing through the stenotic orifice. Continuity of flow is commonly applied in aortic stenosis with the calculation of aortic valve area. Once SV_{LVOT} is equated to SV_{AV}, aortic valve area (CSA_{AV}) can be calculated. Because the shape and timing of the velocity curves are similar, the ratio of peak velocities is proportional to the ratio of VTI_{FLOW}. Peak velocities obtained in the LVOT and at the aortic valve can be substituted for the VTI_{LVOT} and VTI_{AV} measurements. CSA—cross-sectional area; D—diameter; LVOT—LV outflow tract; VTI—velocity time integral.

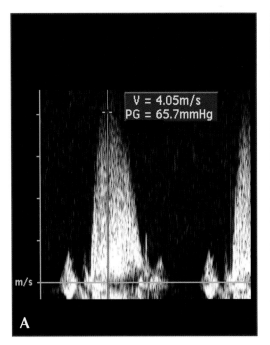

$V = 4.05$ m/s
$PG = 65.7$ mmHg

m/s

A

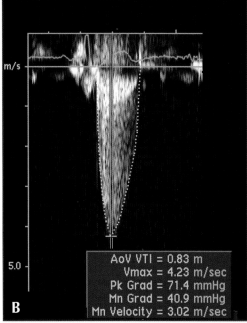

m/s

5.0

AoV VTI = 0.83 m
Vmax = 4.23 m/sec
Pk Grad = 71.4 mmHg
Mn Grad = 40.9 mmHg
Mn Velocity = 3.02 m/sec

B

Figure 3-7. A clinical example of severe aortic stenosis with continuous wave Doppler flow directed towards the transducer (**A**) (from a suprasternal notch window) and flow directed away from the transducer (**B**) (from an apical window). The highest velocity obtained from all views should be used in pressure calculations as this corresponds to the gradient when ultrasound beam alignment is most parallel with flow. In this case, the highest peak velocity was obtained from the apical position (4.23 m/s). Peak transaortic pressure gradient is calculated using the simplified Bernoulli equation (see Fig. 3-9).

$\Delta P = 4V^2$
$\Delta P = 4(4.2)^2 = 70.6$ mm Hg, peak transvalvular gradient, severe aortic stenosis.

Aortic valve area (CSA_{AV}) is calculated using the continuity equation. **B**, the $VTI_{AV} = 83$ cm. Aortic valve annulus diameter is 2.3 cm, and the $VTI_{LVOT} = 20$ cm (see Fig. 3-5). Aortic valve area calculates to 1 cm², consistent with severe stenosis.

$SV_{LVOT} = SV_{AV}$
$CSA_{LVOT} \times VTI_{LVOT} = CSA_{AV} \times VTI_{AV}$
$CSA_{AV} = CSA_{LVOT} \times VTI_{LVOT}/VTI_{AV}$
$CSA_{AV} = \pi(D/2)^2 \times VTI_{LVOT}/VTI_{AV} = (\pi[2.3\ cm/2]^2 \times 20\ cm)/(83\ cm) = 82\ cm^3/83\ cm = 1\ cm^2$

The equation can be simplified by substituting peak velocities for VTI_{FLOW} because the ratio (VTI_{LVOT}/VTI_{AV}) is approximately equal to (V_{LVOT}/V_{AV}).

$CSA_{AV} = (CSA_{LVOT} \times V_{LVOT})/V_{AV}$
$CSA_{AV} = (\pi[2.3\ cm/2]^2) \times (1\ m/s)/(4.2\ m/s) = 4.1\ cm^2/(4.2\ m/s) = 1\ cm^2$

AoV—aortic valve; CSA—cross-sectional area; D—diameter; LVOT—LV outflow tract; PG—pressure gradient; SV—stroke volume; VTI—velocity time integral.

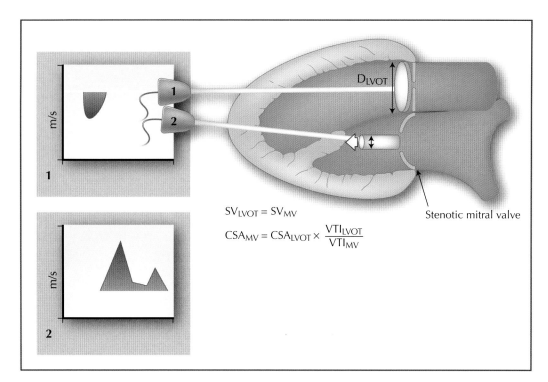

$$SV_{LVOT} = SV_{MV}$$

$$CSA_{MV} = CSA_{LVOT} \times \frac{VTI_{LVOT}}{VTI_{MV}}$$

Figure 3-8. Mitral valve area in mitral stenosis can be calculated using the continuity equation (*see* Fig. 3-7). For continuity mitral valve area calculations, SV_{MV} is compared to SV_{LVOT}. In contrast with aortic valve area, the ratio of peak velocities cannot be substituted for the ratio of VTI_{FLOW} for mitral valve area calculations because ratio proportion at the mitral valve and LV outflow tract (LVOT) are not equal. CSA—cross-sectional area; D—diameter; SV—stroke volume; VTI—velocity time integral.

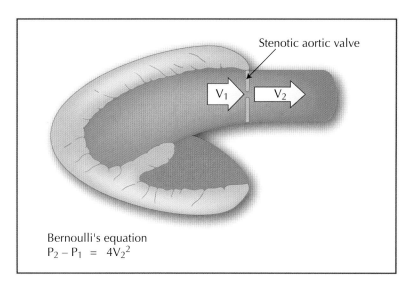

Bernoulli's equation
$$P_2 - P_1 = 4V_2^2$$

Figure 3-9. Pressure-velocity relationship: Bernoullis equation. This equation is used to calculate the pressure gradient across a region with blood velocities measured just proximal and at the region of interest. Assuming that the effects of viscous friction and local acceleration of blood cells are negligible, the pressure-velocity relationship is described as: $P_2 - P_1 = 1/2\rho(V_2^2 - V_1^2)$ where ρ represents the mass density of blood (1.06×10^3 kg/m³). When blood flow traverses through a stenotic valve, blood flow velocity significantly increases, and the poststenotic blood velocity (V_2) is much greater than the prestenotic blood velocity (V_1). In clinical practice, V_1 is ignored, making the simplified Bernoulli equation: $P_2 - P_1 = 4V_2^2$. Application of the simplified Bernoulli equation is most commonly used for transvalvular gradients of stenotic valves and to estimate intracardiac pressures, such as pulmonary arterial systolic pressure.

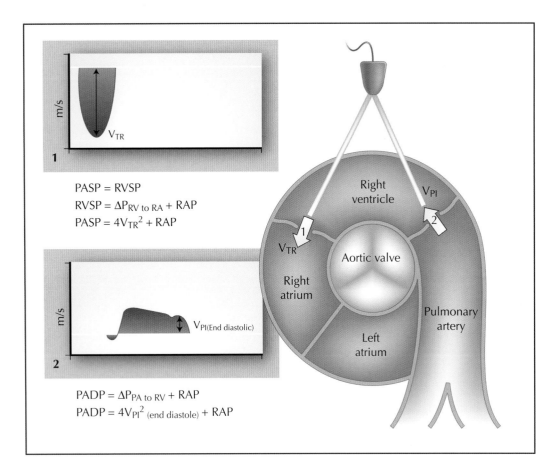

PASP = RVSP
RVSP = $\Delta P_{RV\ to\ RA}$ + RAP
PASP = $4V_{TR}^2$ + RAP

PADP = $\Delta P_{PA\ to\ RV}$ + RAP
PADP = $4V_{PI}^2$ (end diastole) + RAP

Figure 3-10. Using measured blood velocities obtained from Doppler ultrasound, intracardiac and intrapulmonary pressures can be calculated using the simplified Bernoullis equation (*see* Fig. 3-9). A common application is the estimation of pulmonary arterial systolic pressure (PASP). If PASP and RV systolic pressure (RVSP) are equal (significant pulmonic stenosis should be absent), the systolic pressure gradient between the RV and the right atrium is estimated from the tricuspid regurgitant jet. RVSP is then obtained by adding a right atrial pressure (RAP) estimate to the pressure gradient. RAP is estimated based on the evaluation of inferior vena cava dimension at rest and after inspiratory "sniff." Pulmonary arterial diastolic pressure (PADP) can similarly be calculated from the pulmonic regurgitant jet where the pressure gradient from the end-diastolic jet velocity is added to the RAP estimate.

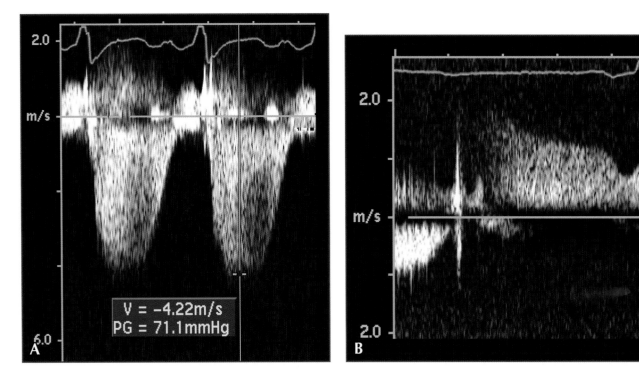

Figure 3-11. Severe pulmonary hypertension in a patient with primary pulmonary hypertension (**A**) is shown. The inferior vena cava (IVC) diameter was 2.3 cm with less than 50% inspiratory collapse, consistent with a right atrial pressure (RAP) of 10 to 15 mm Hg. Based on the simplified Bernoulli equation, pulmonary artery systolic pressure (PASP) calculated from the tricuspid regurgitant jet velocity (V_{TR}) is:

PASP = RVSP = $4V_{TR}^2$ + RAP
PASP = $4(4.2\ m/s)^2$ = 71 mm Hg + 10 to 15 mm Hg = 81 to 86 mm Hg

In a different patient, pulmonary artery diastolic pressure (PADP) is calculated from the pulmonic regurgitant jet end-diastolic velocity (**B**). The PADP is equal to the calculated pressure gradient added to the RAP estimate. In this case, IVC diameter was 1.8 cm with more than 50% inspiratory collapse, consistent with RAP of 5 to 10 mm Hg.

PADP = $4V_{PI\ at\ end\text{-}diastole}^2$ + RAP
PADP = $4(0.9\ m/s)^2$ = 3.2 mm Hg + 5 to 10 mm Hg = 8 to 13 mm Hg, normal range.

RVSP—RV systolic pressure.

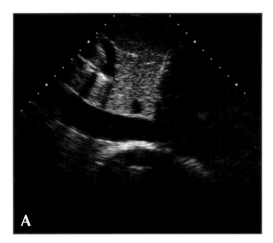
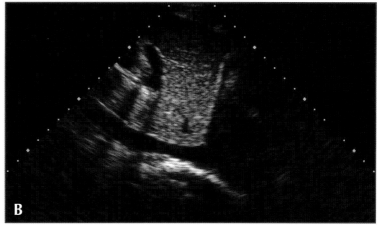

Figure 3-12. Estimating right atrial pressure: two-dimensional echocardiographic images obtained of the inferior vena cava (IVC) diameter from the subcostal window. **A**, A normal caliber IVC. **B**, The same patient following an inspiratory "sniff" demonstrating a reduction in IVC diameter.

Right Atrial Pressure Estimation Using IVC Diameter, Measured 2 cm From the Junction to the Right Atrium

IVC diameter, cm	Change in diameter with inspiratory "sniff," %	Right atrial pressure estimation, mm Hg
< 1.5	Collapse	0–5
1.5–2.5	Decrease in diameter > 50	5–10
1.5–2.5	Decrease in diameter < 50	10–15
> 2.5	Decrease in diameter < 50	15–20
> 2.5	No change	> 20

Figure 3-13. Right atrial pressure estimation using inferior vena cava (IVC) diameter, measured 2 cm from the junction to the right atrium.

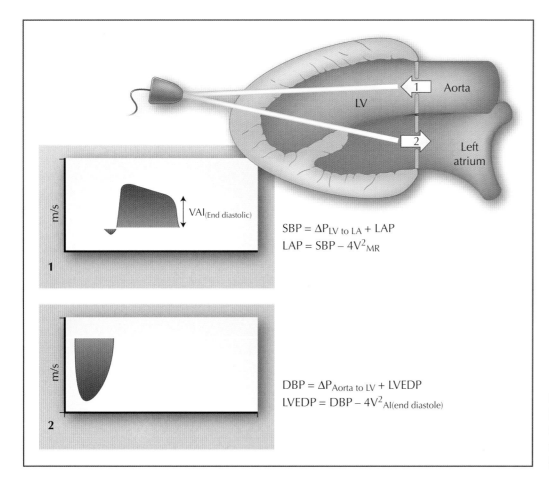

$$SBP = \Delta P_{LV\ to\ LA} + LAP$$
$$LAP = SBP - 4V^2_{MR}$$

$$DBP = \Delta P_{Aorta\ to\ LV} + LVEDP$$
$$LVEDP = DBP - 4V^2_{AI(end\ diastole)}$$

Figure 3-14. Calculation of left atrial pressure (LAP) and LV end-diastolic pressure (LVEDP) using the simplified Bernoulli equation is shown. Systemic systolic (SBP) and diastolic blood pressures (DBP) are needed for these calculations.

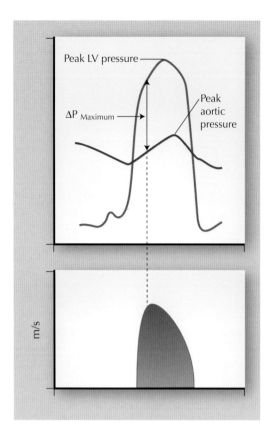

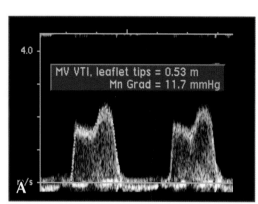

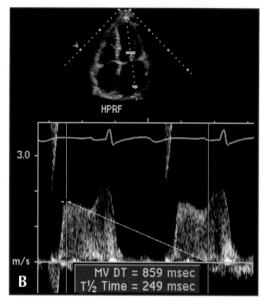

Figure 3-16. Mitral valve (MV) stenosis is shown. Optimal Doppler interrogation at the MV opening is increased with use of high-pulse repetition frequency (HPRF) pulsed wave Doppler over continuous wave Doppler. Mean transvalvular gradient of 11.7 mm Hg (**A**) is obtained from tracing the mitral inflow Doppler envelope, and mitral valve area (MVA) is calculated using the continuity equation. Measurement of LV outflow tract (LVOT) diameter at the aortic valve annulus is 2.4 cm, and VTI$_{LVOT}$ is 13 cm (not shown). VTI$_{MV}$ was 53 cm.

Figure 3-15. Aortic stenosis evaluation. Doppler assessment of transvalvular gradients provides instantaneous pressure gradients. There is a discrepancy between instantaneous gradients and those obtained from direct manometry measurement in the catheterization laboratory, where pressure catheters are placed just proximal and distal to the stenotic valve. Catheterization laboratory reported peak LV to peak aortic, or "peak to peak," gradients will always be less than Doppler-derived maximum instantaneous pressure gradients because of the temporal delay in aortic peak pressure relative to LV peak systolic pressure.

$$SV_{LVOT} = SV_{MV}$$
$$CSA_{LVOT} \times VTI_{LVOT} = CSA_{MV} \times VTI_{MV}$$
$$CSA_{MV} = (CSA_{LVOT} \times VTI_{LVOT})/VTI_{MV}$$
$$CSA_{MV} = \pi(D/2)^2 \times VTI_{LVOT}/VTI_{MV} = (\pi(2.4 \text{ cm}/2)^2 \times 13 \text{ cm})/(53 \text{ cm}) = 58 \text{ cm}^3/53 \text{ cm} = 1.1 \text{ cm}^2$$

MVA can also be calculated from the empirically derived equation: MVA = 220/pressure half time (PHT) where PHT (or T$_{1/2}$) is the time interval for the peak pressure gradient to drop by half. Because of the quadratic relationship described in the Bernoulli equation, in which pressure change is equal to $4V_{max}^2$, PHT is also equal to the time for the peak early mitral inflow velocity to decrease to $V_{max}/\sqrt{2}$, or approximately 30%. Prolongation of PHT is associated with delayed early LV filling and smaller MVA. In this case, PHT = 249 ms so that MVA = 0.9 cm^2 (**B**), which is compatible with the prior calculation. Pulmonary arterial systolic pressure estimation from the tricuspid regurgitant jet is 46 mm Hg, which is consistent with moderate to severe mitral stenosis. CSA—cross-sectional area; D—diameter; SV—stroke volume; VTI—velocity time integral.

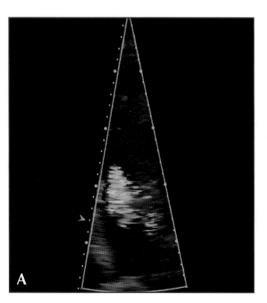

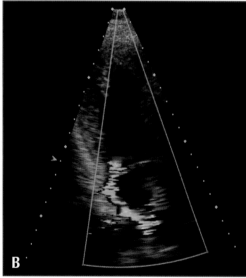

Figure 3-17. Color Doppler allows the direct visualization of regurgitant jet area into the receiving chamber, allowing for a semiquantitative evaluation of regurgitation severity. Color Doppler is particularly helpful in characterizing the flow characteristics of the regurgitant jet, such as differentiating central regurgitant (**A**) and eccentric (**B**) jets.

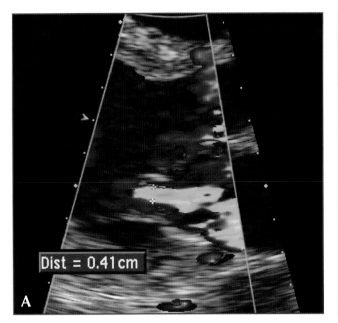

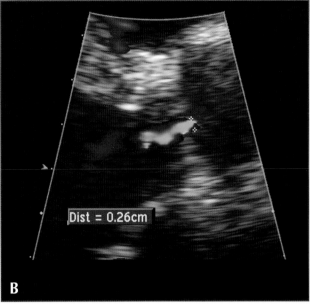

Figure 3-18. With color Doppler imaging, the vena contracta (VC) is the narrowest portion of the jet just distal to the regurgitant orifice. This measurement is generally performed in the parasternal long-axis view. Measurement of VC approximates diameter measurement of the effective regurgitant orifice, and it is correlated with regurgitation severity. Assessment of regurgitation severity with the VC is not affected by eccentric regurgitant jets. VC measurements for mitral valve (**A**) and aortic valve (**B**) regurgitation are provided. Accuracy in measuring the VC is crucial as small errors lead to inaccurate assessment of regurgitation severity.

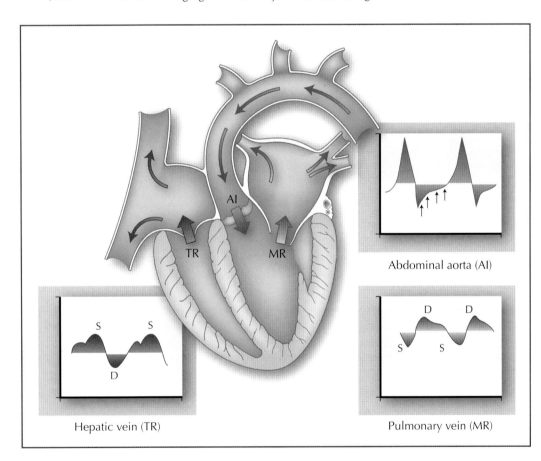

Hepatic vein (TR)

Abdominal aorta (AI)

Pulmonary vein (MR)

Figure 3-19. Doppler signals from upstream adjacent vessels with significant valvular regurgitation. Mitral regurgitation (MR) (*blue*), tricuspid regurgitation (TR) (*green*), and aortic regurgitation (AR) (*purple*) are simultaneously shown along with representative Doppler signals of respective valvular lesions. For example, with significant MR, systolic flow through the incompetent valve is directed retrograde towards the pulmonary veins, and the pulmonary vein Doppler interrogation demonstrates systolic flow reversal. However, absence of flow reversal does not preclude significant regurgitation. If regurgitant flow is perpendicular to the ultrasound beam, the Doppler signal may not demonstrate flow reversal. Analogous findings would be seen with moderate or greater TR (*ie*, systolic flow reversal in the hepatic veins) and significant AR (*ie*, holodiastolic flow reversal in the descending and abdominal aorta [AI]).

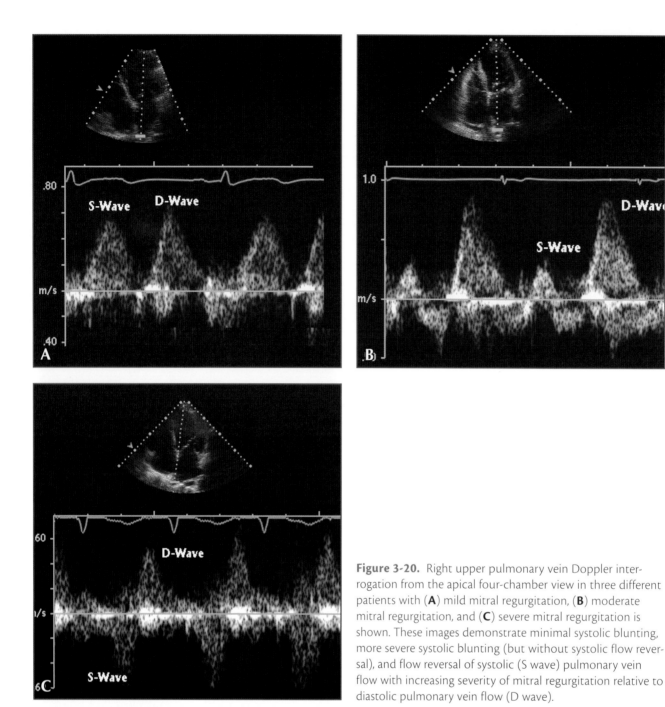

Figure 3-20. Right upper pulmonary vein Doppler interrogation from the apical four-chamber view in three different patients with (**A**) mild mitral regurgitation, (**B**) moderate mitral regurgitation, and (**C**) severe mitral regurgitation is shown. These images demonstrate minimal systolic blunting, more severe systolic blunting (but without systolic flow reversal), and flow reversal of systolic (S wave) pulmonary vein flow with increasing severity of mitral regurgitation relative to diastolic pulmonary vein flow (D wave).

Figure 3-21. Hepatic vein Doppler interrogation in two different patients with (**A**) trace tricuspid regurgitation and no systolic flow reversal and (**B**) severe tricuspid regurgitation showing flow reversal during systole.

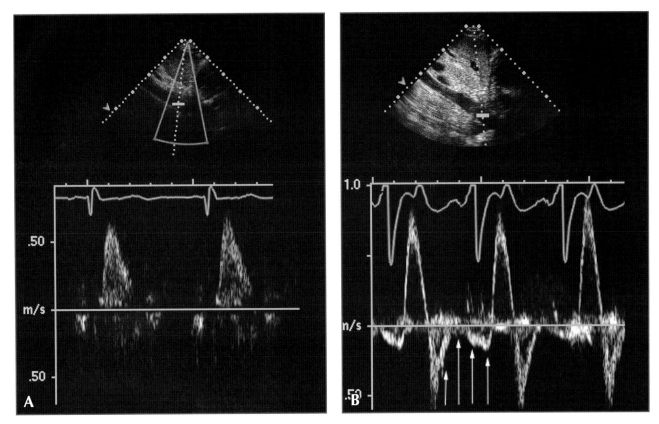

Figure 3-22. Doppler interrogation of the abdominal aorta in two different patients with (**A**) no aortic regurgitation and no flow reversal during diastole and (**B**) severe aortic regurgitation and holodiastolic flow reversal (*arrows*).

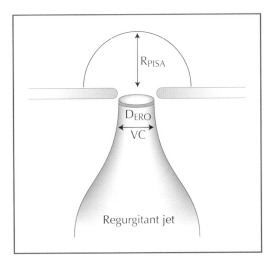

Figure 3-23. Regurgitation severity quantification by the flow convergence method, or proximal iso-velocity surface area (PISA), is shown. As blood flow approaches a regurgitant orifice, velocity increases, forming progressively smaller and concentric isovelocity hemispheres around the orifice. At equidistant points on any hemisphere, velocity is equal. Once the aliasing blood velocity is measured at the margin of an isovelocity hemisphere, and the hemisphere radius (R_{PISA}) is measured, the regurgitant maximal instantaneous flow rate (principle of flow quantification) and the effective regurgitant orifice area (EROA) (continuity equation) can be calculated. Because the PISA calculation provides the maximal instantaneous flow rate, the calculated EROA may be slightly larger than the area calculated by other methods. The PISA calculation for EROA is less accurate with eccentric regurgitant jets and flow that is nonholosystolic, such as mitral valve prolapse with late systolic regurgitation. VC—vena contracta.

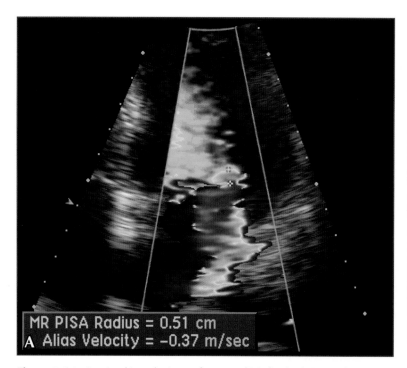

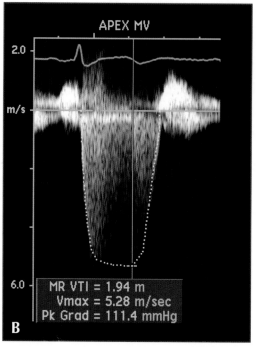

Figure 3-24. Proximal isovelocity surface area (PISA) calculation is shown. The PISA radius is 0.5 cm with an aliasing velocity of 37 cm/s (**A**). Doppler interrogation of the mitral regurgitant (MR) jet demonstrates a peak jet velocity of 5.3 m/s with a VTI$_{MR}$ of 194 cm (**B**). VTI—velocity time integral.

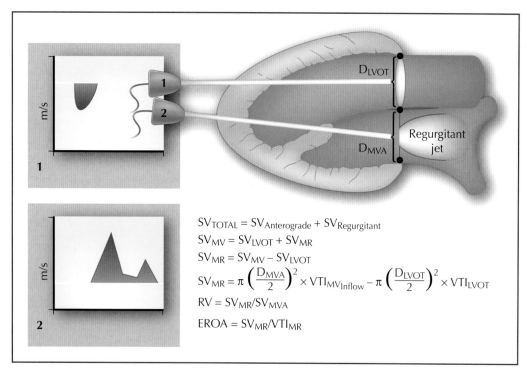

$$SV_{TOTAL} = SV_{Anterograde} + SV_{Regurgitant}$$
$$SV_{MV} = SV_{LVOT} + SV_{MR}$$
$$SV_{MR} = SV_{MV} - SV_{LVOT}$$
$$SV_{MR} = \pi \left(\frac{D_{MVA}}{2}\right)^2 \times VTI_{MV_{Inflow}} - \pi \left(\frac{D_{LVOT}}{2}\right)^2 \times VTI_{LVOT}$$
$$RV = SV_{MR}/SV_{MVA}$$
$$EROA = SV_{MR}/VTI_{MR}$$

Figure 3-25. Doppler quantification of regurgitation severity by comparison at two sites is shown. Total stroke volume (SV$_T$) across a regurgitant valve includes anterograde and regurgitant flow. Stroke volume (SV) from a regurgitant valve is compared with transvalvular SV at a different cardiac site where all flow is anterograde. By comparing SV$_T$ of the regurgitant valve with the SV$_T$ across a competent valve, the difference is the regurgitant SV and the regurgitant fraction can be calculated. For example, for mitral regurgitation (MR), mitral valve (MV) SV can be compared with SV for the LV outflow tract (LVOT) (assuming that significant aortic regurgitation is absent). This method is more reliable than proximal isovelocity surface area (PISA) with eccentric regurgitant jets. D—diameter; EROA—effective regurgitant orifice area; MVA—mitral valve area; VTI—velocity time integral.

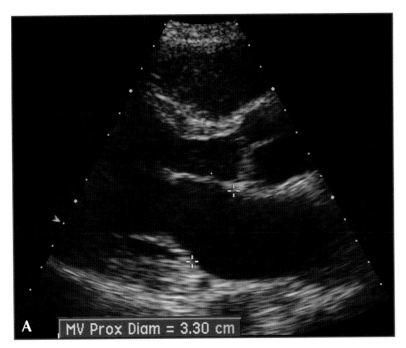

A — MV Prox Diam = 3.30 cm

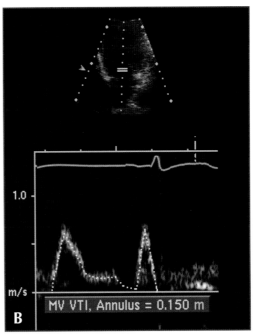

B — MV VTI, Annulus = 0.150 m

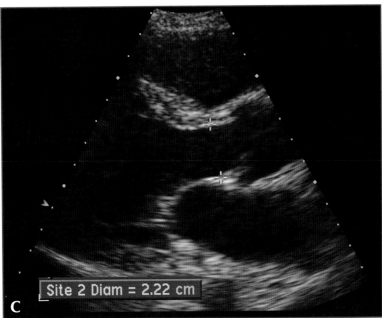

C — Site 2 Diam = 2.22 cm

D — Site 2 VTI = 0.24 m

Figure 3-26. Evaluation of mitral regurgitation (MR) is shown. Proximal isovelocity surface area (PISA) calculations are provided (aliasing velocity 37 cm/s) (*see* Fig 3-24).

PISA area = $2\pi(r)^2 = 2\pi(0.5)^2 = 1.6$ cm^2
MR instantaneous flow rate = 1.6 cm^2 × 37 cm/s = 60.3 cm^3/s

Effective regurgitant orifice area (EROA) is calculated by equating stroke volume (SV) (regurgitant maximal instantaneous flow) at the isovelocity hemisphere to EROA SV. Regurgitant SV (SV$_{MR}$) is obtained by multiplying EROA by VTI$_{MR}$. Transmitral flow is calculated from mitral annular area and VTI$_{MV\ INFLOW}$ (**A** and **B**). The regurgitant fraction (RF) is the fraction of SV$_{MV}$ represented by regurgitant volume (SV$_{MR}$).

MR jet velocity (*see* Fig. 3-24) = 5.3 m/s
EROA = MR instantaneous flow rate/V$_{MR}$ = (60.3 cm^3/s)/(530 cm/s) = 0.11 cm^2
SV$_{MR}$ = EROA × VTI$_{MR}$ = 0.11 cm^2 × 194 cm = 21 cm^3
SV$_{MV}$ = CSA$_{MV}$ × VTI$_{MV\ INFLOW}$ = $\pi(D_{MV}/2)^2$ × VTI$_{MV\ INFLOW}$
SV$_{MV}$ = $\pi(3.3/2)^2$ × 15 cm = 127cm^3
RF = SV$_{MR}$/SV$_{MV}$ = 21 mL/127 mL = 16.5%

Comparing transmitral flow (anterograde and regurgitant flow) with LV outflow (anterograde flow), cross-sectional areas (CSA) (**A** and **C**), and VTI$_{FLOW}$ (**B** and **D**) are needed. SVs are calculated by multiplying CSA and the velocity time integral (VTI). SV$_{MR}$ is the difference between calculated flows. EROA is calculated by dividing regurgitant SV by VTI at the mitral valve annulus.

SV$_{MV}$ = CSA$_{MV}$ × VTI$_{MV\ INFLOW}$ = $\pi(D_{MV}/2)^2$ × VTI$_{MV\ INFLOW}$
SV$_{MV}$ = $\pi(3.3/2)^2$ × 15 cm = 127 cm^3
SV$_{LVOT}$ = CSA$_{LVOT}$ × VTI$_{LVOT}$ = $\pi(D_{LVOT}/2)^2$ × VTI$_{LVOT}$
SV$_{LVOT}$ = $\pi(2.2/2)^2$ × 24 cm = 90 cm^3
SV$_{MR}$ = SV$_{MV}$ − SV$_{LVOT}$ = 127 cm^3 − 90 cm^3 = 37 cm^3 or 37 mL
RF = SV$_{MR}$/SV$_{MV}$ = 37 mL/127 mL = 29.1%
EROA = SV$_{MR}$/VTI$_{MR}$ = 37 cm^3/194 cm = 0.19 cm^2

These calculations are consistent with mild to moderate mitral regurgitation. D—diameter; LVOT—LV outflow tract; MV—mitral valve.

Doppler Assessment of Mitral and Aortic Regurgitation

Mitral Regurgitation	Mild	Severe
Color Doppler flow area	< 20% LA area	> 40% LA area
Vena contracta	< 0.30 cm	≥ 0.70 cm
Upstream Doppler flow: systolic pulmonary vein flow	None	Reversal
EROA	< 0.20 cm²	≥ 0.40 cm²
Regurgitant volume, mL/beat	< 30 mL	≥ 60 mL
Regurgitant fraction	< 30%	≥ 50%
Aortic Regurgitation	**Mild**	**Severe**
Color Doppler jet width: (% of the LVOT filled)	< 25% LVOT width	≥ 65% LVOT width
Vena contracta	< 0.30 cm	> 0.60 cm
Upstream Doppler flow: diastolic descending aorta flow	Limited early diastole only	Holodiastolic flow reversal: descending thoracic and abdominal aorta
Pressure half time (T1/2)	> 500 ms	< 200 ms
EROA	< 0.10 cm²	≥ 0.30 cm²
Reguritant volume (mL/beat)	< 30 mL	≥ 60 mL
Regurgitant fraction	< 30%	≥ 50%

Figure 3-27. EROA—effective regurgitant orifice area; LA—left atrium; LVOT—LV outflow tract.

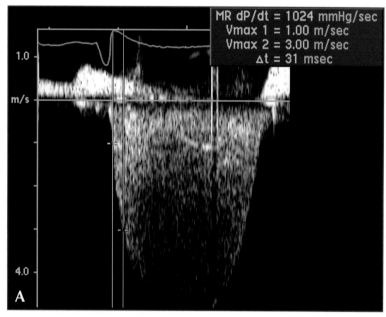

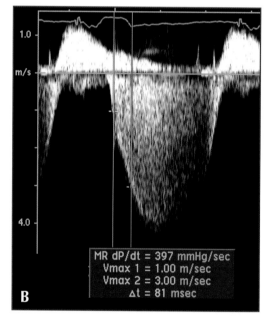

Figure 3-28. Quantitative evaluation of LV systolic function obtained by evaluating the rate of rise of LV pressure is shown. If mitral regurgitation (MR) is present, continuous wave Doppler interrogation of the regurgitant jet provides the instantaneous pressure difference between the left atrium and LV. With normal systolic function, there is a rapid rate of rise of LV pressure and a rapid rate of rise in MR jet velocities. The rate of change in pressure over time (dP/dt) is quantitated from the MR jet by measuring the time interval between measured velocities of 1 m/s and 3 m/s. By using the simplified Bernoulli equation, dP/dt equals:

$$dP/dt = (4[3\ m/s])^2 - 4(1\ m/s)^2)/\text{time interval} = 32\ mm\ Hg/\text{time interval}$$

With normal systolic function, the change in rate of rise in pressure over time should be more than 1000 mm Hg/s. **A,** A patient with an ejection fraction of 52% (low to normal systolic function) and a dP/dt of 1024 mm Hg/s. **B,** A mitral regurgitation continuous wave Doppler signal from a patient with decompensated congestive heart failure and ejection fraction of 12%. The dP/dt of 397 mm Hg/s is consistent with severe systolic dysfunction.

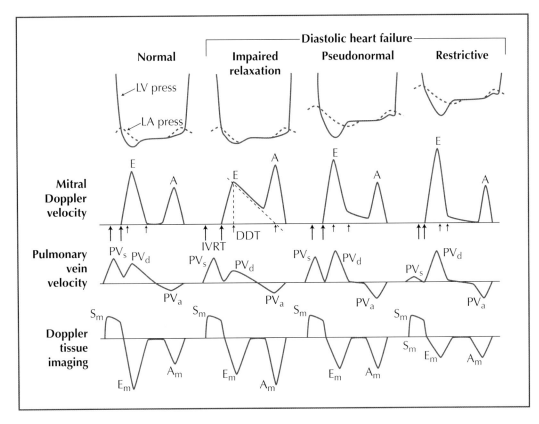

Figure 3-29. Echocardiographic Doppler indices for diastolic function are shown. With normal diastolic function, the mitral inflow E:A ratio is approximately 1 with a pulmonary venous systolic to diastolic velocity ratio over 1. Left atrial (LA) size is normal, with PV_{a-dur} less than MV_{a-dur} and an $E:E_M$ ratio less than 8. With impaired ventricular relaxation, peak early mitral inflow velocity is decreased with prolonged deceleration time (DT) and isovolumic relaxation time (IVRT). There is increased reliance on atrial contribution to ventricular filling with reversal of the E:A ratio. With advanced diastolic dysfunction (restrictive filling), there is decreased ventricular compliance. Higher LA pressures drive transmitral filling with a higher, early peaked E wave and E:A ratio over 2. The decrease in relative transmitral pressure gradient shortens DT and IVRT, and the E:E' ratio is over 12 with prolongation and higher peak velocities of the pulmonary venous A wave. Moderate diastolic dysfunction ("pseudonormal") is the intermediate step between impaired relaxation and restrictive filling. The mitral inflow pattern is in transition and may resemble the "normal" state. a—atrial duration; d—diastole; m—tissue Doppler velocity; MV—mitral valve; s—systole. (*From* Zile and Brutsaert [25]; with permission.).

Echocardiographic Diastolic Indices

	Normal	Mild-Moderate Impaired Relaxation	Severe Decreased Compliance
Mitral inflow E:A ratio	1–2	< 1	> 2
MV E: Tissue Doppler E_m E:E_m ratio	< 8	-	> 15
LA size	Normal	Enlarged	Enlarged
Isovolumic relaxation time	~ 50–100	Longer	Shorter
Deceleration time	~150–200	Longer	Shorter
PVa peak velocity	< 0.35 m/s	> 0.35 m/s	> 0.35 m/s
PV systolic: diastolic ratio	> 1	< 1	< 1
PVa - MVa duration	< 20	> 20	> 20

Figure 3-30. Echocardiographic diastolic indices. LA—left atrium; MV—mitral valve; MV_a—mitral valve atrial wave duration; PV—pulmonary vein; PV_a—pulmonary venous atrial wave duration

References

1. Quinones MA Otto CM, Stoddard M, *et al.*: Recommendations for quantification of Doppler echocardiography: a report from the Doppler Quantification Task Force of the Nomenclature and Standards Committee of the American Society of Echocardiography. *J Am Soc Echocardiogr* 2002, 15:167–184.

2. Otto CM. *Textbook of Clinical Echocardiography*, edn 3. Philadelphia; WB Saunders; 2004.

3. Zoghbi WA, Quinones MA: Determination of cardiac output by Doppler echocardiography: a critical appraisal. *Herz* 1986, 11:258–268.

4. Bouchard A, Blumlein S, Schiller NB, *et al.*: Measurement of left ventricular stroke volume using continuous-wave Doppler echocardiography of the ascending aorta and M-mode echocardiography of the aortic valve. *J Am Coll Cardiol* 1987, 9:75–83.

5. Lewis JF, Kuo LC, Nelson JG, *et al.*: Pulsed Doppler echocardiographic determination of stroke volume and cardiac output: clinical validation of two new methods using the apical window. *Circulation* 1984, 70:425–431.

6. Otto CM, Pearlman AS, Comess KA, *et al.*: Determination of the stenotic aortic valve area in adults using Doppler echocardiography. *J Am Coll Cardiol* 1986, 7:509–517.

7. Galan A, Zoghbi WA, Quinones MA: Determination of severity of valvular aortic stenosis by Doppler echocardiography and relation of findings to clinical outcome and agreement with hemodynamic measurements determined at cardiac catheterization. *Am J Cardiol* 1991, 67:1007–1012.

8. Currie PJ, Seward JB, Chan KL, *et al.*: Continuous wave Doppler determination of right ventricular pressure: a simultaneous Doppler-catheterization study in 127 patients. *J Am Coll Cardiol* 1985, 6:750–756.

9. Kircher BJ, Himelman RB, Schiller NB: Noninvasive estimation of right atrial pressure from the inspiratory collapse of the inferior vena cava. *Am J Cardiol* 1990, 66:493–496.

10. Smith MD, Handshoe R, Handshoe S, *et al.*: Comparative accuracy of two-dimensional echocardiography and Doppler pressure half-time methods in assessing severity of mitral stenosis in patients with and without prior mitral commissurotomy. *Circulation* 1986, 73:100–107.

11. Nakatani S, Masuyama T, Kodama K, *et al.*: Value and limitations of Doppler echocardiography in the quantification of stenotic mitral valve area: comparison of the pressure half-time and the continuity equation methods. *Circulation* 1988, 77:78–85.

12. Heinle SK, Hall SA, Brickner ME, *et al.*: Comparison of vena contracta width by multiplane transesophageal echocardiography with quantitative Doppler assessment of mitral regurgitation. *Am J Cardiol* 1998, 81:175–179.

13. Tribouilloy CM, Enriquez-Sarano M, Bailey KR, *et al.*: Assessment of severity of aortic regurgitation using the width of the vena contracta: a clinical color Doppler imaging study. *Circulation* 2000, 102:558–564.

14. Zoghbi WA, Enriquez-Sarano M, Foster E, *et al.*: Recommendations for evaluation of the severity of native valvular regurgitation with two-dimensional and Doppler echocardiography: a report from the Doppler Quantification Task Force of the Nomenclature and Standards Committee of the American Society of Echocardiography. *J Am Soc Echocardiogr* 2003, 16:777–802.

15. Sakai K, Nakamura K, Satomi G, *et al.*: Hepatic vein flow measured by Doppler echocardiography as an evaluation of tricuspid valve insufficiency. *J Cardiogr* 1983, 13:33–43.

16. Pu M, Griffin BP, Vandervoort PM, *et al.*: The value of assessing pulmonary venous flow velocity for predicting severity of mitral regurgitation: a quantitative assessment integrating left ventricular function. *J Am Soc Echocardiogr* 1999, 12:736–743.

17. Teague SM, Heinsimer JA, Anderson JL, *et al.*: Quantification of aortic regurgitation utilizing continuous wave Doppler ultrasound. *J Am Coll Cardiol* 1986, 8:592–599.

18. Bargiggia GS, Tronconi L, Sahn DJ, *et al.*: A new method for quantitation of mitral regurgitation based on color flow Doppler imaging of flow convergence proximal to the regurgitant orifice. *Circulation* 1991, 84:1481–1489.

19. Enriquez-Sarano M, Miller FA Jr, Hayes SN, *et al.*: Effective mitral regurgitant orifice area: clinical use and pitfalls of the proximal isovelocity surface area method. *J Am Coll Cardiol* 1995, 25:703–709.

20. Pu M, Prior DL, Fan X, *et al.*: Calculation of mitral regurgitant orifice area with use of a simplified proximal convergence method: initial clinical application. *J Am Soc Echocardiogr* 2001, 14:180–185.

21. Rokey R, Sterling LL, Zoghbi WA, *et al.*: Determination of regurgitant fraction in isolated mitral or aortic regurgitation by pulsed Doppler two-dimensional echocardiography. *J Am Coll Cardiol* 1986, 7:1273–1278.

22. Bonow RO, Carabello BA, Kanu C, *et al.*: ACC/AHA 2006 guidelines for the management of patients with valvular heart disease: a report of the American College of Cardiology/American Heart Association Task Force on Practice Guidelines (writing committee to revise the 1998 Guidelines for the Management of Patients with Valvular Heart Disease): developed in collaboration with the Society of Cardiovascular Anesthesiologists: endorsed by the Society for Cardiovascular Angiography and Interventions and the Society of Thoracic Surgeons. *Circulation* 2006, 114:e84–e231.

23. Chen C, Rodriguez L, Guerrero JL, *et al.*: Noninvasive estimation of the instantaneous first derivative of left ventricular pressure using continuous-wave Doppler echocardiography. *Circulation* 1991, 83:2101–2110.

24. Chung N, Nishimura RA, Holmes DR Jr, Tajik AJ, *et al.*: Measurement of left ventricular dP/dt by simultaneous Doppler echocardiography and cardiac catheterization. *J Am Soc Echocardiogr* 1992, 5:147–152.

25. Zile MR, Brutsaert DL: New concepts in diastolic dysfunction and diastolic heart failure: part I: diagnosis, prognosis, and measurements of diastolic function. *Circulation* 2002, 105:1387–1393.

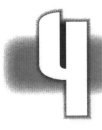

Assessment of Systolic Function

Scott D. Solomon and Bernard E. Bulwer

The echocardiographic assessment of ventricular systolic function plays a critically important role in the diagnosis, risk stratification, prognosis, and guide to therapy and intervention in patients with suspected or established cardiovascular disease.

Assessment of ventricular systolic function routinely begins with a qualitative evaluation; however, more precise measurements of global and regional ventricular systolic function are necessary in order to accurately assess, risk stratify, and prognosticate. Linear and volumetric measures of ventricular wall thicknesses, mass, and volumes are clinically useful parameters used in landmark clinical trials. These are based primarily on M-mode, two-dimensional, and Doppler hemodynamic measures. Derived B-mode indices have important limitations. They are based on comparisons of frames and measures obtained at the beginning and end of the contractile cycle. They are load dependent and do not measure dynamic myocardial behavior and contractility directly. Additionally, the geometric assumptions and derived LV measures have inherent inaccuracies. The advent of real-time three-dimensional echocardiography, however, has overcome some of these inaccuracies. Nevertheless, continuing challenges such as endocardial border delineation remain.

The gross contractile mechanics of ventricular systole is now made easier by recent advances in myocardial velocity and deformation imaging, primarily by tissue Doppler and two-dimensional speckle tracking imaging. These have not only provided new insights into regional ventricular mechanics, but they may also be more sensitive measures of preclinical and clinical insults to the myocardium. Current evidence indicates their use in providing superior prognostic and incremental information over traditional systolic measures. Their derived indices—myocardial velocities, displacement, strain, and strain rate—are becoming increasingly available for use during real-time imaging, as well as for off line (postprocessing) analyses.

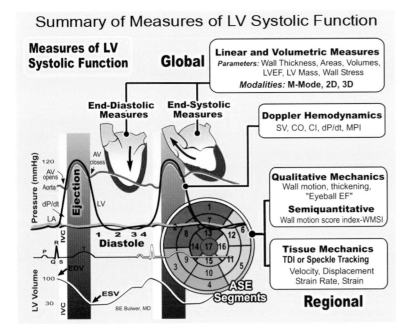

Figure 4-1. Echocardiographic assessment of ventricular systolic function includes measures of both global and regional systolic function [1,2]. The primary measures of systolic function include 1) measurement of ventricular dimensions (eg, distances between opposite walls, ventricular areas, and volumes), in which ejection fraction (EF) can be easily calculated from ventricular volumes; 2) Doppler hemodynamic measures of stroke volumes and cardiac output—the myocardial performance index (MPI); and 3) measures of regional ventricular systolic function, which are based primarily on qualitative assessment and offer promising new automated techniques. ASE—American Society of Echocardiography; CI—cardiac index; CO—cardiac output; dP/dt—rate of change of pressure during ejection; IVC—isovolumetric contraction; LVEF—left ventricular ejection fraction; SV—stroke volume; TDI—tissue Doppler imaging; WMSI—wall motion score index.

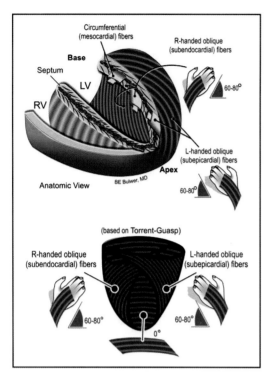

Figure 4-2. The myocardium consists of three macroscopically discernible layers. The first is an obliquely oriented subepicardial left-handed helical layer, which winds into a more horizontal middle layer and then an oppositely wound right-handed, subendocardial, helical layer. This arrangement of myocardial fibers contributes to the heart's ability to contract efficiently [3–5].

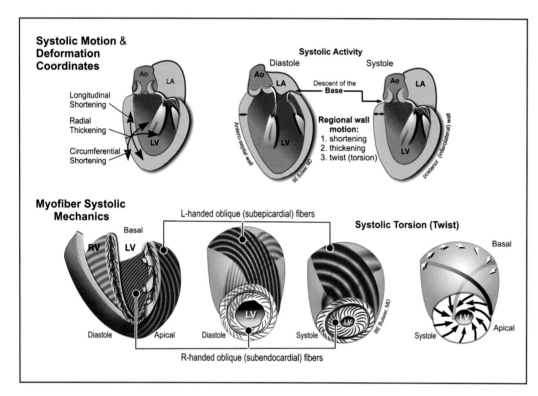

Figure 4-3. During systole, three-dimensional deformation of the LV occurs along three principal coordinates. These include 1) longitudinal shortening, which occurs along the cardiac long-axis and is attributed primarily to contraction of the LV obliquely oriented myocardial fibers; 2) radial thickening, which occurs along the cardiac short axis and is attributed primarily to contraction of the LV circumferential myocardial fibers; and 3) circumferential shortening, which is shortening that occurs in a direction perpendicular to the cardiac-long axis.

Torsion: This is a gradient of rotation along the cardiac long axis. When viewed from the apex, the LV apex and apical segments rotate counter clockwise whereas the base rotates in the opposite direction. Apical rotation is typically greater in magnitude than the clockwise basal rotation. The overall pattern has been termed systolic "twisting" or "wringing" [6–8]. Ao—Aorta.

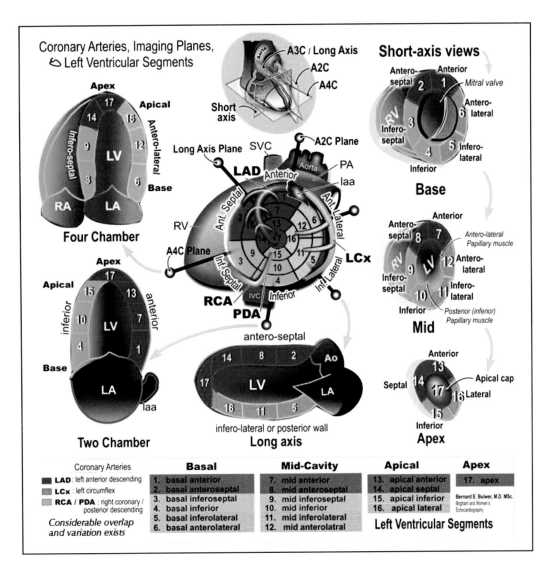

Figure 4-4. Regional wall motion is generally assessed qualitatively based on a 16- or 17-segment model (healthcare professionals from the Cardiac Imaging Committee of the Council on Clinical Cardiology of the American Heart Association). Specific regions from various views can then be depicted in a "bull's eye" polar plot. There are six basal segments (1–6) beginning with the antero-basal segment and numbering in a counter clockwise direction. The next six middle segments (7–12) follow the same pattern followed by the next four apical segments (13–16). The last segment (17) occupies the tip. The corresponding coronary artery territories with LV myocardial segments are depicted, but there is considerable overlap and variation [9]. LA—left atrium; laa—left atrial appendage; LAD—left anterior descending; LCx—left circumflex; MV—mitral valve; PA—pulmonary artery; RCA/PDA—right coronary/posterior descending; SVC—superior vena cava. (*Adapted from* Cerqueria et al. [9].)

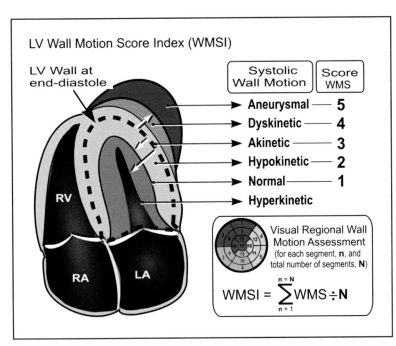

Figure 4-5. Grading of systolic wall motion of the ventricles is described as shown and should be assessed using multiple standard views on two-dimensional echocardiography. Visualization of endocardial motion (radial thickening) is critical because movement of this region normally exceeds that of the epicardial region. Inadequate visualization of the endocardium can lead to underestimation of ventricular wall motion, especially in the LV. Tissue harmonic imaging, LV opacification using contrast agents, and Doppler-based tissue tracking methods can be used when endocardial border delineation is suboptimal [10,11].

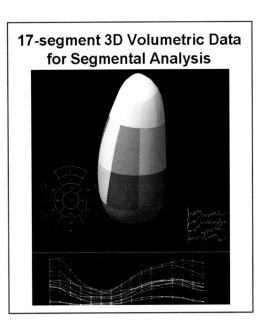

Figure 4-6. Volumetric three-dimensional echocardiography can potentially assess regional and global contractile function accurately and has shown excellent correlation with standard techniques for assessment of the regional wall motion ($r = 0.89$, $P < 0.001$) [12].

Noncoronary Causes of Regional Wall Motion Abnormalities

Pseudodyskinesis*

Postcardiac surgery

Ascites

Pregnancy

Hiatus hernia (large)

Ventricular interdependence

Pericardial tamponade

Constrictive pericarditis

Pulmonary hypertension

Right ventricular pressure overload

Right ventricular volume overload

Abnormal heart rhythm

LBBB

PVCs

Ventricular pacing

WPW

*Constrained wall movement, but normal thickening.

Figure 4-7. Care must be taken in assessing ventricular wall thickening as well as motion because abnormal ventricular wall movement is often seen in clinical practice. The LV posterior wall may be constrained with any condition that causes marked abdominal distension (eg, ascites or pregnancy), causing pseudoskinesis. However, wall thickening is preserved despite the pseudodyskinesis. Abnormal electromechanical coupling occurs in patients with rhythm disorders or left bundle branch block, which results in dys-synchronous wall movements. Ventricular interdependence often causes a septal "bounce." This can be seen in constrictive pericarditis, which is a physiologic consequence of respiratory hemodynamics. Any surgical breach to the pericardium (eg, post open heart surgery) can lead to abnormal septal motion; however, thickening is preserved [13]. LBBB—left bundle branch block; PVC—premature ventricular contractions; WPW—Wolf-Parkinson-White syndrome.

2D guided M-mode measurements and derived indices

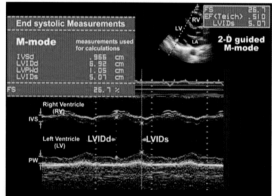

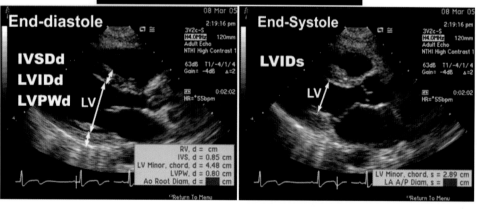

Figure 4-8. Two-dimensional M-mode measurements and derived indices. M-mode is simple, reproducible, and provides excellent temporal resolution of the endocardial border. It retains utility in the assessment of LV dimensions (eg, cavity size, wall thicknesses, and fractional shortening). Its reliability is diminished with abnormal LV geometry, even when guided two-dimensionally. A number of formulas can be used to calculate volumes from M-mode–based ventricular cavity diameter measures. The primary method used is the Teichholz method [Teichholz formula: volume = [7.0/(2.4 + LVIDd)] (LVIDd) 3]. This method is only useful, however, when ventricular geometry is relatively normal [14]. The American Society of Echocardiography recommends two-dimensional measurements of linear dimensions using the leading-edge-to-leading-edge method as shown [14–16]. LVIDd—LV internal diameter at end-diastole; LVIDs—LV internal diameter at end-systole; LVPWd—LV posterior wall thickness at end-diastole.

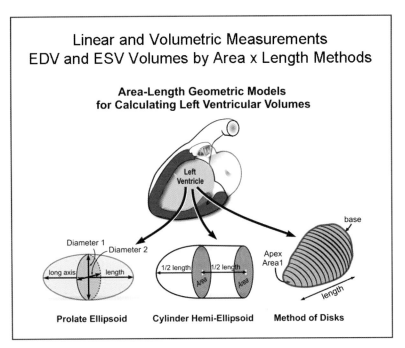

Figure 4-9. Linear and volumetric measurements EDV and ESV volumes by area x length methods. Area-length geometric models used to estimate LV volumes and ejection fraction by two-dimensional echocardiography require measurements of short-axis areas multiplied by long-axis lengths. When poor endocardial border delineation occurs, the area-length based methods (eg, cylinder hemi-ellipse or bullet formula) can be employed in order to calculate end-diastolic and systolic volumes, and hence ejection fraction. The following formula is used: (V = [5 (Area) (Length)] / 6) [15]. EDV—end-diastolic volume; ESV—end-systolic volume.

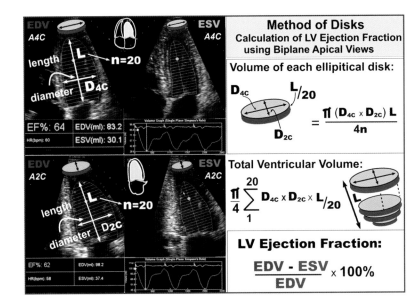

Figure 4-10. The most common and accepted method for assessing ventricular volumes (and from these, ejection fraction) is the Simpson's rule method. This method assumes that the ventricle is composed of a stacked series of elliptical disks. By knowing the major and minor diameters of each disk, an ellipse can be defined and the area of each ellipse is then multiplied by the slice thickness. When these discs are summated, as in the formula, the overall volume of the ventricle can be determined [15]. A4C—apical four chamber; A2C—apical two chamber; EDV—end-diastolic volume; ESV—end-systolic volume.

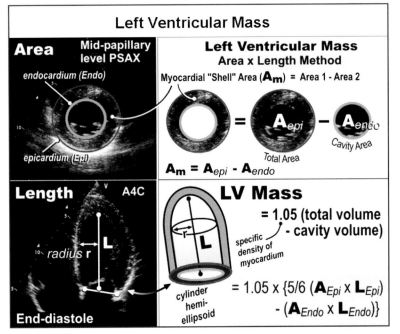

Figure 4-11. LV mass. The area-length method for using a cylinder hemi-ellipsoid of the left ventricle (LV) is the recommended method for measuring LV mass. It is a simple formula with easily obtainable measurements. End-diastolic measurements using parasternal short-axis (PSAX) and apical four chamber (A4C) views at the mid- or high-papillary muscle levels are made and then inserted into the equation as shown. L_1—end-diastolic LV cavity length. A_1—total planimetered PSAX area at the mid- or high-papillary muscle level; A_2—LV cavity planimetered PSAX area; A_m—myocardial "shell" area; A_{epi}—total planimetered PSAX area at the mid- or high-papillary muscle level; A_{endo}—LV cavity planimetered PSAX area; b—minor axis radius; t—wall thickness [15,17,18].

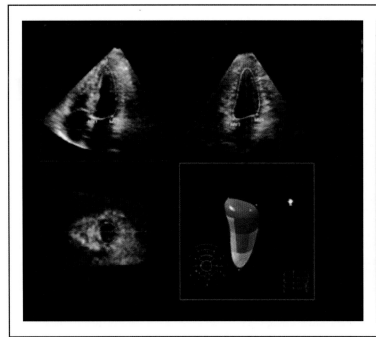
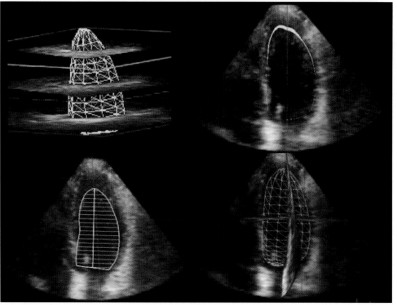

Figure 4-12. Volumetric three-dimensional echocardiography can potentially give the most accurate assessment of ventricular volumes and function because these methods do not rely on geometric assumptions about the ventricle (*left panel*) [19,20]. Semiautomatic border detection with multiplanar reconstruction in three-dimensional echocardiography is also shown (*right panel*).

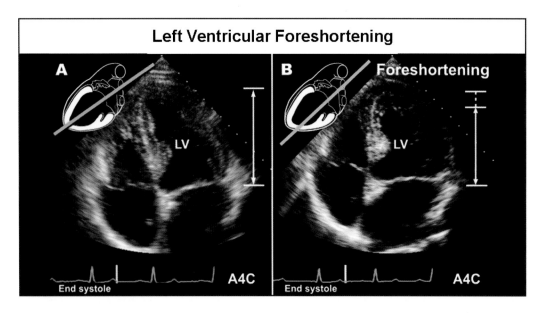

Figure 4-13. LV foreshortening. One of the greatest pitfalls in accurately assessing ventricular volumes and ejection fraction is foreshortening of the ventricle. Foreshortening (**B**) occurs when the imaging plane does not transect the center of left ventricular apex (**A**). This is a common source of error in LV quantification in two-dimensional echocardiography [15]. A4C—apical four chamber.

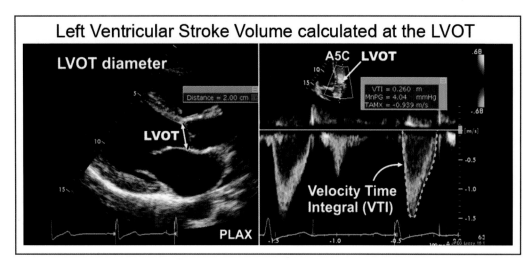

Figure 4-14. LV stroke volume calculated at the LV outflow tract (LVOT). Doppler echocardiography can be used to assess stroke volume. The cross-sectional area of the LVOT is multiplied by the velocity time integral (VTI) of flow at the same location in order to obtain the stroke volume. Typically, the LVOT diameter is measured in the parasternal long-axis (PLAX) view, and the LVOT Doppler is obtained in the apical five-chamber view (A5C) [21].

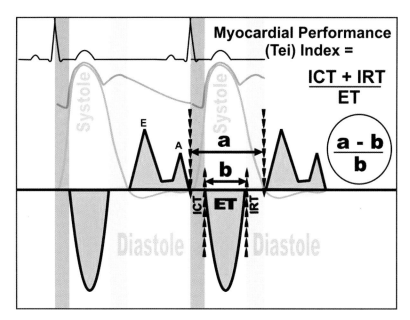

Figure 4-15. The myocardial performance index, also known as the "Tei" index, is a dimensionless index based on the sum of the isovolumic contraction and relaxation times (ICT and IRT, respectively) divided by the ejection time (ET). This index incorporates assessment of both systolic and diastolic function and has been related to prognosis in a variety of disease states [22,23].

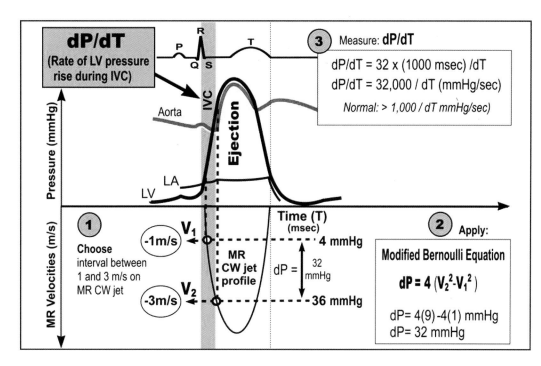

Figure 4-16. The rate of LV pressure rise (dP/dT) during the isovolumetric contraction (IVC) phase of systole is a useful measure of LV contractility. In patients with mitral regurgitation (MR), estimates of dP/dT can be derived from the time interval it takes for the LV pressure to rise by 32 mmHg (ie, from 1 m/sec to 3 m/sec). The Bernoulli equation is used to estimate LV pressures from the MR CW spectral Doppler velocities [24,25]. CW—continuous wave spectral Doppler; LA—left atrium.

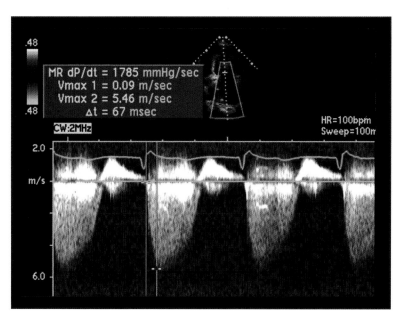

Figure 4-17. Estimation of dP/dt (rate of change of pressure during ejection) from the mitral regurgitation (MR) CW spectral Doppler profile. This can be compared with Fig. 4-16. CW—continuous wave.

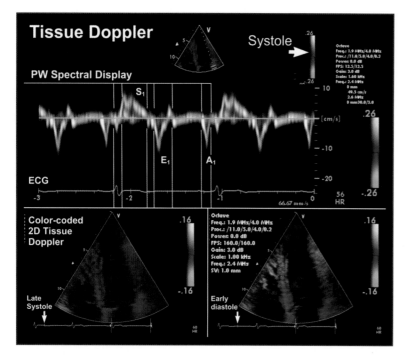

Figure 4-18. Tissue Doppler imaging (TDI) spectral and TDI color two-dimensional display. TDI uses the same Doppler principles to assess the velocity of myocardial motion. The Doppler sample volume placed at either the septal or lateral mitral annulus (MA) will record longitudinal myocardial velocities during the cardiac cycle. This typically reveals three primary waveforms. The first is the S_1, representing the systolic contraction velocity; the second is E_1, representing the diastolic relaxation velocity during early mitral inflow; the third is A_1, representing the late diastolic relaxation velocity during atrial contraction [26,27]. The same TDI data can be color coded (*blue away–red toward transducer*) to assess ventricular wall movements (*color-coded two-dimensional tissue Doppler*).

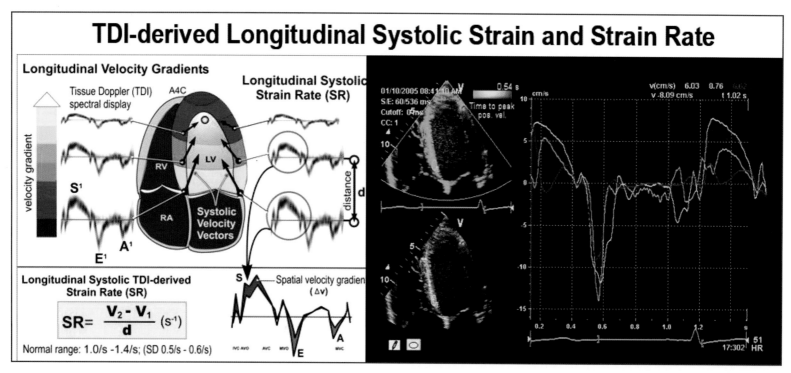

Figure 4-19. Tissue Doppler imaging (TDI) derives longitudinal systolic strain and strain rate (SR). TDI can be used to assess myocardial velocity, as well as myocardial strain and SR using the apical four-chamber views. SR is derived directly from the velocity measured at two different points; strain represents the integration of SR with respect to time. The instantaneous A-velocity gradient exists from LV apex to base as measured by TDI, with higher velocities at the base compared to the relatively stationary apex. Note the color-coded velocity depiction and differential tissue Doppler velocities at different levels within the LV (*upper left panel*). The difference or velocity gra-

dient within two adjacent points within the sample volume of myocardium (during ventricular systolic shortening) can be quantified using a regression calculation from the velocity data obtained by TDI (*lower left panel* and *right panel*). This spatial velocity gradient is called the SR, and the SR curve reflects the rate of longitudinal deformation or LV systolic shortening and lengthening during the cardiac cycle. By convention, SR shortening is negative during systole and positive during diastolic lengthening. The total amount of shortening or lengthening during the cardiac cycle or strain (S or ε) is obtained by the integration of this curve [28,29]. 4AC—apical four chamber.

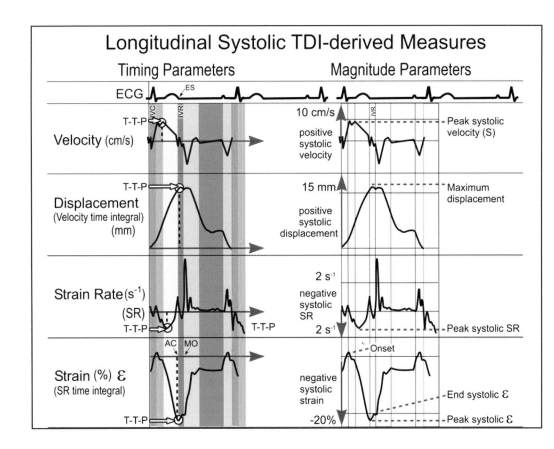

Figure 4-20. Tissue Doppler imaging (TDI) derived data: 1) tissue velocity, 2) displacement (velocity x time), 3) strain (myocardial deformation), and 4) strain rate (SR) (rate of myocardial deformation) [28,29]. These same TDI-derived data can provide incremental measures of myocardial behavior in clinical states. Tissue velocity data merely reflect movement at one site relative to the transducer and do not distinguish normal myocardium from nonviable myocardium that moves along with healthy myocardium due to tethering. Strain and SR measures provide site specificity along the line of Doppler interrogation, thereby distinguishing true contractile motion from that caused by tethering. This has promising use in patients with coronary artery disease [28,29,30]. ε—strain; AC—aortic valve closure; ES—end systole; IVC—isovolumetric contraction; IVR—isovolumetric relaxation; MO—mitral valve opening; S—peak systolic velocity.

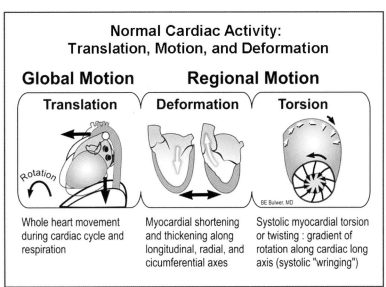

Figure 4-21. Normal cardiac activity: translation, motion, and deformation. Cardiac motion is complex, with much heterogeneity present in normal hearts. Movements are active and passive, global and regional, and occur in three dimensions over time, even within at a single location. During ventricular systole, the heart shortens, thickens, and twists. Ventricular wall motion assessment is the basis for a number of qualitative, semi-quantitative, and quantitative measures of ventricular systolic function [1–8].

Assessment of gross contractile mechanics of LV systole is now possible due to recent advances in myocardial velocity and deformation imaging, primarily by tissue Doppler imaging (TDI) and two-dimensional speckle tracking imaging (STI). These advances have not only provided new insights into regional ventricular mechanics, but they can also be more sensitive in their measurements of preclinical and clinical insults to the myocardium [5]. Early evidence suggests that they can provide superior prognostic and incremental information over traditional systolic measures [6,7]. Their derived indices—myocardial velocities, displacement, strain, and strain rate (SR)—are increasing in availability for use during real-time imaging, as well as for offline (post-processing) analyses.

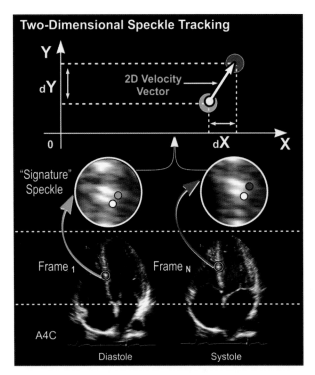

Figure 4-22. Speckle tracking imaging (STI). Tissue Doppler derived measures—velocities, displacement, strain, and strain rate (SR)—are angle-dependent. STI can overcome some of these limitations by assessing myocardial motion and deformation using multiple windows in addition to providing insights into LV torsion, which is an important component of LV systolic performance.

Two-dimensional speckle tracking techniques harness speckle artifacts on B-mode images in order to assess myocardial motion and deformation parameters (velocity, displacement, strain rate (SR), and strain). Their advantage over Doppler-derived methods is that they are angle independent. Algorithms can track "signature" speckle patterns during the cardiac cycle, thereby deriving velocity vectors. The composite images from the interventricular septum in these apical four-chamber (A4C) views depict two-dimensional velocity vectors derived from motion of speckle patterns obtained from frame to frame. *Green dots* represent the initial diastolic location and the *red dot* represents the subsequent systolic location. Relative changes in distances between the speckles reflect deformation (longitudinal shortening) [28,30]. dX—derivative change in X; dY—derivative change in Y; X—x-axis; Y—y-axis;

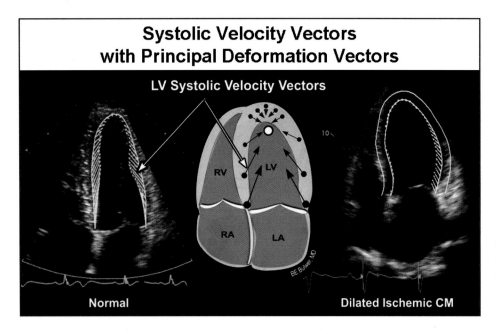

Figure 4-23. Systolic velocity vectors with principal deformation vectors. Schema of LV systolic velocity vectors in the normal and dilated LV. These images were obtained from a speckle tracking based algorithm called velocity vector imaging (VVI) [28,30,31]. CM—cardiomyopathy.

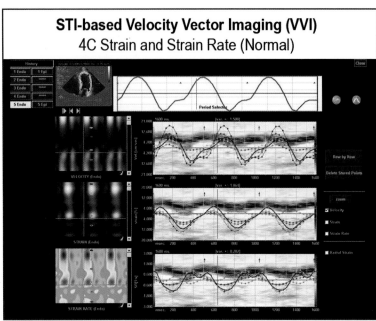

Figure 4-24. Speckle tracking imaging (STI)-based velocity vector imaging (VVI) 4C strain and strain rate (SR) (normal). Speckle tracking algorithm uses one set of data in order to derive LV myocardial velocities, two-dimensional strain, and two-dimensional SR. This method shows promise in the assessment of ventricular dyssynchrony [31].

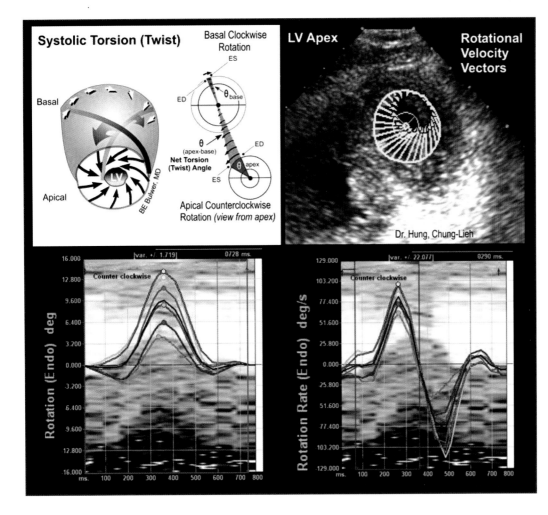

Figure 4-25. LV systolic torsion by speckle tracking imaging (STI). Speckle tracking can be used to assess LV ventricular systolic torsion, which is a gradient of rotation extending from LV apex to LA base. Systolic torsion represents a "wringing" of the ventricle, akin to twisting a towel, with apex twisting up to 15 degrees counter clockwise and the base twisting up to 5 degrees clockwise when viewed from the apex [32,33]. **Upper left**: schema showing LV torsion with a predominantly counter clockwise apical rotation and a smaller, systolic clockwise rotation at the base. **Upper right**: systolic velocity vectors at the left ventricular apex. **Lower left**: graph showing systolic rotation at left ventricular apex (in degrees), superimposed on M-mode image. **Lower right**: Systolic torsional velocities measured at the LV apex. (*Velocity vector images courtesy of Dr. Hung, Chung-Lieh, Brigham and Women's Hospital, Boston, and Mackay Hospital, Taipei.*) ED—end diastole; ES—end systole.

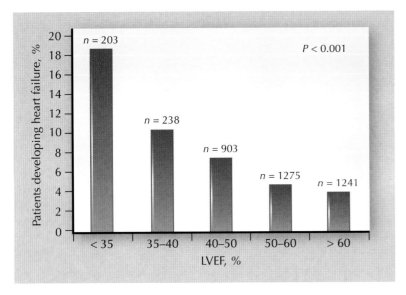

Figure 4-26. The impact of ejection fraction on the development of heart failure after myocardial infarction (MI). Ejection fraction is a strong predictor of outcome following myocardial infarction. The data from the Cardiac Angiography in Renally Impaired Patients (CARE) trial demonstrate the relationship between ejection fraction over a broad range of patients and the development of heart failure [34]

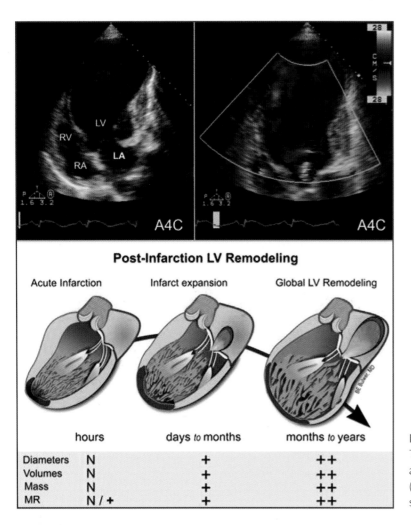

Post-Infarction LV Remodeling

Acute Infarction   Infarct expansion   Global LV Remodeling

	hours	days *to* months	months *to* years
Diameters	N	+	++
Volumes	N	+	++
Mass	N	+	++
MR	N / +	+	++

Figure 4-27. The LV can dilate or "remodel" following a myocardial infarction. This figure shows advanced post-infarction remodeling in a 74-year-old man admitted with congestive heart failure 2 months after myocardial infarction (MI) (*upper panel*) [35]. Schema depicting postinfarction ventricular remodeling is shown (*lower panel*). A4C—apical four chamber; MR—mitral regurgitation.

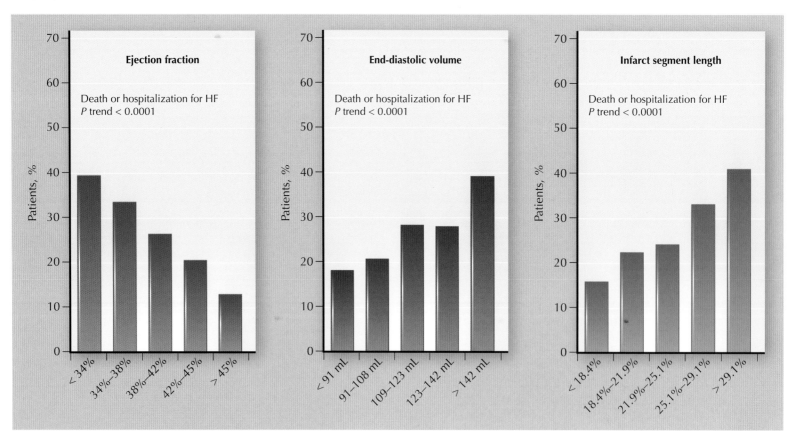

Figure 4-28. In addition to ejection fraction (EF), end-diastolic volume (EDSV) and infarct segment length are predictive of outcome after infarction. These data from the Valsartan in Acute Myocardial Infarction (VALIANT) trial [36] demonstrate the relationship between the echocardiographic findings and the outcome of death or development of heart failure.

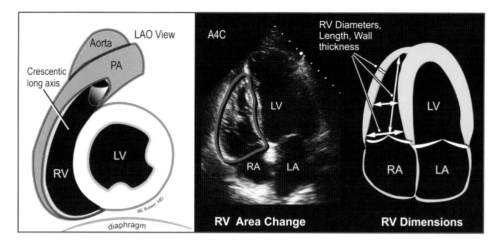

Figure 4-29. RV shortening occurs along its long or crescentic axis, but interventricular dependence results from LV systole assisting RV systole. The complex geometry of the RV remains a challenge to quantification of RV systolic function [8]. Though its assessment in clinical practice remains largely qualitative, selected RV dimensions and hemodynamic measures are of diagnostic and prognostic significance [37]. LAO—left anterior oblique; PA—pulmonary artery.

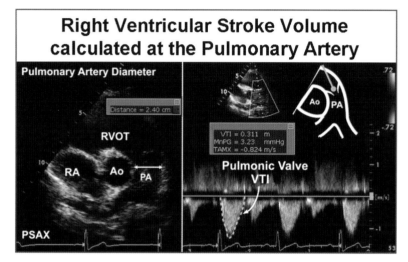

Figure 4-30. RV stroke volume calculated at the pulmonary artery (PA). RV stroke volume can be calculated in a similar manner as LV stroke volume in using the pulsed-wave Doppler from the pulmonary outflow tract. Ao—aorta; PSAX— parasternal short axis; RVOT—right ventricular outflow tract; VTI—velocity time integral.

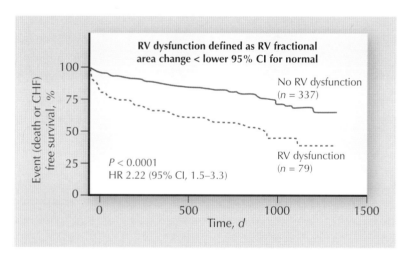

Figure 4-31. RV dysfunction and risk of heart failure and mortality after myocardial infarction. RV function is an important determinant of outcome after myocardial infarction. These data from the Survival and Ventricular Enlargement (SAVE) trial demonstrate how patients with RV dysfunction are at increased risk for death or development of heart failure, even after adjusting for LV function [38]. CHF—congestive heart failure; HR—heart rate; CI—cardiac index.

References

1. Thomas JD, Popovic ZB: Assessment of left ventricular function by cardiac ultrasound. *J Am Coll Cardiol* 2006, 48:2012–2025.

2. Kirkpatrick JN, Vannan MA, Narula J, Lang RM: Echocardiography in heart failure: applications, utility, and new horizons. *J Am Coll Cardiol* 2007, 50:381–396.

3. Buckberg GD, Weisfeldt ML, Ballester M, *et al.*: Left ventricular form and function: scientific priorities and strategic planning for development of new views of disease. *Circulation* 2004, 110:e333–e336.

4. Torrent-Guasp F, Ballester M, Buckberg GD, *et al.*: Spatial orientation of the ventricular muscle band: physiologic contribution and surgical implications. *J Thorac Cardiovasc Surg* 2001, 122:389–392.

5. Sengupta PP, Korinek J, Belohlavek M, *et al.*: Left ventricular structure and function: basic science for cardiac imaging. *J Am Coll Cardiol* 2006, 48:1988–2001.

6. Opie LH: Mechanisms of cardiac contraction and relaxation. In *Heart Disease*. Edited by Braunwald E, edn. 6. Philadelphia: Saunders; 2005:457–490.

7. Moore CC, Lugo-Olivieri CH, McVeigh ER, Zerhouni EA: Three-dimensional systolic strain patterns in the normal human left ventricle: characterization with tagged MR imaging. *Radiology* 2000, 214:453–466.

8. Buckberg GD, Mahajan A, Jung B, *et al.*: MRI myocardial motion and fiber tracking: a confirmation of knowledge from different imaging modalities. *Eur J Cardiothorac Surg* 2006, 29(Suppl 1):S165–S177.

9. Cerqueira MD, Weissman NJ, Dilsizian V, *et al.*: Standardized myocardial segmentation and nomenclature for tomographic imaging of the heart: a statement for healthcare professionals from the Cardiac Imaging Committee of the Council on Clinical Cardiology of the American Heart Association. *Circulation* 2002, 105:539–542.

10. Myers JH, Stirling MC, Choy M, *et al.*: Direct measurement of inner and outer wall thickening dynamics with epicardial echocardiography. *Circulation* 1986, 74:164–172.

11. Carluccio E, Tommasi S, Bentivoglio M, *et al.*: Usefulness of the severity and extent of wall motion abnormalities as prognostic markers of an adverse outcome after a first myocardial infarction treated with thrombolytic therapy. *Am J Cardiol* 2000, 85:411–415.

12. Collins M, Hsieh A, Ohazama CJ, *et al.*: Assessment of regional wall motion abnormalities with real-time 3-dimensional echocardiography. *J Am Soc Echocardiogr* 1999, 12:7–14.

13. Feigenbaum H, Armstrong WF, Ryan T, eds: *Echocardiography*, edn 6. Philadelphia: Lippincott Williams & Wilkins; 2004.

14. Teichholz LE, Kreulen T, Herman MV, Gorlin R: Problems in echocardiographic volume determinations: echocardiographic-angiographic correlations in the presence of absence of asynergy. *Am J Cardiol* 1976, 37:7–11.

15. Lang RM, Bierig M, Devereux RB, *et al.*: Recommendations for chamber quantification: a report from the American Society of Echocardiography's Guidelines and Standards Committee and the Chamber Quantification Writing Group, developed in conjunction with the European Association of Echocardiography, a branch of the European Society of Cardiology. *J Am Soc Echocardiogr* 2005, 18:1440–1463.

16. Sahn DJ, DeMaria A, Kisslo J, Weyman A: Recommendations regarding quantitation in M-mode echocardiography: results of a survey of echocardiographic measurements. *Circulation* 1978, 58:1072–1083.

17. Devereux RB, Wachtell K, Gerdts E, *et al.*: Prognostic significance of left ventricular mass change during treatment of hypertension. *JAMA* 2004, 292:2350–2356.

18. Verdecchia P, Schillaci G, Borgioni C, *et al.*: Prognostic significance of serial changes in left ventricular mass in essential hypertension. *Circulation* 1998, 97:48–54.

19. Sugeng L, Mor-Avi V, Weinert L, *et al.*: Quantitative assessment of left ventricular size and function: side-by-side comparison of real-time three-dimensional echocardiography and computed tomography with magnetic resonance reference. *Circulation* 2006, 114:654–661.

20. Kirkpatrick JN, Vannan MA, Narula J, Lang RM: Echocardiography in heart failure: applications, utility, and new horizons. *J Am Coll Cardiol* 2007, 50:381–396.

21. Cho GY, Park WJ, Han SW, *et al.*: Myocardial systolic synchrony measured by Doppler tissue imaging as a role of predictor of left ventricular ejection fraction improvement in severe congestive heart failure. *J Am Soc Echocardiogr* 2004, 17:1245–1250.

22. Tei C, Ling LH, Hodge DO, *et al.*: New index of combined systolic and diastolic myocardial performance: a simple and reproducible measure of cardiac function—a study in normals and dilated cardiomyopathy. *J Cardiol* 1995, 26:357–366.

23. Gillebert TC, Van de Veire N, De Buyzere ML, De Sutter J: Time intervals and global cardiac function: use and limitations. *Eur Heart J* 2004, 25:2185–2186.

24. Yamamoto K, Masuyama T, Doi Y, *et al.*: Noninvasive assessment of left ventricular relaxation using continuous-wave Doppler aortic regurgitant velocity curve: its comparative value to the mitral regurgitation method. *Circulation* 1995, 91:192–200.

25. Chen C, Rodriguez L, Lethor JP, *et al.*: Continuous wave Doppler echocardiography for noninvasive assessment of left ventricular dP/dt and relaxation time constant from mitral regurgitant spectra in patients. *J Am Coll Cardiol* 1994, 23:970–976.

26. Sohn DW, Chai IH, Lee DJ, *et al.*: Assessment of mitral annulus velocity by Doppler tissue imaging in the evaluation of left ventricular diastolic function. *J Am Coll Cardiol* 1997, 30:474–480.

27. Gorcsan J III: Assessment of left ventricular systolic function using color-coded tissue doppler echocardiography. *Echocardiography* 1999, 16:455–463.

28. Teske AJ, De Boeck BW, Melman PG, *et al.*: Echocardiographic quantification of myocardial function using tissue deformation imaging, a guide to image acquisition and analysis using tissue Doppler and speckle tracking. *Cardiovasc Ultrasound* 2007, 5:27.

29. Pislaru C, Abraham TP, Belohlavek M: Strain and strain rate echocardiography. *Curr Opin Cardiol* 2002, 17:443–454.

30. Marwick TH: Measurement of strain and strain rate by echocardiography: ready for prime time? *J Am Coll Cardiol* 2006, 47:1313–1327.

31. Cannesson M, Tanabe M, Suffoletto MS, *et al.*: Velocity vector imaging to quantify ventricular dyssynchrony and predict response to cardiac resynchronization therapy. *Am J Cardiol* 2006, 98:949–953.

32. Notomi Y, Popovic ZB, Yamada H, *et al.*: Ventricular untwisting: a temporal link between left ventricular relaxation and suction. *Am J Physiol Heart Circ Physiol* 2008, 294:H505–H513.

33. Notomi Y, Martin-Miklovic MG, Oryszak SJ, *et al.*: Enhanced ventricular untwisting during exercise: a mechanistic manifestation of elastic recoil described by Doppler tissue imaging. *Circulation* 2006, 113:2524–2533.

34. Lewis EF, Moye LA, Rouleau JL, *et al.*: Predictors of late development of heart failure in stable survivors of myocardial infarction: the CARE study. *J Am Coll Cardiol* 2003, 42:1446–1453.

35. St John Sutton M, Pfeffer MA, Plappert T, *et al.*: Quantitative two-dimensional echocardiographic measurements are major predictors of adverse cardiovascular events after acute myocardial infarction—the protective effects of captopril. *Circulation* 1994, 89:68–75.

36. Solomon SD, Skali H, Anavekar NS, *et al.*: Changes in ventricular size and function in patients treated with valsartan, captopril, or both after myocardial infarction. *Circulation* 2005, 111:3411–3419.

37. Gorcsan J III, Murali S, Counihan PJ, *et al.*: Right ventricular performance and contractile reserve in patients with severe heart failure: assessment by pressure-area relations and association with outcome. *Circulation* 1996, 94:3190–3197.

38. Zornoff LA, Skali H, Pfeffer MA, *et al.*: Right ventricular dysfunction and risk of heart failure and mortality after myocardial infarction. *J Am Coll Cardiol* 2002, 39:1450–1455.

5

Assessment of Diastolic Function

James Thomas and Ron Jacob

Diastolic heart failure is an important clinical entity that affects between 30% to 50% of all patients with congestive cardiac failure [1]. Diastole is a complex sequence of events, which can be divided into the following stages (*see* Fig. 5-1).

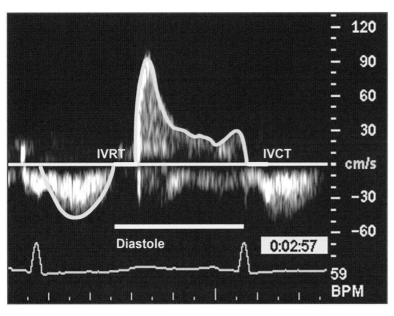

Figure 5-1. Doppler evaluation of the mitral valve, demonstrating the various stages of diastole. 1) Isovolumic relaxation, which is an energy-dependent process during which there is no ventricular filling (*yellow line*, isovolumic relaxation time [IVRT]) [2]. 2) Rapid filling, which accounts for approximately 80% of ventricular filling in a normal individual. This stage of diastole is affected by multiple factors, including left atrial pressure and LV minimum pressure, compliance, and suction. The gradient generated between the left atrium and the LV by the complex interaction between these factors determines the rate and the amount of filling that occurs in this stage. 3) Diastasis or slow filling makes a minor contribution to end diastolic volume. 4) Atrial contraction, which accounts for approximately 15% of diastolic filling volume in normal individuals. 5) Isovolumic contraction time (IVCT) (*yellow line*, IVCT).

Echocardiography is a valuable tool when making the diagnosis and evaluation of diastolic dysfunction.

A comprehensive assessment of diastolic function by echocardiography should include assessment of the structure and function of the heart using M-mode and two-dimensional echocardiography. LV hypertrophy is often associated with decreased tissue elastance and diastolic dysfunction [3]. Patients with pathologic LV hypertrophy operate on a different pressure volume curve and will have increased pressures for any given volume when compared with a normal ventricle. Normal diastolic filling patterns may be seen in patients with severe LV hypertrophy despite advanced diastolic dysfunction (the pseudonormal pattern). Left atrial volume indexed to body surface area [4] increases with worsening diastolic dysfunction as adequate LV filling is accomplished at the expense of raised left atrial pressures. Conversely, a diagnosis of diastolic dysfunction with elevated pressures should be questioned in a patient with normal left atrial volume indexed to body surface area. BPM—beats per min.

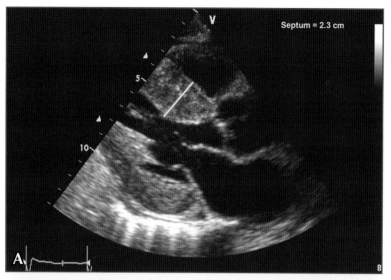

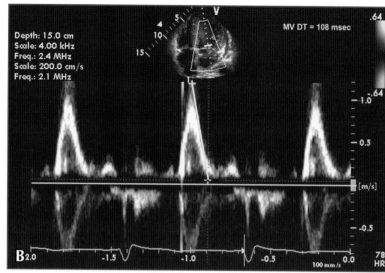

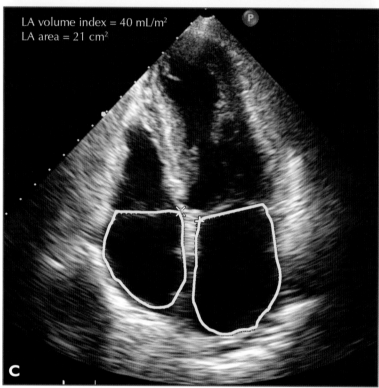

Figure 5-2. The patient is a 73-year-old man with biopsy-confirmed amyloid with progressive dyspnea on exertion. **A,** Parasternal long-axis views demonstrate severe LV wall thickening. **B,** Mitral deceleration time (DT) demonstrates a restrictive filling pattern with severe diastolic dysfunction. LV hypertrophy present on two-dimensional images should prompt a thorough assessment of diastolic function [5]. **C,** The patient, an 89-year-old woman with a body surface area of 1.5 m² and an ischemic cardiomyopathy, has a markedly abnormal left atrial volume index of 40 mL/m². Her left atrial area measured 21 cm². If the left atrial area were used, then she would be erroneously classified as having mild left atrial dilation. LA—left atrium; MV—mitral valve; V—volume.

Assessment of Ventricular Relaxation, Compliance, and Filling Pressures Using Doppler and Color M-Mode

The ventricle relaxes with the onset of diastole, causing the LV pressure to fall below left atrial pressure. The pressure gradient generated causes the volume of blood in the left atrium to be accelerated across the mitral valve, with a mitral inflow pattern that can be seen with Doppler echocardiography. A widely accepted invasive standard for measuring LV relaxation is the isovolumic relaxation time constant τ, which is derived from the descending limb of the LV pressure curve obtained in the cardiac catheterization laboratory. A steep curve will yield a lower number (normal relaxation), whereas delayed relaxation will result in a more gradual slope and a higher number. The mitral inflow on Doppler echocardiography is strongly influenced by τ [6]. The growth in the pressure gradient, which primarily determines E wave acceleration and peak velocity, is roughly proportional to left atrial pressure (LAP)/τ. In other words, E velocity is lowered when τ is prolonged (delayed relaxation) and raised by elevated LAP, the latter effect termed "preload compensation." This dual determination of peak E velocity is the fundamental limitation when using transmitral profile alone to assess diastolic function.

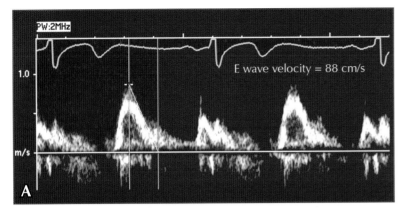

E wave velocity = 88 cm/s

A

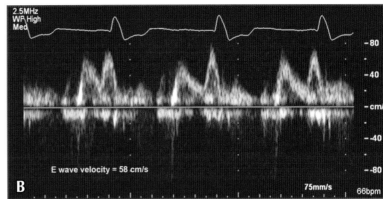

E wave velocity = 58 cm/s

B

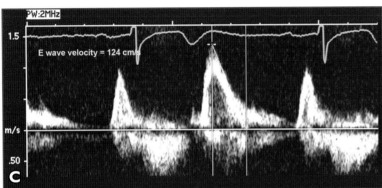

E wave velocity = 124 cm/s

C

Figure 5-3. The transmitral profile from three patients. **A**, Normal patient with low left atrial pressure (LAP) and low τ (normal relaxation) leading to a normal E velocity of 88 cm/s. **B**, Mitral inflow from a healthy elderly patient with low LAP and elevated τ (delayed relaxation) producing a lower peak E velocity of 58 cm/s. **C**, Patient with advanced diastolic dysfunction with both elevated LAP and prolonged τ (markedly delayed relaxation), producing an E velocity of 124 cm/s. Thus, the first patient has a normal filling pattern, the second patient shows a delayed relaxation pattern, and the third patient is termed the "pseudonormal" pattern; one of the principal tasks in assessing diastolic function is to distinguish normal from pseudonormal.

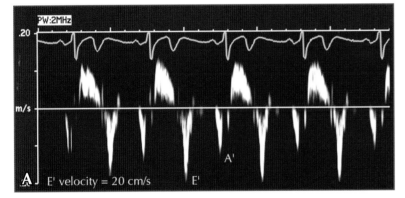

A   E' velocity = 20 cm/s   E'   A'

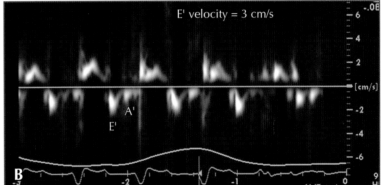

E' velocity = 3 cm/s

A'
E'

B

Figure 5-4. In order to distinguish normal from pseudonormal, one seeks independent evidence of delayed relaxation. One of the simplest approaches is by using tissue Doppler imaging (TDI) in order to measure early relaxation velocity of the mitral annulus. A sample volume placed over the septal or lateral annulus of the mitral valve in the four-chamber view yields an early diastolic velocity correlating with rapid diastolic filling (E') and a late diastolic velocity (A'), correlating with atrial contraction. In normal subjects, the onset of E' precedes the onset of the mitral E wave tracing, indicating that basal displacement of the annulus helps to drive mitral filling rather than vice versa, which is often observed in patients with diastolic dysfunction. In normal individuals, an increase in the rate of LV relaxation allows stroke volume to be augmented without an increase in left atrial pressures during exercise. Studies have shown that E' velocity is roughly inversely proportional to the relaxation time constant, τ. The E' velocity

becomes less sensitive to preload and provides a key parameter in assessing diastolic function with impaired relaxation [7]. In general, the lateral annulus has higher velocities (approximately 15 cm/s) than the medial annulus (typically 10 cm/s). E' velocities should always be assessed with the age of the patient in mind. With progressive aging, the E' velocities decrease; eg, a septal annular velocity of 10 cm/s in a 15-year-old boy would be cause for concern, even though it is in the "normal" range. A normal annular pattern with an E' of 20 cm/s is shown (**A**) compared with a patient with advanced diastolic dysfunction and an E' of only 3 cm/s (**B**). Although it was initially hoped that TDI annular velocities would be completely independent of preload (left atrial pressure in this context), it is now clear that they are merely less preload dependent than transmitral flow, particularly for pathologic cases. Thus, they provide a very useful way in which to distinguish normal from pseudonormal [8].

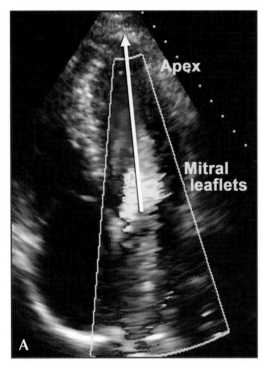

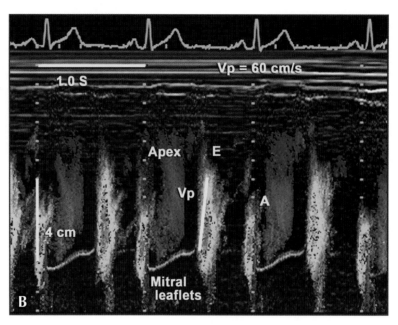

Figure 5-5. Another type of data available to distinguish normal from pseudonormal is the transmitral flow propagation velocity (Vp) assessed by Doppler color M-mode. This is measured by imaging the ventricle from the apical four-chamber window using color Doppler (**A**). An M-mode cursor is directed from the mid left atrium through the middle of the mitral valve to the LV apex, and color M-mode data are obtained. Two waves of flow are seen passing from the atrium to the ventricle, representing early rapid filling and atrial contraction (**B**). Flow propagation is measured as the slope of the dominant E-wave flow. Unfortunately, this is not completely standardized; however, it can conveniently be done by baseline shifting the color in order to highlight an aliasing contour with a velocity about 30% to 40% of the peak E-wave velocity. Vp can be measured by a linear approximation of this color M-mode contour by drawing a line from the mitral leaflets to the apex with information about both distance (y-axis) and time (x-axis), and therefore velocity. It is important to not measure the leading edge of the flow, because this often reflects redistribution of LV blood during isovolumic relaxation.

A Vp of 60 cm/s in a 42-year-old man is shown (**B**). Normal ventricles create a suction force during diastole, which accelerates blood through the distance between the mitral orifice and the apex. In normal ventricles, the slope will be steep (> 55 cm/s), reflecting normal suction with a rapid

acceleration of blood from the leaflets to the apex. An abnormal ventricle with impairment in relaxation will have a reduced acceleration of blood and a lower value for Vp [9] and can thus be a useful discriminant between normal and pseudonormal. Like tissue Doppler imaging annular velocity, Vp is roughly inversely related to τ and is relatively independent of left atrial pressure.

Another key aspect of diastolic function is ventricular compliance (or its converse, stiffness, defined by the change in LV pressure for a given change in volume, $\Delta p/\Delta V$). Unfortunately, this is a gross simplification of the physiologic situation. First, the LV pressure volume (PV) relationship is not linear, but roughly exponentially shaped so that stiffness increases with increasing volume. Even more confounding, the PV relationship itself changes dramatically during diastole, from the extremely stiff end systolic relationship to fully relaxed end diastole. LV pressure continues to fall from early diastole; even as its volume increases, the effective stiffness of the ventricle is actually negative at this time. Thus, any attempt to characterize ventricular compliance is bound to be imperfect. One useful analogue, however, is the deceleration time of the transmitral E wave, which has been shown theoretically and in animal and clinical studies to be inversely proportional to the operating stiffness of the LV. In general, a deceleration time of less than 150 ms is indicative of abnormal stiffness and is commonly found in restrictive cardiomyopathies.

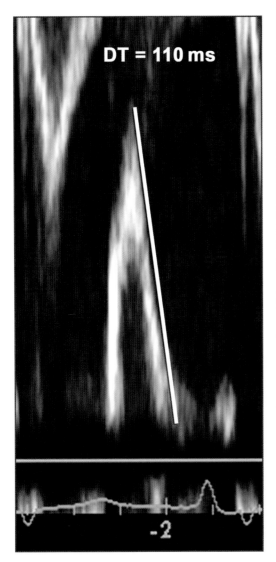

DT = 110 ms

-2

Figure 5-6. The figure shows a very rapid mitral deceleration time (DT) of 110 ms in a patient with an infiltrative cardiomyopathy. Assessment of filling pressures using E/E' and E/propagation velocity (Vp) is explained. These ratios rely on using a relatively preload-independent parameter (E', Vp) compared with a preload-dependent parameter like the mitral inflow velocity. E/E' ratios have been shown to correlate with filling pressures estimated by cardiac catheterization [10]. Unlike abnormal ventricles, E/E' should be used with caution in normal ventricles in order to estimate filling pressures as in these individuals
tissue annular velocities are preload dependent [11]. If E/E' is less than 10, it suggests normal pulmonary capillary wedge pressures; if it is greater than 15, it suggests elevated pulmonary capillary wedge pressures. If the values fall between 10 and 15, other echocardiographic parameters have to be used to estimate filling pressures. An E/Vp greater than 1.5 suggests elevated pulmonary capillary wedge pressures.

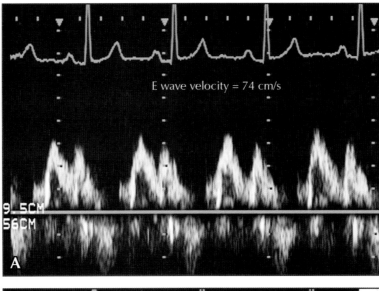

E wave velocity = 74 cm/s

9.5CM

56CM

A

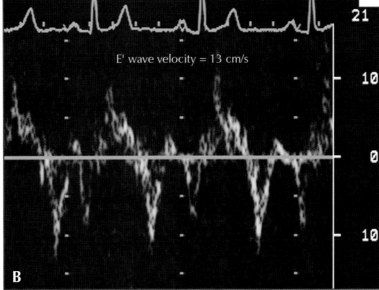

E' wave velocity = 13 cm/s

21

10

0

10

B

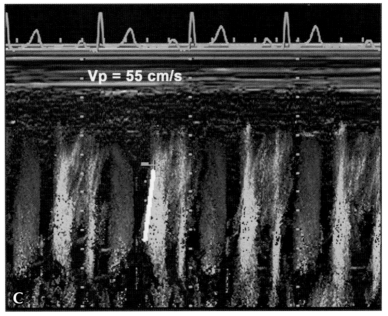

Vp = 55 cm/s

C

Figure 5-7. A, Mitral inflow Doppler with a peak velocity of 74 cm/s. **B**, Tissue Doppler velocity of 13 cm/s at the septal annulus suggesting normal relaxation. **C**, Color M-mode with a normal propagation velocity (Vp) of 55 cm/s. Normal filling pressures, suggested by an E/E' ratio less than 10 (74/13) and an E/Vp less than 1.5 (74/55) is shown.

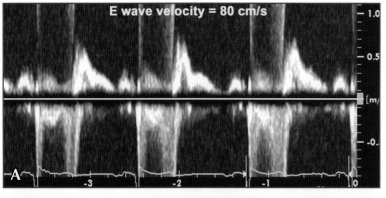

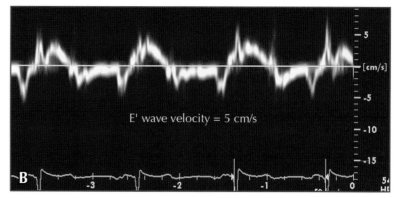

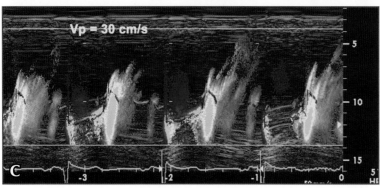

Figure 5-8. A, Mitral inflow Doppler with a peak velocity of 80 cm/s. **B**, Abnormal tissue Doppler velocity of 5 cm/s at the septal annulus. **C**, Abnormal propagation velocity (Vp) of 30 cm/s. Elevated filling pressures suggested by an E/E' ratio of more than 15 (80/5) and an E/Vp of more than 1.5 (80/30).

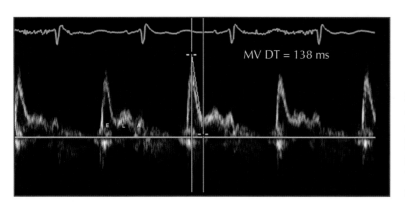

Figure 5-9. A mitral L wave represents transmitral flow during diastasis. An L wave on the transmitral flow pattern in patients with structural heart disease may represent elevated end diastolic pressures and a higher risk for future hospitalizations for heart failure [12]. Diastolic relaxation can be graded using mitral inflow, tissue Doppler, pulmonary vein, and color M-mode, with grade 1 representing a normal filling pattern and grade 4 representing an irreversible restrictive filling pattern. MV DT—mitral valve deceleration time.

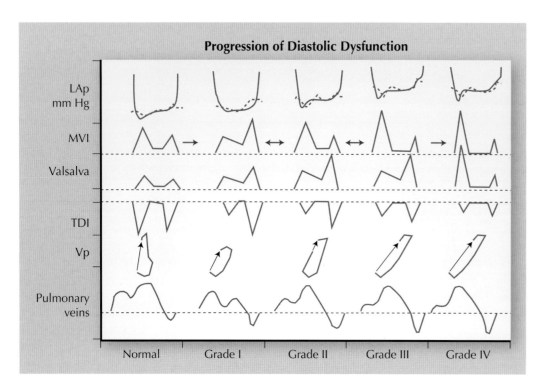

Figure 5-10. Progressive degrees of diastolic dysfunction (grades 1–4), as evaluated by the mitral inflow pattern, mitral annular velocities (tissue Doppler imaging [TDI]), flow propagation velocity (Vp) (color M-mode or Vp), and pulmonary vein velocities. Normal diastolic function is suggested by a mitral inflow with an E/A ratio greater than 1.5, predominant diastolic flow in the pulmonary veins, a color M-mode velocity greater than 55 cm/s, and normal tissue annular velocities. The mitral deceleration time should be between 160 to 240 ms in normal middle-aged individuals [13]. The deceleration slope should always be interpreted with the age of the patient in mind, as younger patients have a short deceleration time because of rapid ventricular relaxation. Grade 1 diastolic dysfunction is characterized by an E/A ratio of less than 1, with a prolonged deceleration time of the E wave. There is a reduction in the velocity of the diastolic segment of the pulmonary vein tracing and the tissue annular velocity.

Continued on the next page

Figure 5-10. *(Continued)* The mitral flow propagation velocity will be less than 55 cm/s. Grade 2 diastolic dysfunction can be confused with normal diastolic function if one just looks at the mitral inflow. The E/A ratio will be 1 to 1.5, and the deceleration time of the E wave may be in the normal range. Careful examination of the tissue annular velocities, pulmonary veins, and color M-mode values will reveal abnormal values, making the diagnosis of grade 2 diastolic dysfunction. Performing a Valsalva maneuver will decrease the preload, causing the ventricle to operate on a different position on the pressure volume loop and convert the grade 2 mitral inflow pattern to a grade 1 mitral inflow pattern.

Grade 3–4 diastolic dysfunction, or a restrictive filling pattern, represents a decrease in compliance and an increase in left atrial pressure (LAp). It can result from many causes, such as systolic heart failure, severe mitral regurgitation, restrictive cardiomyopathy, and pericardial constriction. The mitral inflow will have an E/A ratio of more than 2 with a short deceleration time, usually below 150 ms. The pulmonary vein tracing will reveal very little flow during systole with a blunting of the S wave and dominant flow in early diastole. The values for tissue annular velocities and color M-mode are also markedly abnormal. If changing the preload using the Valsalva maneuver or diuretics fails to alter the restrictive pattern on the mitral inflow, the pattern is considered irreversible or grade 4. Patients with systolic heart failure who have a persistent restrictive pattern in the mitral inflow despite optimal medical therapy tend to do poorly when compared with patients with grade 1 or 2 patterns on the mitral inflow [14]. MVI—mitral valve inflow.

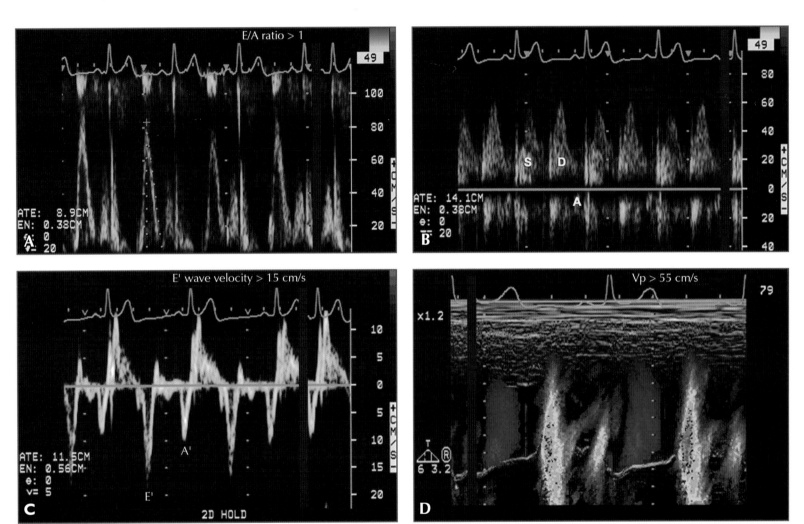

Figure 5-11. Patient with normal diastolic function. Note that the E/A ratio is greater than 1.0 (**A**). The S wave is smaller than the D wave due to prominent diastolic flow (**B**). This reflects vigorous diastolic relaxation with normal filling pressures and should not be mistaken for raised left atrial pressures and blunting of the S wave. Normal diastolic function is reinforced by the normal tissue annular velocities of more than 15 cm/s (**C**), and color M-mode Doppler, with propagation velocity (Vp) more than 55 cm/s (**D**). A′—late diastolic annulus velocity; E′—early diastolic velocity.

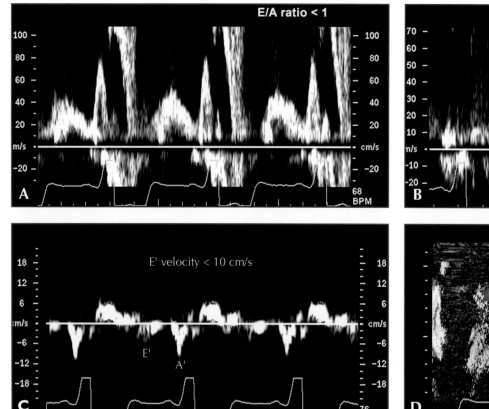

E/A ratio < 1

E' velocity < 10 cm/s

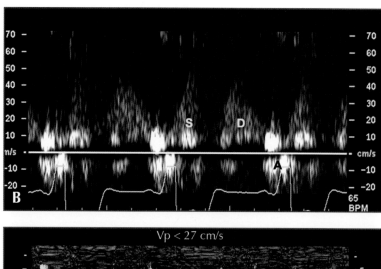

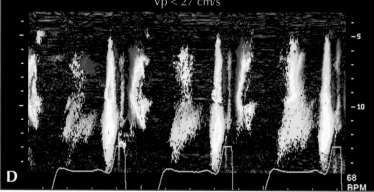

Vp < 27 cm/s

Figure 5-12. Stage I diastolic dysfunction in a patient with Fabry's disease. In stage I diastolic dysfunction, the E/A ratio is less than 1 (**A**). The pulmonary veins do not reveal significant blunting (**B**); however, the patient has low tissue annular velocities of 10 cm/s (**C**) and an abnormal color M-mode slope of 27 cm/s (**D**). A'—late diastolic velocity; D—D wave; E'—rapid diastolic filling; S—S wave.

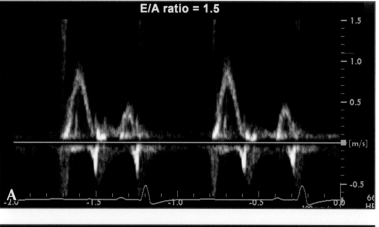

E/A ratio = 1.5

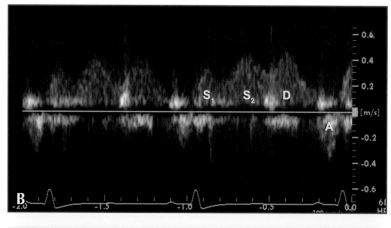

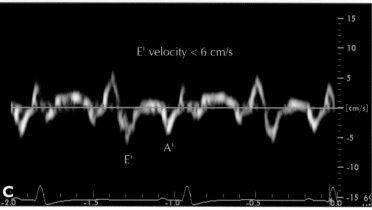

E' velocity < 6 cm/s

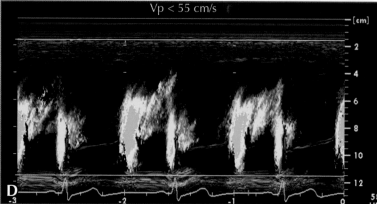

Vp < 55 cm/s

Figure 5-13. Stage II diastolic dysfunction. This patient demonstrates a pseudonormal pattern on the mitral inflow with an E/A ratio of 1 to 1.5 (**A**). The pulmonary vein pattern demonstrates two systolic waves (S_1, S_2) and two diastolic waves (D, A) (**B**). The S_1 and S_2 waves represent changes that occur during left atrial filling, corresponding to the time between the peak of the A wave on the jugular venous pulse to the peak of the V wave. The D wave represents early diastolic filling of the ventricle and mirrors changes in the E wave on the mitral inflow. The S_1 wave is a marker of left atrial relaxation [15] and occurs shortly after the Q wave. The S_2 wave is related temporally to ventricular contraction and the descent of the mitral annulus.

Continued on the next page

Figure 5-13. *(Continued)* It is also reduced in patients with mitral regurgitation (MR), which may be reversed with severe MR. The systolic component of the pulmonary venous Doppler in patients with impaired LV function decreases with increasing wedge pressure [16]. This may be due to a decrease in left atrial compliance, related to the left atrium operating on a steeper portion of its pressure volume curve. The ratio between the systolic flow velocities of the pulmonary vein tracing to the diastolic flow velocities is helpful in the different stages of diastolic dysfunction.

In stage I diastolic dysfunction, the systolic flow velocities are typically greater than the diastolic flow velocities (*see* Fig. 5-12), whereas in stage III, systolic flow velocities are even more blunted relative to diastolic flow velocities than they are in this example (*see* Fig. 5-14). There is a prominent atrial reversal wave, suggesting increased LV stiffness at the time of atrial contraction. Tissue annular velocities are markedly abnormal with 6 cm/s at the lateral annulus (**C**). The E/E′ ratio is more than 15, suggesting elevated filling pressures. The color M-mode velocity slope is less than 55 cm/s (**D**), which is consistent with slow propagation velocity (Vp), supporting the diagnosis. This case highlights the importance of analyzing all the information available through echocardiography and not focusing on any one parameter (the pulmonary veins with no obvious blunting of the S wave, for instance) to arrive at an accurate estimation of diastolic function. A′—late diastolic annular velocity; E′—early diastolic annular filling.

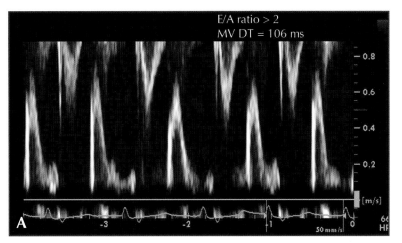

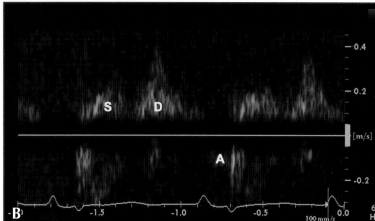

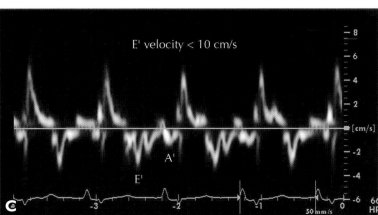

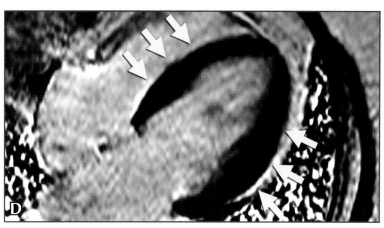

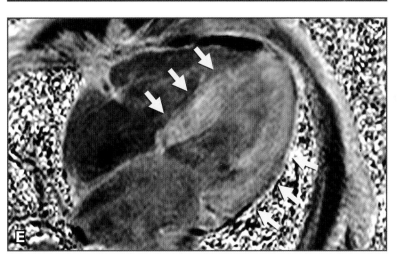

Figure 5-14. Stage III diastolic dysfunction. Patient is a 52-year-old man with cardiac amyloidosis. The mitral inflow pattern reveals an E/A ratio of more than 2 (**A**). The deceleration slope of the E wave is less than 150 ms and the peak E wave velocity is 80 cm/s (**B**). The pulmonary veins are blunted, with the area of the S wave being less than 40% of the D wave. The filling pressures are elevated with an E/E′ ratio greater than 15 (E/E′ or 80/5). The tissue annular velocities are markedly abnormal at 5 cm/s (**C**). Normal myocardium is "nulled," and appears black (*yellow arrows*) after administration of gadolinium (**D**). The MRI from the patient demonstrates significant hyperenhancement of the myocardium, which appears white (*yellow arrows*), consistent with an infiltrative cardiomyopathy (**E**). The patient had an RV biopsy that confirmed amyloidosis as the diagnosis. This patient had a persistence of the restrictive pattern on the mitral inflow despite optimal medical therapy, portending a poor prognosis. A′—late diastolic velocity; E′—rapid diastolic filling; MV DT—mitral valve deceleration time.

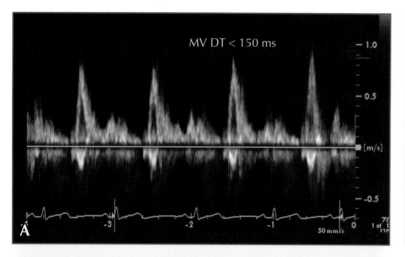

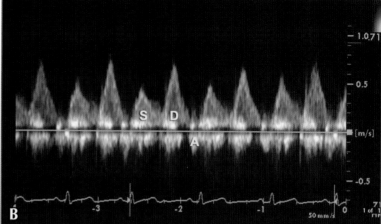

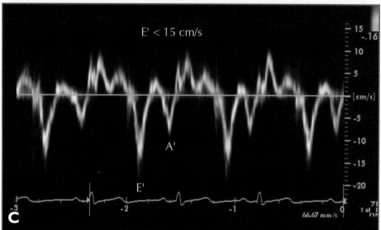

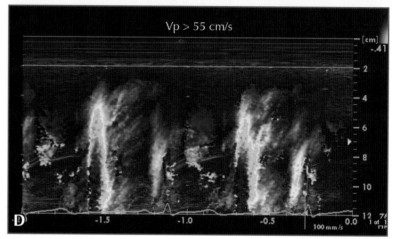

Figure 5-15. Mitral inflow from a normal 15-year-old boy with a rapid deceleration time, reflecting vigorous relaxation with a compliant ventricle [17]. **A**, Mitral inflow with a normal E wave velocity and a deceleration time, which is less than 150 ms. **B**, The pulmonary vein flows demonstrates dominant flow in diastole with blunting in systole. Interpreting the pulmonary vein flow in isolation would lead to an incorrect diagnosis of diastolic dysfunction. **C**, The tissue annular velocities are normal, reflecting normal relaxation. **D**, The flow propagation velocities are normal once again reinforcing normal relaxation. The constellation of findings would indicate normal diastolic function in this young adult. MV DT—mitral valve deceleration time; Vp—propagation velocity.

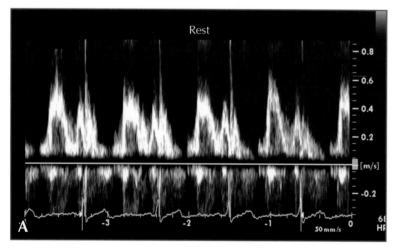

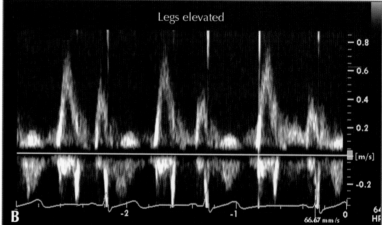

Figure 5-16. The effect of preload on mitral E wave velocity. Patient has grade 2 pattern on the mitral inflow at rest (**A**); there is an increase in the E wave velocity and a shorter deceleration slope with the legs up and increased preload (**B**).

Continued on the next page

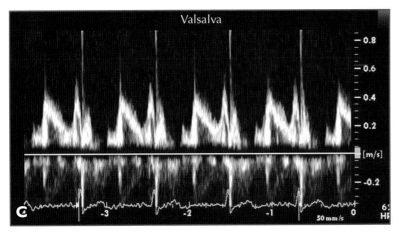

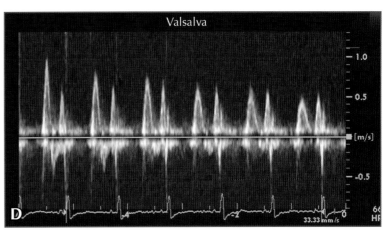

Figure 5-16. (*Continued*) There is a decrease in the preload and a decrease in E wave velocity and reversion to a grade 1 mitral inflow pattern with the Valsalva maneuver (**C**) [18,19]. Preload affects the peak velocity and mitral deceleration time (**D**). By reducing venous return, Valsalva maneuver changes the atrioventricular pressure gradient and affects the E wave velocity and slope [19,20].

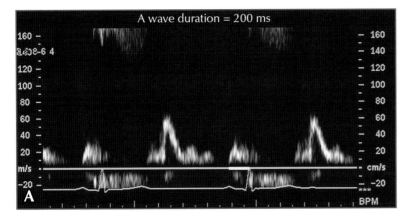

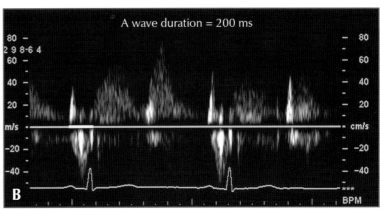

Figure 5-17. A noncompliant ventricle will prolong the duration of the left atrial Doppler tracing in the pulmonary veins relative to the mitral inflow. In this 60-year-old man with hypertension who has grade 2 diastolic dysfunction, the duration of the pulmonary vein atrial reversal wave is greater than the mitral A wave duration (**A** and **B**), a Doppler finding that correlates with an elevated end diastolic pressure [21]. With progressive elevation of LV end diastolic pressure, the mitral A wave will shorten in duration with an increase in the duration of the pulmonary atrial reversal wave [22]. Pulmonary vein atrial reversal wave that exceeds the duration of the mitral A wave duration by more than 30 ms predicts an LV end diastolic pressure greater than 20 mm Hg [18]. BPM—beats per min.

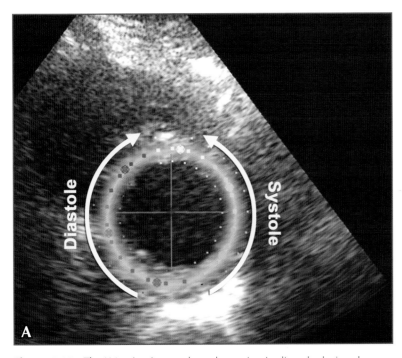

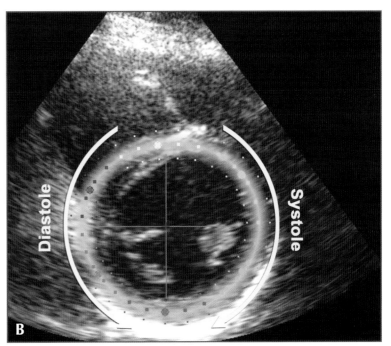

Figure 5-18. The LV twists in systole and untwists in diastole during the cardiac cycle [23]. The untwisting of the ventricle during diastole starts during isovolumic relaxation with the apex rotating in a clockwise direction (**A**) and the base rotating in a counter clockwise direction [24] (**B**).

Continued on the next page

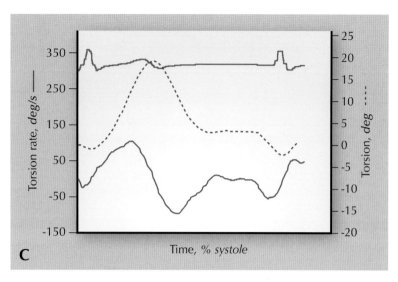

Figure 5-18. *(Continued)* This untwisting of the LV in diastole can be abnormal in disease states or with aging [25,26]. Motion analysis by speckle tracking imaging allows the rate of untwisting to be analyzed by providing values for LV rotation at the base and the apex. The *pink line* represents torsion in degrees, whereas the *blue line* represents torsional rate in degrees per second (**C**). The ECG is also indicated (*green line*).

Intraventricular Pressure Gradient

The rapid phase of diastolic filling is facilitated by an intraventricular pressure gradient (IVPG) from the base to the apex [27]. This IVPG is related to the force from elastic recoil of the LV [28]. Color M-mode provides data regarding the spatiotemporal velocity distribution between the base and the apex of the ventricle. IVPG can be derived by application of the Euler equation to color M-mode data along a streamline of flow [29]. The Euler equation is closely related to the Bernoulli equation, and it is commonly used in Doppler echocardiography to estimate pressure drop across a fixed stenosis. The Euler equation yields the gradual pressure drop in nonstenotic flow. The ability of the ventricle to augment IVPG with increased preload is impaired with the aging process and structural heart disease.

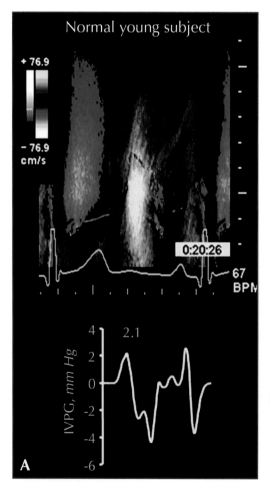

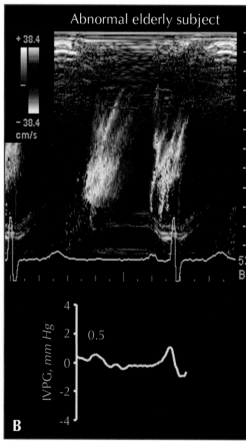

Figure 5-19. Intraventricular pressure gradient (IVPG) in a young healthy subject measuring 2.1 mm Hg is higher than IVPG in the healthy elderly subject measuring 0.5 mm Hg (**A** and **B**). BPM—beats per min.

Stress Echocardiography

Stress echocardiography can be used in order to assess diastolic function during exercise [30]. During exercise, the ventricle accommodates in part to increased blood flow by enhancing relaxation. Patients with significant diastolic dysfunction purchase increased flow at the expense of elevated filling pressures. The E′ gives a reasonable estimate of ventricular relaxation, and the mitral E wave provides a reasonable correlation with left atrial pressures. Filling pressures assessed from these two variables (E/E′) can be used to determine whether a patient's symptoms are caused by an increase in the pulmonary capillary wedge pressure during exercise [31].

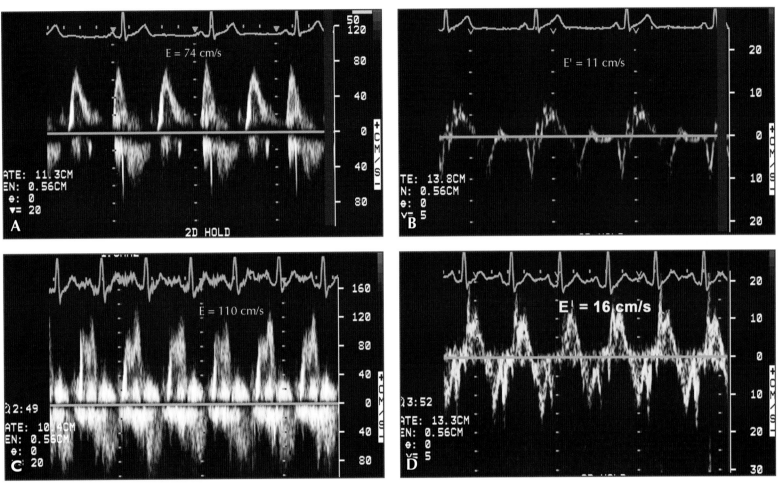

Figure 5-20. The patient is a 53-year-old obese hypertensive who was found to have stage I diastolic dysfunction with normal filling pressures at rest (E = 74 cm/s, E′ = 11 cm/s, E/E′ = < 10) (**A** and **B**). With exercise, there is an increase in E wave velocities and annular velocities (without exercise), and increase in filling pressures (E = 110 cm/s, E′ = 16 cm/s, E/E′ = < 10) (**C** and **D**). The patient's shortness of breath is unlikely to have been caused by diastolic dysfunction with elevated filling pressures.

References

1. Redfield MM, Jacobsen SJ, Burnett JC Jr, *et al.*: Burden of systolic and diastolic ventricular dysfunction in the community: appreciating the scope of the heart failure epidemic. *JAMA* 2003, 289:194–202.

2. Zile MR, Brutsaert DL: New concepts in diastolic dysfunction and diastolic heart failure: part I: diagnosis, prognosis, and measurements of diastolic function. *Circulation* 2002, 105:1387–1393.

3. de Simone G, Kitzman DW, Palmieri V, *et al.*: Association of inappropriate left ventricular mass with systolic and diastolic dysfunction: the HyperGEN study. *Am J Hypertens* 2004, 17:828–833.

4. Pritchett AM, Mahoney DW, Jacobsen SJ, *et al.*: Diastolic dysfunction and left atrial volume: a population-based study. *J Am Coll Cardiol* 2005, 45:87–92.

5. Wachtell K, Smith G, Gerdts E, *et al.*: Left ventricular filling patterns in patients with systemic hypertension and left ventricular hypertrophy (the LIFE study). Losartan Intervention For Endpoint. *Am J Cardiol* 2000, 85:466–472.

6. Thomas JD, Weyman AE: Echocardiographic Doppler evaluation of left ventricular diastolic function. Physics and physiology. *Circulation* 1991, 84:977–990.

7. Nagueh SF, Sun H, Kopelen HA, *et al.*: Hemodynamic determinants of the mitral annulus diastolic velocities by tissue Doppler. *J Am Coll Cardiol* 2001, 37:278–285.

8. Prasad A, Popovic ZB, Arbab-Zadeh A, *et al.*: The effects of aging and physical activity on Doppler measures of diastolic function. *Am J Cardiol* 2007, 99:1629–1636.

9. Takatsuji H, Mikami T, Urasawa K, *et al.*: A new approach for evaluation of left ventricular diastolic function: spatial and temporal analysis of left ventricular filling flow propagation by color M-mode Doppler echocardiography. *J Am Coll Cardiol* 1996, 27:365–371.

10. Nagueh SF, Middleton KJ, Kopelen HA, *et al.*: Doppler tissue imaging: a noninvasive technique for evaluation of left ventricular relaxation and estimation of filling pressures. *J Am Coll Cardiol* 1997, 30:1527–1533.

11. Firstenberg MS, Levine BD, Garcia MJ, et al.: Relationship of echocardiographic indices to pulmonary capillary wedge pressures in healthy volunteers. *J Am Coll Cardiol* 2000, 36:1664–1669.

12. Lam CS, Han L, Ha JW, et al.: The mitral L wave: a marker of pseudonormal filling and predictor of heart failure in patients with left ventricular hypertrophy. *J Am Soc Echocardiogr* 2005, 18:336–341.

13. Nishimura RA, Tajik AJ: Evaluation of diastolic filling of left ventricle in health and disease: Doppler echocardiography is the clinician's Rosetta Stone. *J Am Coll Cardiol* 1997, 30:8–18.

14. Traversi E, Pozzoli M, Cioffi G, et al.: Mitral flow velocity changes after 6 months of optimized therapy provide important hemodynamic and prognostic information in patients with chronic heart failure. *Am Heart J* 1996, 132:809–819.

15. Appleton CP: Hemodynamic determinants of Doppler pulmonary venous flow velocity components: new insights from studies in lightly sedated normal dogs. *J Am Coll Cardiol* 1997, 30:1562–1574.

16. Castello R, Vaughn M, Dressler FA, et al.: Relation between pulmonary venous flow and pulmonary wedge pressure: influence of cardiac output. *Am Heart J* 1995, 130:127–134.

17. Schmitz L, Koch H, Bein G, Brockmeier K: Left ventricular diastolic function in infants, children, and adolescents. Reference values and analysis of morphologic and physiologic determinants of echocardiographic Doppler flow signals during growth and maturation. *J Am Coll Cardiol* 1998, 32:1441–1448.

18. Tabata T, Thomas JD, Klein AL: Pulmonary venous flow by Doppler echocardiography: revisited 12 years later. *J Am Coll Cardiol* 2003, 41:1243–1250.

19. Dumesnil JG, Gaudreault G, Honos GN, Kingma JG Jr.: Use of Valsalva maneuver to unmask left ventricular diastolic function abnormalities by Doppler echocardiography in patients with coronary artery disease or systemic hypertension. *Am J Cardiol* 1991, 68:515–519.

20. Triulzi MO, Castini D, Ornaghi M, Vitolo E: Effects of preload reduction on mitral flow velocity pattern in normal subjects. *Am J Cardiol* 1990, 66:995–1001.

21. Rossvoll O, Hatle LK: Pulmonary venous flow velocities recorded by transthoracic Doppler ultrasound: relation to left ventricular diastolic pressures. *J Am Coll Cardiol* 1993, 21:1687–1696.

22. Yamamoto K, Nishimura RA, Burnett JC Jr, Redfield MM: Assessment of left ventricular end-diastolic pressure by Doppler echocardiography: contribution of duration of pulmonary venous versus mitral flow velocity curves at atrial contraction. *J Am Soc Echocardiogr* 1997, 10:52–59.

23. Notomi Y, Lysyansky P, Setser RM, et al.: Measurement of ventricular torsion by two-dimensional ultrasound speckle tracking imaging. *J Am Coll Cardiol* 2005, 45:2034–2041.

24. Notomi Y, Popovic ZB, Yamada H, et al.: Ventricular untwisting: a temporal link between left ventricular relaxation and suction. *Am J Physiol Heart Circ Physiol* 2008, 294:H505–H513.

25. Oxenham H, Sharpe N: Cardiovascular aging and heart failure. *Eur J Heart Fail* 2003, 5:427–434.

26. Stuber M, Scheidegger MB, Fischer SE, et al.: Alterations in the local myocardial motion pattern in patients suffering from pressure overload due to aortic stenosis. *Circulation* 1999, 100:361–368.

27. Ling D, Rankin JS, Edwards CH II, et al.: Regional diastolic mechanics of the left ventricle in the conscious dog. *Am J Physiol* 1979, 236:H323–H330.

28. Nikolic SD, Feneley MP, Pajaro OE, et al.: Origin of regional pressure gradients in the left ventricle during early diastole. *Am J Physiol* 1995, 268(2 Pt 2):H550–H557.

29. Popovic ZB, Prasad A, Garcia MJ, et al.: Relationship among diastolic intraventricular pressure gradients, relaxation, and preload: impact of age and fitness. *Am J Physiol Heart Circ Physiol* 2006, 290:H1454–H1459.

30. Ha JW, Lulic F, Bailey KR, et al.: Effects of treadmill exercise on mitral inflow and annular velocities in healthy adults. *Am J Cardiol* 2003, 91:114–115.

31. Ha JW, Oh JK, Pellikka PA, et al.: Diastolic stress echocardiography: a novel noninvasive diagnostic test for diastolic dysfunction using supine bicycle exercise Doppler echocardiography. *J Am Soc Echocardiogr* 2005, 18:63–68.

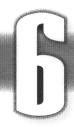

Stress Echocardiography

Patricia A. Pellikka

Stress echocardiography was initially proposed as a means of detecting coronary artery disease (CAD) in 1979. Advances in ultrasound technology and refinements in stress testing protocols have since made the technology highly feasible. Myocardial contrast for LV endocardial border detection is used if two or more segments cannot be adequately visualized at rest [1]. The basic premise of stress echocardiography is that with some form of stress, abnormalities of wall motion and thickening will occur in areas subtended by a stenosed coronary artery. These can be appreciated echocardiographically. Side-by-side comparison of rest and stress images permits detailed assessment of stress-induced changes [2].

Exercise stress echocardiography with supine or upright bicycle exercise or treadmill exercise is preferred for patients who are able to perform an exercise test. Although most patients can achieve a higher workload with treadmill exercise, bicycle stress testing has the advantage in that imaging can be performed during exercise as opposed to in immediate recovery. Bicycle exercise is preferred if additional Doppler data are to be obtained in conjunction with regional wall motion assessment [3]. For patients who are unable to exercise, pharmacologic stress testing may be performed with dobutamine or with the vasodilators, such as dipyridamole or adenosine. These agents are often combined with atropine in order to augment the heart rate. Dobutamine echocardiography is most widely used. A standard protocol begins with a starting dose of 5 μg/kg/min, increasing at 3 minutes to 10 μg/kg/min, and then increasing at 3-minute intervals to 20, 30, and 40 μg/kg/min. Atropine is administered at a starting dose of 0.25 to 0.5 mg and repeated as needed to a total dose of 2 mg. The target heart rate is an achievement of 85% of the age-predicted maximum heart rate [4].

The accuracy of stress echocardiography in demonstrating angiographic CAD has been shown to be equivalent to other stress imaging techniques [5–7]. A normal stress echocardiogram is characterized by the absence of wall motion abnormalities at rest and with stress. Fixed abnormalities are wall motion abnormalities present at rest, which are unchanged with stress, and are considered to present regions of infarction. Ischemia is characterized by new or worsening wall motion abnormalities with stress.

The prognostic value of stress echocardiography for identifying patients at risk of death and cardiac events has also been demonstrated at various centers in thousands of patients [8–10]. Stress echocardiography has been shown to be prognostically useful in both men and women [10], the elderly [11], patients with diabetes mellitus [12], and after coronary revascularization [13,14]. A normal study identifies a patient with an excellent prognosis [15]. In addition to baseline LV systolic function, variables associated with poor outcomes include extensive ischemia (characterized by a decrease in ejection fraction with stress), an increase in end-systolic volume with stress [16], wall motion abnormalities in a multivessel distribution, or a low heart rate, at which ischemia develops [17].

Stress echocardiography also permits accurate assessment of myocardial viability. Viable myocardium is that which is hypokinetic or akinetic at rest, but augments its contractility with a low level of exercise or low dose of dobutamine. In an area subtended by a severely stenosed vessel (*ie*, hibernating myocardium), reworsening of function occurs with continued infusion of higher doses of dobutamine [18].

Stress echocardiography has been shown to be versatile and cost effective [19]. Compared with other forms of stress imaging, it can generally be performed at a lower cost. Also compared with other forms, there is no radiation involved, and the safety of the test is well established. The versatility of stress echocardiography is well recognized. In addition to its recognition of CAD, the test provides a screening assessment of valves, chamber sizes, and wall thicknesses. Other causes of chest pain, including pericarditis, aortic dissection, and valvular heart disease, can be readily recognized [2]. Future developments in stress echocardiography will include quantitative assessment [20]. Myocardial contract perfusion imaging appears promising as a means of assessing perfusion and wall motion simultaneously [21].

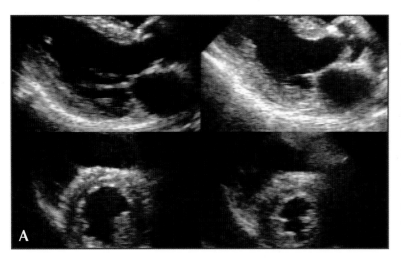

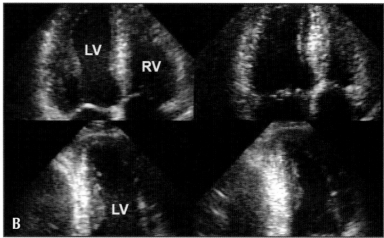

Figure 6-1. Normal exercise echocardiograms are presented. The patient exercised maximally on a treadmill (according to the Bruce protocol) to the development of fatigue [2]. Parasternal (**A**) and apical (**B**) views show the normal response to exercise stress. Rest images (**A** and **B**, *left panels*) and postexercise images (**A** and **B**, *right panels*) are shown. There was a decrease in end-systolic volume and an increase in ejection fraction. Contractility of all wall segments increased appropriately. Wall thicknesses and chamber sizes were normal. The aortic valve was mildly thickened. The exercise echocardiogram was otherwise normal. The event rate after a normal exercise echocardiogram is less than 1% per year [15].

Normal and Ischemic Responses for Various Modalities of Stress

| Stress Method | Regional | | Global | |
	Normal Response	Ischemic Response	Normal Response	Ischemic Response
Treadmill	Postexercise ↑ in function compared with rest	Postexercise ↓ in function compared with rest	↓ in ESV; ↑ in EF	↑ in ESV; ↓ in EF in multivessel or left main disease
Supine bicycle	Peak exercise ↑ in function compared with rest	Peak exercise ↓ in function compared with rest	↓ in ESV; ↑ in EF	↑ in ESV; ↓ in EF in multivessel or left main disease
Dobutamine	↑ in function, velocity of contraction compared with rest and usually to low dose	↓ in function; velocity of contraction compared with low dose; may be less compared with rest	Greater ↓ in ESV; marked ↑ in EF	Often same as normal response. Ischemia infrequently produces ↓ EF; cavity dilatation rarely occurs
Vasodilator	↑ in function compared with rest	↓ in function compared with rest	↓ in ESV; ↑ in EF	Often same as normal response. Occasionally, ischemia produces ↓ EF; cavity dilatation rarely occurs
Atrial pacing	No change or ↑ in function compared with rest	↓ in function compared with rest	↓ in ESV; no change in EF	No change or ↑ ESV, ↓ in EF

Figure 6-2. The normal and ischemic responses for various modalities of stress echocardiography are listed, including treadmill and supine bicycle exercise, dobutamine, and vasodilator stress and atrial pacing stress. (*From* Pellikka *et al.* [1]; with permission.) EF—ejection fraction; ESV—end-systolic volume.

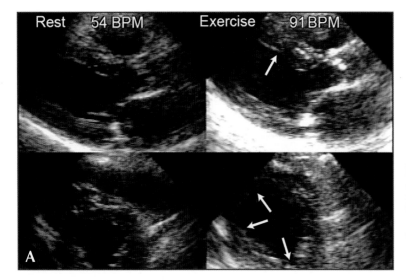

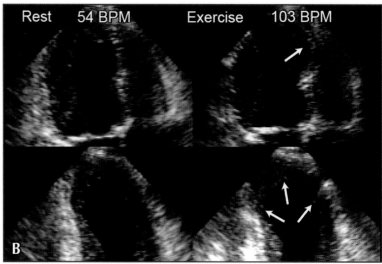

Figure 6-3. Marked ischemia with exercise in a patient with a normal exercise electrocardiogram. In this patient who presented with exertional dyspnea, LV systolic function appeared normal at rest, but there was marked worsening of function with exercise. This is shown in both the parasternal (**A**) and apical (**B**) views. Heart rate response to exercise was attenuated because of β–blocker therapy for hypertension. Regions of akinesis or dyskinesis (*arrows*) are shown in all four views and are manifested in end-systolic images as bulging. This patient had multivessel coronary artery disease. This illustrates the incremental value of exercise echocardiography. The test provides information beyond that available from clinical, rest echocardiographic, or exercise electrocardiogram predictors of prognosis [10].

Summary of Studies Evaluating the Value of Stress Echocardiography in Predicting Outcome

Author	Patients, *n*	Patient characteristics	Stress type	Mean or median follow-up, *y*	End point	Echocardiographic predictors
Arruda-Olson *et al.* [10]	5798	Known or suspected CAD	Exercise	3.2	Cardiac death/MI	Exercise WMSI
Marwick *et al.* [8]	5375	Known or suspected CAD	Exercise	5.5	All deaths	Extent of resting WMA; extent of ischemia
Biagini *et al.* [9]	3381	Known or suspected CAD	Dobutamine	7	Cardiac death/MI	Resting WMA; ischemia
Marwick *et al.* [22]	3156	Known or suspected CAD	Dobutamine	3.8	Cardiac death	Resting WMA; ischemia
Chuah *et al.* [16]	860	Known or suspected CAD	Dobutamine	2	Cardiac death/MI	Stress WMA; end-systolic volume response
Shaw *et al.* [23]	11132	Known or suspected CAD	Exercise or dobutamine	5	Cardiac death	Extent of resting WMA; extent of ischemia
Sicari *et al.* [24]	7333	Known or suspected CAD	Dipyridamole or dobutamine	2.6	Cardiac death/MI	Resting EF; change in WMSI
Tsutusi *et al.* [25]	788	Known or suspected CAD	Dobutamine myocardial contrast perfusion	1.7	Death/MI	Contrast perfusion defects
Bergeron *et al.* [26]	3260	Chest pain or dyspnea	Exercise	3.1	Mortality/morbidity	Change in WMSI
Elhendy *et al.* [12]	563	Diabetes	Exercise	3	Cardiac death/MI	EF; extent of ischemia
Sozzi *et al.* [27]	396	Diabetes	Dobutamine	3	Cardiac death/MI	EF; extent of ischemia
Marwick *et al.* [28]	937	Diabetes	Exercise or dobutamine	3.9	All deaths	Extent of resting WMA; extent of ischemia
Chaowalit *et al.* [29]	2349	Diabetes	Dobutamine	5.4	Mortality/morbidity; (MI, late coronary revascularization)	Extent of ischemia and failure to reach target heart rate
Arruda *et al.* [11]	2632	Elderly (≥ 65 y)	Exercise	2.9	Cardiac death/MI	Changes of EF and end-systolic volume
Biagini [30]	1434	Elderly (> 65 y)	Dobutamine	6.5	Cardiac death/MI	Resting WMA; ischemia
Carlos *et al.* [31]	214	Acute MI	Dobutamine	1.4	Cardiac death, MI, arrhythmias, heart failure	Resting WMSI; remote abnormalities
Elhendy *et al.* [32]	528	Heart failure	Dobutamine	3.2	Cardiac death	Resting EF; ischemia
Elhendy *et al.* [33]	483	LVH by echo criteria	Exercise	3	Cardiac death/MI	Resting WMSI; EF response
Arruda *et al.* [34]	718	Previous CABG	Exercise	2.9	Cardiac death/MI	Changes of EF and end-systolic volume
Bountioukos *et al.* [14]	331	Previous CABG or PCI	Dobutamine	2	Cardiac death/MI/late revascularization	Ischemia
Biagini *et al.* [35]	136	Pacemaker recipients	Pacing	3.5	Cardiac death	Ischemia
Das *et al.* [17]	530	Before nonvascular surgery	Dobutamine	Hospital stay	Cardiac death/MI	Ischemic threshold
Poldermans *et al.* [36]	360	Before vascular surgery	Dobutamine	1.6	Perioperative and late	Ischemia
Sicari *et al.* [37]	509	Before vascular surgery	Dipyridamole	Hospital stay	Death, MI, unstable angina	Ischemia

CAD—coronary artery disease; CABG—coronary artery bypass grafting; EF—ejection fraction; LVH—LV hypertrophy; MI—myocardial infarction; PCI—percutaneous intervention; WMA—wall motion abnormalities; WMSI—wall motion score index.

Figure 6-4. Studies evaluating the value of stress echocardiography in predicting outcome are summarized. Extensive data for multiple institutions show the prognostic value of various types of stress echocardiography in thousands of patients. Larger studies are included. Stress echocardiography results were predictive of cardiac death, myocardial infarction, and all-cause mortality. Echocardiographic predictors of events included not only rest wall motion abnormalities and the presence of ischemia, but stress wall motion score index, the change in wall motion score index, and stress-induced changes in ejection fraction and end-systolic volume, which are indicators of the extent and severity of ischemia [22—37]. (*From* Pellikka *et al.* [1]; with permission.)

Stress Echocardiography Predictors of Risk

Very Low-Risk* MI (Cardiac Events < 1% Per Year)	Low-Risk* MI (Cardiac Death < 2% Per Year)	Factors Increasing Risk[†]	High-Risk[‡] MI (RR ≥ 4-Fold Over Low Risk)
Normal exercise echocardiogram with good exercise capacity 7 MET men 5 MET women	Normal pharmacologic stress exhocardiogram with adequate stress, defined as achievement of HR ≥ 85% age-predicted maximum for dobutamine stress, and low to intermediate pretest probability of CAD	Increasing age	Extensive rest WMA (4–5 segments of LV)
		Male gender	Baseline EF < 40%
		Diabetes	Extensive ischemia (4–5 segments of LV)
		High pretest probability	Multivessel ischemia
		History of dyspnea or CHF	Rest WMA and remove ischemia
		History of myocardial infarction	Low ischemic threshold
		Limited exercise capacity	Ischemia with 0.56 μg/kg/min dipyridamole or 20 μg/kg/min dobutamine or based on heart rate[¶]
		Inability to exercise	Ischemic WMA, no change or decrease in exercise
		Stress electrocardiogram with ischemia	
		Rest WMA	
		LV hypertrophy	
		Stress echocardiography with ischemia	
		Reduced baseline EF	
		No change or increase ESV with stress[§]	
		No change or decrease EF with stress[§]	
		Increasing wall motion score with stress	

*High pretest probability of CAD, poor exercise capacity, or low rate pressure product, increased age, angina during stress, LV hypertrophy, history of infarction, history of CHF, and anti-ischemic therapy are factors known to increase risk in patients with normal stress echocardiograms.

[†]Cutoff values for high-risk group are approximate values derived from available studies. Studies have shown that increased rest and low and peak dose wall motion scores can identify high-risk subjects, especially those with reduced global LV function; however, threshold values used to define high-risk patients have been variable (eg, peak exercise scores range from 1.4 to > 1.7).

[‡]The degree to which each factor increases risk is variable.

[§]For treadmill and dobutamine stress.

[¶]Low ischemic threshold, based on HR for dobutamine stress, has been defined in various studies as ischemia with HR less than 60% of age-predicted max, less than 70% of age-predicted max, or at heart rate of less than 120/min.

CAD—coronary artery disease; CHD—congestive heart disease; EF—ejection fraction; ESV—end-systolic volume; HR—heart rate; MET—metabolic equivalent; MI—myocardial infarction; RR—relative risk; WMA—wall motion abnormalities.

Figure 6-5. Stress echocardiographic predictors of risk of cardiac events during follow-up are shown. These are divided into characteristics that describe a very low-risk population, factors associated with low and increasing risk, and factors associated with high risk of cardiac events during follow-up. Although a normal exercise echocardiogram in a patient with a good exercise capacity predicts an excellent outcome, inability to exercise, failure to achieve target heart rate, reduced ejection fraction, ischemia occurring at a low heart rate (ischemic threshold), and extensive ischemia (characterized by a multivessel pattern of wall motion abnormalities, worsening of systolic function of many segments, and abnormal responses of ejection fraction and end-systolic volume to stress), characterizes the patient at increased risk. Clinical parameters, including increasing age, diabetes mellitus, male sex, and a history of heart failure or myocardial infarction are also associated with increased risk. (*From* Pellikka *et al.* [1]; with permission.)

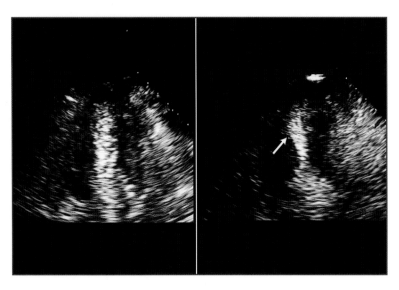

Figure 6-6. Apical ischemia in the setting of mild dynamic intracavitary obstruction with exercise is shown. In this patient, the LV cavity size was somewhat small, and LV systolic function was vigorous. Contrast was used for endocardial border detection because two or more segments could not be adequately visualized at rest. With exercise, there was hypokinesis of a small region of the apex, as best seen in the apical long-axis view (*arrow, right panel*). Doppler revealed a dynamic late peaking intracavitary velocity profile, which peaked at 3 m/s. This corresponds to a maximum instantaneous pressure of 36 mm Hg. This contributed to the development of apical ischemia. Dynamic obstruction with exercise has also been observed in patients with hypertrophic cardiomyopathy and may contribute to wall motion abnormalities in the absence of coronary artery disease [38].

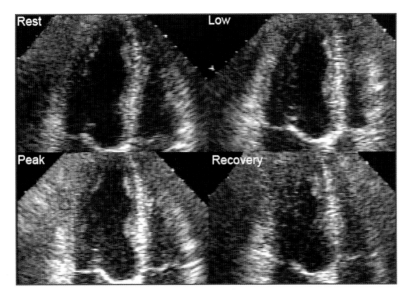

Figure 6-7. Supine bicycle exercise echocardiography is shown. This examination provides the opportunity to perform stress imaging during peak exercise rather than in recovery. Images obtained at peak exercise may reveal ischemia that is not appreciated in recovery. This was the case in the example shown. Quad screen images show the apical four-chamber view with the LV on each panel (*left-hand side*). Images displayed are from rest (*upper left*), low-level exercise (*upper right*), peak exercise (*lower left*), and recovery (*lower right*). With exercise in this patient, there was mild global hypokinesis, with two-vessel coronary artery disease. By the time of early recovery images, ischemic wall motion abnormalities had recovered. Although workload, heart rate, and double product are higher with treadmill exercise, blood pressure is higher with supine bicycle exercise [39]. Bicycle exercise is advantageous if additional Doppler information (*ie*, assessment of mitral regurgitation, tricuspid regurgitation velocity, valve gradients) is desired during exercise.

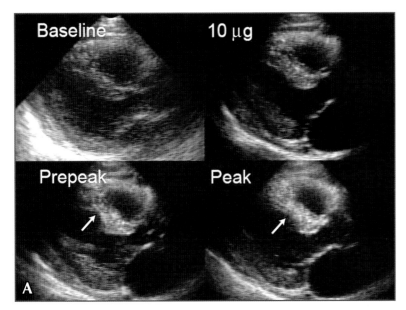

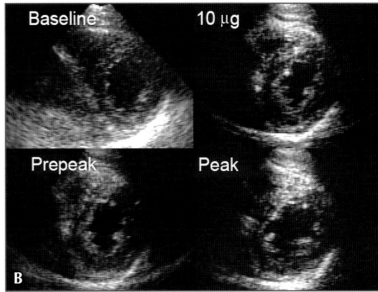

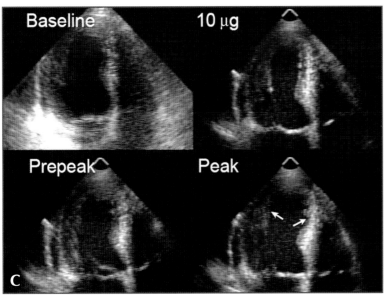

Figure 6-8. Dobutamine stress echocardiography for preoperative risk stratification is shown. Beginning with an intermediate dose of dobutamine, there was ischemia involving the mid to distal septum (*arrows*), as seen in the parasternal long-axis view (**A**). In the short-axis view, ischemia was represented by a slight increase in end-systolic volume and deformity in the LV contour (**B**). In the apical four-chamber view, there is significant ischemia involving the apex (**C**, *arrows*). Pharmacologic stress echocardiogram has been shown to be very useful for cardiac risk stratification before vascular [27,28] and nonvascular [36,37] surgery. Ischemia occurring at a low heart rate identifies patients at the highest risk of perioperative cardiac events.

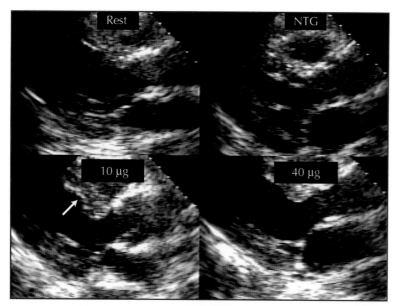

Figure 6-9. A demonstration of viability by dobutamine stress echocardiography is shown. Parasternal long-axis images in this patient showed baseline hypokinesis with an ejection fraction of 40%. The patient had a recent anterior wall myocardial infarction. A dobutamine viability study showed augmentation of contractility with nitroglycerin. Beginning at the 10 μg/kg/min dose of dobutamine, there was reworsening of function of the anteroseptum (*arrow*). At the peak dose, there was near global worsening. The patient was found to have severe three-vessel coronary artery disease and underwent revascularization. At 2 months postoperatively, his LV systolic function had almost completely recovered.

Dobutamine augments myocardial blood flow. Thus, regions of hibernating myocardium (*ie*, regions that are severely hypokinetic or akinetic because of markedly compromised blood supply) will augment contractility with low doses of dobutamine [18]. A similar response occurs with an administration of nitroglycerin [40]. With higher doses of dobutamine, heart rate increases and ischemia supervenes, resulting in reworsening of function in areas subtended by a stenotic coronary artery.

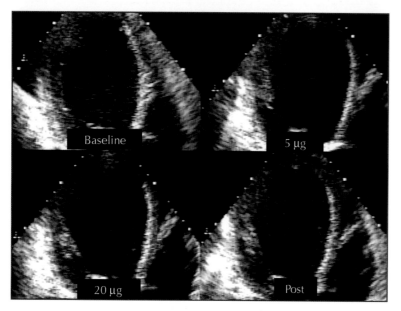

Figure 6-10. Dobutamine stress echocardiography in end-stage ischemic cardiomyopathy. In this case, the apical four-chamber view shows severe LV hypokinesis associated with wall thinning. There was no augmentation of contractility with increasing doses of dobutamine; thus, no significant viability was present in this patient.

Use of Dobutamine Stress Echocardiography in Low-Output, Low-Gradient Aortic Stenosis

	Baseline	Stress
LVOT velocity, *m/s*	0.6	1
LVOT TVI, *cm*	12	17
Aortic valve velocity, *m/s*	3	4.6
Aortic valve TVI, *cm*	55	78
Aortic valve area, *cm²*	0.9	0.9

Figure 6-11. This patient had cardiomyopathy, ejection fraction of 30%, and calcific aortic stenosis. With a total of 20 μg/kg/min of dobutamine, there was an increase in LV outflow tract (LVOT) velocity and time velocity interval (TVI) with a corresponding increase in velocity and TVI across the aortic valve. The aortic valve area was recalculated using both sets of values and was measured both times at 0.9 cm². This was consistent with severe aortic stenosis. This patient would be expected to benefit from aortic valve surgery [41].

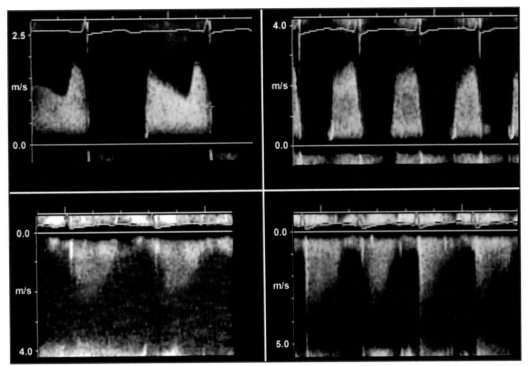

Figure 6-12. Exercise Doppler hemodynamics in a patient with mitral stenosis shows a resting mean gradient across the mitral valve of 9 mm Hg (*upper left*), which increased to 32 mm Hg with exercise (*upper right*). Tricuspid regurgitant velocity increased from 2.5 (*lower left*) to 3.7 m/s (*lower right*). The patient was symptomatic, and her symptoms were relieved with mitral balloon valvuloplasty. In sedentary patients with exertional dyspnea, an exertional increase in mean mitral valve gradient to more than 15 mm Hg and pulmonary artery systolic pressure to more than 60 mm Hg identifies those who may benefit from percutaneous valvuloplasty if there is little or no mitral regurgitation and valve anatomy is appropriate [42,43].

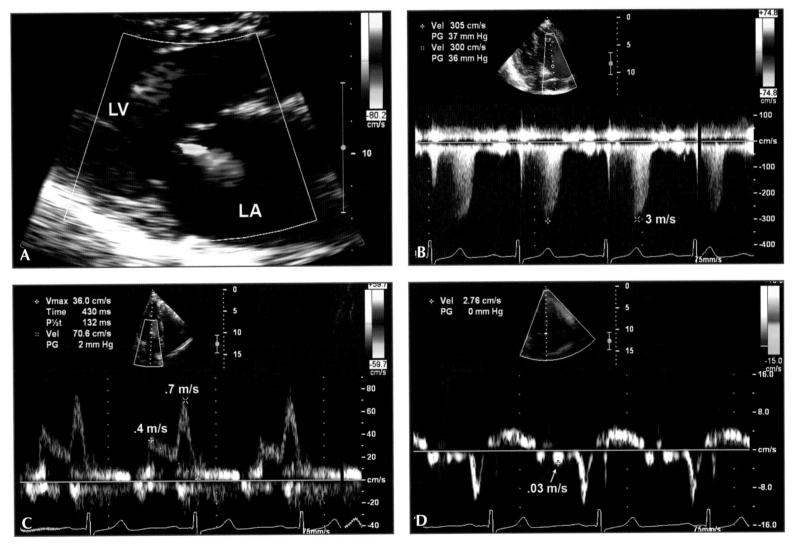

Figure 6-13. Demonstration of diastolic dysfunction and pulmonary hypertension in a patient presenting with dyspnea is shown. In this patient, stress echocardiographic images were negative for ischemia. The screening echocardiographic images performed prior to the stress test showed left atrial (LA) enlargement and mild mitral regurgitation (**A**), as well as pulmonary hypertension with a tricuspid regurgitant velocity of 3 m/s (**B**) and grade 1 diastolic dysfunction, as demonstrated by the mitral inflow pattern (**C**) and tissue Doppler assessment of the mitral annulus (**D**). E' velocity was reduced at .03 m/s (*arrow*). Diastolic dysfunction and mild pulmonary hypertension likely contributed to this patient's symptoms. A limited screening examination is recommended at the time of stress echocardiography unless other imaging has already been performed.

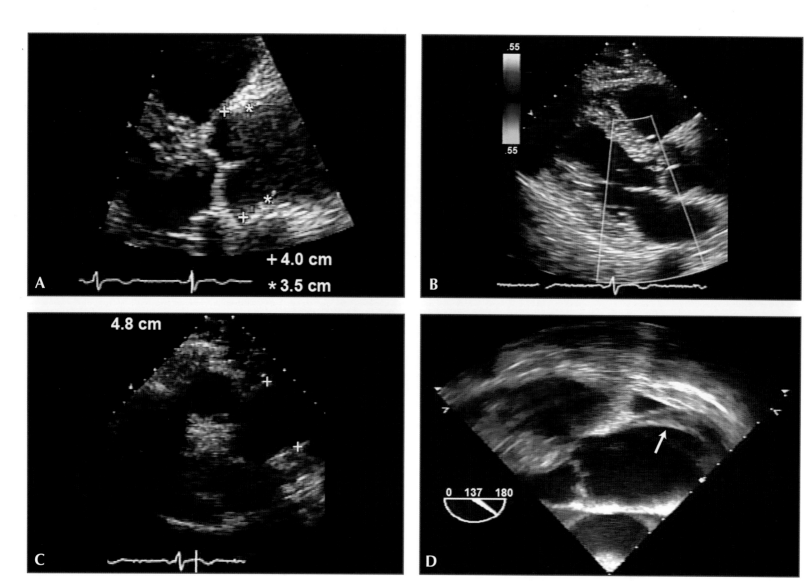

Figure 6-14. Patient with atypical chest pain referred for exercise echocardiography is shown. A parasternal long-axis view obtained at the screening examination prior to the beginning of exercise showed a mildly dilated aortic root (**A**), which measured 4.0 cm at the sinus of Valsalva and 3.5 cm at the sinotubular junction. There was trivial aortic regurgitation (**B**), and the proximal aorta measured 4.8 cm in diameter as indicated (**C,** *markers*). Instead of performing exercise testing, transesophageal echocardiography was performed and revealed an aortic dissection, with the image depicting the dissection flap (*arrow*) as the etiology of this patient's chest pain (**D**). This illustrates the versatility of stress echocardiography.

References

1. Pellikka PA, Nagueh SF, Elhendy AA, *et al.*: American Society of Echocardiography recommendations for performance, interpretation, and application of stress echocardiography. *J Am Soc Echocardiogr* 2007, 20:1021–1041.

2. Roger VL, Pellikka P, Oh JK, *et al.*: Stress echocardiography. Part I. Exercise echocardiography: techniques, implementation, clinical applications, and correlations. *Mayo Clin Proc* 1995, 70:5–15.

3. Modesto K, Rainbird A, Klarich K, *et al.*: Comparison of supine bicycle exercise and treadmill exercise Doppler echocardiography in evaluation of patients with coronary artery disease. *Am J Cardiol* 2003, 91:1245–1248.

4. Pellikka P, Roger VL, Oh JK, *et al.*: Stress echocardiography. Part II. Dobutamine stress echocardiography: techniques, implementation, clinical applications, and correlations. *Mayo Clin Proc* 1995, 70:16–27.

5. Quinones M, Verani M, Haichin R, *et al.*: Exercise echocardiography versus 201Tl single-photon emission computed tomography in evaluation of coronary artery disease. Analysis of 292 patients. *Circulation* 1992, 85:1217–1218.

6. Fleischmann KE, Hunink MG, Kuntz KM, Douglas PS: Exercise echocardiography or exercise SPECT imaging? A meta-analysis of diagnostic test performance. *JAMA* 1998, 280:913–920.

7. Schinkel AF, Bax JJ, Geleijnse ML, *et al.*: Noninvasive evaluation of ischaemic heart disease: myocardial perfusion imaging or stress echocardiography? *Eur Heart J* 2003, 24:789–800.

8. Marwick TH, Case C, Vasey C, *et al.*: Prediction of mortality by exercise echocardiography: a strategy for combination with the Duke treadmill score. *Circulation* 2001, 103:2566–2571.

9. Biagini E, Elhendy A, Bax JJ, *et al.*: Seven-year follow-up after dobutamine stress echocardiography: impact of gender on prognosis. *J Am Coll Cardiol* 2005, 45:93–97.

10. Arruda-Olson AM, Juracan EM, Mahoney DW, *et al.*: Prognostic value of exercise echocardiography in 5,798 patients: is there a gender difference? *J Am Coll Cardiol* 2002;39:625-631.

11. Arruda AM, Das MK, Roger VL, *et al.*: Prognostic value of exercise echocardiography in 2,632 patients > or = 65 years of age. *J Am Coll Cardiol* 2001, 1036–1041.

12. Elhendy A, Arruda AM, Mahoney DW, Pellikka PA: Prognostic stratification of diabetic patients by exercise echocardiography. *J Am Coll Cardiol* 2001, 37:1551–1557.

13. Arruda AM, McCully RB, Oh JK, *et al.*: Prognostic value of exercise echocardiography in patients after coronary artery bypass surgery. *Am J Cardiol* 2001, 87:1069–1073.

14. Bountioukos M, Elhendy A, van Domburg RT, *et al.*: Prognostic value of dobutamine stress echocardiography in patients with previous coronary revascularization. *Heart* 2004, 90:1031–1035.

15. McCully RB, Roger VL, Mahoney DW, *et al.*: Outcome after normal exercise echocardiography and predictors of subsequent cardiac events: follow-up of 1,325 patients. *J Am Coll Cardiol* 1998, 31:144–149.

16. Chuah SC, Pellikka PA, Roger VL, *et al.*: Role of dobutamine stress echocardiography in predicting outcome in 860 patients with known or suspected coronary artery disease. *Circulation* 1998, 97:1474–1480.

17. Das MK, Pellikka PA, Mahoney DW, *et al.*: Assessment of cardiac risk before nonvascular surgery: dobutamine stress echocardiography in 530 patients. *J Am Coll Cardiol* 2000, 35:1647–1653.

18. Nagueh SF, Mikati I, Weilbaecher D, *et al.*: Relation of the contractile reserve of hibernating myocardium to myocardial structure in humans. *Circulation* 1999, 100:490–496.

19. Shaw LJ, Marwick TH, Berman DS, *et al.*: Incremental cost-effectiveness of exercise echocardiography vs. SPECT imaging for evaluation of stable chest pain. *Eur Heart J* 2006, 27:2448–2458.

20. Voigt JU, Nixdorff U, Bogdan R, *et al.*: Comparison of deformation imaging and velocity imaging for detecting regional inducible ischaemia during dobutamine stress echocardiography. *Eur Heart J* 2004, 25:1517–1525.

21. Elhendy A, O'Leary EL, Xie F, *et al.*: Comparative accuracy of real-time myocardial contrast perfusion imaging and wall motion analysis during dobutamine stress echocardiography for the diagnosis of coronary artery disease. *J Am Coll Cardiol* 2004, 44:2185–2191.

22. deFilippi CR, Willett DL, Brickner ME, *et al.*: Usefulness of dobutamine echocardiography in distinguishing severe from nonsevere valvular aortic stenosis in patients with depressed left ventricular function and low transvalvular gradients. *Am J Cardiol* 1995, 75:191–194.

23. Aviles RJ, Nishimura RA, Pellikka PA, *et al.*: Utility of stress Doppler echocardiography in patients undergoing percutaneous mitral balloon valve valvotomy. *J Am Soc Echocardiogr* 2001, 14:676–681.

24. Bonow R, Carabello B, Chatterjee K, *et al.*: ACC/AHA 2006 guidelines for the management of patients with valvular heart disease: a report of the American College of Cardiology/American Heart Association Task Force on Practice Guidelines (Writing Committee to Revise the 1998 Guidelines for the Management of Patients with Valvular Heart Disease) developed in collaboration with the Society of Cardiovascular Anesthesiologist endorsed by the Society for Cardiovascular Angiography and Interventions and the Society of Thoracic Surgeons. *J Am Coll Cardiol* 2006, 48:e1–e148. [Published erratum appears in *J Am Coll Cardiol* 2007, 49:1014.]

25. Bunch TJ, Chandrasekaran K, Ehrsam JE, *et al.*: Prognostic significance of exercise induced arrhythmias and echocardiographic variables in hypertrophic cardiomyopathy. *Am J Cardiol* 2007, 99:835–838.

26. Modesto KM, Rainbird A, Klarich KW, *et al.*: Comparison of supine bicycle exercise and treadmill exercise Doppler echocardiography in evaluation of patients with coronary artery disease. *Am J Cardiol* 2003, 91:1245–1248.

27. Sicari R, Ripoli A, Picano E, *et al.*: Perioperative prognostic value of dipyridamole echocardiogram in vascular surgery: a large-scale multicenter study in 509 patients. EPIC (Echo Persantine International Cooperative) study group. *Circulation* 1999, 100:269–274.

28. Poldermans D, Fioretti PM, Forster T, *et al.*: Dobutamine stress echocardiogram for assessment of perioperative cardiac risk in patients undergoing major vascular surgery. *Circulation* 1993, 87:1506–1512.

29. Ling LH, Christian TF, Mulvagh SL, *et al.*: Determining myocardial viability in chronic ischemic left ventricular dysfunction: a prospective comparison of rest-redistribution thallium 201 single-photon emission computed tomography, nitroglycerin-dobutamine echocardiography, and intracoronary myocardial contrast echocardiography. *Am Heart J* 2006, 151:882–889.

22. Marwick TH, Case C, Sawada S: Prediction of mortality using dobutamine echocardiography. *J Am Coll Cardiol* 2001, 37:754–760.

23. Shaw LJ, Vasey C, Sawada S, et al.: Impact of gender on risk stratification by exercise and dobutamine stress echocardiography: long-term mortality in 4234 women and 6898 men. *Eur Heart J* 2005, 26:447–456.

24. Sicari R, Pasanisi E, Venneri L, et al.: Stress echo results predict mortality: a large-scale multicenter prospective international study. *J Am Coll Cardiol* 2003, 41:589–595.

25. Tsutsui JM, Elhendy A, Anderson JR, et al.: Prognostic value of dobutamine stress myocardial contrast perfusion echocardiography. *Circulation* 2005, 112:1444–1450.

26. Bergeron S, Ommen SR, Bailey KR, et al.: Exercise echocardiographic findings and outcome of patients referred for evaluation of dyspnea. *J Am Coll Cardiol* 2004, 43:2242–2246.

27. Sozzi FB, Elhendy A, Roelandt JR: Prognostic value of dobutamine stress echocardiography in patients with diabetes. *Diabetes Care* 2003, 26:1074–1078.

28. Marwick TH, Case C, Sawada S, et al.: Use of stress echocardiography to predict mortality in patients with diabetes and known or suspected coronary artery disease. *Diabetes Care* 2002, 25:1042–1048.

29. Chaowalit N, Arruda A, McCully R, et al.: Dobutamine stress echocardiography in patients with diabetes mellitus: enhanced prognostic prediction using a simple risk score. *J Am Coll Cardiol* 2006, 47:1029–1036.

30. Biagini E, Elhendy A, Schinkel AF, et al.: Long-term prediction of mortality in elderly persons by dobutamine stress echocardiography. *J Gerontol A Biol Sci Med Sci* 2005, 60:1333–1338.

31. Carlos ME, Smart SC, Wynsen JC, Sagar KB: Dobutamine stress echocardiography for risk stratification after myocardial infarction. *Circulation* 1997, 95:1402–1410.

32. Elhendy A, Sozzi F, van Domburg RT, et al.: Effect of myocardial ischemia during dobutamine stress echocardiography on cardiac mortality in patients with heart failure secondary to ischemic cardiomyopathy. *Am J Cardiol* 2005, 96:469–473.

33. Elhendy A, Modesto K, Mahoney D, et al.: Prediction of mortality in patients with left ventricular hypertrophy by clinical, exercise stress, and echocardiographic data. *J Am Coll Cardiol* 2003, 41:129–135.

34. Arruda AM, McCully RB, Oh JK, et al.: Prognostic value of exercise echocardiography in patients after coronary artery bypass surgery. *Am J Cardiol* 2001, 87:1069–1073.

35. Biagini E, Schinkel AF, Elhendy A, et al.: Pacemaker stress echocardiography predicts cardiac events in patients with permanent pacemaker. *Am J Med* 2005, 118:1381–1386.

36. Poldermans D, Arnese M, Fioretti PM, et al.: Sustained prognostic value of dobutamine stress echocardiography for late cardiac events after major noncardiac vascular surgery. *Circulation* 1997, 95:53–58.

37. Sicari R, Ripoli A, Picano E, et al.: Perioperative prognostic value of dipyridamole echocardiography in vascular surgery: a large-scale multicenter study in 509 patients. EPIC (Echo Persantine international cooperative) Study Group. *Circulation* 1999, 100(19 Suppl):II269–II274.

38. Bunch TJ, Chandrasekaran K, Ehrsam JE, et al.: Prognostic significance of exercise induced arrhythmias and echocardiographic variables in hypertrophic cardiomyopathy. *Am J Cardiol* 2007, 99:835–838.

39. Modesto KM, Rainbird A, Klarich KW, et al.: Comparison of supine bicycle exercise and treadmill exercise Doppler echocardiography in evaluation of patients with coronary artery disease. *Am J Cardiol* 2003, 91:1245–1248.

40. Ling LH, Christian TF, Mulvagh SL, et al.: Determining myocardial viability in chronic ischemic left ventricular dysfunction: a prospective comparison of rest-redistribution thallium 201 single-photon emission computed tomography, nitroglycerin-dobutamine echocardiography, and intracoronary myocardial contrast echocardiography. *Am Heart J* 2006, 151:882–889.

41. deFilippi CR, Willett DL, Brickner ME, et al.: Usefulness of dobutamine echocardiography in distinguishing severe from nonsevere valvular aortic stenosis in patients with depressed left ventricular function and low transvalvular gradients. Am J Cardiol 1995, 75:191–194.

42. Aviles RJ, Nishimura RA, Pellikka PA, et al.: Utility of stress Doppler echocardiography in patients undergoing percutaneous mitral balloon valve valvotomy. J Am Soc Echocardiogr 2001, 14:676–681.

43. Bonow R, Carabello B, Chatterjee K, et al.: ACC/AHA 2006 guidelines for the management of patients with valvular heart disease: a report of the American College of Cardiology/American Heart Association Task Force on Practice Guidelines (Writing Committee to Revise the 1998 Guidelines for the Management of Patients with Valvular Heart Disease) developed in collaboration with the Society of Cardiovascular Anesthesiologist endorsed by the Society for Cardiovascular Angiography and Interventions and the Society of Thoracic Surgeons. J Am Coll Cardiol 2006, 48: e1–e148. [Published erratum appears in J Am Coll Cardiol 2007, 49:1014.]

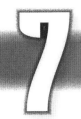

7

Transesophageal Echocardiography

Amil M. Shah, Bernard E. Bulwer, and Scott D. Solomon

Transesophageal echocardiography (TEE) has become an important adjunct to the transthoracic echocardiography (TTE) examination since its introduction in the late 1980s. TEE utilizes an electronically steered high-frequency ultrasound transducer (5–7 MHz) mounted on an endoscope. The higher resolution, coupled with anatomic proximity of the transducer to the posterior cardiac structures, delivers superior image quality when compared with TTE, particularly of posterior cardiac structures.

TEE has become the definitive diagnostic cardiac imaging modality for the evaluation of patients with suspected endocarditis and intracardiac thrombus. It is also central to the evaluation of cardiac source of embolus in patients with cryptogenic stroke, valvular dysfunction, and acute aortic syndromes. This chapter introduces the indications, patient preparation, standard TEE views, and examples of TEE's use in selected patients. The chapter concludes with a primer on comparative two-dimensional and real time three-dimensional TEE.

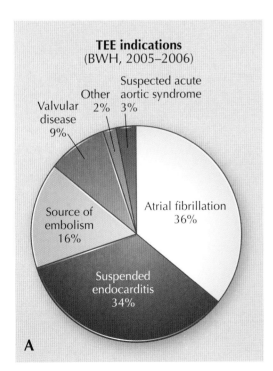

TEE indications
(BWH, 2005–2006)

- Suspected acute aortic syndrome 3%
- Other 2%
- Valvular disease 9%
- Source of embolism 16%
- Atrial fibrillation 36%
- Suspended endocarditis 34%

A

B ACCF/ASE/ACEP/ASNC/SCAI/SCCT/SCMR 2007 Appropriateness Criteria For TEE as an Initial Study

Possibly appropriate as initial test

Evaluation of suspected acute aortic pathology including dissection/transection

Guidance for percutaneous noncoronary cardiac interventions including, but not limited to, septal ablation in patients with hypertrophic cardiomyopathy, mitral valvuloplasty, PFO/ASD closure, radiofrequency ablation

To determine mechanism of regurgitation and determine suitability of valve repair

To diagnose/manage endocarditis with a moderate or high pretest probability (*eg*, bacteremia, especially *Staphylococcus aureus* bacteremia or fungemia)

Persistent fever in patient with intracardiac device

Evaluation of patients with atrial fibrillation/flutter to facilitate clinical decision making with regards to anticoagulation and/or cardioversion and/or radiofrequency ablation

Inappropriate as initial test

Evaluation of patients with atrial fibrillation/flutter for left atrial thrombus or spontaneous contrast when a decision has been made to anticoagulate and not to perform cardioversion

Appropriateness unknown

Evaluation of cardiovascular source of embolic event in a patient who has had a normal TTE and normal ECG and no history of atrial fibrillation/flutter

Figure 7-1. A, Indications for transesophageal echocardiography (TEE) examinations performed in a university hospital setting during the past year. Atrial fibrillation, suspected endocarditis, cardiac source of embolism, and valvular disease are the most common indications for TEE. TEE is also particularly useful in the assessment of acute aortic syndromes, interatrial shunts, and cardiac masses. **B**, The American Society of Echocardiography, in conjunction with the American College of Cardiology, recently published appropriateness guidelines for the use of transthoracic echocardiography (TTE) and TEE [1]. The TEE examination was assumed to be appropriate as an adjunct to or following TTE when adequate diagnostic information could not be obtained from the surface study. The writing group published seven indications in which TEE may be appropriate as an initial test. (*Adapted from* Douglas *et al.* [1].) ASD—atrial septal defect; PFO—patent foramen ovale.

Potential Risks and Contraindications to TEE

A. Potential Risks for TEE
   Probe insertion
   Dental trauma
   Oropharyngeal trauma
   Esophageal/gastric bleeding
   Esophageal laceration/perforation
   Vagal reaction
   Conscious Sedation
   Hypoventilation and hypoxia
   Hypotension
   Aspiration
   Topical anesthetic
   Methemoglobinemia (benzocaine)
   Allergic reaction
B. Contraindications to TEE
   Absolute contraindications
   Recent esophageal/gastric trauma or surgery
   Esophageal stricture, diverticulum, or tumor
   Active upper gastrointestinal bleeding
   Relative contraindications
   Recent upper gastrointestinal bleeding
   Dysphagia or odynophagia
   Esophageal varices
   Excessive anticoagulation (INR > 4)
   Poorly cooperative patient

Figure 7-2. Risks and contraindications for transesophageal echocardiography (TEE) (**A**). Although TEE is generally a safe procedure, there are risks associated with both probe insertion and conscious sedation administered to facilitate the examination. In multiple large multicenter registries, the reported incidence of oropharyngeal and esophageal trauma has been low [2,3]. The reported incidence of esophageal perforation is roughly 0.03% [2]. Conscious sedation is administered to facilitate patient tolerance of the examination at most centers. Although this is often invaluable for patient comfort and examination quality, it also introduces the risk associated with conscious sedation. Mortality related to TEE has been reported, but is quite rare. As the TEE probe is blindly introduced into the esophagus, anatomic esophageal abnormalities increase the procedural risks. For this reason, known significant esophageal anatomic abnormalities or trauma are contraindications to TEE (**B**). A preprocedural gastroenterology evaluation is suggested in patients with preexisting dysphagia, odynophagia, or esophageal varices. INR—international normalized ratio.

Transesophageal Echocardiography: Preprocedural Preparation

1. **History**
   Evaluate for contraindications
   Esophageal pathology
   Dysphagia, odynophagia, recent esophageal bleeding
   Evaluate for factors affecting intravenous conscious sedation risk:
   Poor ability to cooperate
   Impaired ability to protect airway
   Sleep apnea
   Systemic illness
   Nothing by mouth for 4–6 h
2. **Examination**
   Evaluate oropharynx for airway patentcy
3. **Consider anesthesia consult for patients at increased risk from conscious sedation**
4. **Informed consent**
5. **Establish peripheral IV with 3-way stopcock**
6. **Topical anesthesia**
   Benzocaine 20% topical spray (Hurricaine*, Topex†)
   For treatment of methemoglobinemia: methylene blue, 1–2 mg/kg IV
   Lidocaine 2% viscous solution or spray
   Cetacaine‡ spray (14% benzocaine, 2% tetracaine, 2% butamben)
7. **Conscious sedation**
   Administered by nurse specifically trained in conscious sedation in concert with a conscious sedation trained physician
   Commonly used agents:
   Sedation: midazolam hydrochloride (versed): 1–6 mg IV
   Reversal: flumazenil: 0.2–0.4 mg IV
   Analgesia: fentanyl: 25–200 µg IV
   Reversal: naloxone: up to 0.1 mg/kg IV

*Beutlich Pharmaceuticals, Waukegan, Il
†Sultan Dental Products Ltd, Englewood, NJ
‡Cetyline Industries Inc., Pennsauken, NJ

Figure 7-3. Transesophageal echocardiography: preprocedural preparation; including history, examination, informed consent, and use of anesthesia. IV—intravenous.

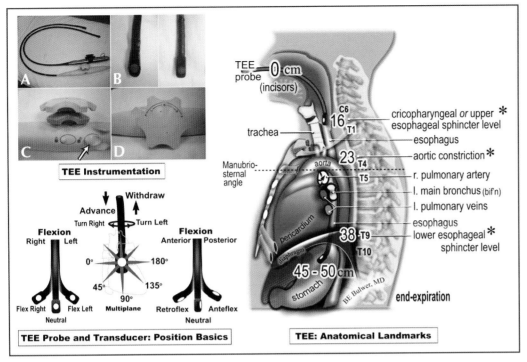

Figure 7-4. Transesophageal echocardiography (TEE) equipment. Instrumentation of TEE. **Upper left, A,** Two models of TEE probes. **B, upper left,** Miniature multiplanar transducer and housing located at the tip of the TEE probe. **C, upper left,** Profile of TEE probe controls. The multiplane (omni) control button is indicated (*arrow*). **D, upper left,** View from the top showing TEE probe control positions as indicated.

Lower left, TEE probe and multiplanar transducer: position basics. Mechanical movements of the transesophageal probe include anterior and posterior flexion and flexion to the right or left. The entire probe can also be manually rotated to the right or to the left. Arrays of piezoelectric crystals permit visualization along multiple planes.

Right, Anatomic relationship between the esophagus and other mediastinal structures. The aortic arch arches over the right pulmonary artery (RPA) and the left main bronchus as it enters the posterior mediastinum. The RPA is located immediately behind the ascending aorta and inferior to the aortic arch. In the superior mediastinum, the air-filled trachea is interposed between the aortic arch and the esophagus. This is the basis of the TEE "blind spot" because air is a poor conductor and major reflector of ultrasound waves. As it descends into the posterior mediastium, the esophagus lies to the right of the aorta, but then moves anteriorly on its way to the stomach.

The Standard Examination

The American Society of Echocardiography, in association with the Society of Cardiovascular Anesthesiologists, has published guidelines of standard recommended views for the transesophageal echocardiography (TEE) examination [4]. Although the focus of any given TEE examination will depend on the indication, the goal of these views is to image each cardiac structure in an efficient and standardized fashion, ideally in multiple tomographic planes. Although these views were initially published as recommendations for intraoperative TEE examinations, they have become the standard for TEEs performed outside the intraoperative setting as well.

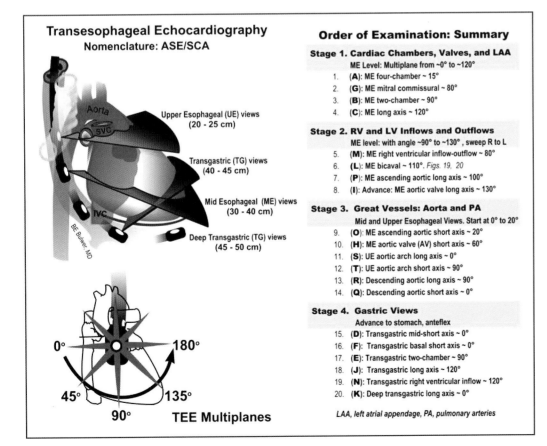

Figure 7-5. Anatomic reference schematic and nomenclature, adopted by the Society of Echocardiography and the Society of Cardiovascular Anesthesiologists. The fundamental parts of the transesophageal echocardiography (TEE) multiplanar examination are represented by a set of 20 cross-sectional imaging planes represented by letters of the alphabet [4].

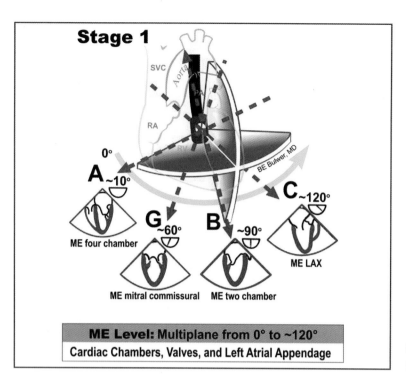

Figure 7-6. Schematic of stage 1 of the transesophageal echocardiography (TEE) examination. LAX—long-axis; ME—midesophageal.

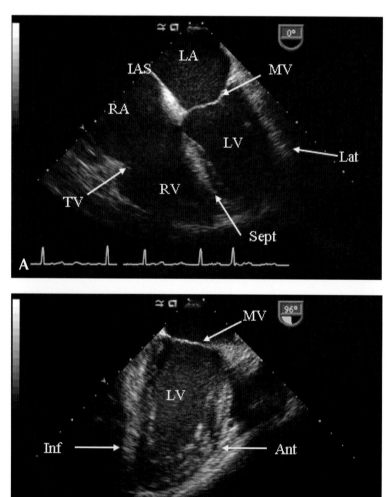

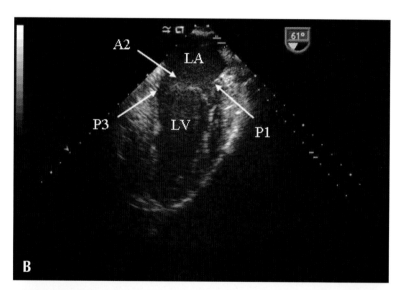

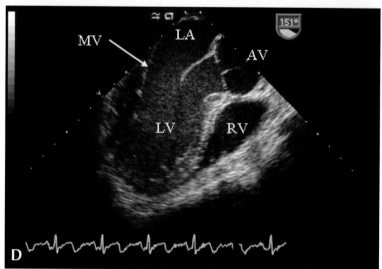

Figure 7-7. Stage 1 of the standard transesophageal (TEE) examination. **A,** Midesophageal four-chamber view. **B,** Midesophageal mitral bicommissural view. **C,** Midesophageal two-chamber view. **D,** Midesophageal long-axis view.

Ant—anterior wall of the LV; AV—aortic valve; IAS—interatrial septum; Inf—inferior wall of the LV; LA—left atrium; Lat—lateral wall of the LV; MV—mitral valve; RA—right atrium; Sept—interventricular septum; TV—tricuspid valve.

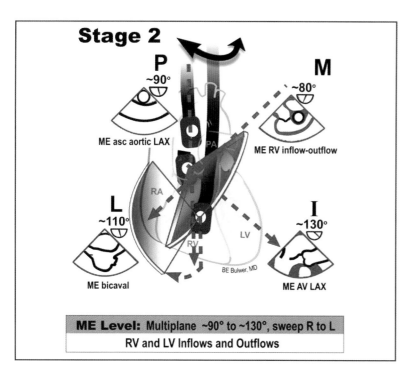

Figure 7-8. Schematic of stage 2 of the transesophageal echocardiography examination. Asc—ascending; AV—aortic valve; LAX—long-axis; ME—midesophageal.

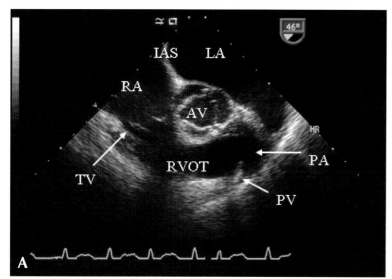

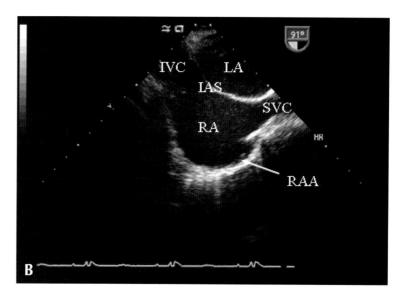

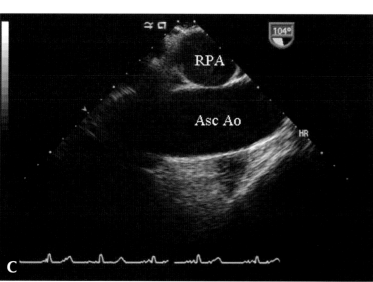

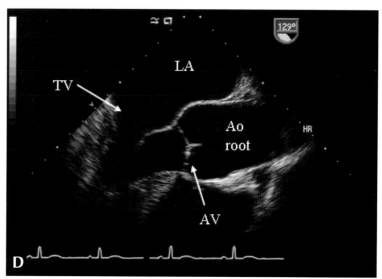

Figure 7-9. Stage 2 of the standard transesophageal echocardiography examination, focusing on RV and LV inflow and outflow. **A**, Midesophageal RV inflow-outflow view. **B**, Midesophageal bicaval view. **C**, Midesophageal ascending aorta in long axis. **D**, Midesophageal aortic valve in long axis. Asc Ao—ascending aorta; Ao root—aortic root; AV—aortic valve; IAS—interatrial septum; IVC—inferior vena cava; LA—left atrium; PA—pulmonary artery; PV—pulmonic valve; RA—right atrium; RAA—right atrial appendage; RPA—right pulmonary artery; RVOT—RV outflow tract; SVC—superior vena cava; TV—tricuspid valve.

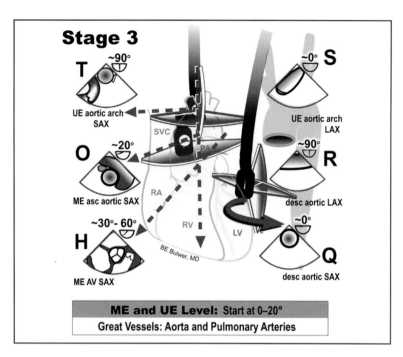

Stage 3

ME and UE Level: Start at 0–20°
Great Vessels: Aorta and Pulmonary Arteries

Figure 7-10. Schematic of stage 3 of the transesophageal echocardiography examination. AV—aortic valve; LAX—long-axis; ME—midesophageal; PA—pulmonary artery; RA—right atrium; SAX—short-axis; SVC—superior vena cava; UE—upper esophageal.

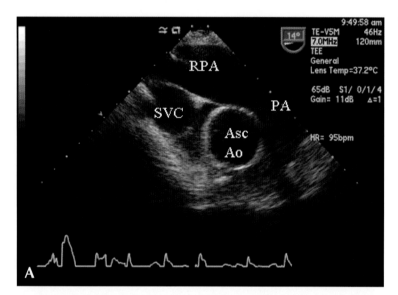

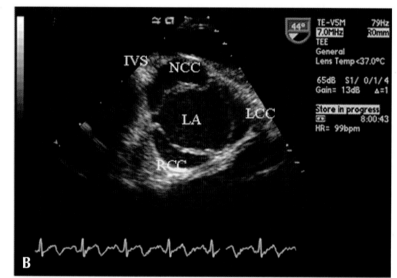

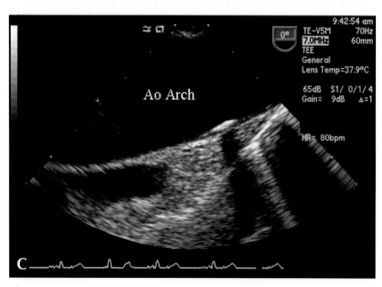

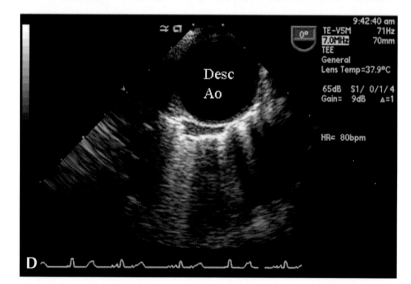

Figure 7-11. Stage 3 of the standard transesophageal echocardiography examination, focusing on the great vessels. **A**, Midesophageal view of the ascending aorta in short axis. **B**, Midesophageal view of the aortic valve in short axis. **C**, Upper esophageal view of the aortic arch in long axis. **D**, Descending thoracic aorta in short axis. Asc Ao—ascending aorta; Desc Ao—descending aorta; IVS—interventricular septum; LA—left atrium; LCC—left coronary cusp; NCC—noncoronary cusp; PA—main pulmonary artery; RCC—right coronary cusp; RPA—right pulmonary artery; SVC—superior vena cava.

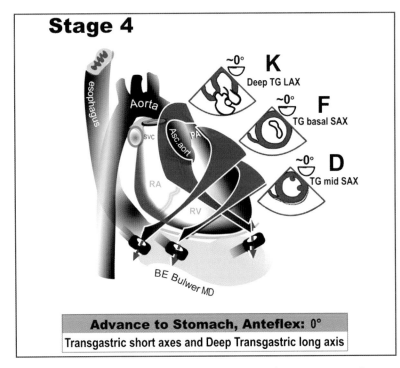

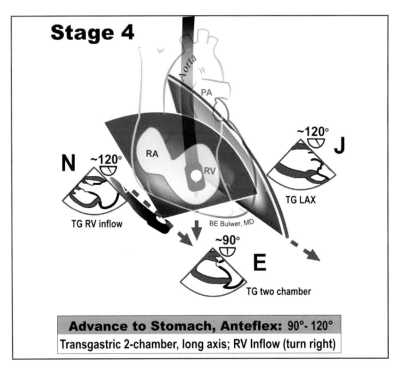

Figure 7-12. Schematic of stage 4. Asc aort—ascending aorta; LAX—long axis; PA—pulmonary artery; RA—right atrium; SAX—short axis; SVC—superior vena cava; TG—transgastric.

Figure 7-13. Schematic of stage 4, rotated views. LAX—long axis; PA—pulmonary artery; RA—right atrium; TG—transgastric.

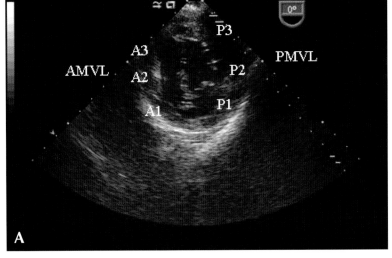

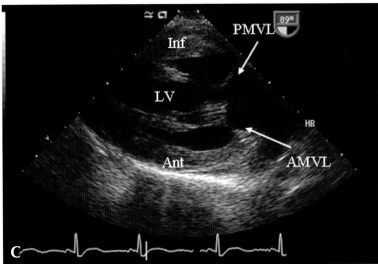

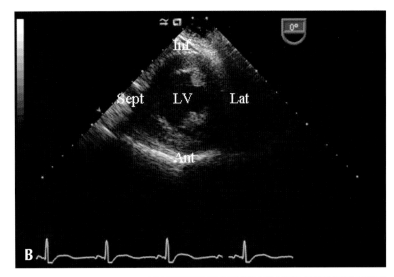

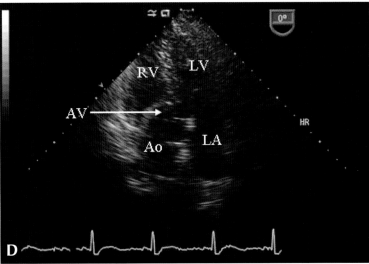

Figure 7-14. Stage 4 of the standard transesophageal echocardiography examination, focusing on transgastric views. **A**, Transgastric basal short-axis view of the LV at the level of the mitral valve. **B**, Transgastric short-axis view of the LV at the midpapillary level. **C**, Transgastric two-chamber view. **D**, Deep transgastric five-chamber view. AMVL—anterior mitral valve leaflet; Ant—anterior wall; Ao—aorta; AV—aortic valve; Inf—inferior wall; LA—left atrium; Lat—lateral wall; PMVL—posterior mitral valve leaflet; Sept—septal wall.

Transesophageal Echocardiography in Atrial Fibrillation

The presence of left atrial (LA) or left atrial appendage (LAA) thrombus, dense spontaneous echocontrast (SEC), and a reduced peak LAA emptying velocity (PLAAEV) of less than 20 cm/s are significantly associated with increased stroke incidence in patients with atrial fibrillation [5–7]. The presence of complex aortic atherosclerotic plaque is also significantly associated with stroke. All of these features are better imaged by transesophageal echocardiography (TEE) compared with transthoracic echocardiography. With

regards to thromboembolic events, studies support TEE-guided early cardioversion as being equivalent to standard therapy with 3 weeks of therapeutic anticoagulation prior to cardioversion [8]. TEE-guided early cardioversion is recommended by the American College of Cardiology/American Heart Association guidelines on the management of atrial fibrillation as a reasonable alternative to 3 weeks of anticoagulation precardioversion (class IIa, level of evidence B). This is now a standard practice [9].

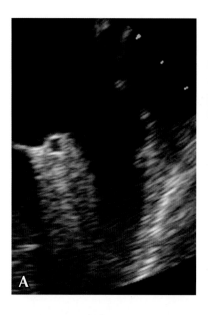 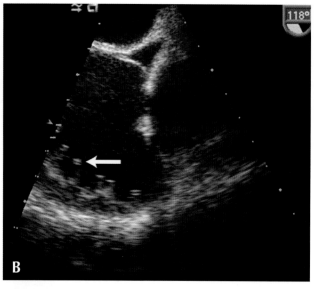

Figure 7-15. Normal left atrial appendage (LAA). The LAA is best visualized from the midesophageal position (**A**). It is a complex anatomic structure and is multilobed in up to 80% of the general population [10]. The walls of the appendage are lined by pectinate muscles (**B**, *arrow*). In the evaluation for thrombus, the appendage must be meticulously examined in multiple planes in order to assure that all aspects and lobes are visualized. One approach is to center the LAA in the imaging field at the 0° position and scan through to 180°, keeping the appendage centered in the field. Two-dimensional imaging of the appendage also allows for visual estimation of the appendage size and contractile function.

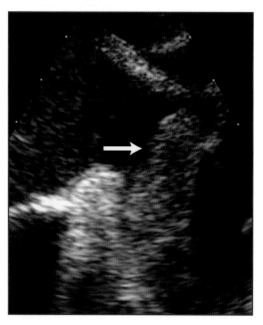

Figure 7-16. Left atrial appendage (LAA) thrombus (*arrow*). The presence of left atrial (LA) or LAA thrombus is a contraindication to immediate cardioversion [9]. The presence of LA or LAA thrombus is associated with a significantly increased risk of stroke (relative risk 2.7 in the Stroke Prevention in Atrial Fibrillation III [SPAF III] TEE substudy [5]). At least 3 weeks of therapeutic anticoagulation prior to, and at least 4 weeks of therapeutic anticoagulation following, cardioversion is recommended (class IIa, level of evidence C) in the 2006 American College of Cardiology (ACC) and the American Heart Association (AHA) guidelines on the management of atrial fibrillation [9].

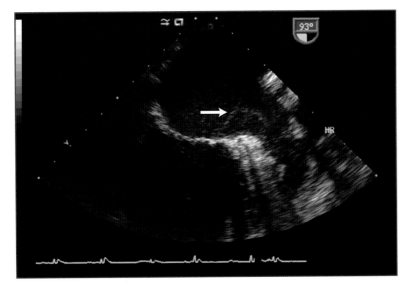

Figure 7-17. Dense spontaneous echocontrast in the left atrial appendage (LAA) (*arrow*). Spontaneous echocontrast (SEC) is due to backscatter of ultrasound from red blood cell aggregates or low-velocity blood flow [10]. It is characterized by a swirling pattern of increased echogenicity at standard settings, and is often identified in the left atrium (LA). Data regarding the optimal management of patients with atrial fibrillation and dense SEC are lacking. Multiple studies have demonstrated an association between dense SEC and stroke risk [7]. In the Stroke Prevention and Atrial Fibrillation III (SPAF III) transesophageal echocardiography substudy, dense SEC was present in 89% of patients with thrombus, and 24% of patients with dense SEC had LAA thrombus [5]. In published studies that reported the presence of SEC without associated thrombus in patients undergoing cardioversion, the reported incidence of adverse events is extremely low [7]. Although this finding is not an absolute contraindication to early cardioversion, it should prompt a meticulous search for thrombus.

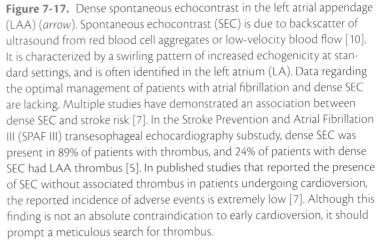

Figure 7-18. Normal left atrial appendage (LAA) spectral pulse wave Doppler pattern. The pulse wave sample is placed 1 cm into the appendage from its orifice. Normal LAA Doppler flow pattern demonstrates a late diastolic flow towards the transducer, representing LAA emptying (*horizontal arrow*). This signal occurs after the P wave on the surface electrocardiogram, and it is contemporaneous with the mitral inflow A wave. The peak LAA ejection velocity reflects appendage contractile function. LAA filling results in a signal away from the transducer in early systole (*arrowhead*). Following LAA filling there is often a variable number of low amplitude inflow and outflow signals termed systolic reflection waves (*verticle arrow*).

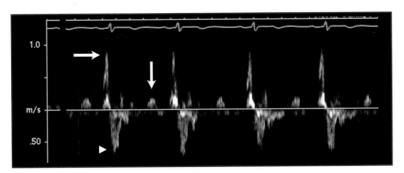

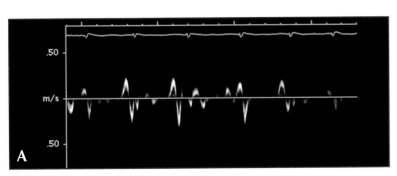

Figure 7-19. Left atrial appendage (LAA) pulse wave Doppler patterns in atrial fibrillation. Spectral Doppler pattern demonstrates high-frequency alternating saw-tooth appearing signals of varying velocities (**A**). Velocities tend to be lower during ventricular systole and at higher ventricular response rates. Markedly diminished peak LAA emptying velocity (PLAAEV) (**B**) reflects markedly impaired appendage contractility. Multiple studies have found an association between low peak LAA emptying velocity (< 20 cm/s) and incidence of stroke in patients with atrial fibrillation. In the SPAF III TEE substudy, patients with low PLAAEV were more likely to have thrombus (17% vs. 5%) [5]. Like dense spontaneous echocontrast, low LAA velocities are a marker of poor LAA function.

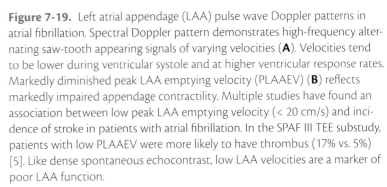

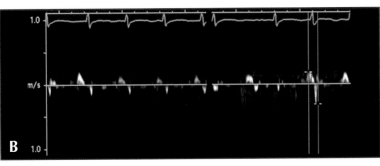

Figure 7-20. Left atrial appendage pulse wave Doppler pattern in atrial flutter. Spectral Doppler pattern demonstrates more consistent high-frequency alternating saw-tooth appearing signals. As with atrial fibrillation, the peak ejection velocity is generally lower during ventricular systole when compared with ventricular diastole.

Transesophageal Echocardiography and Evaluation of Embolic Events

The evaluation for cardiac source of embolism includes assessment of LV global systolic function, regional systolic function (hypo- or akinetic segments), intracardiac thrombus or tumors, valvular abnormalities such as endocarditis or severe calcification, atrial septal abnormalities, and aortic atherosclerosis. Many of these are adequately assessed by transthoracic imaging. Transesophageal echocardiography (TEE) is best suited for evaluation of atrial septal abnormalities, atrial thrombus, aortic atherosclerosis, and valvular abnormalities, such as endocarditis.

Atrial septal abnormalities include patent foramen ovale (PFO), atrial septal aneurysm, atrial septal defect, and right-to-left shunts. Atrial septal abnormalities are common, with PFOs identified in 26% of the general population [11]. Atrial septal abnormalities have been associated with cerebrovascular events, particularly cryptogenic strokes in young patients. However, this association remains controversial, and data regarding the risk of first or recurrent stroke in patients with atrial septal abnormalities are inconsistent [11–22]. The American Academy of Neurology practice parameters conclude that although the prevalence of PFO may be increased in patients with cryptogenic stroke, there is not compelling evidence that its presence increases the risk of a subsequent stroke over that experienced by patients with cryptogenic stroke and no PFO [23]. In patients less than 55 years of age, the presence of a PFO and atrial septal abnormalities may increase the risk of subsequent stroke. The ACC/AHA guidelines for the prevention of stroke in patients with ischemic stroke or TIA recommend antiplatelet therapy as reasonable preventative action (Class IIa, level of evidence B) [24]. In spite of imperfect data, atrial septal abnormalities and right-to-left shunts represent potential sources of embolism. Assessment for these conditions is a standard part of the TEE examination in any patient with a cryptogenic cerebrovascular or embolic event.

Thoracic aortic atherosclerosis is common, with a prevalence of over 50% in a randomly selected asymptomatic population [11]. Multiple retrospective and prospective studies have documented the association between complex aortic atheroma and stroke, recurrent stroke, coronary events, postcardiopulmonary bypass strokes, and mortality postcardiopulmonary bypass [5,25–33]. Although causality has not been demonstrated, complex aortic atheroma is clearly associated with other risk factors for vascular disease and with an increased risk of stroke and vascular events. Thorough imaging of the full ascending aorta, aortic arch, and descending thoracic aorta, with determination of plaque presence, thickness, and morphology, is essential in the examination of any patient presenting with an arterial embolic event.

Multiple case reports have described valvular abnormalities such as papillary fibroelastoma or Lambl's excrescence in patients presenting with cerebrovascular events [34,35]. These are uncommon, and there are no reliable data demonstrating a firm relationship between these findings and embolic events. However, in patients presenting with embolism, a thorough investigation of the valves for any abnormal masses or structures is essential.

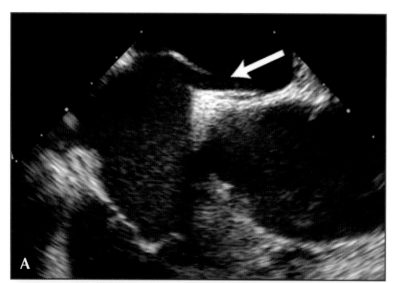

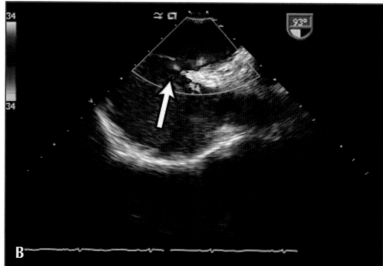

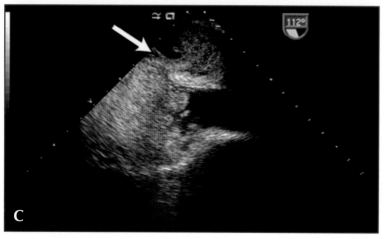

Figure 7-21. Midesophageal bicaval view demonstrating a patent foramen ovale (PFO) with two-dimensional imaging (**A**, *arrow*). There is left-to-right shunting demonstrated by color Doppler imaging (**B**, *arrow*). **C** demonstrates agitated saline contrast injection ("bubble study") with transit of bubbles through the PFO into the left atrium, consistent with intermittent right-to-left shunting through the PFO (*arrow*). Agitated saline contrast studies should be performed both at rest and with maneuvers to increase right atrial pressure (Valsalva strain and release phase). Adequate increase in right atrial pressure is reflected by bowing of the interatrial septum towards the left atrium. Some studies suggest that the degree of right-to-left shunting through the PFO is associated with stroke risk, although data are conflicting [21].

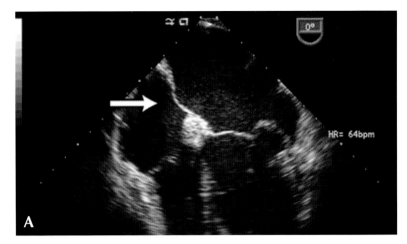 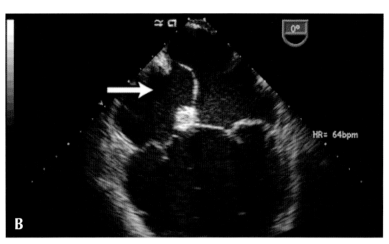

Figure 7-22. Atrial septal aneurysm (ASA). The interatrial septum in this midesophageal four-chamber view demonstrates a total excursion of greater than 15 mm (**A** and **B**, *arrows*). ASAs are characterized by excessive excursion of the interatrial septum from midline. Commonly accepted criteria for ASA include septal hypermobility with maximal excursion of 15 mm or more, or of 10 mm from midline in either direction [11]. ASAs have been identified in 1.9% of a large unselected population and up to 11% of patients with cryptogenic stroke [11,18]. In large published cohort and randomized trials, patent foramen ovale (PFO) is present in 54% to 84% of patients with ASA [11,17–19]. Multiple studies have suggested that ASAs, either alone or in combination with PFO, are significantly associated with primary or recurrent stroke [11,16,17,21].

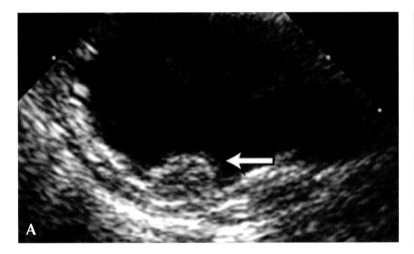 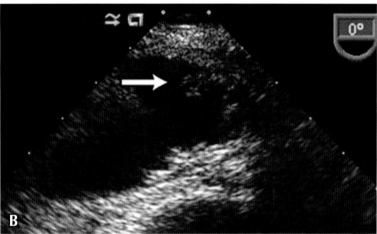

Figure 7-23. High-esophageal image of the aortic arch, demonstrating significant atherosclerotic plaque. Features of aortic atheroma associated with stroke or recurrent stroke (complex atheroma) include plaque thickness of greater than 4 mm, mobility, and ulceration. **A**, Demonstration of plaque measuring greater than 4 mm in thickness (*arrow*). **B**, Demonstration of complex plaque greater than 4 mm thick with a mobile component (*arrow*).

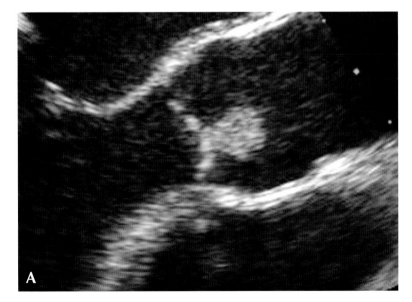 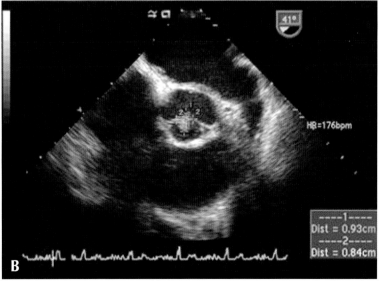

Figure 7-24. Midesophageal long-axis (**A**) and short-axis (**B**) views demonstrating a large fibroelastoma found in a 40-year-old woman complaining of palpitations. This papillary fibroelastoma is attached to the aortic aspect of the right coronary leaflet toward the leaflet tip. It measured 1.1 cm in length and was mobile. Although firm data are lacking, large case series suggest that the size (> 1 cm) and mobility of this lesion are risk factors for embolism [34,35].

Transesophageal Echocardiography in Infective Endocarditis

Transesophageal echocardiography (TEE) plays a central role in the diagnosis of infective endocarditis (IE). IE is a clinical diagnosis, and the modified Duke criteria are the most widely used diagnostic schema [36]. Multiple studies have demonstrated the high sensitivity and specificity of the Duke criteria [37]. Major echocardiographic criteria for the diagnosis of IE include 1) an oscillating intracardiac mass on a valve or supporting structure in the path of a regurgitant jet, or on implanted material in the absence of an alternative anatomic explanation; 2) abscess; 3) new partial dehiscence of a prosthetic valve; 4) new valvular regurgitation. TEE has been shown to be superior to transtho-

racic echocardiography in the detection of native valvular vegetations [38], prosthetic valve endocarditis [39,40], abscesses [41,42], subaortic complications of aortic valve endocarditis [43], and pacemaker lead infections [44].

Recent studies also suggest that echocardiographic features of endocarditis, visualized by TEE, have prognostic significance. Large well-designed multicenter studies have demonstrated that vegetation size, vegetation mobility, and the presence of periannular complications are significant predictors of embolic events and mortality [45–48].

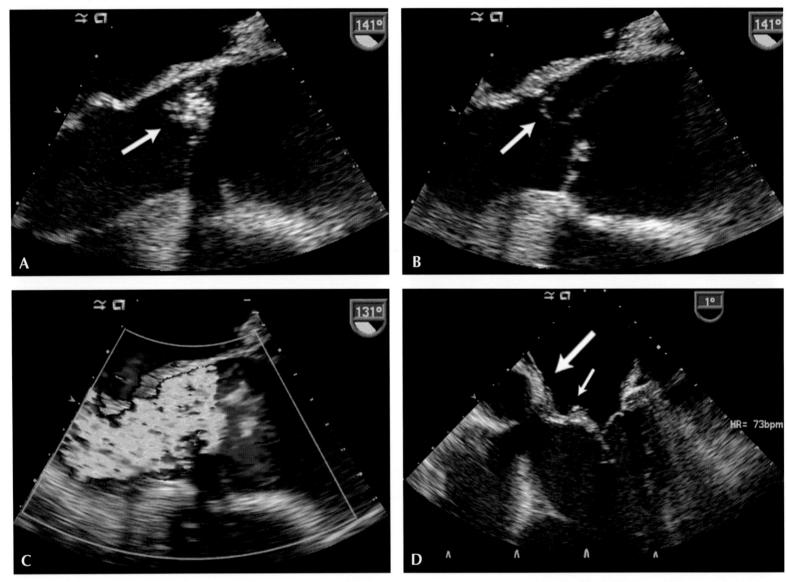

Figure 7-25. Native aortic valve endocarditis with subaortic complications. Multiple studies have demonstrated the superiority of transesophageal echocardiography (TEE) compared with transthoracic echocardiography (TTE) in identifying left-sided valvular vegetations (sensitivity as low as 55%) [38, 49,50]. TEE is especially more sensitive than TTE in diagnosing subaortic complications of aortic valve endocarditis, as seen in these images. Midesophageal long-axis view of the aortic valve (**A**) demonstrates a vegetation on the ventricular aspect of the aortic valve. This was a bicuspid aortic valve. This infection also caused leaflet aneurysm with prolapse (**B**, *arrow*) just adjacent

to the vegetation. Aortic valve leaflet perforation was present in this same location (**C**) with severe associated aortic insufficiency. In the midesophageal five-chamber view, abnormal thickening of the intervalvular fibrosa consistent with abscess is present (**D**, *long arrow*). This view also demonstrates abnormal thickening of the anterior mitral valve leaflet with a small vegetation present on its atrial aspect (**D**, *short arrow*). This patient also had evidence of an anterior mitral leaflet aneursym with leaflet perforation. Compared with TEE, the sensitivity of TTE in diagnosing intervalvular fibrosa abscess, aneurysm, or perforation is reported to be as low as 21% [43].

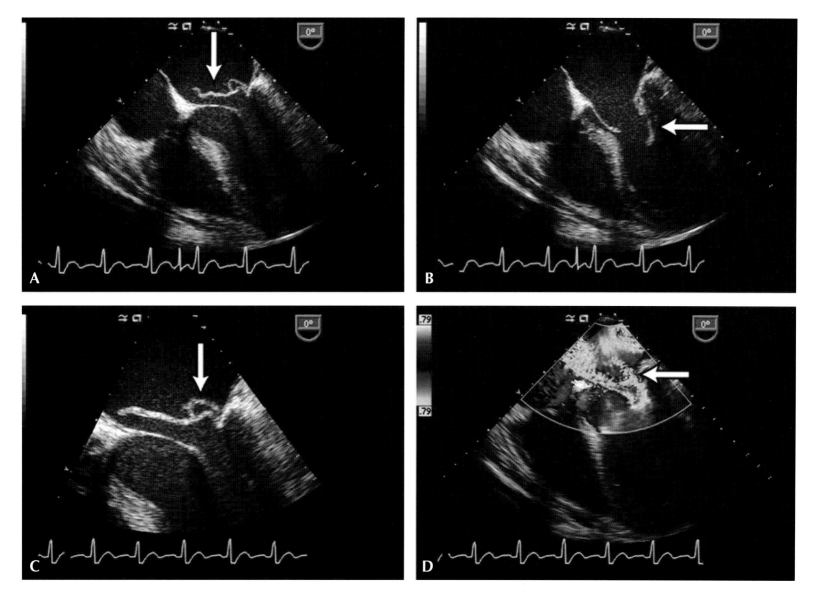

Figure 7-26. Native mitral valve endocarditis. This young woman presented with altered mental status and heart failure and was found to have *Staphylococcus aureus* bacteremia. Transesophageal echocardiography (TEE) demonstrated a large vegetation on the posterior mitral valve leaflet measuring 2.8 cm in length (**A**, *arrow*). The vegetation was also severely mobile, with prolapse into the LV in diastole (**B**, *arrow*). There is evidence of leaflet disruption with forma- tion of a posterior leaflet aneurysm and posterior leaflet flail (**C**, *arrow*). Color Doppler examination confirmed the presence of severe eccentric anteriorly directed mitral regurgitation due to the flail posterior leaflet (**D**). A second regurgitant jet is seen through a perforation in the posterior leaflet aneurysm (**D**, *arrow*). In addition to heart failure, the size and mobility of this vegetation are associated with a high risk of embolic events and mortality in this patient.

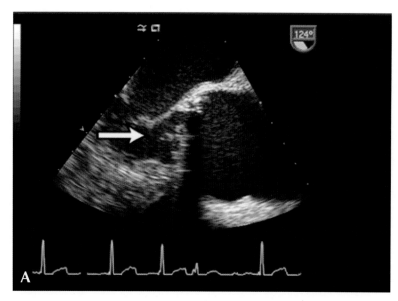

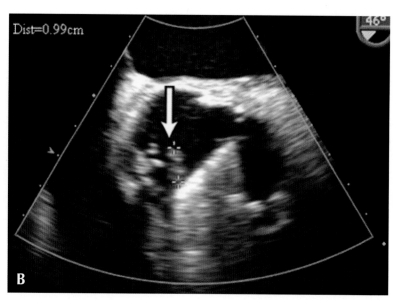

Figure 7-27. Mechanical prosthetic aortic valve vegetation. This elderly man presented with fever and bacteremia several years following aortic valve replacement with a single leaflet tilting disk mechanical prosthesis. A vegetation was identified on the prosthetic valve, seen in the midesophageal long-axis (**A**, *arrow*) and short-axis (**B**, *arrow*) views. The vegetation measured nearly 1 cm. In a large multicenter registry of 2670 definite endocarditis cases, 556 (20.1%) involved prosthetic valves [51]. Patients with prosthetic valve infective endocarditis (IE) had a significantly higher in-hospital mortal- ity compared with native valve IE (22.8% and 16.4%, respectively), less commonly had vegetation (89.9% and 73.0%, respectively) or new regurgitation (71.0% and 46.2%, respectively) identified, and more frequently had abcesses identified (29.7% and 11.7%, respectively). Compared with surgical findings, the sensitivity of transesophageal echocardiography is 86% to 93% and appears to be higher for mitral valve prostheses compared with aortic valve prostheses (97% and 77%, respectively) [39,40]. In contrast, the sensitivity of TTE is only 43% to 57%.

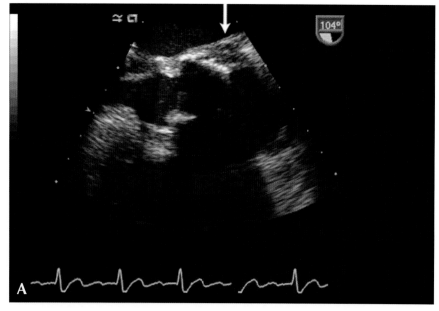

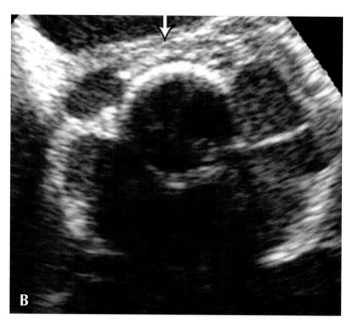

Figure 7-28. Mechanical prosthetic aortic valve with perivalvular abscess. Thickening of the intervalvular fibrosa and the posterior wall of the aortic root is seen in the midesophageal long-axis (**A**, *arrow*) and short-axis (**B**, *arrow*) images. There is a heterogeneous echotexture in this region, consistent with a perivalvular abscess. A vegetation is also seen on the ventricular aspect of the annulus anteriorly. Aneurysmal dilatation of the aortic root is also present. Severe valvular regurgitation was also present by color Doppler. The reported sensitivity of transesophageal echocardiography in identifying abscess compared with surgical findings or autopsy is 87% to 88% [40,41]. In contrast, the reported sensitivity for transthoracic echocardiography is 18% to 28%. The presence of abscess has been shown to be a predictor of in-hospital mortality in both native and prosthetic valve infective endocarditis (IE) [48,51]. In a series of 118 cases of IE, the in-hospital mortality of patients with abscess was 52.3% versus 16.2% in patients without abscess [41].

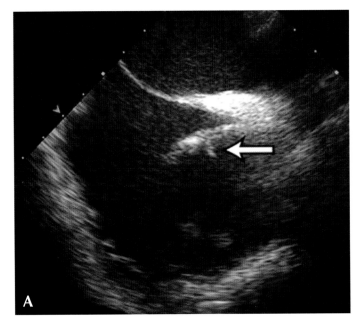

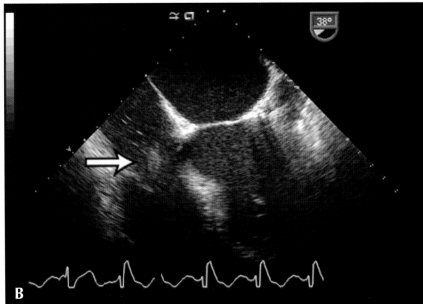

Figure 7-29. A, Pacemaker lead vegetation. An 81-year-old man who had had a pacemaker implanted presented with an infected diabetic foot ulcer complicated by persistent fevers and *Staphylococcus aureus* bacteremia. This midesophageal bicaval view demonstrates multiple small mobile echodensities attached to the pacemaker lead in the right atrium (*arrow*). There was no evidence of tricuspid valve involvement. The sensitivity of transesophageal echocardiography (TEE) for vegetations of intracardiac devices is superior to transthoracic echocardiography (TTE). In a series of 52 patients with pacemaker lead infection, TEE identified vegetations on the lead in 94% of patients while TTE demonstrated vegetations in only 23% [44]. **B**, Tricuspid valve vegetation. The patient underwent lead extraction. He continued to experience persistent fever and bacteremia for a week following lead extraction. A repeat TEE was performed (**B**). This midesophageal four-chamber view demonstrates a new vegetation on the tricuspid valve (*arrow*). This vegetation was large (measuring up to 23 mm long) and severely mobile. Data regarding the sensitivity of TEE versus TTE for tricuspid valve endocarditis are sparse [52]. In this case, TTE performed the previous day failed to demonstrate the tricuspid valve vegetation.

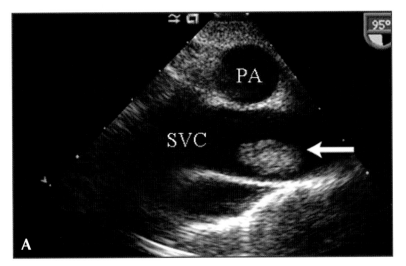

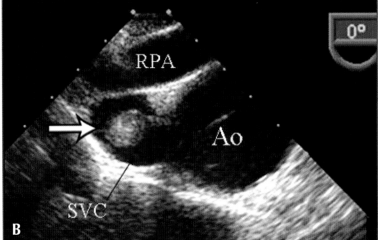

Figure 7-30. Vegetation on a central venous catheter. This 45-year-old man was admitted with a suspected bowel perforation. Following stabilization, a peripherally inserted central catheter was placed for total parenteral nutrition. He subsequently developed persistent fevers and fungemia. This high-esophageal long-axis view of the superior vena cava (SVC) at 95° demonstrates a large mobile mass (**A** and **B**, *arrow*) attached to the central venous catheter in the proximal SVC (**A**). This mass is also seen in the short axis and is consistent with a vegetation or thrombus with super imposed vegetation (**B**). This case highlights the importance of fully visualizing all intracardiac devices along their full course. Ao—aorta; PA—pulmonary artery; RPA—right pulmonary artery.

Transesophageal Echocardiography and Valvular Dysfunction

Transesophageal echocardiography (TEE) has proven to be a useful adjunct to transthoracic imaging in the assessment of valvular disease. In our experience, TEE is most commonly employed in the evaluation of mitral valve disease. The ACC/AHA 2006 Guidelines on the Management of Patients with Valvular Heart Disease recommend TEE in patients with severe mitral regurgitation in whom surgery is recommended to define the valve anatomy and the feasibility of valve repair (class I indication) [53]. Given the proximity of the mitral valve to the transducer, TEE can provide detailed information regarding the valvular and subvalvular anatomy, the etiology of the regurgitation, and the severity of regurgitation. TEE has also been particularly useful in the assessment of suspected prosthetic valve dysfunction.

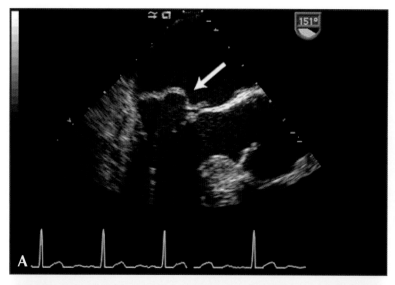

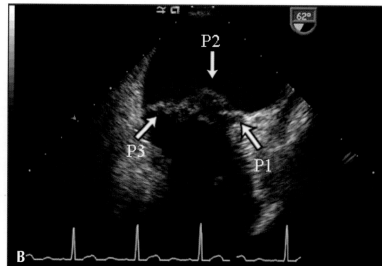

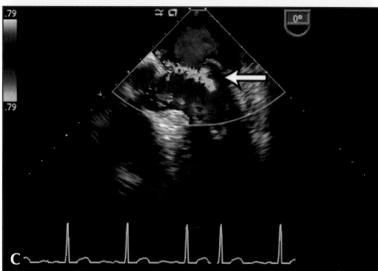

Figure 7-31. Transesophageal echocardiography (TEE) in the assessment of mitral regurgitation etiology and severity. This patient was referred for assessment of the etiology of mitral regurgitation in anticipation of possible surgery. In the midesophageal three-chamber view (**A**), there is clear prolapse of the posterior mitral valve leaflet with a flail segment (*arrow*). Imaging in the midesophageal bicommissural view at 60° (**B**) with slight rotation to the left confirms that the prolapse predominantly involves the middle scallop of the posterior leaflet (P2). Color Doppler assessment in the midesophageal five-chamber view (**C**) again demonstrates the posterior leaflet prolapse with partial flail and a highly eccentric anteriorly directed jet of mitral regurgitation. Color Doppler tends to underestimate the severity of regurgitation that is this eccentric, although the width of the vena contracta seen here (*arrow*) suggests that this is severe regurgitation.

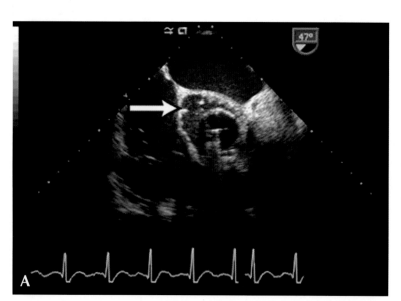

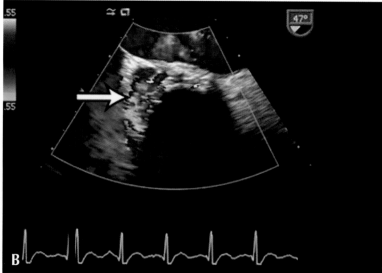

Figure 7-32. Transesophageal echocardiography (TEE) in the assessment of prosthetic valve dysfunction. This elderly patient was referred for TEE for evaluation of mechanical prosthetic aortic valve insufficiency. Neither the cause nor the severity of regurgitation was discernible on transthoracic echocardiography due to acoustic shadowing from the prosthesis. TEE demonstrated dehiscence of the posteromedial aspect of the prosthesis (**A**, *arrow*). There was resulting severe paravalvular insufficiency through this region of dehiscence (**B**, *arrow*). No valvular vegetation or paravalvular abscess was identified. The finding of prosthetic valve dehiscence is highly suggestive of endocarditis and as a general rule is due to endocarditis until proven otherwise.

Transesophageal Echocardiography and Acute Aortic Syndromes

Aortic dissection is a clinical emergency that is challenging to diagnose. Data from the International Registry of Acute Aortic Dissection demonstrate that despite advances in diagnostic imaging and surgical intervention, the in-hospital mortality remains high at approximately 27% [54]. Transesophageal echocardiography (TEE) and CT angiography are the two most commonly employed imaging modalities for aortic dissection. Multiple studies have demonstrated the high sensitivity and specificity of both modalities for diagnosing type A dissections. The sensitivity and specificity of TEE have been reported as 90% to 100% and 94%, respectively [55,56]. TEE offers the additional advantage of assessing for complications of dissection including pericardial effusion, aortic insufficiency, and regional LV wall motion abnormalities that suggest coronary involvement. One limitation of TEE is the inability to image the distal portion of the ascending aorta and the proximal transverse aorta due to interposition of the tracheal air column. Intramural hematomas and penetrating atherosclerotic ulcers share many risk factors, presenting features, and complications with classic aortic dissection. A careful search for these entities should be performed in any patient undergoing assessment for aortic dissection.

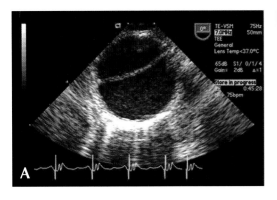 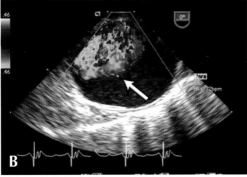

Figure 7-33. Midesophageal short-axis view of the descending thoracic aorta demonstrating a dissection flap separating the true and false lumens (**A**). The true lumen is often the smaller of the two lumens. The true lumen often expands in systole due to pulsatile flow. Color Doppler demonstrates flow in the true lumen (**B**). The small amount of color flow visualized over the dissection flap in early diastole demonstrates a site of communication between the true and false lumens (*arrow*).

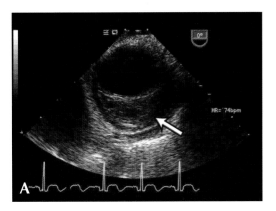 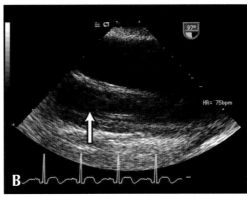

Figure 7-34. Short-axis view (**A**) and long-axis view (**B**) of a chronic Stanford type B descending thoracic aortic dissection with thrombosis of the false lumen (*arrows*). Studies suggest that false lumen thrombosis is associated with improved long-term survival in patients with aortic dissection [57,58]. Among patients with Stanford type B dissections in the International Registry of Acute Aortic Dissection registry, the presence of partial thrombosis of the false lumen (defined as thrombus and evidence of flow in the false lumen) was associated with significantly higher 3-year morality compared with patients with either a patent or fully thrombosed false lumen [59].

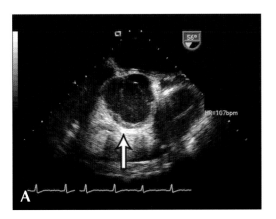 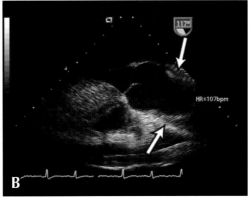

Figure 7-35. Intramural hematoma involving the aortic root and ascending aorta. Intramural hematoma results from hemorrhage into the medial layer of the aortic wall without evidence of an intimal tear. On echocardiography, intramural hematoma is characterized by crescentic thickening of the aortic wall, seen in short axis along the anterior wall of the aortic root (**A**, *arrow*). In the long-axis view (**B**), there is linear thickening of the aortic wall (*arrows*). It can be difficult to distinguish from classic dissection with thrombosed false lumen. However, with intramural hematoma, the shape of the aortic lumen is preserved. Multiple cohort studies suggest that mortality from intramural hematoma is similar to frank dissection with high early mortality in patients with ascending aorta involvement treated medically (47%–80%) versus surgically (8%–24%) [60–62]. Mortality from distal intramural hematoma is significantly lower (14%–17%) and is not significantly different between those managed medically versus surgically. Although some studies have suggested a more benign prognosis for proximal intramural hematoma [63], intramural hematoma involving the aortic root or ascending aorta is generally managed surgically.

Real Time Three-dimensional "Live 3D" Transesophageal Echocardiography

Real-time three-dimensional "live 3D" transesophageal echocardiography (TEE) is based on volumetric three-dimensional technology. By providing true three-dimensional acquisition, real-time three-dimensional TEE can provide more anatomically accurate views of the cardiac structures, including views that mimic those that a surgeon will see. This technology is currently used primarily in the operating department during cardiac surgery, but its use is likely to expand over the next several years.

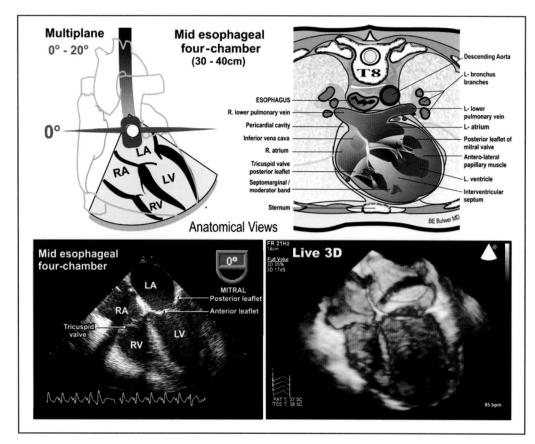

Figure 7-36. Midesophageal four-chamber views. **Top left**, For best assessment of the midesophageal four-chamber views, multiplane to 15°, and examine cardiac chambers and valvular structures and function. **Top right**, Illustration showing the relationships of important mediastinal structures at the level of the eighth thoracic vertebra. Note the close relationship of the esophagus to the left atrium (LA). As the transducer is confined to the esophagus at this level, understanding this relationship helps in the interpretation of many images acquired at this level. **Bottom left**, The midesophageal four-chamber view on two-dimensional echocardiography. **Bottom right**, Real time full volume three-dimensional transesophageal echocardiography of the midesophageal four-chamber view. (*Bottom images couresty of* S. Shernan, MD). RA—right atrium.

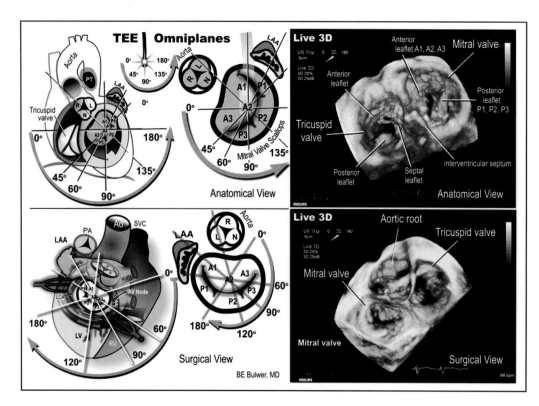

Figure 7-37. Transesophageal echocardiography (TEE) omniplanes on two-dimensional echocardiography with "live 3D" anatomic and surgical correlates. (*Right-sided images courtesy of* S. Shernan, MD). Ao—aorta; AV node—aortic valve node; L—left coronary cusp; LAA—left atrial appendage; LCA—left coronary artery; N—noncoronary cusp; PA—pulmonary artery; PT—pulmonary trunk; R—right coronary cusp; SVC—superior vena cava.

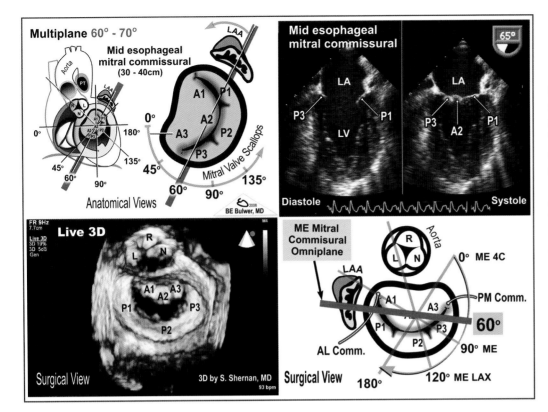

Figure 7-38. Mid esophageal (ME) mitral commissural 80° (G). Multiplane 60° to 80° while examining mitral valve structure and function. Note anterolateral and posteromedial mitral valve commissures and lateral (A1, P1), middle (A2, P2), and medial (A3, P3) scallops of both anterior and posterior leaflets. **Top right**, ME mitral commissural views showing the scallops visualized on 2D TEE. **Bottom left**, "Live 3D" surgical view of the mitral valve scallops. **Bottom right,** illustration depicting the surgeon's view of the mitral valve and scallops corresponding to the ME mitral commissural view (omniplane 60°, *bold red line*) on 2D TEE. (*Top right/bottom left images courtesy of* S. Shernan, MD). AL Comm—anterolateral commissure; L—left coronary cusp; LA—left atrium; LAA—left atrial appendage; LAX—long axis; N—noncoronary cusp; PT—pulmonary trunk; R—right coronary cusp; 4C—four chamber; 2C—two chamber.

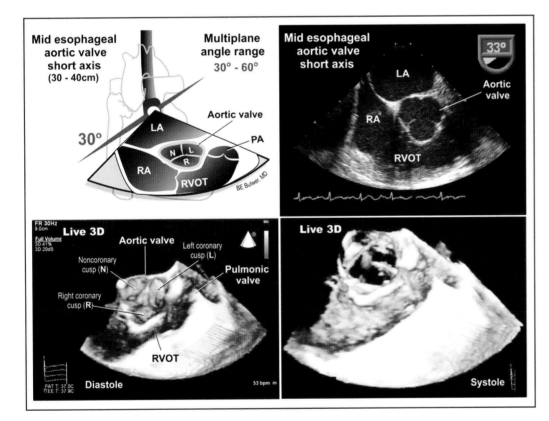

Figure 7-39. Multiplane 60°. Mid esopageal aortic valve short-axis views on 2D (*top*) and 3D (*bottom images*) echocardiography . (*Top right/ bottom images courtesy of* S. Shernan, MD). L—left coronary cusp; LA—left atrium; N—noncoronary cusp; PA—pulmonary artery; R—right coronary cusp; RA—right atrium; RVOT—RV outflow tract.

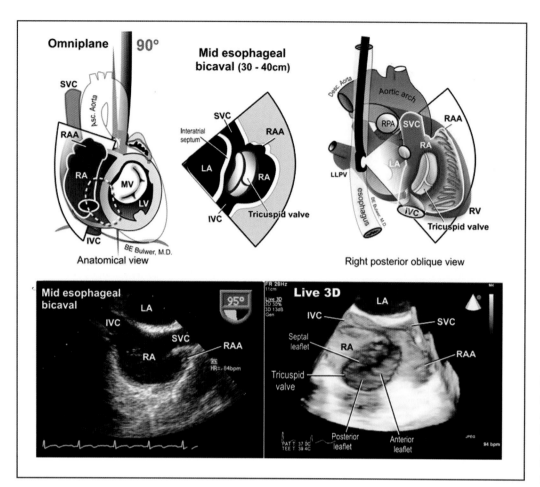

Figure 7-40. Mid esophageal bicaval view. (*Bottom images courtesty of* S. Shernan, MD). Asc Aorta—ascending aorta; IVC—inferior vena cava; LA—left atrium; LLPV—left lower pulmonary vein; MV—mitral valve; RA—right atrium; RAA—right aortic arch; RPA—right pulmonary artery; SVC—superior vena cava.

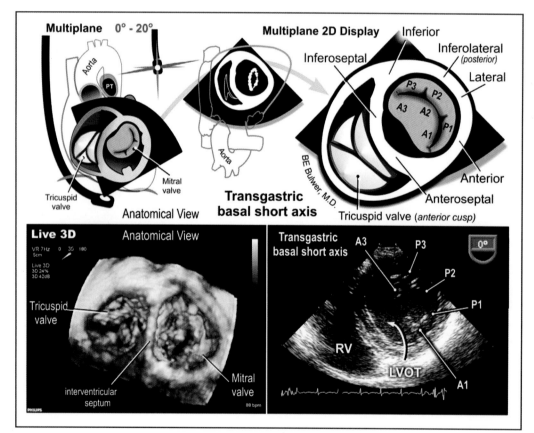

Figure 7-41. Transgastric basal short-axis view. (*Bottom images courtesy of* S. Shernan, MD). LVOT—LV outflow tract; PT—pulmonary trunk/main pulmonary artery.

References

1. Douglas PS, Khandheria B, Stainback RF, *et al.*: ACCF/ASE/ACEP/ASNC/SCAI/SCCT/SCMR 2007 appropriateness criteria for transthoracic and transesophageal echocardiography. *J Am Coll Cardiol* 2007, 50:187–204.

2. Min JK, Spencer KT, Furlong KT, *et al.*: Clinical features of complications from transesophageal echocardiography: a single center case series of 10,000 consecutive examinations. *J Am Soc Echocardiogr* 2005, 18:925–929.

3. Daniel WG, Erbel R, Kasper W, *et al.*: Safety of transesophageal echocardiography: a multicenter survey of 10,419 examinations. *Circulation* 1991, 83:817–821.

4. Shanewise JS, Cheung AT, Aronson S, *et al.*: ASE/SCA guidelines for performing a comprehensive intraoperative multiplane transesophageal echocardiography examination: recommendations of the American Society of Echocardiography Council for intraoperative echocardiography and the Society of Cardiovascular Anesthesiologists task force for certification in perioperative transesophageal echocardiography. *J Am Soc Echocardiogr* 1999, 12:884–900.

5. Transesophageal echocardiographic correlates of thromboembolism in high-risk patients with nonvalvular atrial fibrillation. The Stroke Prevention in Atrial Fibrillation Investigators Committee on Echocardiography. *Ann Intern Med* 1998, 128:639–639.

6. Bernhardt P, Schmidt H, Hammerstingl C, *et al.*: Patients with atrial fibrillation and dense spontaneous echo contrast at high risk: a prospective and serial follow-up over 12 months with transesophageal echocardiography and cerebral magnetic resonance imaging. *J Am Coll Cardiol* 2005, 45:1807–1812.

7. Patel SV, Flaker G: Is early cardioversion for atrial fibrillation safe in patients with spontaneous echocardiographic contrast? *Clin Cardiol* 2007, [Epub ahead of print.]

8. Klein AL, Grimm RA, Murray RD, *et al.*: Use of transesophageal echocardiography to guide cardioversion in patients with atrial fibrillation. *N Engl J Med* 2001, 344:1411–1420.

9. Fuster V, Ryden LE, Cannom DS, *et al.*: ACC/AHA/ESC 2006 guidelines for the management of patients with atrial fibrillation. *Circulation* 2006, 114:e257–e354.

10. Agmon Y, Khandheria BK, Gentile F, Seward JB: Echocardiographic assessment of the left atrial appendage. *J Am Coll Cardiol* 1999, 34:1867–1877.

11. Meissner I, Khandheria BK, Heit JA, *et al.*: Patent foramen ovale: innocent or guilty? Evidence from a prospective population-based study. *J Am Coll Cardiol* 2006, 47:440–445.

10. Strandberg M, Raatikainen MJP, Niemela M, *et al.*: Clinical practicality and predictive value of transoesophageal echocardiography in early cardioversion of atrial fibrillation. *Europace* 2006, 8:408–412.

11. Seidl K, Rameken M, Drogemuller A, *et al.*: Embolic events in patients with atrial fibrillation and effective anticoagulation: value of transesophageal echocardiography to guide direct-current cardioversion. *J Am Coll Cardiol* 2002, 39:1436–1442.

12. de Belder MA, Tourikis L, Leech G, Camm AJ: Risk of patent foramen ovale for thromboembolic events in all age groups. *Am J Cardiol* 1992, 69:1316–1320.

13. Labovitz AJ, Camp A, Castello R, *et al.*: Usefulness of transesophageal echocardiography in unexplained cerebral ischemia. *Am J Cardiol* 1993, 72:1448–1452.

14. Cabanes L, Mas JL, Cohen A, *et al.*: Atrial septal aneurysm and patent foramen ovale as risk factors for cryptogenic stroke in patients less than 55 years of age. A study using transesophageal echocardiography. *Stroke* 1993, 24:1865–1873.

15. Jones EF, Calafiore P, Donnan GA, Tonkin AM: Evidence that patent foramen ovale is not a risk factor for cerebral ischemia in the elderly. *Am J Cardiol* 1994, 74:596–599.

16. Overell JR, Bone I, Lees KR: Interatrial septal abnormalities and stroke: a meta-analysis of case-control studies. *Neurology* 2000, 55:1172–1179.

17. Mas JL, Arquizan C, Lamy C, *et al.*: Recurrent cerebrovascular events associated with patent foramen ovale, atrial septal aneurysm, or both. *N Engl J Med* 2001, 345:1740–1746.

18. Homma S, Sacco RL, Di Tullio MR, *et al.*: Effect of medical treatment in stroke in patients with patent foramen ovale: patent foramen ovale in Cryptogenic Stroke Study. *Circulation* 2002, 105:2625–2631.

19. Lamy C, Giannesini C, Zuber M, *et al.*: Clinical and imaging findings in cryptogenic stroke patients with and without patent foramen ovale: the PFO-ASA study. *Stroke* 2002, 33:706–711.

20. Petty GW, Khandheria BK, Meissner I, *et al.*: Population-based study of the relationship between patent foramen ovale and cerebrovascular ischemic events. *Mayo Clin Proc* 2006, 81:602–608.

21. De Castro S, Cartoni D, Fiorelli M, *et al.*: Morphological and functional characteristics of patent foramen ovale and their embolic implications. *Stroke* 2000, 31:2407–2413.

22. Bogousslavsky J, Garazi S, Jeanrenaud X, *et al.*: Stroke recurrence in patients with patent foramen ovale: the Lausanne study. *Neurology* 1996, 46:1301–1305.

23. Messe SR, Silverman IE, Kizer JR, *et al.*: Practice parameter: recurrent stroke with patent foramen ovale and atrial septal aneurysm: report of the Quality Standards Subcommittee of the American Academy of Neurology. *Neurology* 2004, 62:1042–1050.

24. Sacco RL, Adams R, Albers G, *et al.*: Guidelines for prevention of stroke in patients with ischemic stroke or transient ischemic attack: a statement for healthcare professionals from the American Heart Association/American Stroke Association Council on Stroke. *Circulation* 2006, 113:e409–e449.

25. Amarenco P, Duyckaerts C, Tzourio C, *et al.*: The prevalence of ulcerated plaques in the aortic arch in patients with stroke. *N Engl J Med* 1992, 326:221–225.

26. Horowitz DR, Tuhrim S, Budd J, Goldman ME: Aortic plaque in patients with brain ischemia: diagnosis by transesophageal echocardiography. *Neurology* 1992, 42:1602–1604.

27. Tunick PA, Rosenzweig BP, Katz ES, *et al.*: High risk for vascular events in patients with protruding aortic atheromas: a prospective study. *J Am Coll Cardiol* 1994, 23:1085–1090.

28. Atherosclerotic disease of the aortic arch as a risk factor for recurrent ischemic stroke. The French Study of Aortic Plaques in Stroke Group. *N Engl J Med* 1996, 334:1216–1221.

29. Wareing TH, Davila-Roman VG, Barzilai B, *et al.*: Management of the severely atherosclerotic ascending aorta during cardiac operations: a strategy for detection and treatment. *J Thorac Cardiovasc Surg* 1992, 103:453–462.

30. Gardner TJ, Horneffer PJ, Manolio TA, *et al.*: Stroke following coronary artery bypass grafting: a ten-year study. *Ann Thorac Surg* 1985, 40:574–581.

31. Katz ES, Tunick PA, Rusinek H, *et al.*: Protruding aortic atheromas predict stroke in elderly patients undergoing cardiopulmonary bypass: experience with intraoperative transesophageal echocardiography. *J Am Coll Cardiol* 1992, 20:70–77.

32. Davila-Roman VG, Murphy SF, Nickerson NJ, *et al.*: Atherosclerosis of the ascending aorta is an independent predictor of long-term neurologic events and mortality. *J Am Coll Cardiol* 1999, 33:1308–1316.

33. Mackensen GB, Ti LK, Phillips-Bute BG, *et al.*: Cerebral embolization during cardiac surgery: impact of aortic atheroma burden. *Br J Anaesth* 2003, 91:656–661.

34. Sun JP, Asher CR, Yang XS, *et al.*: Clinical and echocardiographic characteristics of papillary fibroelastomas: a retrospective and prospective study in 162 patients. *Circulation* 2001, 103:2687–2693.

35. Gowda RM, Khan IA, Nair CK, *et al.*: Cardiac papillary fibroelastoma: a comprehensive analysis of 725 cases. *Am Heart J* 2003, 146:404–410.

36. Li JS, Sexton DJ, Mick N, *et al.*: Proposed modifications to the Duke criteria for the diagnosis of infective endocarditis. *Clin Infect Dis* 2000, 30:633–638.

37. Baddour LM, Wilson WR, Bayer AS, *et al.*: Infective endocarditis: diagnosis, antimicrobial therapy, and management of complications: a statement for healthcare professionals from the Committee on Rheumatic Fever, Endocarditis, and Kawasaki Disease, Council on Cardiovascular Disease in the Young, and the Councils on Clinical Cardiology, Stroke, and Cardiovascular Surgery and Anesthesia, American Heart Association. *Circulation* 2005, 111:e393–e433. [Published erratum appears in *Circulation* 2005, 112:2373; *Circulation* 2007, 115:e408; *Circulation* 2007, 116:e547.]

38. Reynolds HR, Jagen MA, Tunick PA, Kronzon I: Sensitivity of transthoracic versus transesophageal echocardiography for the detection of native valve vegetation in the modern era. *J Am Soc Echocardiogr* 2003, 16:67–70.

39. Daniel WG, Mugge A, Grote J, *et al.*: Comparison of transthoracic and transesophageal echocardiography for detection of abnormalities of prosthetic and bioprosthetic valves in the mitral and aortic positions. *Am J Cardiol* 1993, 71:210–215.

40. Mohr-Kahaly S, Kupferwasser I, Erbel R, *et al.*: Value and limitations of transesoph- ageal echocardiography in the evaluation of aortic prostheses. *J Am Soc Echocar- diogr* 1993, 6:12–20.

41. Daniel WG, Mugge A, Martin RP, *et al.*: Improvement in the diagnosis of abscesses associated with endocarditis by transesophageal echocardiography. *N Engl J Med* 1991, 324:795–800.

42. Cicioni C, Di Luzio V, Di Emidio L, *et al.*: Limitations and discrepancies of trans- thoracic and transesophageal echocardiography compared with surgical findings in patients submitted to surgery for complications of infective endocarditis. *J Cardiovasc Med (Hagerstown)* 2006, 7:660–666.

43. Karalis DG, Bansal RC, Hauck AJ, *et al.*: Transesophageal echocardiographic recog- nition of subaortic complications in aortic valve endocarditis: clinical and surgical implications. Clinical and surgical implications. *Circulation* 1992, 86:353–362.

44. Klug D, Lacroix D, Savoye C, *et al.*: Systemic infection related to endocarditis on pacemaker leads: clinical presentation and management. *Circulation* 1997, 95:2098–2107.

45. Thuny F, Disalvo G, Belliard O, *et al.*: Risk of embolism and death in infective endocarditis: prognostic value of echocardiography: a prospective multicenter study. *Circulation* 2005, 112:69–75. [Published erratum appears in *Circulation* 2005, 112:e125.]

46. Di Salvo G, Habib G, Pergola V, *et al.*: Echocardiography predicts embolic events in infective endocarditis. *J Am Coll Cardiol* 2001, 37:1069–1076.

47. Cabell CH, Pond KK, Peterson GE, *et al.*: The risk of stroke and death in patients with aortic and mitral valve endocarditis. *Am Heart J* 2001, 142:75–80.

48. San Roman JA, Lopez J, Vilacosta I, *et al.*: Prognostic stratification of patients with left-sided endocarditis determined at admission. *Am J Med* 2007, 120:369.e1–369.e7.

49. Erbel R, Rohmann S, Drexler M, *et al.*: Improved diagnostic value of echocardiog- raphy in patients with infective endocarditis by transoesophageal approach: a prospective study. *Eur Heart J* 1988, 9:43–53.

50. Mugge A, Daniel WG, Frank G, Lichtlen PR: Echocardiography in infective endocar- ditis: reassessment of prognostic implications of vegetation size determined by the transthoracic and the transesophageal approach. *J Am Coll Cardiol* 1989, 14:631–638.

51. Wang A, Athan E, Pappas PA, *et al.*: Contemporary clinical profile and outcome of prosthetic valve endocarditis. *JAMA* 2007, 297:1354–1361.

52. San Roman JA, Vilacosta I, Zamorano JL, *et al.*: Transesophageal echocardiography in right-sided endocarditis. *J Am Coll Cardiol* 1993, 21:1226–1230.

53. Bonow RO, Carabello BA, Chatterjee K, *et al.*: ACC/AHA 2006 guidelines for the management of patients with valvular heart disease: a report of the Ameri- can College of Cardiology/American Heart Association Task Force on Practice Guidelines (writing committee to revise the 1998 guidelines for the management of patients with valvular heart disease). *J Am Coll Cardiol* 2006, 48:e1–e148. [Pub- lished erratum appears in *J Am Coll Cardiol* 2007, 49:1014.]

54. Hagan PG, Nienaber CA, Isselbacher EM, *et al.*: The International Registry of Acute Aortic Dissection (IRAD): new insights into an old disease. *JAMA* 2000, 283:897–903.

55. Moore AG, Eagle KA, Bruckman D, *et al.*: Choice of computed tomography, trans- esophageal echocardiography, magnetic resonance imaging, and aortography in acute aortic dissection: International Registry of Acute Aortic Dissection (IRAD). *Am J Cardiol* 2002, 89:1235–1238.

56. Sommer T, Fehske W, Holzknecht N, *et al.*: Aortic dissection: a comparative study of diagnosis with spiral CT, multiplanar transesophageal echocardiography, and MR imaging. *Radiology* 1996, 199:347–352.

57. Erbel R, Oelert H, Meyer J, et al.: Effect of medical and surgical therapy on aortic dissection evaluated by transesophageal echocardiography: implications for prog- nosis and therapy. The European Cooperative Study Group on Echocardiography. Circulation 1993, 87:1604–1615.

58. Bernard Y, Zimmermann H, Chocron S, et al.: False lumen patency as a predictor of late outcome in aortic dissection. Am J Cardiol 2001, 87:1378–1382.

59. Tsai TT, Evangelista A, Nienaber CA, et al.: Partial thrombosis of the false lumen in patients with acute type B aortic dissection. N Engl J Med 2007, 357:349–359.

60. Nienaber CA, von Kodolitsch Y, Petersen B, et al.: Intramural hemorrhage of the tho- racic aorta: diagnostic and therapeutic implications. Circulation 1995, 92:1465–1472.

61. Sawhney NS, DeMaria A, Blanchard DG: Aortic intramural hematoma: an increas- ingly recognized and potentially fatal entity. Chest 2001, 120:1340–1346.

62. von Kodolitsch Y, Csosz SK, Koschyk DH, et al.: Intramural hematoma of the aorta: predictors of progression to dissection and rupture. Circulation 2003, 107:1158–1163.

63. Song JK, Kim HS, Kang DH, et al.: Different clinical features of aortic intramural hematoma versus dissection involving the ascending aorta. J Am Coll Cardiol 2001, 37:1604–1610.

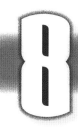

Mitral Valve Disease

Judy Hung and Robert A. Levine

Echocardiography first demonstrated its quantitative strength in the direct planimetry of cross-sectional mitral valve area (MVA), and it remains the standard today. The diagnosis of mitral stenosis (MS) is based on the restriction of area available for inflow from one of two mechanisms. The first is leaflet doming (ie, concavity toward the left atrium [LA]) in rheumatic MS, which is caused by thickening and fusion of the leaflet commissures, and in congenital MS by tethering of the leaflets to an asymmetrically predominant papillary muscle (PM). The second is predominant annular calcification extending into the leaflet bodies, which tend to produce milder MS and are typically associated with inflow limitation due to associated LV hypertrophy. Doming magnifies the stenosis because the resulting flow convergence creates a smaller vena contracta beyond the anatomic orifice. Ischemic leaflet tethering limits diastolic leaflet excursion, generally without stenosis, and without the abrupt cessation of motion and doming of rheumatic MS. Posterior leaflet immobility alone can indicate a rheumatic deformity associated with mitral regurgitation (MR).

MVA planimetry requires careful attention to beam position and angulation to intersect the limiting orifice because of the funnel shape of the valve. The process is now facilitated by biplane and three-dimensional acquisition, so the limiting orifice can be identified in a long-axis view, automatically ensuring the correct short-axis area.

The challenges of orifice visualization led to the MVA calculation by the Doppler pressure half time method as 220/Doppler-derived mitral pressure half time (time for pressure gradient to fall by half equals the time for velocity to fall to 71% of the peak velocity). Although the technique has been successfully applied by several groups, including in the presence of atrial fibrillation and MR, it does not work well when following percutaneous mitral valvotomy. This suggests that changes in hemodynamic variables other than MVA also affect the half time. The half time reflects the rate at which left atrial and ventricular pressures move toward equilibrium in diastole. The half time then depends on ventricular and atrial compliance and left atrial pressure as well as the orifice area. Therefore, the half time will be shortened (overestimating valve area) for a given MVA if: 1) LV diastolic pressure rises faster than expected based on valve area alone due to aortic insufficiency or a noncompliant LV. If aortic insufficiency is mild or chronic with a compliant LV, the effect may not be important. A dilated LV (ie, poor systolic function) may also be in a "stiff" region of its compliance curve; 2) LA pressure falls faster than expected because of depressurization through an atrial septal defect (eg, postvalvotomy) or a noncompliant LA. Converse changes can prolong the half time, which underestimates valve area (eg, a chronically dilated and very compliant atrial cavity). In the case of such discrepancies, the directly planimetered orifice area is used. Three-dimensional imaging has been recently shown to enhance MVA measurement in MS, just as a simultaneous display of orthogonal views can aid in planimetry measurement.

Continuity can also provide MVA as flow/velocity, but the nonuniform velocity across the mitral annulus in MS requires that forward flow be calculated across the aortic or pulmonary valves, assuming minimal MR, aortic insufficiency, or pulmonary regurgitation. The proximal flow convergence method provides MVA from peak flow rate/peak orifice velocity, where the flow rate is calculated from the proximal flow convergence image, starting with flow rate equaling the area of a hemispherical shell at the aliasing velocity ($2\pi r^2$) times the aliasing velocity, then taking into account the angle made by the leaflets ($\alpha/180°$).

Mitral valve morphology is used to guide valvuloplasty based on a score comprising mitral valve mobility, thickness, calcification, and subvalvular thickening (0–4 each), where a total score of 8 or less predicts a good chance of success and 12 or greater predicts a poorer chance. The procedure is also contraindicated by moderate or greater MR, LA thrombus, a localized thin leaflet with calcification elsewhere (predisposing to leaflet tear), and severe tricuspid regurgitation, which often persists despite successful balloon valvuloplasty, leaving the patient with adverse outcome and prognosis.

Quantitation and Mechanism of Mitral Regurgitation

The quantitation and mechanism of MR is of growing importance, with greater reliance on mitral valve repair versus replacement. The clinical challenge is in deciding when MR is severe enough to warrant surgery before the development of LV dysfunction, pulmonary hypertension, or symptoms—indicators previously used in making this decision.

Clinical tools currently in use include jet extent in the receiving chamber (maximal jet/LA area ratio), which has the advantage of being rapid and routine and providing reasonable assessment of mild and severe lesions. Its limitations include the fact that it is weak in differentiating moderate MR from mild or severe, and it has a variable relationship between jet size and regurgitant volume because of technical factors (eg, "dial-a-jet," color gain, frequency), variation among views, physical factors (eg, jet area determined by momentum flux at the orifice as it depends on driving pressure), and biological factors (eg, effect of wall jets, which appear thinner in views perpendicular to the wall then free jets, pulmonary venous counterflow, and timing - same jet area but shorter or longer duration). There is growing recog-

nition of the proximal jet size (vena contracta) as a stronger measure. Its advantages include the fact that it reflects the basic size of the defect, and it is relatively independent of flow rate, driving pressure, or wall jet character. It is rapid in clinical practice and can be made routine and standard windows can measure jet height (parasternal long-axis) and cross-sectional area (parasternal short-axis). Jet height > 5 mm corresponds to moderate to severe MR. Cross-sectional area ranges from .1-.2 (trace-mild) up to 1.2 cm^2 (severe).

MR volume can be quantitated using pulsed Doppler integrative techniques (mitral valve inflow minus aortic outflow) or by the proximal flow convergence technique (PISA, proximal isovelocity surface area continuity method that can be made routine with a relatively simple calculation that assumes a hemispherical velocity surface through a circular orifice in a flat plate). However, isovelocity contours are generally not hemispherical, orifices are often not circular and in nonplanar leaflets, so that three-dimensional assessment of the PISA surface will improve the calculation.

Mechanism of Mitral Regurgitation

The mechanism of MR can be classified by Carpentier's method into excessive leaflet motion, restricted leaflet motion due to rheumatic thickening and shortening, restricted leaflet motion due to functional leaflet tethering, and neither excessive nor restricted leaflet motion (ie, intrinsic changes).

MR relates to a deficiency in leaflet free-edge apposition and effective coaptation, with the exception being in fenestration, which is rare. A general principle is that this deficiency results from an alteration in the three-dimensional geometry of the valve and its attachments, which in turn alter the relations of the leaflets to the surrounding flow field. Unifying concepts relate systolic anterior motion (SAM), mitral valve prolapse (MVP), and ischemic or functional MR. The first concept is that SAM and MVP are both excessive superior motions of the mitral leaflets. MVP occurs posteriorly because the PMs and leaflets are normally posterior. In SAM, anterior malposition of the PMs and leaflets positions their ends into the outflow tract; leaflet elongation provides a slack "sail" that is "blown" into the LV outflow tract. Patients can transition from MVP to SAM spontaneously (this is occasional) or after mitral valve repair. This complication can be reduced by diminishing posterior leaflet height (eg, sliding leaflet technique) so that coaptation must occur posteriorly, and the leaflets are not entrained into the outflow. The second concept is ischemic MR, which can also be understood based on PM displacement, restricting the ability of the leaflets to close at the level of the mitral annulus. Such tethering will therefore

not always respond to annular ring reduction, and new approaches targeting PM position and LV remodeling may be more effective.

MR is a common complication of ischemic heart disease that conveys adverse prognosis after both myocardial infarction and coronary revascularization, and more than doubles the risk of death. Such functional ischemic MR is now receiving increased attention as one of the last frontiers in surgical mitral valve repair as well as a therapeutic opportunity in heart failure. Valve repair has proved more challenging for ischemic MR than for degenerative mitral valve prolapse, in which surgery is tailored to the detailed anatomy displayed by echocardiography and inspection. Successful valve repair must target the mechanism of dysfunction in the individual patient. Until recently, however, both understanding of mechanism and targeting of therapy were elusive for ischemic MR.

Extensive work has now confirmed the relation of ischemic MR to remodeling and distortion of the ischemic LV and the PMs to which the mitral leaflets are attached. Ischemic MR occurs in the setting of normal mitral leaflets, but with abnormal LV function and geometry. Displacement of the PMs away from the mitral annulus tethers the leaflets into the LV and restricts their ability to close effectively at the level of the annulus. The leaflets are caught between the dilated annulus and deformed ventricle. This problem is compounded by LV contractile dysfunction, which decreases the force available to close the leaflets in opposition to the increased tethering.

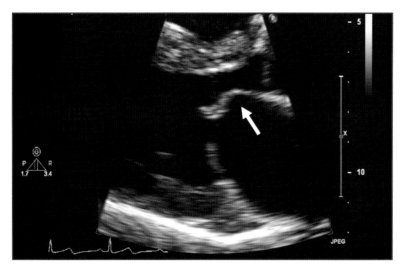

Figure 8-1. A parasternal long-axis view of rheumatic mitral stenosis is shown. The anterior mitral leaflet develops a characteristic doming appearance (*arrow*) concave toward the left atrium, with the leaflet tips restricted from opening because of rheumatic scarring and commissural fusion.

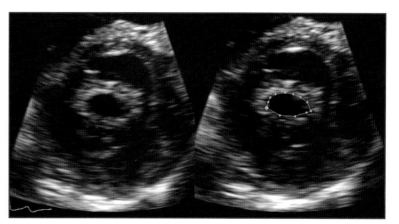

Figure 8-2. A planimetry of the mitral valve area is performed in these short-axis images of the rheumatic valve orifice during diastole. The smallest orifice is determined by scanning back and forth in the short-axis views, and can be facilitated by biplane and three-dimensional acquisition. The planimetered orifice area is indicated (*dotted blue line*)

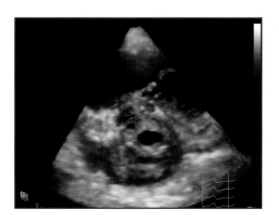

Figure 8-3. Three-dimensional data set of rheumatic mitral valve as viewed from the left atrium, showing the characteristic "fish mouth" appearance of the rheumatic mitral orifice. This appearance results from fusion of the mitral commissures, with mediolateral narrowing of the orifice.

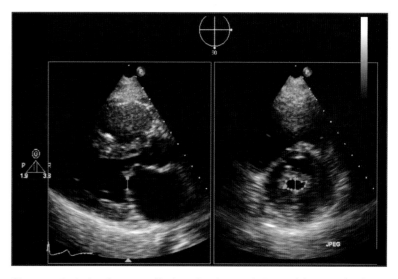

Figure 8-4. A simultaneous display of orthogonal views of the mitral valve is possible by slicing into a three-dimensional data set or, in this instance, by biplane acquisition. This allows alignment along the mitral leaflet tips for accurate planimetry. Note the anteroposterior diameters of the orifice are equal in both views.

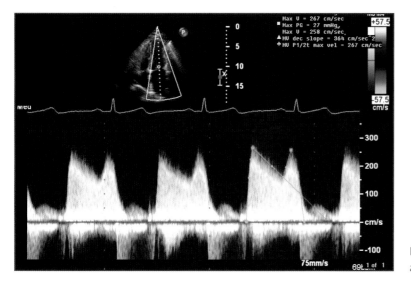

Figure 8-5. Pressure half time measurement for calculation of mitral valve area in mitral stenosis is shown.

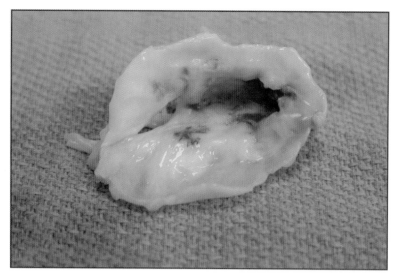

Figure 8-6. An excised rheumatic mitral valve is shown, as viewed from the left atrium. There has been extensive fibrosis of the orifice, especially from the posteromedial commissure (*right side*), resulting in significant narrowing of the mitral orifice.

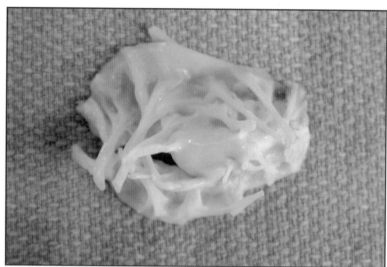

Figure 8-7. An excised rheumatic mitral valve as viewed from the LV is shown. The subvalvular chords are thickened and fibrotic.

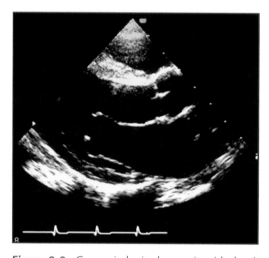

Figure 8-8. Congenital mitral stenosis, with doming of long unthickened leaflets is shown.

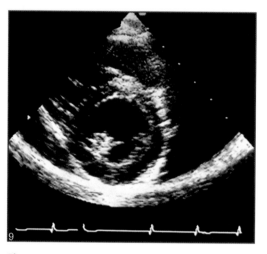

Figure 8-9. Congenital mitral stenosis is shown, with asymmetry of the papillary muscles. This causes the leaflets to be drawn to one side, which in turn causes the diastolic doming.

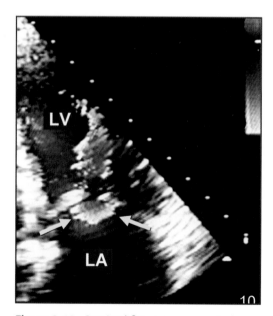

Figure 8-10. Proximal flow convergence is shown, with aliased accelerating mitral inflow. The flow converging towards the orifice area through the valvular funnel is shown (*arrows*) LA—left atrium.

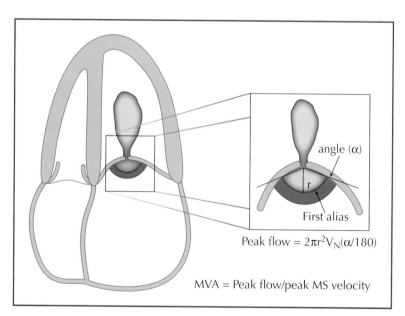

Figure 8-11. Proximal isovelocity surface area calculation of the mitral valve area by continuity is shown, taking into account the angle (α) between the converging leaflets.

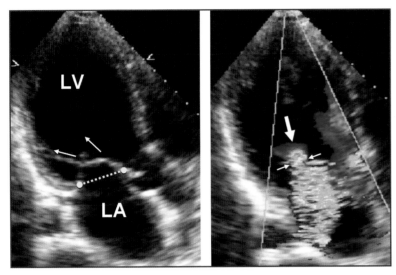

Figure 8-12. Three main flow domains of a mitral regurgitant jet used for quantitative and semiquantitative assessment are shown. Proximal flow convergence (*large arrow*) and vena contracta (*small arrows*) is shown. (*From* Levine and Schwammenthal [1]; with permission). LA—left atrium.

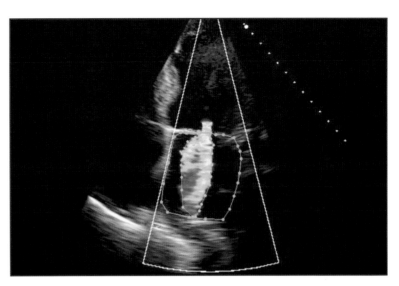

Figure 8-13. Distal jet area and left atrial area measurements for mitral regurgitation assessment is shown.

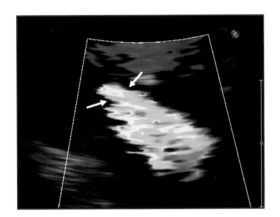

Figure 8-14. Vena contracta measurement for mitral regurgitation assessment: long-axis measure at narrowest neck. Vena contracta width is shown (*arrows*).

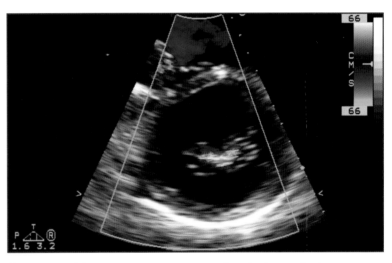

Figure 8-15. Vena contracta measurement for mitral regurgitation assessment: short-axis area.

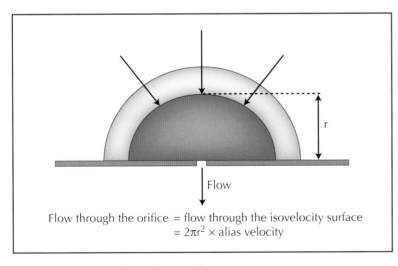

Flow through the orifice = flow through the isovelocity surface
= $2\pi r^2 \times$ alias velocity

Figure 8-16. Proximal isovelocity surface area concept.

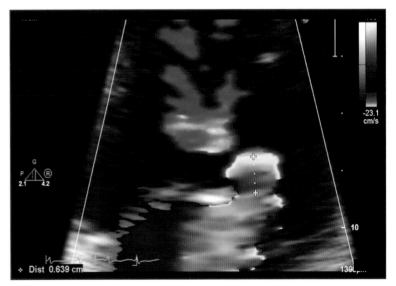

Figure 8-17. The proximal isovelocity surface area (PISA) region has been magnified and baseline shifted to optimize measurement of the radius of the PISA region.

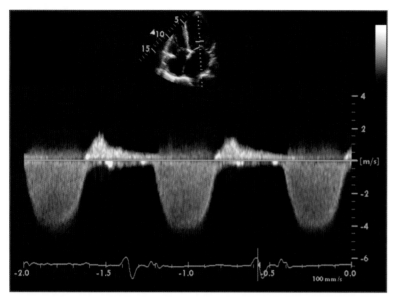

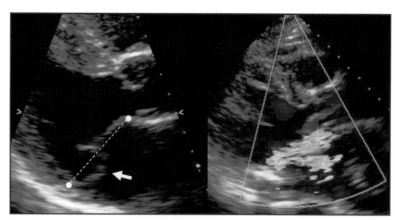

Figure 8-18. Peak instantaneous velocity of the mitral regurgitation jet is obtained by continuous wave velocity for use in calculating effective orifice area.

Figure 8-19. A posterior leaflet mitral valve prolapse in parasternal long-axis views is shown. Posterior mitral leaflet prolapsing (*left panel*, *arrow*) across mitral annular line (*dashed line*), defined by the annular hinge points (*circles*) is shown. Anteriorly directed mitral regurgitation jet due to posterior leaflet prolapse is shown (*right panel*) with another jet, suggesting multiple valve lesions giving rise to multiple areas of coaptation. Mitral valve prolapse is best diagnosed in the parasternal long or apical long-axis views as these views show the most superior points of the saddle-shaped mitral annulus.

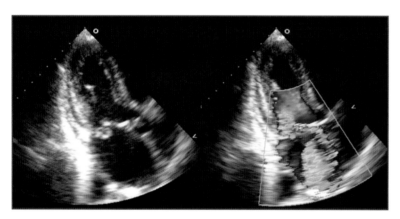

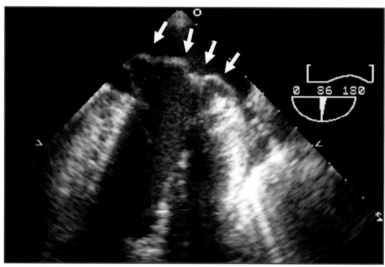

Figure 8-20. Posterior leaflet prolapse in the apical long-axis view is shown.

Figure 8-21. A transesophageal image of a bileaflet mitral valve prolapse is shown. All segments of the mitral leaflets in this view are redundant and billow into the left atrium (*arrows*).

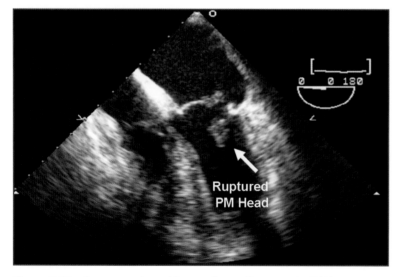

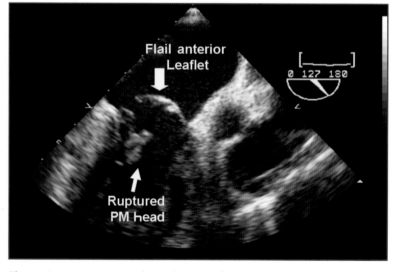

Figure 8-22. A transesophageal image of a papillary muscle (PM) rupture (*arrow*) due to occlusion of the right coronary artery is shown.

Figure 8-23. A transesophageal image of partial flail of the anterior mitral leaflet (*arrow*), which has resulted from papillary muscle (PM) rupture, is shown.

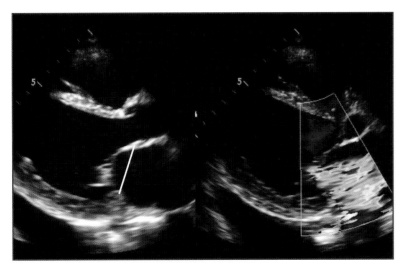

Figure 8-24. Tethering of the mitral leaflets in a dilated LV is shown in the parasternal long-axis view. The leaflet coaptation line occurs apically, apical to the mitral annulus (*left panel, solid line*). Moderate severe mitral regurgitation is also shown (*right panel*).

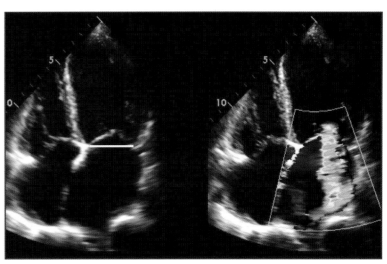

Figure 8-25. Tethering of the mitral leaflets in the apical four-chamber view is shown. The leaflets close apical to the mitral annulus (*left panel, solid line*). Moderate to severe mitral regurgitation extending toward the pulmonary veins is also depicted (*right panel*).

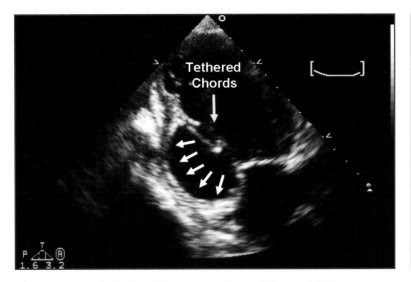

Figure 8-26. An inferobasal LV aneurysm (*arrows*) from an inferior myocardial infarction, which results in papillary muscle displacement and tethering of the mitral chords and leaflets, preventing mitral valve closure, is shown.

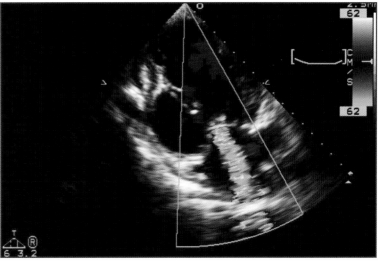

Figure 8-27. Moderate to severe mitral regurgitation that has developed from tethering of the mitral leaflets is shown.

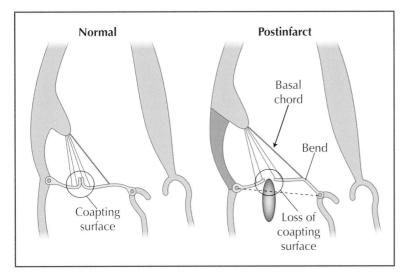

Figure 8-28. The mechanism of functional ischemic mitral regurgitation is shown, with papillary muscle displacement, possibly combined with annular enlargement, tethering the leaflets to restrict their closure.

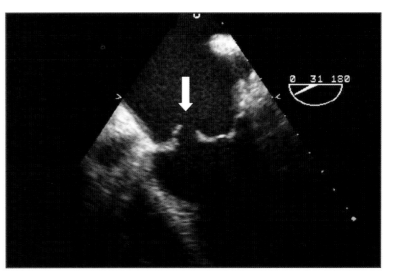

Figure 8-29. A mitral valve anterior leaflet perforation is shown (*arrow*).

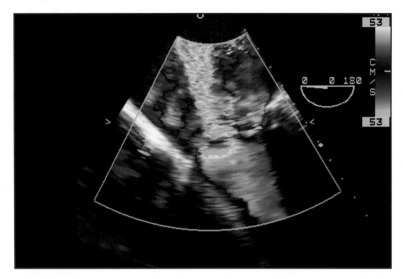

Figure 8-30. Severe mitral regurgitation originating through the leaflet perforation.

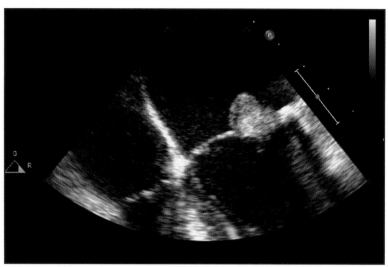

Figure 8-31. A mitral valve tumor on the posterior mitral leaflet is shown.

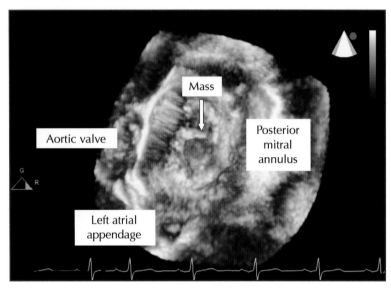

Figure 8-32. A mitral valve tumor as viewed using a three-dimensional dataset is shown. The mitral valve is viewed from the left atrium. The tumor (seen within the orifice) is localized to the middle scallop of the posterior mitral leaflet.

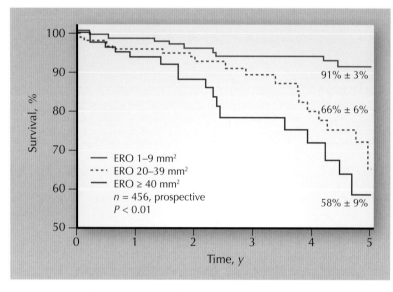

Figure 8-33. Adverse prognosis of asymptomatic mitral regurgitation (MR) quantitatively relates to severity of MR by effective orifice area (ERO). (*Adapted from* Enriquez-Sarano *et al.* [2].)

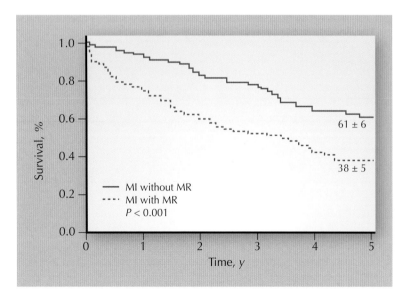

Figure 8-34. Adverse prognosis of ischemic mitral regurgitation (MR) relative to that of myocardial infarction (MI) alone is shown. (*Adapted from* Grigioni *et al.* [3].)

References

1. Levine RA, Schwammenthal E: Ischemic Mitral regurgitation on the threshold of a solution: from paradoxes to unifying concepts. *Circulation* 2005, 112:745–758.

2. Enriquez-Sarano M, Avierinos JF, Messika-Zeitoun D, *et al.*: Quantitative determinants of the outcome of asymptomatic mitral regurgitation. *N Engl J Med* 2005, 352:875–883.

3. Grigioni F, Enriquez-Sarano M, Zehr KJ, *et al.*: Ischemic mitral regurgitation: long-term outcome and prognostic implications with quantitative Doppler assessment. *Circulation* 2001, 103:1759–1764.

Suggested Reading

Aklog L, Filsoufi F, Flores KQ, *et al.*: Does coronary artery bypass grafting alone correct moderate ischemic mitral regurgitation? *Circulation* 2001, 104(Suppl I):68–75.

Buck T, Mucci RA, Guerrero JL, *et al.*: The power-velocity integral at the vena contracta: a new method for direct quantification of regurgitant volume flow. *Circulation* 2000, 102:1053–1061.

Cape EG, Yoganathan AP, Weyman AE, Levine RA: Adjacent solid boundaries alter the size of regurgitant jets on color Doppler flow maps. *J Am Coll Cardiol* 1991, 17:1094–1102.

Enriquez-Sarano M, Bailey KR, Seward JB, *et al.*: Quantitative Doppler assessment of valvular regurgitation. *Circulation* 1993, 87:841–848.

Enriquez-Sarano M, Seward JB, Bailey KR, Tajik AJ: Effective regurgitant orifice area: a noninvasive Doppler development of an old hemodynamic concept. *J Am Coll Cardiol* 1994, 23:443–451.

Grayburn PA, Smith MD, Gurley JC, *et al.*: Effect of aortic regurgitation on the assessment of mitral valve orifice area by Doppler pressure half time in mitral stenosis. *Am J Cardiol* 1987, 60:322–326.

Grigioni F, Enriquez-Sarano M, Zehr KJ, *et al.*: Ischemic mitral regurgitation: long-term outcome and prognostic implications with quantitative Doppler assessment. *Circulation* 2001, 103:1759–1764.

Hall SA, Brickner ME, Willett DL, *et al.*: Assessment of mitral regurgitation severity by Doppler color flow mapping of the vena contracta. *Circulation* 1997, 95:636–642.

Hatle L, Angelsen B, Tromsdal A: Non-invasive assessment of atrioventricular pressure half time by Doppler ultrasound. *Circulation* 1979, 60:1096–1104.

He S, Fontaine AA, Schwammenthal E, *et al.*: An integrated mechanism for functional mitral regurgitation: leaflet restriction vs. coapting force: in vitro studies. *Circulation* 1997, 96:1826–1834.

Helmcke F, Nanda NC, Hsiung MC, *et al.*: Color Doppler assessment of mitral regurgitation with orthogonal planes. *Circulation* 1987, 75:175–183.

Hung J, Guerrero JL, Handschumacher MD, *et al.*: Reverse ventricular remodeling reduces ischemic mitral regurgitation: echo-guided device application in the beating heart. *Circulation* 2002, 106:2594–2600.

Komeda M, Glasson JR, Bolger AF, *et al.*: Geometric determinants of ischemic mitral regurgitation. *Circulation* 1997, 96(9 Suppl):II128–II133.

Kono T, Sabbah HN, Rosman H, *et al.*: Mechanism of functional mitral regurgitation during acute myocardial ischemia. *J Am Coll Cardiol* 1992, 19:1101–1105.

Kron IL, Green GR, Cope JT: Surgical relocation of the posterior papillary muscle in chronic ischemic mitral regurgitation. *Ann Thorac Surg* 2002, 74:600–601.

Kumanohoso T, Otsuji Y, Yoshifuku S, *et al.*: Mechanism of higher incidence of ischemic mitral regurgitation in patients with inferior myocardial infarction: quantitative analysis of left ventricular and mitral valve geometry in 103 patients with prior myocardial infarction. *J Thorac Cardiovasc Surg* 2003, 125:1135–1143.

Lancellotti P, Lebrun F, Pierard LA: Determinants of exercise-induced changes in mitral regurgitation in patients with coronary artery disease and left ventricular dysfunction. *J Am Coll Cardiol* 2003, 42:1921–1928.

Lancellotti P, Troisfontaines P, Toussaint AC, Pierard LA: Prognostic importance of exercise-induced changes in mitral regurgitation in patients with chronic ischemic left ventricular dysfunction. *Circulation* 2003, 108:1713–1717.

Levine RA, Lefebvre X, Guerrero JL, *et al.*: Unifying concepts of mitral valve function and disease: SAM, prolapse and ischemic mitral regurgitation. *J Cardiol* 1994, 24(Suppl 38):157–169.

Liel-Cohen N, Guerrero JL, Otsuji Y, *et al.*: Design of a new surgical approach for ventricular remodeling to relieve ischemic mitral regurgitation: insights from 3-dimensional echocardiography. *Circulation* 2000, 101:2756–2763.

Llaneras MR, Nance ML, Streicher JT, *et al.*: Pathogenesis of ischemic mitral insufficiency. *J Thorac Cardiovasc Surg* 1993, 105:439–443.

Mele D, Vandervoort P, Palacios I, *et al.*: Proximal jet size by Doppler color flow mapping predicts the severity of mitral regurgitation: clinical studies. *Circulation* 1995, 91:746–754.

Menicanti L, Di Donato M, Frigiola A, *et al.*: Ischemic mitral regurgitation: intraventricular papillary muscle imbrication without mitral ring during left ventricular restoration. *J Thorac Cardiovasc Surg* 2002, 123:1041–1050.

Messas E, Guerrero JL, Handschumacher MD, *et al.*: Chordal cutting: a new therapeutic approach for ischemic mitral regurgitation. *Circulation* 2001, 104:1958–1963.

Messas E, Guerrero JL, Handschumacher MD, *et al.*: Paradoxic decrease in ischemic mitral regurgitation with papillary muscle dysfunction: insights from three-dimensional and contrast echocardiography with strain rate measurement. *Circulation* 2001, 104:1952–1957.

Messas E, Pouzet B, Touchot B, *et al.*: Efficacy of chordal cutting to relieve chronic persistent ischemic mitral regurgitation. *Circulation* 2003, 108(Suppl 1):II111–II115.

Miyatake K, Izumi S, Okamoto M, *et al.*: Semiquantitative grading of severity of mitral regurgitation by real-time two-dimensional Doppler flow imaging technique. *J Am Coll Cardiol* 1986, 7:82–88.

Moainie SL, Guy TS, Gorman JH III, *et al.*: Infarct restraint attenuates remodeling and reduces chronic ischemic mitral regurgitation after postero-lateral infarction. *Ann Thorac Surg* 2002, 74:444–449.

Otsuji Y, Handschumacher MD, Schwammenthal E, *et al.*: Insights from three-dimensional echocardiography into the mechanism of functional mitral regurgitation: direct in vivo demonstration of altered leaflet tethering geometry. *Circulation* 1997, 96:1999–2008.

Recusani F, Bargiggia GS, Yoganathan AP, *et al.*: A new method for quantification of regurgitant flow rate using color flow imaging of the flow convergence region proximal to a discrete orifice: an in vitro study. *Circulation* 1991, 83:594–604.

Sagie A, Freitas N, Chen MH, *et al.*: Echocardiographic assessment of mitral stenosis and its associated valvular lesions in 205 patients and lack of association with mitral valve prolapse. *J Am Soc Echocardiogr* 1997, 10:141–148.

Sagie A, Freitas N, Padial LR, *et al.*: Doppler echocardiographic assessment of long-term progression of mitral stenosis in 103 patients: valve area and right heart disease. *J Am Coll Cardiol* 1996, 28:472–479.

Sagie A, Schwammenthal E, Newell JB, *et al.*: Significant tricuspid regurgitation is a marker for adverse outcome in patients undergoing percutaneous balloon mitral valvuloplasty. *J Am Coll Cardiol* 1994, 24:696–702.

Sagie A, Schwammenthal E, Palacios IF, *et al.*: Significant tricuspid regurgitation does not resolve after percutaneous balloon mitral valvotomy. *J Thorac Cardiovasc Surg* 1994, 108:727–735.

Schwammenthal E, Chen C, Benning F, *et al.*: Dynamics of mitral regurgitant flow and orifice area in different forms of mitral regurgitation: physiologic application of the proximal flow convergence method: clinical data and experimental testing. *Circulation* 1994, 90:307–322.

Schwammenthal E, Chen C, Giesler M, *et al.*: New method for accurate calculation of regurgitant flow rate based on analysis of Doppler color flow maps of the proximal flow field: validation in a canine model of mitral regurgitation with initial application in patients. *J Am Coll Cardiol* 1996, 27:161–172.

Schwammenthal E, Nakatani S, He S, *et al.*: Mechanism of mitral regurgitation in hypertrophic cardiomyopathy: mismatch of posterior to anterior leaflet length and mobility. *Circulation* 1998, 98:856–865.

Shiota T, Jones M, Teien DE, *et al.*: Evaluation of mitral regurgitation using a digitally determined color Doppler flow convergence "centerline" acceleration method: studies in an animal model with quantified mitral regurgitation. *Circulation* 1994, 89:2879–2887.

Tahta SA, Oury JH, Maxwell JM, *et al.*: Outcome after mitral valve repair for functional ischemic mitral regurgitation. *J Heart Valve Dis* 2002, 11:11–18.

Thomas JD, Wilkins GT, Choong CY, *et al.*: Inaccuracy of mitral pressure half time immediately after percutaneous mitral valvotomy: dependence on transmitral gradient and left atrial and ventricular compliances. *Circulation* 1988, 78:980–983.

Utsunomiya T, Ogawa T, Doshi R, *et al.*: Doppler color flow "proximal isovelocity surface area" method for estimating volume flow rate: effects of orifice shape and machine factors. *J Am Coll Cardiol* 1991, 17:1103–1111. [Published erratum appears in *J Am Coll Cardiol* 1993, 21:1537.]

Vandervoort PM, Rivera JM, Mele D, *et al.*: Application of color Doppler flow mapping to calculate effective regurgitant orifice area: an in vitro study with initial clinical observations. *Circulation* 1993, 88:1150–1156.

Yoshida K, Yoshikawa J, Yamaura Y, *et al.*: Value of acceleration flows and regurgitant jet direction by color Doppler flow mapping in the evaluation of mitral valve prolapse. *Circulation* 1990, 81:879–885. [Published erratum appears in *Circulation* 1990, 82:1547.]

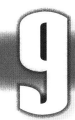

Echocardiography in Valvular Heart Disease: Aortic Valve Disease

Hector I. Michelena, Sunil V. Mankad, and Maurice Enriquez-Sarano

Diseases of the heart valves are frequent, with a national prevalence of 2.5% [1]. They are strongly linked to aging, affecting 13% of patients 75 years of age or older and being driven primarily by aortic stenosis and mitral regurgitation. Patients affected with moderate or severe valve diseases have less than expected long-term survival [1]. Natural history studies indicate that over 80% of patients presenting with symptoms from severe aortic stenosis will be dead within 4 years [2] without surgical intervention. Asymptomatic patients presenting with severe aortic stenosis have a risk of sudden death of 1% per year and most become symptomatic within 5 years [3]. The most common form of aortic stenosis is calcification with prominent calcium deposition in the cusps, which renders them restricted to opening in systole. This so called degenerative form originates as an active inflammatory process with similarities to atherosclerosis [4], which eventually lead to bone formation through an active regulated process associated with an osteoblast-like phenotype [5]. Furthermore, classic cardiovascular risk factors are associated with the development of calcific aortic stenosis [6]. Congenitally abnormal aortic valves, such as unicuspid and bicuspid aortic valves, incur accelerated aortic degeneration, leading to stenosis. Conversely, rheumatic diseases result in commissural fusion followed by valve stenosis, but a common pattern of all forms of aortic stenosis in the adult is the valve calcification, which leads to increased valve rigidity and obstruction to flow.

Similarly, three-fourths of patients with significant aortic regurgitation incur death or corrective surgery within 10 years [7], particularly those with symptoms, decreased ejection fraction, or LV enlargement. Aortic regurgitation results from primary abnormalities of the aortic cusps (ie, bicuspid aortic valve) or secondary to dilatation of the aortic root (ie, Marfan's syndrome), rendering cusp coaptation insufficient. Rheumatic aortic regurgitation results from postinflammatory retraction of leaflets, causing incomplete coaptation. Endocarditic lesions result in aortic regurgitation through the destruction of valvular tissue, which causes perforation or loss of valve support and flail leaflet.

Currently, the sole available definitive treatment for severe aortic valve dysfunction is surgical intervention by repair or replacement. Timely surgical correction in appropriate patients prevents mortality and limits morbidity. Thus, accurate stratification of severity and identification of indicators for intervention are paramount, not only in selecting appropriate patients and procedures, but also in preventing unnecessary interventions. Surgery is not devoid of risk. Echocardiography offers high temporal spatial resolution imaging, which allows noninvasive and comprehensive real time evaluation of aortic valve morphology and function, and of the cardiac consequences of valve dysfunction. Continuous and pulsed-wave Doppler interrogation renders qualitative and quantitative assessment of valve hemodynamics highly accurate and reproducible. Thus, echocardiography represents the primary mode of aortic valve disease evaluation. This chapter contains a series of figures that illustrate the key morphological features and hemodynamic principles of the echocardiographic assessment of aortic valve disease.

Morphology and Congenital Abnormalities

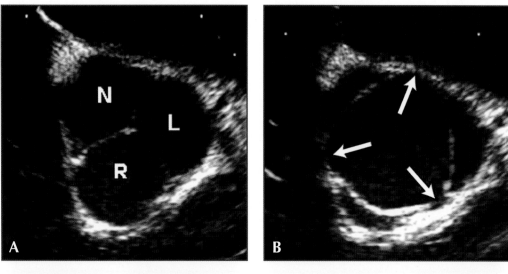

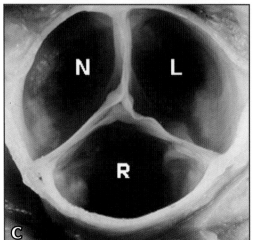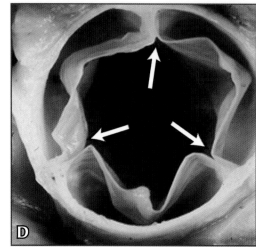

Figure 9-1. Normal tricuspid aortic valve. The figures show transesophagel echocardiographic (**A** and **B**) and anatomic (**C** and **D**) basal short-axis images in diastole (**A** and **C**) and systole (**B** and **D**) of a morphologically normal tricuspid aortic valve. Note that the normal aortic valve cusps are thin, pliable, have excellent coaptation during diastole, and demonstrate wide excursion in systole. The aortic valve commissures are indicated (*arrows*). The functional geometry of the trileaflet aortic valve allows for the total length of the free edges to equal the circumference and be greater than the inter-commissural distances. This permits the coaptation to be wrinkle-free, with even pressure distribution in systole and diastole [8]. L—left coronary cusp; N—noncoronary cusp; R—right coronary cusp.

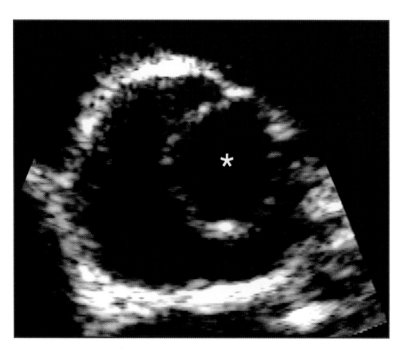

Figure 9-2. Unicuspid aortic valve. The figure is a short-axis transesophageal echocardiographic image of a unicuspid, acommissural aortic valve during systole. The orifice of the aortic valve is indicated (*asteric*). Unicuspid aortic valve was the underlying etiology of aortic valve stenosis in 1.5% of cases resulting in surgical aortic valve replacement in a large published series from a tertiary medical center [9] and 6% in a large surgical pathology study [10]. Patients with a unicuspid aortic valve may develop stenosis of the valve, requiring surgical intervention within the first few decades of life [10].

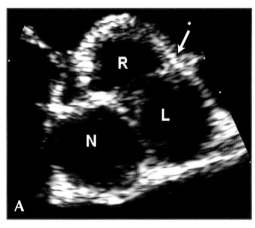
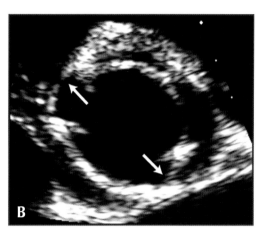
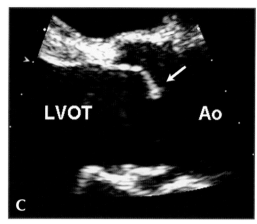

Figure 9-3. Typical bicuspid aortic valve. Corresponding short-axis transthoracic echocardiographic images depicting a normal functioning, minimally degenerated typical bicuspid aortic valve in diastole (**A**) and systole (**B**). This represents the typical anteroposterior orientation of the cusps (**B**), with right coronary cusp (R) and left coronary cusp (L) fusion and a visible raphe between them (**A**, *arrow*). The commissures (hinge points) are depicted by the arrows (**B**, *arrows*) and are usually at "10 o'clock and 4 o'clock." The long-axis transthoracic echocardiographic image of a typical bicuspid aortic valve is shown (**C**) with characteristic doming in systole of the cojoined cusp (*arrow*). A bicuspid aortic valve is a common congenital heart abnormality, affecting 0.5% to 2% of the population [11–13], with male predominance. The most common complication is stenosis of the valve, especially in men [14], but aortic regurgitation [15], endocarditis [16], and complications of the aorta also occur [12]. Ao—aorta; LVOT—LV outflow tract; N—noncoronary cusp.

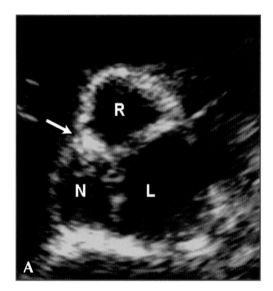
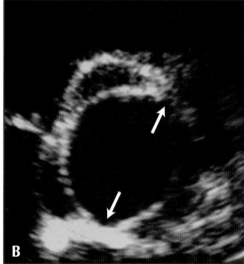

Figure 9-4. Atypical bicuspid aortic valve. Short-axis transthoracic echocardiographic images of a normally functioning, minimally degenerated atypical bicuspid aortic valve in diastole (**A**) and systole (**B**) with fusion of the right coronary cusp (R) and noncoronary cusp (N) and a visible raphe (**A**, *arrow*) in diastole. The raphe may lead to confusion with a tricuspid valve in diastole [17,18]. The combination of eccentric valve closure in long-axis M-mode and "football" shape opening in systole, as well as eccentric posteriorly directed aortic regurgitation are clues to the diagnosis. Note the commissures at "1 o'clock and 7 o'clock" (**B**, *arrows*), typical of an atypical bicuspid valve. There is a third type of bicuspid aortic valve with fusion of the left coronary cusps (L) and N; however, it is very rare [19].

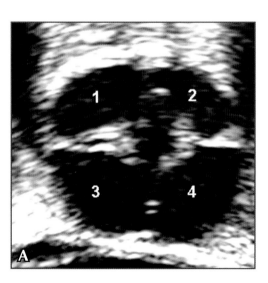
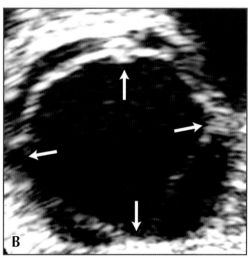

Figure 9-5. Transesophageal short-axis images of a quadricuspid aortic valve in diastole (**A**) and systole (**B**). Note the "four-leaf clover" appearance of the leaflets (numbered in **A**) and the commissures marked (**B**, *arrows*). Although the prevalence by autopsy review is approximately 0.008% [20], a recent echocardiographic database review identified the prevalence to be 0.013% to 0.043%, depending on the years studied [21]. Although rare by either review method, significant aortic regurgitation due to cusp malcoaptation may not be uncommon, and valve replacement may be necessary by the fifth or sixth decade of life [22].

Valve Attachments

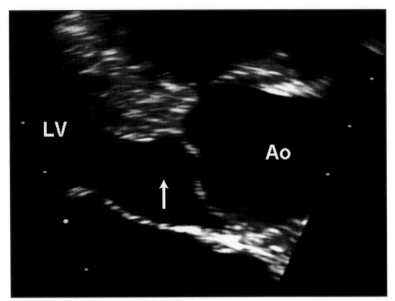

Figure 9-6. Transesophageal echocardiographic long-axis image of the aortic valve, demonstrating a Lambl's excrescence (fibrous strand) on the aortic valve (*arrow*) in diastole. Described in 1856 by Lambl, these excrescences are fine thread-like strands arising on the line of closure or contact surface of heart valves. They usually measure 2 mm or less in width and 10 mm or less in length and are most commonly present in left heart valves [23]. When present in the aortic valve, they are typically seen in the LV outflow tract in diastole, as shown. Pathologically, they are acellular strands of collagen and elastic fibrils covered by a single layer of endothelium. Most often, they are of no clinical consequence and are not associated with cardioembolic events, although this is not completely understood [23,24]. Ao—aorta.

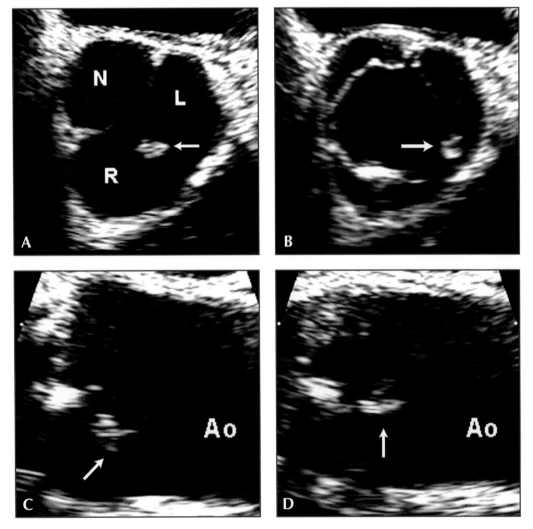

Figure 9-7. Transesophageal echocardiographic images of a papillary fibroelastoma attached to the free edge of the left coronary cusp (L) of the aortic valve. The upper panels depict short-axis images during diastole (**A**) and systole (**B**), with the head of the fibroelastoma (*arrows*). Most often these benign tumors are solitary and of small size (usually < 10 mm diameter but can be up to 21 mm) and their pathology is similar to the Lambl's excrescence [25]. The tumor typically arises from the middle portion of the valve leaflets, as opposed to the closure line, as is the case with fibrous strands [26]. These tumors may be highly mobile when a stalk is present. The lower panels (**C** and **D**) depict the motion during diastole and discernible stalk, usually displaying a "frond-like" appearance (pom-pom or sea anemone) with high-frequency oscillations during the cardiac cycle. Cardioembolic events are associated with the presence of these attachments [25–27]. Surgical removal is generally recommended for large fibroelastomas (> 10 mm), which are highly mobile [27].

Endocarditis and Its Complications

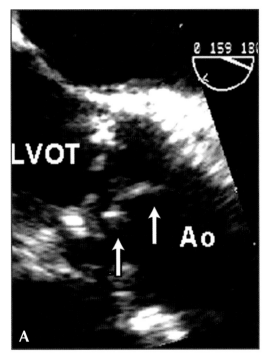

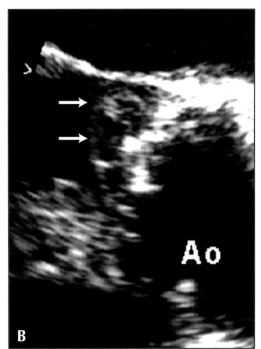

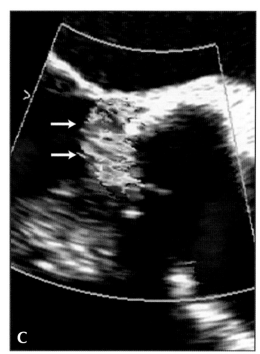

Figure 9-8. Transesophageal images of aortic valve endocarditis. Systolic protrusion of "fresh" vegetations (**A**, *arrows*) into the aorta (Ao) in systole is shown. Cusp-associated mycotic aneurysm that prolapses (**B**, *arrows*) into the LV outflow tract (LVOT) in diastole, and offers containment for aortic regurgitation, is shown (**C**, *arrows*). Vegetations are discrete masses of echogenic material adherent at some point to a leaflet and distinct in character from it [28]. Their texture is that of gray scale reflectance of myocardium, especially when fresh as opposed to healed (*ie*, when they are usually calcified). These vegetations are usually lobulated and amorphous, displaying chaotic and "orbiting" movement, and can cause multiple complications, such as fistula, abscess, pseudoaneurysm, and aneurysm of surrounding structures and valves. Highly mobile vegetations that are greater than 15 mm in size have been strongly associated with embolization potential, as defined by echocardiography [29]. Sensitivity of transthoracic echocardiography for detection of vegetations is 30% to 63%, whereas transesophageal sensitivity is 87% to 100% [30]. This phenomenon is mostly related to the higher resolution of transesophageal echocardiography. The specificity is greater than 90% for both modalities.

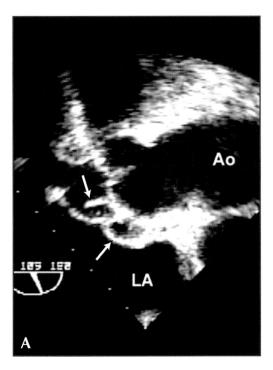

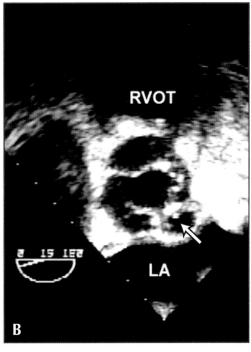

Figure 9-9. Aortic endocarditis with abscess of the intervalvular fibrosa. Shown are transesophageal images of a patient with a healed vegetation calcified (**A**, *upper arrow*) and aorto-mitral curtain abscess cavity (**A**, *lower arrow*) as sequelae of infective endocarditis in the long-axis plane (**A**) and short-axis plane (**B**, *arrow*). Endocarditis of the aortic valve is most commonly associated with abscess formation, which carries a poor prognosis and is usually caused by *Staphylococcus aureus* infection [31]. A transesophageal echocardiogram has a sensitivity of 87% for detection of abscess versus 29% for a transthoracic echocardiogram. Complications of aortic valve endocarditis as detected by transesophageal echocardiography have been reported and include intervalvular fibrosa abscess, aneurysm, and perforation, often with prominent involvement of the anterior mitral valve leaflet [32]. Ao—aorta; LA—left atrium; RVOT—RV outflow tract. (*Images courtesy of* J Oh, MD.)

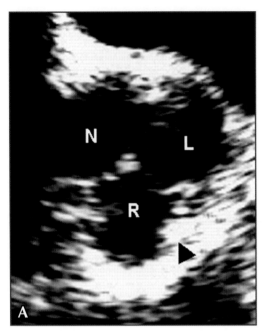
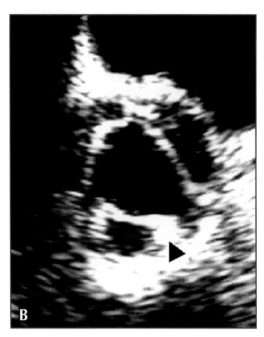

Figure 9-10. Shown are short-axis transesophageal echocardiographic images in diastole (**A**) and systole (**B**) depicting aortic sclerosis. A focal calcification nodule is indicated (*arrowheads*). Note the thickening of the cusp edges in systole and the wide opening of the valve. Aortic sclerosis is defined as focal areas of increased echogenicity and thickening of the aortic valve leaflets without restriction of leaflet motion [33]. Approximately one out of four patients over 65 years of age is affected and, although it does not cause symptoms, it often produces a soft systolic ejection heart murmur. Because risk factors for coronary artery disease (*eg*, smoking, hypertension, dyslipidemia) appear to also be risk factors for the development of aortic sclerosis, it is not surprising that its presence is associated with an increased risk of heart attack and death [33]. Thus, identification of aortic sclerosis may be a marker of subclinical atherosclerosis and is important in targeting patients for more aggressive risk factor modification. L—left coronary cusp; N—noncoronary cusp; R—right coronary cusp.

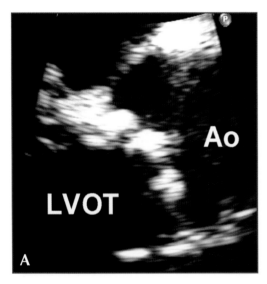
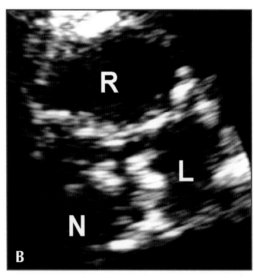
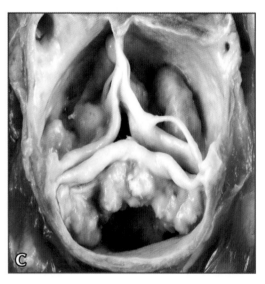

Figure 9-11. Long-axis (**A**) and short-axis (**B**) transthoracic echocardiographic systolic images in severe calcific aortic valve stenosis. Note the heavy calcification and thickening of the leaflets with a markedly reduced orifice during systole, which displays a stellate or "star-like" opening. When there are heavy calcific deposits present on all three aortic valve cusps in an elderly patient, the term *Mönckeberg senile calcific aortic stenosis* has been used. This term suggests degeneration as the primary mechanism underlying the disease; however, an underlying active inflammatory process with similarities to atherosclerosis [4] has been proven to exist. A representative pathologic correlation specimen is displayed, showing large calcific deposits along the body of the leaflets, which tends to spare the free edges, creating a "stellate" opening (**C**). Ao—aorta; L—left coronary cusp; LVOT—LV outflow tract, N—noncoronary cusp; R—right coronary cusp.

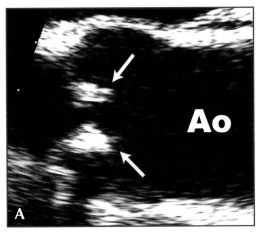 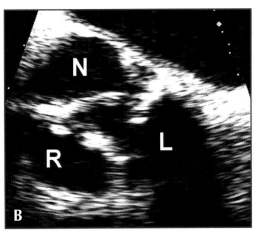 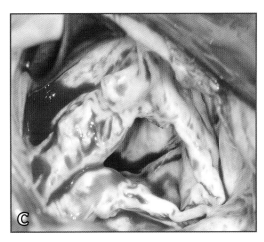

Figure 9-12. Intraoperative transesophageal echocardiographic images of a patient with postinflammatory, rheumatic aortic valve disease. Thickening of the leaflet tips (free edges) is evident in the long-axis view shown in systole (**A**, *arrows*) with marked commissural fusion and thickening demonstrated in the diastolic short-axis image (**B**). Note that commissural fusion creates a triangular ankylosed opening with severe malcoaptation in diastole, which results in severe central aortic regurgitation. The excellent intraoperative pathologic correlation is demonstrated with severely thickened valve and completely fused commissures (**C**). This appearance can be caused by other inflammatory conditions, such as autoimmune diseases. Although rheumatic valvular heart disease has become less frequent in developed countries over the last 50 years, it remains a very important cause of valvular heart disease in developing countries [34]. L—left coronary cusp; N—noncoronary cusp; R—right coronary cusp.

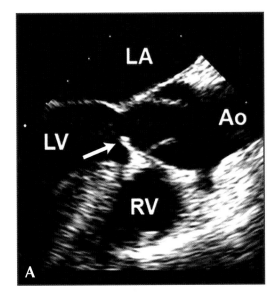 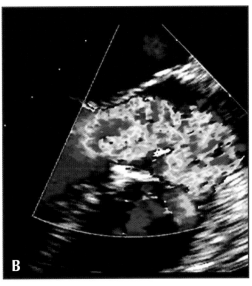

Figure 9-13. Shown are systolic transesophageal images of an 18-year-old patient with symptomatic discrete subaortic membrane (**A**, *arrow*) causing severe subaortic obstruction, which required surgery. Note the color Doppler turbulence that originates at the subaortic membrane site in systole (**B**). Subaortic membranes can be discrete (most commonly short segment), or tunnel type (long segment). They may be congenital or acquired, and they tend to be progressive in severity regardless of their nature. They are also known to cause dysfunction of the aortic valve, especially aortic regurgitation. For that reason, some groups advocate their surgical excision early in the disease process, before severe obstruction occurs [35]. In some cases, subaortic obstruction may recur and this may be prevented by recognizing and surgically treating other associated abnormalities at the time of surgery [36]. Common associated abnormalities are anomalous septal insertion of mitral valve, accessory mitral valve tissue, anomalous papillary muscles and anomalous muscular bands. Ao—aorta; LA—left atrium. (*Images courtesy of P. O'Leary, MD.*)

Aortic Stenosis Severity Assessment

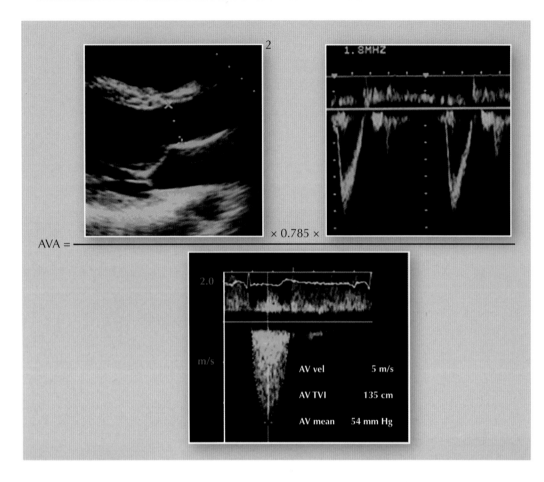

AV vel   5 m/s

AV TVI   135 cm

AV mean   54 mm Hg

Figure 9-14. Conservation of mass principle. In a noncompressible fluid system such as blood, flow is the same at any point. Thus, $area_1 \times$ time velocity integral $(TVI)_1 = area_2 \times TVI_2$. This is the "continuity equation." Flow (cm^3) = area (cm^2) $\times$ length traveled by the volume per beat (cm). The length traveled by the volume per beat is the TVI, obtained by integration of the area under the curve of the Doppler spectral envelope. Area = πr^2 = $\pi \times (diameter/2)^2$ = $diameter^2 \times \pi/4$ = $diameter^2$ $\times$ 0.785. The diagram shows how to calculate the aortic valve area (AVA) by multiplying the square of the LV outflow tract (LVOT) diameter obtained in the parasternal long-axis view by 0.785 and then by the TVI calculated by integrating the area under the curve (black-white interface) of the LVOT pulsed-wave spectral Doppler on the apical three-chamber view. This is then divided by the TVI of the continuous spectral Doppler signal through the aortic valve. Care must be taken when placing the pulse-wave sample volume near the aortic valve to avoid the high velocity flow convergence laminar flow area that precedes the aortic valve. This would cause overestimation of the AVA (underestimation of the severity of stenosis). This is achieved by placing the sample volume 0.5 to 1 cm before the aortic valve [37].

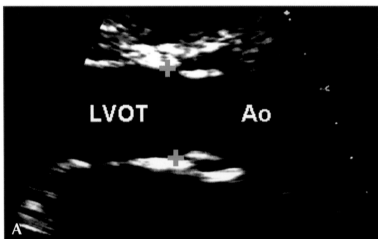

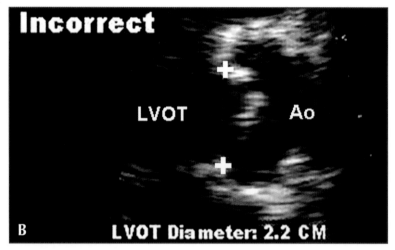

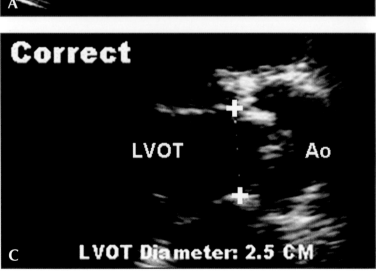

Figure 9-15. Annular diameter measurement. **A,** Appropriate measurement of the LV outflow tract (LVOT) diameter. This is made during early systole from the junction of the aortic leaflets with the septal endocardium to the junction of the leaflet with the mitral valve posteriorly, using inner edge to inner edge, perpendicular to the LVOT (*green calipers*). The largest of three to five measurements should be taken because the inherent error of the tomographic plane is to underestimate the annulus diameter [37]. **B,** Incorrect LVOT diameter measurement is indicated (*white calipers*); poorly optimized image with uncertain visualization of aortic valve cusp insertion points. **C,** Correct measurement of LVOT diameter (*white calipers*) on the same patient with an optimized image that offers adequate visualization of cusp insertion points. There is a tendency to underestimate the LVOT diameter such that the greatest perpendicular measurement should be taken. Because the diameter is squared, small errors in measurement lead to large miscalculations of the aortic valve area. Ao—aorta.

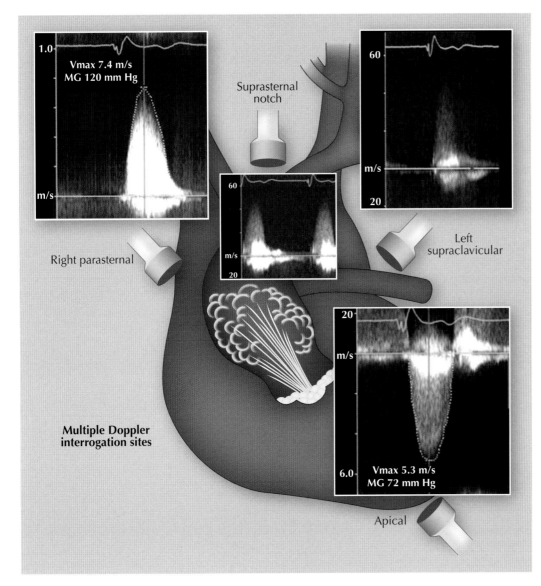

Figure 9-16. The determination of the aortic valve time velocity integral (TVI) should be carried out with a dedicated nonimaging probe with continuous wave Doppler. The shown scheme represents the different anatomic positions to sample for the maximal TVI of the aortic valve. The angle between the systolic flow and the beam should be less than 20° [37] in order to prevent severe underestimation of the aortic valve TVI, which is one the most common errors in stenosis evaluation (underestimation of severity). The case shown is that of an elderly woman with critical calcific aortic stenosis. Note that the maximal mean gradients (MG) are obtained in the apical- and right-parasternal views; however, the right parasternal mean gradient (120 mm Hg) almost doubles the apical gradient (72 mm Hg). Note the suprasternal and left supraclavicular positions. The right supraclavicular position is not depicted.

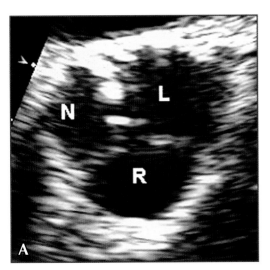
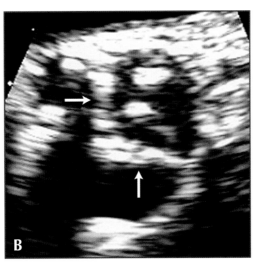
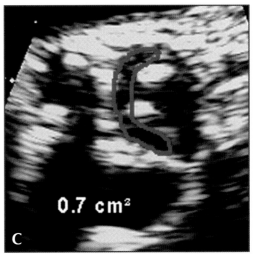

Figure 9-17. Shown are the transesophageal basal short-axis images of a severely calcified aortic valve in diastole (**A**) and systole (**B**). The arrows indicate the immobile border of the fused and ankylosed/immobile right coronary cusp (R) and noncoronary cusp (N). The left coronary cusp (L) shows prominent calcific nodules, and the systolic excursion is severely limited. The planimetry of the anatomic orifice of the valve in systole is represented (**C,** *red outline*), which confirms the critical nature of the stenosis, measuring 0.7 cm². Because of its high image resolution, transesophageal echocardiography (TEE) can assess the anatomical orifice area with direct planimetry of the open valve in systole as shown. However, caution should be exercised when performing this measurement. Previous studies [38,39] have shown an excellent linear correlation between TEE planimetry and valve area calculations by continuity and cardiac catheterization; however, when the Bland-Altman method was applied in a consequent study [40], the agreement between modalities was poor, with systematic overestimation of the orifice by planimetry. Variability in gain settings, degree of valve calcification, and level of tomographic assessment have the potential of causing planimetry measurement errors.

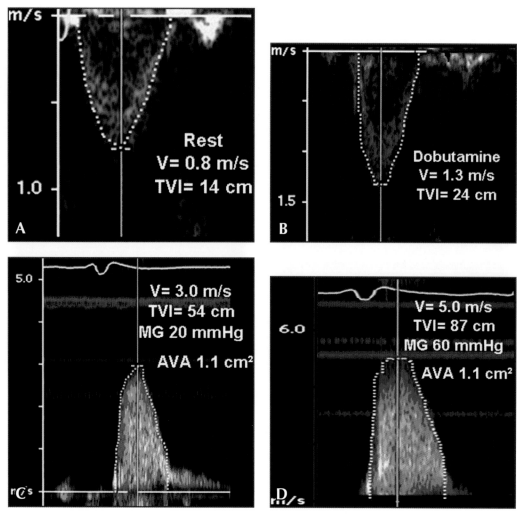

Figure 9-18. LV outflow tract (LVOT) pulsed-wave time velocity integral (TVI) measurements of a patient with low-output low-gradient aortic stenosis at rest and after dobutamine, respectively (**A** and **B**). The patient's ejection fraction (EF) was 25% and increased to 35% during infusion. The increase in TVI from 14 to 24 cm represents more than a 20% increase in stroke volume, which suggests the presence of systolic reserve [41]. The right parasternal nonimaging probe continuous wave Doppler profiles through the aortic valve at rest and after dobutamine, respectively (**C** and **D**). Note that at rest (**C**), the mean gradient (MG) is 20 mm Hg, but this results in a small valve area of 1.1 cm². After dobutamine (**D**), the MG increases to 60 mm Hg and the valve area remains 1.1 cm², confirming the presence of severe aortic stenosis.

The definition of low-gradient low-output aortic stenosis is LV systolic dysfunction (EF ≤ 40%) with a systolic aortic MG of less than 30 to 40 mm Hg and valve area less than or equal to 1 cm² [41–43]. This situation is generally associated with increased operative mortality for aortic valve replacement [42]. If Dobutamine stimulation in up to 20 μg/Kg per min causes an increase in stroke volume greater than 20% with a significant increase in MG and no change in valve area, the aortic stenosis is severe and the systolic dysfunction is likely related to after load mismatch; thus, this patient will derive benefit from aortic valve replacement surgery. When true severe stenosis is present and there is no evidence of systolic reserve, patients still may benefit from aortic valve replacement [44] with improvement of EF after surgery. AVA—aortic valve area; V—velocity.

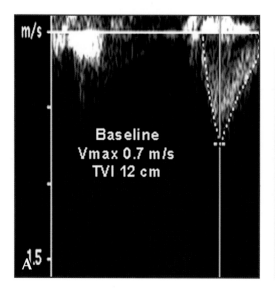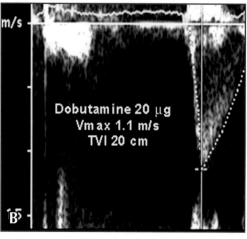

Figure 9-19. Low-output, low-gradient pseudosevere stenosis. Shown are LV outflow tract (LVOT) pulsed-wave time velocity integral (TVI) measurements of a patient with syncope and low-output low-gradient aortic stenosis at rest and after dobutamine, respectively (**A** and **B**). The patient's ejection fraction was 40% and increased to 60% during infusion. The increase in TVI from 14 to 24 cm represents a more than 20% increase in stroke volume, suggesting the presence of systolic reserve [41].

Continued on the next page

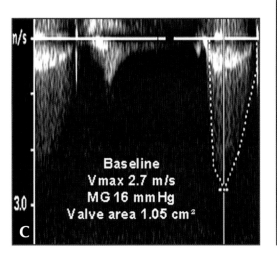

Baseline
Vmax 2.7 m/s
MG 16 mmHg
Valve area 1.05 cm²

C

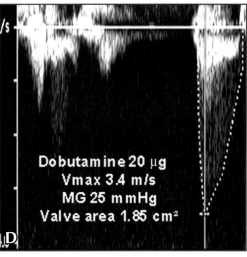

Dobutamine 20 μg
Vmax 3.4 m/s
MG 25 mmHg
Valve area 1.85 cm²

D

E. Aortic Stenosis Severity

Parameter	Mild	Moderate	Severe
Maximal velocity, *m/s*	< 3.0	3.0–4.0	> 4.0
Mean gradient, *mm Hg*	< 25	25–40	> 40
Valve area, *cm²*	> 1.5	1.0–1.5	< 1.0
Valve area index, *cm²/m²*			< 0.6
Dimensionless index			< 0.25
Two-dimensional systolic valve opening	Mildly restricted	Moderately restricted	Severely restricted

Figure 9-19. *(Continued)* The apical nonimaging probe continuous wave Doppler profiles through the aortic valve at rest and after dobutamine, respectively, are represented (**C** and **D**). Note that at rest (**C**), the mean gradient is 16 mm Hg, but results in a small valve area of 1.05 cm². After dobutamine (**D**), the mean gradient increases to 25 mm Hg (nonsignificant increase) and the valve area increases 1.85 cm² (mild stenosis, **E**) confirming the presence of relative or pseudosevere aortic stenosis. This patient's syncope was due to orthostatic hypotension, and his LV dysfunction was due to dilated cardiomyopathy. This patient will clearly not benefit from aortic valve replacement. MG—mean gradient; Vmax—velocity maximum.

Aortic Regurgitation Mechanisms

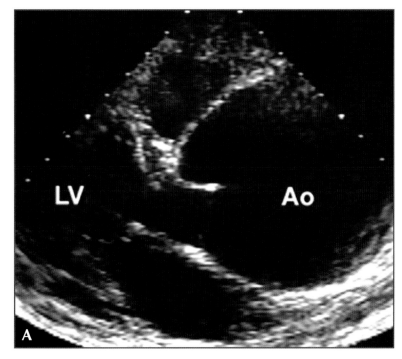

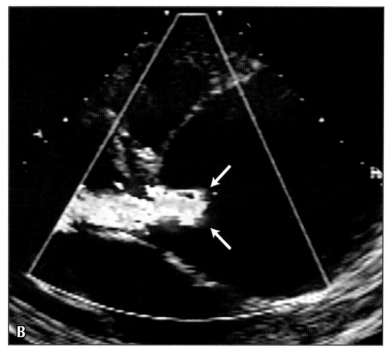

Figure 9-20. Shown are transesophageal echocardiographic images in a patient with severe aortic regurgitation as a result of severe dilatation of the aortic root and ascending aorta in a patient with Marfan's syndrome.

A long-axis image demonstrating complete effacement of the sinotubular ridge secondary to severe dilatation of the ascending aorta is shown (**A**). Color Doppler flow interrogation reveals severe aortic regurgitation (**B**, *arrows*).

Continued on the next page

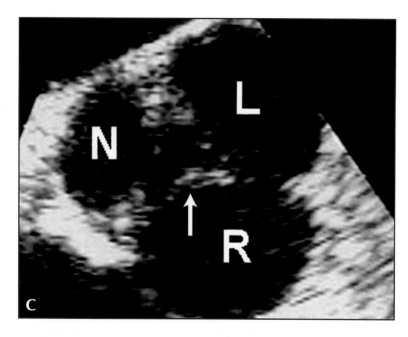

Figure 9-20. (Continued) Complete central failure of leaflet coaptation is shown in the short-axis transesophageal echocardiographic image (**C**, *arrow*). Ao—aorta; L—left coronary cusp; N—noncoronary cusp; R—right coronary cusp.

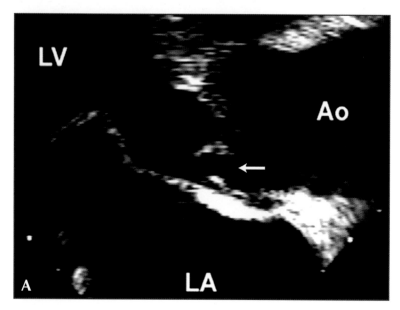

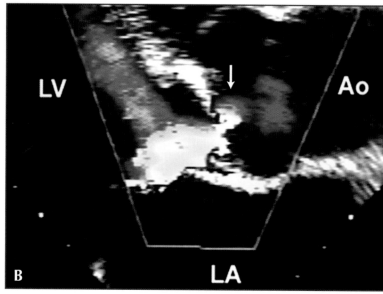

Figure 9-21. Shown is a transesophageal echocardiographic image demonstrating perforation of the aortic valve left coronary leaflet (**A**, *arrow*). Color Doppler flow demonstrates flow through the perforation (**B**), which often results as a complication of previous endocarditis. The color Doppler proximal flow convergence is demonstrated (*arrow*). Ao—aorta; LA—left atrium.

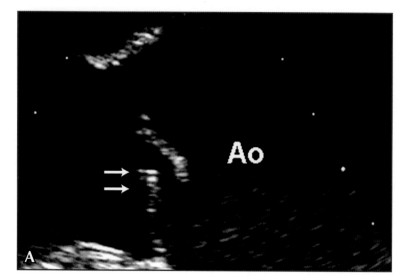

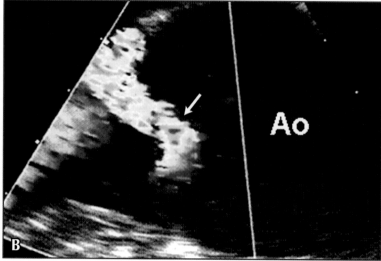

Figure 9-22. This transesophageal long-axis view demonstrates a severely prolapsing right coronary cusp (**A**, *arrows*) as a result of previous endocarditis. The anatomy of the eccentric regurgitant jet is shown (**B**) with its flow convergence, vena contracta area (*arrow*), and eccentric posteriorly directed jet towards the anterior mitral leaflet. Ao—aorta

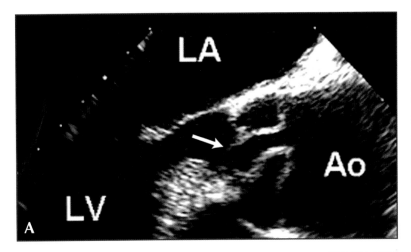

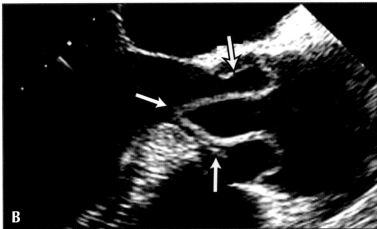

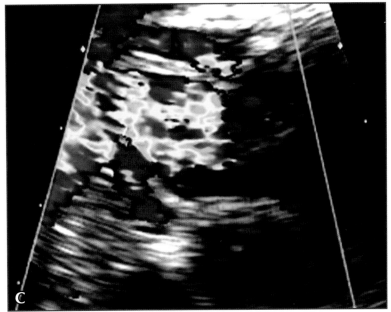

Figure 9-23. Shown are transesophageal echocardiographic long-axis images in a patient with severe aortic regurgitation occurring as a result of a Stanford type A dissection. **A** and **B**, Two-dimensional echocardiographic images demonstrate how the dissection flap (*white arrow*) prevents coaptation and closure of the relatively normal aortic valve leaflets (*yellow arrows*). **C**, The resultant severe aortic regurgitation jet by color Doppler is demonstrated. The mechanism of the patient's severe aortic regurgitation is readily demonstrated by transesophageal echocardiography and may be quite helpful in determining whether aortic valve repair or replacement will be necessary at the time of surgical treatment of the aortic dissection [45]. As in most cases of aortic regurgitation secondary to acute aortic dissection with unremarkable aortic valve leaflet morphology, aortic valve replacement was not necessary in this patient and the aortic regurgitation resolved with replacement of the ascending aorta.

Aortic Regurgitation Severity Assessment

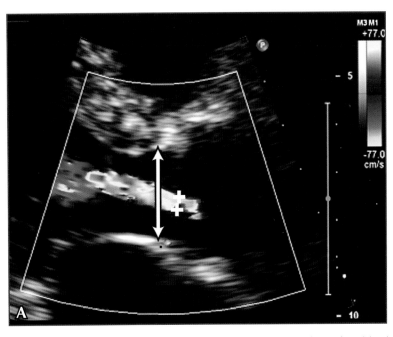

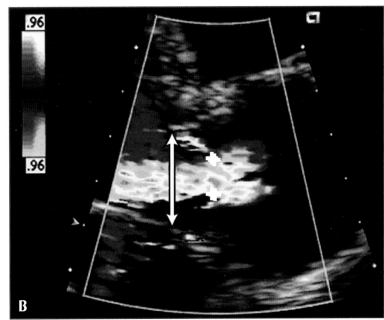

Figure 9-24. Vena contracta and jet width/LV outflow tract (LVOT) width. Shown are parasternal long-axis transthoracic echo images of a patient with mild aortic regurgitation (**A**) and severe regurgitation (**B**).

Continued on the next page

Ⓒ Aortic Regurgitation Severity

Type of echocardiographic information	Mild	Moderate		Severe
Specific and supportive signs	Vena contracta < 0.3 cm	Intermediate values		Vena contracta > 0.6 cm
	Central jet width < 25% of LVOT			Central jet width > 65% of LVOT
	No or brief early diastolic flow reversal in descending aorta			Prominent holodiastolic flow reversal in descending aorta
	Pressure half time > 500 ms			Pressure half time < 200 ms
	Normal LV size			LV enlargement
Quantitative parameters	Mild	Moderate	Moderate–Severe	Severe
ERO, cm²	< 0.1	0.1–0.19·	0.20–0.29	≥ 0.30
	< 30	30–44	45–59	≥ 60

Figure 9-24. (*Continued*) The vena contracta is 0.3 and 0.7 cm (**A** and **B**), respectively (**C**). Note that the central jet width is less than or equal to 25% of the LVOT width (**A**, *two-headed arrow*) and greater than or equal to 65% of the LVOT width (**B**, *two-headed arrow*). The quantification of aortic regurgitation can be a challenging task for the echocardiographer. It is not recommended to rely on one or two measurements, but to combine multiple measurements in a comprehensive manner. A simple reliable method is measurement of the vena contracta; the smallest width of the regurgitant flow at the orifice immediately beyond the flow convergence region (**A** and **B**, *calipers*) and before expansion of the turbulent regurgitant jet, which is a surrogate measure of the effective regurgitant orifice [46]. Measurement of vena contracta is carried out in the parasternal long-axis with a zoomed view and optimized color Doppler settings at early to mid diastole [47]. Vena contracta has been shown to be superior to the jet/LVOT ratio for quantification of aortic regurgitation.

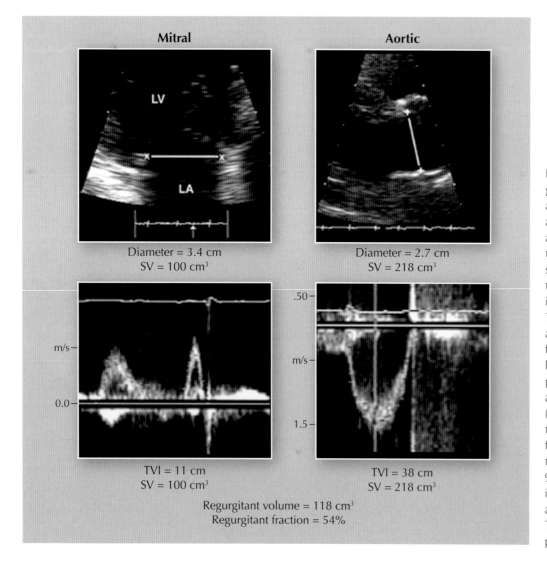

Diameter = 3.4 cm
SV = 100 cm³

Diameter = 2.7 cm
SV = 218 cm³

TVI = 11 cm
SV = 100 cm³

TVI = 38 cm
SV = 218 cm³

Regurgitant volume = 118 cm³
Regurgitant fraction = 54%

Figure 9-25. Continuity equation in aortic regurgitation. In a noncompressible fluid system such as blood, flow is the same at any point and flow = area × time velocity integral (TVI) (*see* Fig. 9-14). In aortic regurgitation, the stroke volume (SV) (flow) through the aortic valve will be greater (normal stroke volume + regurgitant volume) than the one through the mitral valve (normal stroke volume) in the absence of significant mitral regurgitation. Thus, aortic flow volume − mitral flow volume = aortic regurgitation volume. The left aspect of the figure shows the measurement of the mitral annular diameter (*top*) from anterior to posterior hinge point (insertion point of the mitral leaflet into the annulus) in mid diastole and the mitral valve TVI (*bottom*) tracing the modal velocity itself and not the black-white interface [37]. The right side of the figure shows the measurement of the LV outflow tract (LVOT) diameter in its top aspect (*see* Fig. 9-15) and the LVOT TVI, tracing the black-white interface in the lower aspect. The SV through the aortic valve is 218 mL and the mitral is 100 mL. Thus, 218 − 100 = 118 mL of regurgitant volume per beat. LA—left atrium.

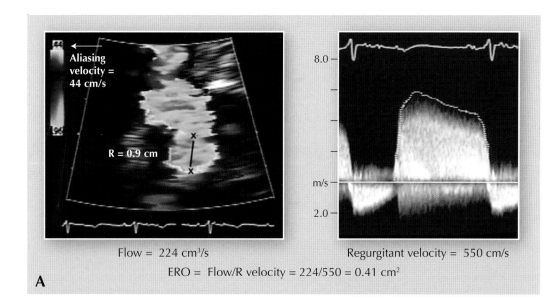

Flow = 224 cm³/s

Regurgitant velocity = 550 cm/s

ERO = Flow/R velocity = 224/550 = 0.41 cm²

A

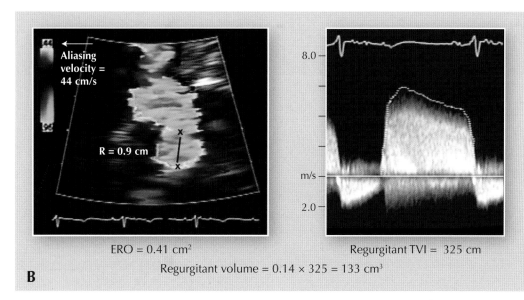

ERO = 0.41 cm²

Regurgitant TVI = 325 cm

Regurgitant volume = 0.14 × 325 = 133 cm³

B

Figure 9-26. The application of proximal isovelocity surface area (PISA) for calculation of the effective regurgitant orifice (ERO) is also based on the principle of conservation of mass. When noncompressible fluid approaches an orifice, it organizes itself in concentric shells that have the same velocity. These shells are hemispheres, which appear more as circles on color Doppler due to the inherent lateral resolution limitations of the technique. If we know the area of the hemisphere and its velocity, we can determine the reguritant flow (R_{flow}) before the orifice ($R_{Flow} = 2\pi \times r^2 \times V_r$), where r is the radius of the hemisphere measured in early diastole, and V_r is the corresponding aliasing velocity. Because ERO × regurgitant velocity (R_{vel}) = flow before the orifice, ERO (PISA) = R_{Flow}/R_{vel} where R_{vel} is the maximal instantaneous velocity of the aortic regurgitation jet [49]. A zoomed view shows the convergence zone of the aortic regurgitation jet on the transthoracic apical three-chamber view (**A**). The radius of the hemisphere is measured from the first aliasing contour (*red–blue interface*) to the incisures that close the circle (r = 0.9 cm). The aliasing velocity is chosen by the operator and it is 44 cm/s (*arrow*). Thus, the flow before the orifice is 224 mL/s. The peak regurgitant velocity is 5.5 m/s, so the ERO = 0.41 cm² (*see* Fig. 9-24C). The calculation of regurgitant volume from the ERO and regurgitant TVI (area × TVI = flow) is shown (**B**).

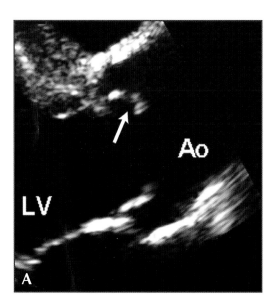

A

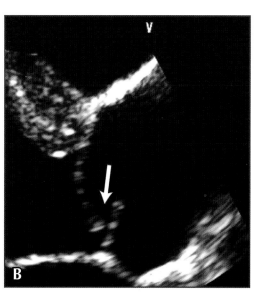

B

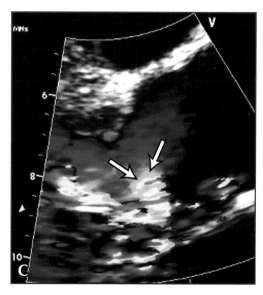

C

Figure 9-27. Eccentric aortic regurgitation proximal isovelocity surface area (PISA) calculation. Shown is the transthoracic parasternal long-axis view in systole of a typical bicuspid aortic valve with doming of the cojoined cusp (**A**, *arrow*) and prominent prolapse of the cojoined cusp in diastole (**B**, *arrow*), which causes a very eccentric, posteriorly directed jet with prominent flow convergence (**C**, *arrows*).

Continued on the next page

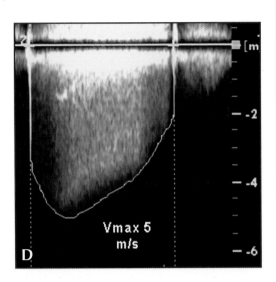

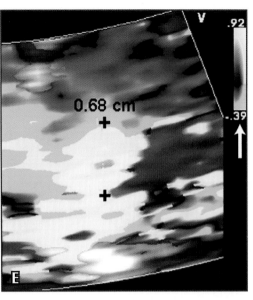

Figure 9-27. *(Continued)* Parasternal nonimaging probe evaluation shows a dense regurgitation Doppler envelope (**D**). Because the direction of the jet is parallel to the ultrasound beam on the parasternal long-axis view and not on the apical three-chamber view, analysis of the regurgitation is best performed in the parasternal view. After improving the frame rate by decreasing the depth and using a small "color-box," a zoomed view of the convergence zone with lowering of the baseline to an aliasing velocity of 39 cm/s (**E**, *arrow*), a PISA hemisphere is elicited and measured (**E**, *calipers*). $R_{flow} = 2 \times r^2 \times Vr$, thus $2 \times 3.1416 \times 0.68^2 \times 39 = 113$ mL/s. ERO (PISA) $= R_{flow}/R_{vel}$, thus 113/500, ERO = 0.2 cm^2 compatible with moderate to severe aortic regurgitation (*see* Fig. 9-24C). Ao—aorta; r—radius; R_{flow}—regurgitant flow; R_{vel}—regurgitant velocity; V_{max}—velocity maximum.

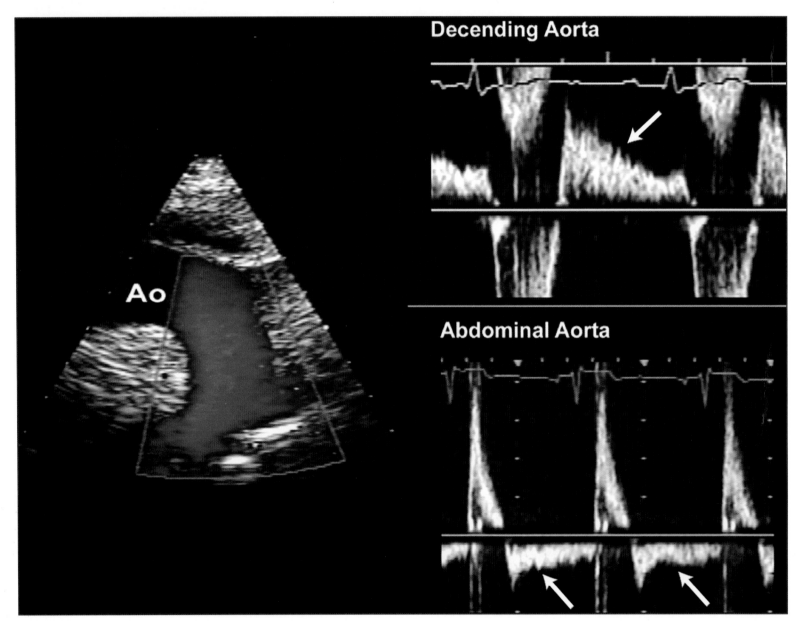

Figure 9-28. Flow reversal in the aorta. Shown is a diastolic still frame of the descending thoracic aorta showing prominent flow reversal (*red*) by color Doppler (*left panel*). There is a pulsed-wave Doppler analysis of the descending thoracic aorta showing prominent holodiastolic reversal of flow (*upper right panel, arrow*). There is also evidence of holodiastolic reversal in the abdominal aorta by pulsed-wave Doppler (*lower right panel, arrows*). This finding is sensitive [50] for the detection of significant/severe aortic regurgitation but lacks specificity (*ie*, reduced compliance of the aorta seen with advancing age may also prolong the normal diastolic reversal in the absence of significant regurgitation). The significance of this sign increases as the time velocity integral (TVI) of the holodiastolic flow approaches the TVI of the forward flow [48]. (*Images courtesy of F. Miller, MD.*)

Mixed Aortic Valve Disease

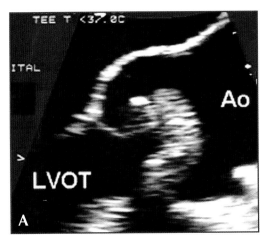
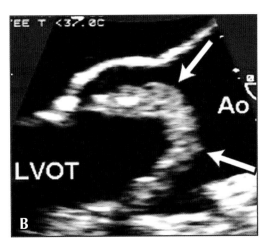
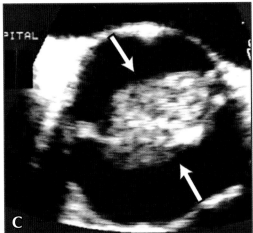
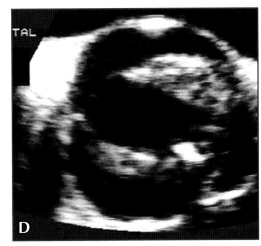

Figure 9-29. Shown are transesophageal long-axis echocardiographic images during diastole (**A**) and systole (**B**) in a patient who presented with acute valvular obstruction secondary to aortic valvulitis. Note the marked globular thickening/deposition on the aortic valve leaflets (**B** and **C**, *arrows*). Subsequent pathologic review of the explanted valve revealed homogenous, tan-red connective tissue with fibrin and inflammatory cells but without thrombus or bacterial vegetations (subsequent cultures also negative). The transesophageal echocardiographic short-axis images in diastole (**C**) and systole (**D**) display the underlying bicuspid aortic valve found at surgery. The differential diagnosis of acute valvulitis includes systemic lupus erythematosus, Wegener's granulomatosis, Kawasaki's disease, anti-phospholipid antibody syndrome, syphilis, and other collagen vascular diseases [51–53]. Ao—aorta; LVOT—LV outflow tract.

References

1. Nkomo VT, Gardin JM, Skelton TN, *et al.*: Burden of valvular heart diseases: a population-based study. *Lancet* 2006, 368:1005–1011.

2. Ross J Jr, Braunwald E: Aortic stenosis. *Circulation* 1968, 38(1 Suppl):61–67.

3. Pellikka PA, Sarano ME, Nishimura RA, *et al.*: Outcome of 622 adults with asymptomatic, hemodynamically significant aortic stenosis during prolonged follow-up. *Circulation* 2005, 111:3290–3295.

4. Otto CM, Kuusisto J, Reichenbach DD, *et al.*: Characterization of the early lesion of 'degenerative' valvular aortic stenosis. Histological and immunohistochemical studies. *Circulation* 1994, 90:844–853.

5. Rajamannan NM, Subramaniam M, Rickard D, *et al.*: Human aortic valve calcification is associated with an osteoblast phenotype. *Circulation* 2003, 107:2181–2184.

6. Peltier M, Trojette F, Sarano ME, *et al.*: Relation between cardiovascular risk factors and nonrheumatic severe calcific aortic stenosis among patients with a three-cuspid aortic valve. *Am J Cardiol* 2003, 91:97–99.

7. Dujardin KS, Enriquez-Sarano M, Schaff HV, *et al.*: Mortality and morbidity of aortic regurgitation in clinical practice: a long-term follow-up study. *Circulation* 1999, 99:1851–1857.

8. Robicsek F, Thubrikar MJ, Cook JW, Fowler B: The congenitally bicuspid aortic valve: how does it function? Why does it fail? *Ann Thorac Surg* 2004, 77:177–185.

9. Davies MJ, Treasure T, Parker DJ: Demographic characteristics of patients undergoing aortic valve replacement for stenosis: relation to valve morphology. *Heart* 1996, 75:174–178.

10. Subramanian R, Olson LJ, Edwards WD: Surgical pathology of pure aortic stenosis: a study of 374 cases. *Mayo Clin Proc* 1984, 59:683–690.

11. Roberts WC: The congenitally bicuspid aortic valve: a study of 85 autopsy cases. *Am J Cardiol* 1970, 26:72–83.

12. Larson EW, Edwards WD: Risk factors for aortic dissection: a necropsy study of 161 cases. *Am J Cardiol* 1984, 53:849–855.

13. Steinberger J, Moller JH, Berry JM, Sinaiko AR: Echocardiographic diagnosis of heart disease in apparently healthy adolescents. *Pediatrics* 2000, 105(4 Pt 1):815–818.

14. Roberts WC, Ko JM: Frequency by decades of unicuspid, bicuspid, and tricuspid aortic valves in adults having isolated aortic valve replacement for aortic stenosis, with or without associated aortic regurgitation. *Circulation* 2005, 111:920–925.

15. Roberts WC, Morrow AG, McIntosh CL, *et al.*: Congenitally bicuspid aortic valve causing severe, pure aortic regurgitation without superimposed infective endocarditis. Analysis of 13 patients requiring aortic valve replacement. *Am J Cardiol* 1981, 47:206–209.

16. Lamas CC, Eykyn SJ: Bicuspid aortic valve—a silent danger: analysis of 50 cases of infective endocarditis. *Clin Infect Dis* 2000, 30:336–341.

17. Tirrito SJ, Kerut EK: How not to miss a bicuspid aortic valve in the echocardiography laboratory. *Echocardiography* 2005, 22:53–55.

18. Brandenburg RO Jr, Tajik AJ, Edwards WD, *et al.*: Accuracy of 2-dimensional echocardiographic diagnosis of congenital bicuspid aortic valve: echocardiographic-anatomic correlation in 115 patients. *Am J Cardiol* 1983, 51:1469–1473.

19. Sabet HY, Edwards WD, Tazelaar HD, Daly RC: Congenitally bicuspid aortic valves: a surgical pathology study of 542 cases (1991 through 1996) and a literature review of 2,715 additional cases. *Mayo Clin Proc* 1999, 74:14–26.

20. Simonds JP: Congenital malformations of the aortic and pulmonary valves. *Am J Med Sci* 1923, 166:584–595.

21. Feldman BJ, Khandheria BK, Warnes CA, *et al.*: Incidence, description and functional assessment of isolated quadricuspid aortic valves. *Am J Cardiol* 1990; 65:937–938.

22. Timperley J, Milner R, Marshall AJ, Gilbert TJ: Quadricuspid aortic valves. *Clin Cardiol* 2002, 25:548–552.

23. Roldan CA, Shively BK, Crawford MH: Valve excrescences: prevalence, evolution and risk for cardioembolism. *J Am Coll Cardiol* 1997, 30:1308–1314.

24. Voros S, Navin NC, Thakur AC, *et al.*: Lambl's excrescences (valvular strands). *Echocardiography* 1999, 16:399–414.

25. Klarich KW, Enriquez-Sarano M, Gura GM, *et al.*: Papillary fibroelastoma: echo-cardiographic characteristics for diagnosis and pathologic correlation. *J Am Coll Cardiol* 1997, 30:784–790.

26. Daveron E, Jain N, Kelley GP, *et al.*: Papillary fibroelastoma and Lambl's excrescences: echocardiographic diagnosis and differential diagnosis. *Echocardiography* 2005, 22:285–287.

27. Sun JP, Asher CR, Yang XS, *et al.*: Clinical and echocardiographic characteristics of papillary fibroelastomas: a retrospective and prospective study in 162 patients. *Circulation* 2001, 103:2687–2693.

28. Sanfilippo AJ, Picard MH, Newell JB, *et al.*: Echocardiographic assessment of patients with infectious endocarditis: prediction of risk for complications. *J Am Coll Cardiol* 1991, 18:1191–1199.

29. Di Salvo G, Habib G, Pergola V, *et al.*: Echocardiography predicts embolic events in infective endocarditis. *J Am Coll Cardiol* 2001, 37:1069–1076.

30. Jacob S, Tong AT: Role of echocardiography in the diagnosis and management of infective endocarditis. *Curr Opin Cardiol* 2002, 17:478–485.

31. Daniel WG, Mugge A, Martin RP, *et al.*: Improvement in the diagnosis of abscesses associated with endocarditis by transesophageal echocardiography. *N Engl J Med* 1991, 324:795–800.

32. Karalis DG, Bansal RC, Hauck AJ, *et al.*: Transesophageal echocardiographic recognition of subaortic complications in aortic valve endocarditis. Clinical and surgical implications. *Circulation* 1992, 86:353–362.

33. Otto CM, Lind BK, Kitzman DW, *et al.*: Association of aortic-valve sclerosis with cardiovascular morbidity and mortality in the elderly. *N Engl J Med* 1999, 341:142–147.

34. Essop MR, Nkomo VT: Rheumatic and nonrheumatic valvular heart disease: epidemiology, management, and prevention in Africa. *Circulation* 2005, 112:3584–3591.

35. Brauner R, Laks H, Drinkwater DC Jr, *et al.*: Benefits of early surgical repair in fixed subaortic stenosis. *J Am Coll Cardiol* 1997, 30:1835–1842.

36. Marasini M, Zannini L, Ussia GP, *et al.*: Discrete subaortic stenosis: incidence, morphology and surgical impact of associated subaortic anomalies. *Ann Thorac Surg* 2003, 75:1763–1768.

37. Quinones MA, Otto, CM, Stoddard M, et al.: American Society of Echocardiography Recommendations for Quantification of Doppler Echocardiography: A Report from the Doppler Quantification Task Force of the Nomenclature and Standards Committee of the American Society of Echocardiography. Accessible at www.asecho.org. Accessed March 24, 2008.

38. Hoffmann R, Flachskampf FA, Hanrath P: Planimetry of orifice area in aortic stenosis using multiplane transesophageal echocardiography. *J Am Coll Cardiol* 1993, 22:529–534.

39. Tribouilloy C, Shen WF, Peltier M, *et al.*: Quantitation of aortic valve area in aortic stenosis with multiplane transesophageal echocardiography: comparison with monoplane transesophageal approach. *Am Heart J* 1994, 128:526–532.

40. Bernard Y, Meneveau N, Vuillemenot A, *et al.*: Planimetry of aortic valve area using multiplane transoesophageal echocardiography is not a reliable method for assessing severity of aortic stenosis. *Heart* 1997, 78:68–73.

41. Bonow RO, Carabello BA, Chatterjee K, *et al.*: ACC/AHA 2006 guidelines for the management of patients with valvular heart disease *J Am Coll Cardiol* 2006, 1:48: e1–e148. [Published erratum appears in *J Am Coll Cardiol* 2007, 49:1014.]

42. Connolly HM, Oh JK, Schaff HV, *et al.*: Severe aortic stenosis with low transvalvular gradient and severe left ventricular dysfunction: result of aortic valve replacement in 52 patients. *Circulation* 2000, 101:1940–1946.

43. Monin JL, Quéré JP, Monchi M, *et al.*: Low-gradient aortic stenosis: operative risk stratification and predictors for long-term outcome: a multicenter study using dobutamine stress hemodynamics. *Circulation* 2003, 108:319–324.

44. Quere JP, Monin JL, Levy F, *et al.*: Influence of preoperative left ventricular contractile reserve on postoperative ejection fraction in low-gradient aortic stenosis. *Circulation* 2006, 113:1738–1744.

45. Movsowitz HD, Levine RA, Hilgenberg AD, Isselbacher EM: Transesophageal echocardiographic description of the mechanisms of aortic regurgitation in acute Type A aortic dissection: implications for aortic valve repair. *J Am Coll Cardiol* 2000, 36:884–890.

46. Enriquez-Sarano M, Tajik AJ: Clinical practice. Aortic regurgitation. *N Engl J Med* 2004, 351:1539–1546.

47. Tribouilloy CM, Enriquez-Sarano M, Bailey KR, *et al.*: Assessment of severity of aortic regurgitation using the width of the vena contracta: a clinical color Doppler imaging study. *Circulation* 2000, 102:558–564.

48. Zoghbi WA, Enriquez-Sarano M, *et al.*: Recommendations for evaluation of the severity of native valvular regurgitation with two-dimensional and Doppler echocardiography. *J Am Soc Echocardiogr* 2003, 16:777–802.

49. Tribouilloy CM, Enriquez-Sarano M, Fett SL, *et al.*: Application of the proximal flow convergence method to calculate the effective regurgitant orifice area in aortic regurgitation. *J Am Coll Cardiol* 1998, 32:1032–1039.

50. Touche T, Prasquier R, Nitenberg A, *et al.*: Assessment and follow-up of patients with aortic regurgitation by an updated Doppler echocardiographic measurement of the regurgitant fraction in the aortic arch. *Circulation* 1985, 72:819–824.

51. Nesher G, Ilany J, Rosenmann D, Abraham AS: Valvular dysfunction in antiphospholipid syndrome: prevalence, clinical features, and treatment. *Semin Arthritis Rheum* 1997, 27:27–35.

52. Yanda RJ, Guis MS, Rabkin JM: Aortic valvulitis in a patient with Wegener's granulomatosis. *West J Med* 1989, 151:555–556.

53. Roldan CA, Shively BK, Crawford MH: An echocardiographic study of valvular heart disease associated with systemic lupus erythematosus. *N Engl J Med* 1996, 335:1424–1430.

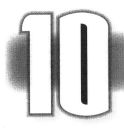

Prosthetic Valve Disease

Hisham Dokainish and William A. Zoghbi

Mechanical and bioprosthetic valves are placed in patients in the aortic, mitral, tricuspid, and pulmonic positions for a variety of conditions. In general, mechanical valves have greater longevity than bioprostheses and are thus used in patients 65 years of age or younger, or in patients who require long-term anticoagulation for other reasons. Bioprosthetic valves are typically used for patients 65 years of age or older, or in those with contraindications to anticoagulation. Transthoracic echocardiography (TTE) is a readily available and important screening modality for prosthetic valve function, especially with Doppler for evaluation of valvular hemodynamics. Transesophageal echocardiography (TEE) provides more definitive morphologic evaluation and is crucial in prosthetic valve management decisions. All prosthetic valves are inherently mildly stenotic, and therefore mildly elevated gradients by Doppler are accepted as normal. When transvalvular velocities and gradients are elevated beyond accepted normal values, valve obstruction, regurgitation, or valve undersizing is suspected.

The common causes of prosthetic valve dysfunction are endocarditis, thrombosis, and pannus formation. In cases of elevated prosthetic valve gradients on transthoracic imaging, TEE is generally recommended to elucidate the mechanism of pathology. For prosthetic valve endocarditis, intravenous antibiotic therapy is standard, with surgical intervention indicated for complications, including abscess, significant prosthetic valve dysfunction, pseudoaneurysm, or fistula formation. Valve thrombosis is generally a problem in mechanical prostheses and can be treated in certain cases with systemic thrombolysis (for which TEE serves as an important guide). Both TTE and TEE are complementary techniques in the evaluation of prosthetic valve function as well as in the management of patients with prosthetic valves. This chapter, by way of echocardiographic images from patients with prosthetic valves, along with tables and graphs, aims at facilitating the evaluation of prosthetic cardiac valve function and the recognition of the spectrum of valvular dysfunction and complications.

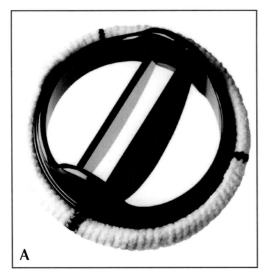

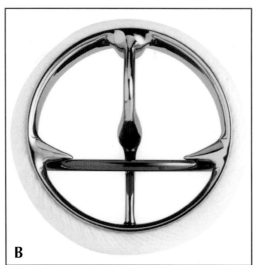

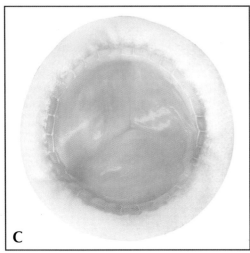

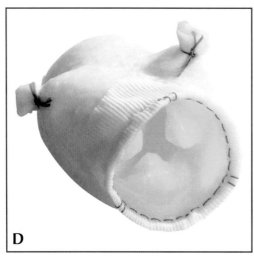

Figure 10-1. A, Normal appearance of a St. Jude mechanical bileaflet prosthetic valve. This mechanical valve, made of pyrolitic carbon, can be used in either the aortic or mitral position and has been in existence since 1977 [1]. It is also the most commonly used mechanical prosthesis currently in the United States. In general, mechanical prostheses have superior durability compared with bioprostheses but require long-term anticoagulation and are therefore associated with warfarin-related complications [2]. Mechanical prostheses are generally preferred for patients younger than 65 years of age, or in patients who require anticoagulation for other indications (*eg*, atrial fibrillation), whereas bioprosthetic valves are preferred for patients older than 65 years of age [2]. Twenty-year follow-up data have been completed on the St. Jude prosthesis [3]. Mechanical failure was rare, and at 20 years, freedom from reoperation was 90% ± 3% in both the aortic and mitral positions. Freedom from thromboembolism at 20 years was 68% ± 8% in the aortic, and 59% ± 7% in the mitral position, whereas freedom from valve-related mortality was 86% ± 4% in the aortic and 76% ± 8% in the mitral position.

B, Normal appearance of a Medtronic Hall mechanical single leaflet prosthetic valve. The Medtronic Hall mechanical valve consists of a carbon-coated disk in a titanium ring and can be used in either the aortic or mitral positions. Twenty-year follow-up have been published for this valve [4], showing good valve durability and relatively low complication rates. Incidence of valve-related late death was 0.8% per year in the aortic position, and 0.9% per year in the mitral position. For the aortic and mitral positions, rates of valve thrombosis were 0.04% and 0.03%, respectively, per year; stroke, 0.6% and 0.8% per year; major hemorrhage, 1.2% and 1.4% per year; prosthetic endocarditis, 0.4% and 0.4% per year.

C, Normal appearance of a Hancock porcine stented bioprosthesis. The Hancock bioprosthetic valve (Medtronic, Inc.) is made of porcine pericardium and is mounted on a stented ring. Fifteen-year follow-up is available on this valve, and reveals good durability [5]. Freedom from structural valve deterioration at 15 years was 71.8% ± 5.6% (88.9% ± 6.2% in the aortic position vs 59.5% ± 3.9% in the mitral position). Freedom from structural valve deterioration was less than that seen in older patients (84.5% ± 3.5% vs 95.0% ± 3.0%) in patients younger than 65 years of age. In terms of complications, freedom from thromboembolism was 78.2% ± 4% and from anticoagulant-related hemorrhage 83.5% ± 3.6% at 15 years.

D, Normal appearance of a Freestyle Medtronic stentless bioprosthesis. Bioprosthetic valves can either be mounted with or without stents, the latter available for use in the aortic position. The theoretical advantage of a stentless design is that it requires less space for mounting in the absence of a stented ring that occupies area, and it may be of value in elderly patients and patients with smaller aortic roots [6]. Because stentless prostheses are relatively new in design, long-term follow-up is not yet available; however, 5-year follow-up has been reported for the Freestyle stentless bioprosthesis in the aortic position [7]. Ninety-five patients with a mean age of 75 years underwent aortic valve replacement with a mean of 44 + 18 months follow-up. The overall actuarial survival rate was 80% ± 6% at 5 years, although only two of the deaths were cardiac related, yielding freedom from cardiac mortality of 94% ± 3% after 5 years. No patient required reoperation on the aortic valve. There were nine thromboembolic and three anticoagulant-related bleeding events, none of which were fatal. The actuarial freedom from valve-related morbidity and mortality was 79% ± 4% at 5 years. (*Images courtesy of* Medtronic, Inc., Minneapolis, MN.)

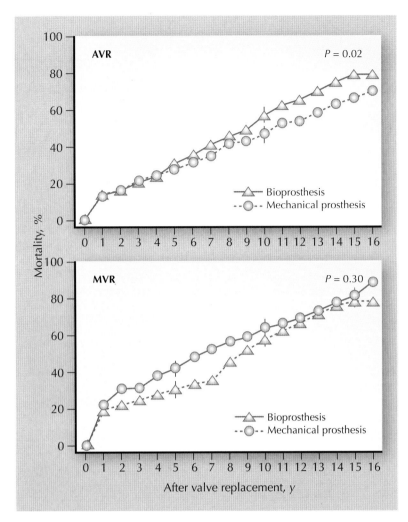

Figure 10-2. Kaplan-Meier mortality curves at 15-year follow-up from the Veterans Affairs randomized trial of mechanical versus bioprosthetic valves [8]. This study randomly assigned 575 men from 1977 to 1982 to bioprosthetic or mechanical valve replacement. The top graph depicts mortality from any cause in the aortic valve replacement group (AVR), with bioprosthetic valves depicted by triangles and mechanical valves by circles. At 15 years, significantly more patients died from any cause in the bioprosthesis group than in the mechanical valve group. Most of this increased death was attributed primarily to valve failure in the bioprosthesis group in patients younger than 65 years of age (26%), a phenomenon virtually nonexistent in the mechanical valve group (0%, $P < 0.001$). However, in patients older than 65 years of age, the valve failure rate was similar in the bioprosthetic group compared with the mechanical valve group (9 ± 6% vs 0% respectively, $P = 0.16$). There was no significant difference in death rates between the two types of valves for mitral valve replacement (MVR) (*bottom*). In addition, there was no significant difference in overall valve-related complications (*ie*, bleeding, endocarditis, systemic embolism, nonthrombotic valve obstruction, valvular regurgitation, or valve thrombosis) for bioprosthetic or mechanical valves in either the aortic valve replacement or MVR groups at 15 years of follow-up. Data from this trial, among others [9], form the basis for current recommendations regarding choice of prosthetic valve type in cardiac patients. (*Adapted from* Hammermeister *et al.* [8].)

Echocardiographic Appearance of Normal Prosthetic Valves

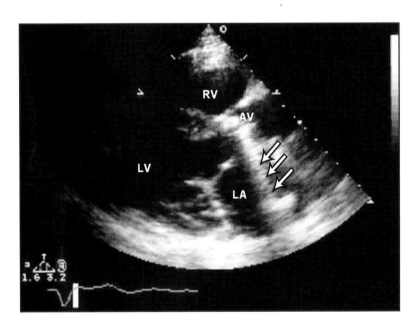

Figure 10-3. Prosthetic valves have characteristic features when imaged with echocardiography, depending upon the type of prosthesis visualized. Mechanical valves reflect ultrasound the most and thus produce the most attenuation and reverberation artifact. This figure depicts transthoracic echocardiography (TTE) of a normal mechanical prosthetic valve in the aortic position. TTE is an important first-line investigation in the evaluation of patients with prosthetic valves [10]. Although transesophageal echocardiography (TEE) provides better resolution and a complementary posterior imaging approach, Doppler interrogation of flow velocity through aortic and pulmonic prostheses by TTE is easier. Displayed in the figure is the parasternal long-axis view on TTE. With the ultrasound beam hitting the mechanical aortic valve (AV) orthogonally in this view, intense reverberations (*arrows*) produced by the metallic leaflets can be seen trailing the valve. These artifacts can be mistaken for abnormal structures in adjacent chambers; in this case, the left atrium (LA).

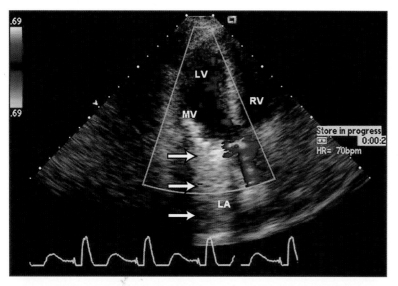

Figure 10-4. Transthoracic echocardiographic (TTE) depiction of a normal mechanical prosthetic valve in the mitral position. Displayed is the apical three-chamber view on TTE, and so the ultrasound beam is hitting the mechanical mitral valve en face. Note the intense reverberations (*arrows*) produced by the metallic leaflets. These reverberation-generated artifacts greatly limit the detection of prosthetic mitral regurgitation by color Doppler in TTE, as the left atrium (LA) is obscured by artifact, and most of the ultrasound energy is reflected by the prosthesis. MV—mitral valve prosthesis.

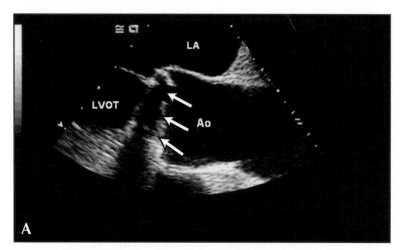

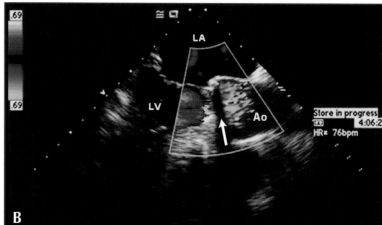

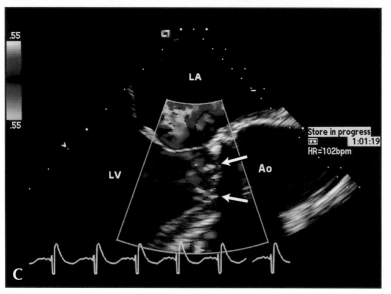

Figure 10-5. Transesophageal echocardiographic (TEE) depiction of a normal mechanical prosthetic valve in the aortic position. The two-dimensional image of the prosthetic aortic valve is depicted in the long-axis view at 119° rotation in the midesophagus (**A**). Note the excellent visualization of the sinuses of Valsalva, the proximal aortic root, and the ascending aorta (Ao). There is prosthesis-generated artifact (*arrows*) shadowing the proximal LV outflow tract (LVOT). Nevertheless, good prosthetic visualization is achieved, allowing exclusion of masses or dehiscence. Color Doppler imaging during systole (**B**) depicts the normal appearance of blood being ejected from the LVOT (laminar red color flow; thus the flow is directed towards the transducer, which lies in the esophagus). Turbulent blue color flow in the aortic root is also shown, as the blood undergoes flow acceleration through the prosthesis, thus exceeding the Nyquist limit set at 0.69 m/s; normal velocities through a prosthetic aortic valve usually reach 3 m/s (*see* Figure 10-9). Note the interruption of color flow visualization by the prosthesis-generated shadowing and artifact (*arrow*). Color Doppler imaging during diastole (**C**) depicts the normal appearance of two physiologic regurgitant jets ("washing jets," *arrows*) in the LV outflow, characteristic of the mechanical bileaflet design. LA—left atrium.

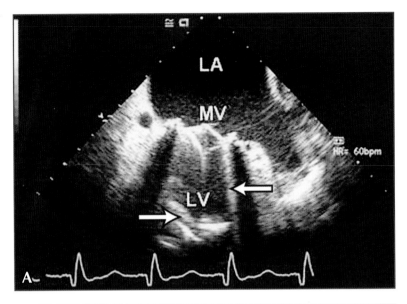

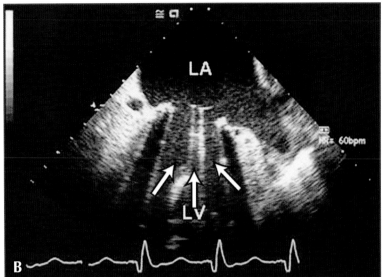

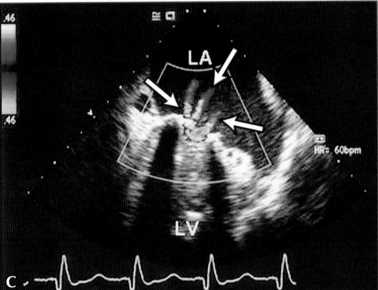

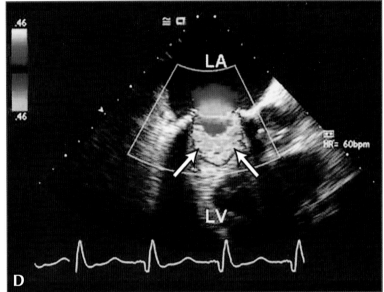

Figure 10-6. Transesophageal echocardiographic (TEE) depiction of a normal bileaflet mechanical prosthetic valve in the mitral position. Note the visualization of both metallic leaflets (MV), which are closed in systole (**A**) and open in diastole (**B**). In the systolic image (**A**), note the artifact (*arrows*) on the LV side, generated by reflections from the prosthetic valve. In the diastolic images (**B**), three parallel echolucent tracts (*arrows*) are visualized, representing the open passages through which blood flows from the left atrium (LA) to LV. During color Doppler imaging in systole (**C**), three physiologic mitral regurgitation "washing" jets (*arrows*) are depicted. This is a normal finding for a bileaflet valve, and should not be mistaken for pathologic prosthetic regurgitation. During color Doppler imaging in diastole (**D**), a column of aliased inflow is visualized (*arrows*), again a normal finding for a mechanical prosthetic mitral valve. MV—prosthetic valve.

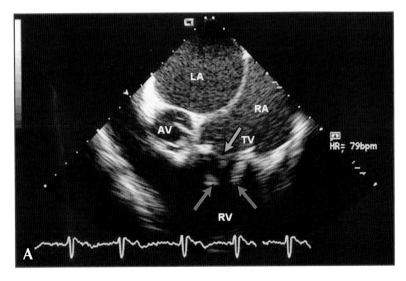

Figure 10-7. Transesophageal echocardiographic (TEE) depiction of a normal stented bioprosthetic valve in the tricuspid position. In the two-dimensional TEE image (**A**) (with left-right inversion of the image), the tricuspid bioprosthesis is well visualized. Note the normal appearance of the two echodense valve struts (*red arrows*), within which two thin, normal-appearing bioprosthetic leaflets (*blue arrow*) are visualized.

Continued on the next page

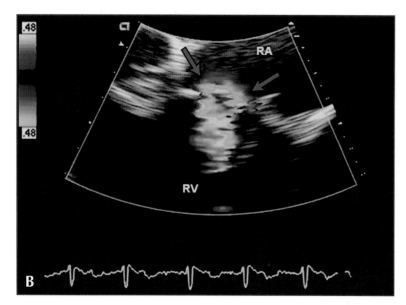 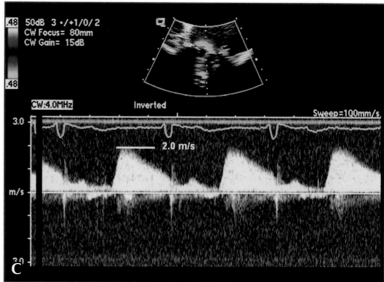

Figure 10-7. *(Continued)* During color Doppler imaging in diastole (**B**), turbulent blood flow into the RV is visualized. Note the proximal isovelocity surface area, which is evidence of flow acceleration (*red arrows*) into the prosthesis. Continuous wave Doppler interrogation of the prosthesis (**C**) demonstrated a peak velocity of 2 m/s, and a mean transvalvular gradient of 8 mm Hg, reflecting elevated velocities for this type of

tricuspid prosthesis (*see* Fig. 10-24 for normal prosthetic tricuspid values). In this case, the prosthesis inserted was likely small for the tricuspid annulus size (the under sizing of which can be appreciated in the two-dimensional imaging (**A**); *see* Fig. 10-14 for discussion of valve undersizing), as there was no evidence of mass or degeneration of the prosthesis. LA—left atrium; RA—right atrium; TV—tricuspid valve.

Echocardiography and Doppler Evaluation of Prosthetic Valve Function: Normal, Stenotic, and Regurgitant Valves

Prosthetic Aortic Valve: Doppler Parameters

Maximal velocity
Mean gradient
Doppler velocity index (V_{LVO}/V_{AVR})
EOA
Contour of the jet velocity

Figure 10-8. Listed are the five Doppler variables useful in evaluating prosthetic aortic valve function, all of which are obtainable by transthoracic echocardiography. Several of these parameters depend on the valve size and flow through the prosthesis. The peak velocity is a useful and relatively accurate screening variable, with normal values generally being less than 3 m/s, assuming preserved LV ejection fraction (LVEF) and normal ($\geq$ 21 mm) valve size of the prosthesis. The mean gradient is easily obtained on most echocardiographic platforms. Generally, in the setting of a normal stroke volume, a mean gradient less than 25 mm Hg is considered within normal limits. The Doppler velocity index (*see* Fig. 10-10) is a useful index that is less dependent on valve size and flow; normal values are more than 0.25. Derivation of effective orifice area (EOA) of a valve can also be measured and should be referenced to the valve size and type (*see* Fig. 10-12). Adjusting the EOA to body surface area provides an estimate of the appropriate prosthetic orifice area for the size of the patient, with normal being more than 0.85 cm² (*see* Fig. 10-13a); however, this value can vary depending on the type of prosthesis used. Finally, an aortic spectral velocity contour on continuous Doppler provides a qualitative evaluation of valve function. Normally, a short acceleration time and early peaking of the velocity occurs, whereas a rounded or late peaking jet morphology (*see* Fig. 10-11, *red arrow*) usually implies prosthetic obstruction. V_{LVO}—peak velocity of the LVOT; V_{AVR}—peak velocity of the aortic valve prosthesis.

Normal Doppler Values in Patients with Various Types of Aortic Valve Prostheses

Valve Type	Peak Velocity, *m/s* Mean ± SD	Mean Gradient, *mm* Hg Mean ± SD	Doppler Velocity Index Mean ± SD
Caged Ball			
Starr Edwards*	3.1 ± 0.5	24 ± 4	0.32 ± 0.09
Tilting disk			
Bjork-Shiley[†]	2.6 ± 0.4	14 ± 5	0.40 ± 0.10
Medtronic-Hall[‡]	2.4 ± 0.2	14 ± 3	0.39 ± 0.09
Omniscience[§]	2.8 ± 0.4	14 ± 3	
Bileaflet			
St. Jude Medical[¶]	2.5 ± 0.6	12 ± 7	0.41 ± 0.12
Heterograft			
Hancock**	2.4 ± 0.3	11 ± 2	0.44 ± 0.21
Carpentier-Edwards[††]	2.4 ± 0.5	14 ± 6	
Ionescu-Shiley[‡‡]	2.5 ± 1.7	14 ± 4	
Homograft	1.9 ± 0.4	7.7 ± 2.7	0.56 ± 0.10

*Edwards Lifesciences, Irvine, CA
[†]Pfizer, Inc., New York, NY
[‡]Medtronic, Inc., Minneapolis, MN
[§]Medical, Inc., Minneapolis, MN
[¶]St. Jude, Inc., St. Paul, MN
** Medtronic, Inc., Minneapolis, MN
[††]Edwards Lifesciences, Irvine, CA
[‡‡]Pfizer, Inc., New York, NY

Figure 10-9. Normal Doppler-derived data in various mechanical and bioprosthetic valves in the aortic position. Doppler echocardiography has become the standard for the detection of prosthetic valve dysfunction, reducing the need for invasive hemodynamics at catheterization [10]. In some valve designs, particularly the bileaflet valve, Doppler leads to an overestimation of gradients compared with invasive hemodynamics. This invasive/Doppler mismatch is due to the ability to localize the maximum velocity between the prosthetic leaflets with the Doppler approach, which is not often possible by invasive techniques, owing to catheter movement in the proximal aorta. Transthoracic echocardiography is well suited in assessing prosthetic valve function because it is readily available, noninvasive, and generally provides suitable angles for accurate Doppler interrogation of aortic, mitral, tricuspid, and pulmonic valves. For prosthetic aortic valves, peak velocity, mean gradient, and the Doppler velocity index are all useful for the assessment of prosthetic valve function. In general (see chart for exact values), a peak velocity across the aortic valve of less than 3 m/s, a mean gradient less than 25 mm Hg, and a Doppler velocity index more than 0.25 are considered normal [11,12]. (*Adapted from* Barbetseas and Zoghbi [11].)

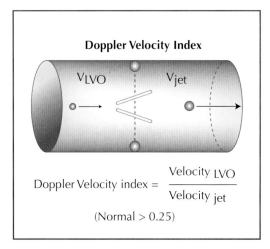

Doppler Velocity Index

V_{LVO} V_{jet}

$$\text{Doppler Velocity index} = \frac{\text{Velocity }_{LVO}}{\text{Velocity }_{jet}}$$

(Normal > 0.25)

Figure 10-10. Derivation of the Doppler velocity index (DVI), a parameter of aortic prosthetic valve function. This index, representing the degree of acceleration of velocity across the prosthesis, is derived as the ratio of blood velocity at the LV outflow (LVO) to the velocity across the prosthesis. The DVI can be derived using the ratio of time velocity integrals (TVI) at these two sites, or simply as the ratio of the respective peak velocities [12]. The LVO velocity is measured from the apical window approximately 1 cm proximal to the prosthetic aortic valve using pulsed Doppler. The velocity through the prosthesis is recorded using continuous wave Doppler from the apical window, right parasternal or suprasternal window, using the highest representative velocity. The tighter the stenosis, the greater the flow acceleration at the prosthesis, and the smaller is the DVI ratio. Thus, in general, normal aortic mechanical prosthetic valve function is present when the DVI is greater than 0.25 [12]. V_{LVO}—peak velocity of the LVOT; V_{jet}—jet velocity.

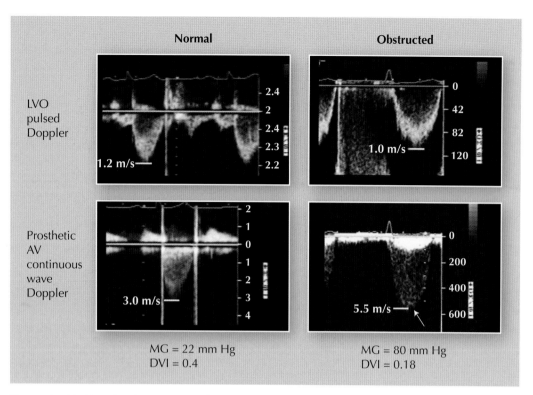

Figure 10-11. Doppler characteristics of normal and obstructed prosthetic mechanical valves in the aortic position. **Left panel**, In the normal side, the LV outflow (LVO) spectral envelope is displayed with a peak velocity of 1.2 m/s. In order to calculate the Doppler velocity index (DVI) in this patient (*see* Fig. 10-10), the LVO peak velocity is divided by the peak velocity of the prosthetic aortic valve spectral tracing obtained by continuous wave Doppler (3 m/s). This results in a DVI of 0.4, which is normal, corroborated by a normal mean gradient of 22 mm Hg. **Right panel**, In the obstructed side, the LVO velocity is 1 m/s and the prosthetic AV velocity is 5.5 m/s, resulting in an abnormally low DVI of 0.18, corroborated by an elevated prosthetic aortic valve gradient of 80 mm Hg. AV—prosthetic aortic valve; MG—mean gradient. (*From* Barbetseas and Zoghbi [11]; with permission.)

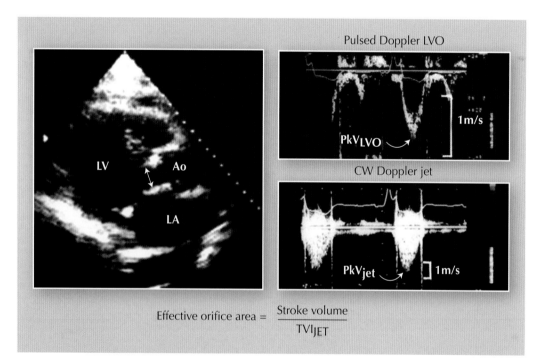

$$\text{Effective orifice area} = \frac{\text{Stroke volume}}{\text{TVI}_{JET}}$$

Figure 10-12. Calculation of the effective orifice area (EOA) of a prosthetic valve in the aortic position using the continuity equation. The EOA is a physiologic estimation of the size of the opening of the prosthetic valve, calculated using Doppler variables readily obtained by transthoracic echocardiography (TTE). **Left panel**, Parasternal long-axis view from which the LV outflow (LVO) diameter is measured in order to calculate the LVO area. Next, the time velocity integral (TVI) of the LVO is obtained by pulsed Doppler in the apical five-chamber view. Multiplying the LVO area by the TVI results in the stroke volume (SV). Using the continuity equation, dividing the SV by the TVI of the prosthetic aortic valve (obtained using continuous wave [CW] in the apical five-chamber view) results in the EOA. Normal values of EOA depend on the size of the prosthesis and have to be referenced to the type and size of the respective valve. On the other hand, DVI is much less dependent on valve size [12]. Ao—aorta; LA—left atrium; PkV—peak velocity; PkV$_{LVO}$—peak velocity of LV outflow; TVI$_{jet}$—time velocity integral of jet. (*From* Barbetseas and Zoghbi [11]; with permission.)

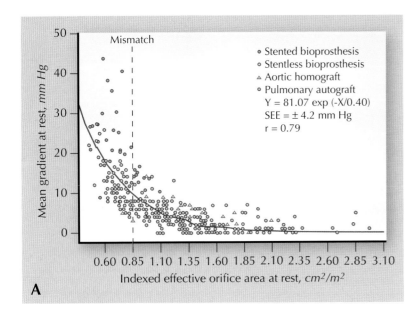

A

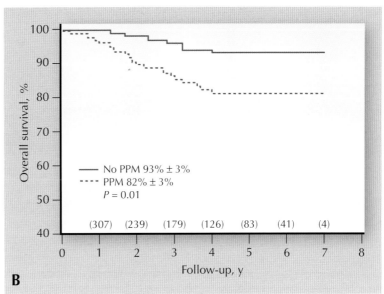

B

Figure 10-13. Relation of prosthetic valve size to patient body surface area and mean valve gradient: the concept of prosthesis-patient mismatch (PPM). PPM is considered to be present when the size of the prosthesis orifice is too small for the patient's body size [13]. PPM can result in high transvalvular gradients through otherwise normally functioning aortic prostheses. One method for detecting the presence of PPM (in addition to an elevated transvalvular gradient in the presence of a normally appearing prosthesis on echocardiography) is calculating the effective prosthetic orifice area (EOA) indexed to body surface area (BSA) [14]. The continuity equation is used to calculate the prosthetic EOA, determined by the product of the LV outflow tract (LVOT) area and the LVOT time velocity integral (TVI), divided by the aortic valve TVI (*see* Fig. 10-12). The EOA is then divided by the patient's BSA, resulting in the EOA index. As depicted (**A**), a prosthetic aortic valve EOA index less than 0.85 cm²/m² in the absence of any identifiable obstructive pathology it is associated with elevated mean gradients at rest, which is suggestive of mismatch. PPM has recently been shown to predict outcome after aortic valve replacement [15]. As depicted (**B**), mortality is significantly lower at 7-year follow-up in the presence (compared with the absence) of significant PPM in the aortic position. (*Adapted from* [**A**] Pibarot and Dumesnil [13] and [**B**] Tasca *et al.* [15]). SEE—standard error estimate.

Prosthetic Mitral Valve: Doppler Parameters

Mean gradient: importance of heart rate
Pressure half time
MVA by pressure half time
EOA (continuity equation)

Figure 10-14. Doppler variables used in the determination of mitral prosthetic valve function. The mean gradient across a mitral prosthesis is a valuable and quick screening tool for prosthetic valve dysfunction. An elevated mean gradient (> 5 mm Hg) in the presence of a normal heart rate may suggest obstruction, significant regurgitation, or valve undersizing. Elevated heart rates (> 85 bpm) can increase the mean gradient in the absence of identifiable pathology due to shortened diastolic time. The pressure half time (PHT) of mitral deceleration may be employed in order to assess prosthetic valve function and longer PHT (> 130 ms), which implies possible valve obstruction as it takes longer for the left atrial and ventricular pressures to equalize. The effective orifice area (EOA) may also be calculated using PHT in the manner used in native rheumatic mitral stenosis (220/PHT). However, this index depends on LV and atrial pressures, among other factors, and it is not well validated for prosthetic valves. EOA may also be calculated using the continuity equation using the mitral valve time velocity integral (TVI) at the mitral annulus level, and the aortic or pulmonary valve areas and TVI (*see* Fig. 10-12). MVA—mitral valve area.

Normal Doppler Values in Patients with Various Types of Mitral Valve Prostheses

Valve Type	Peak Velocity, *m/s* Mean ± SD	Mean Gradient, *mm Hg* Mean ± SD	Pressure Half-Time, *ms* Mean ± SD
Caged Ball			
Starr Edwards*	1.9 ± 0.4	5 ± 2	109 ± 27
Tilting disk			
Bjork-Shiley†	1.6 ± 0.3	3 ± 2	90 ± 22
Medtronic-Hall‡	1.7 ± 0.3	3 ± 0.9	89 ± 19
Omniscience§	1.8 ± 0.3	3 ± 0.9	125 ± 29
Bileaflet			
St. Jude Medical¶	1.6 ± 0.3	3 ± 1	76 ± 17
Heterograft			
Hancock**	1.5 ± 0.3	4 ± 2	129 ± 31
Carpentier-Edwards††	1.8 ± 0.2	6 ± 2	90 ± 25
Ionescu-Shiley‡‡	1.5 ± 0.3	3 ± 1	93 ± 25

*Edwards Lifesciences, Irvine, CA
†Pfizer, Inc., New York, NY
‡Medtronic, Inc., Minneapolis, MN
§Medical Inc., Minneapolis, MN
¶St. Jude Medical, St. Paul, MN
**Medtronic, Inc., Minneapolis, MN
††Edwards Lifesciences, Irvine, CA
‡‡Pfizer, Inc., New York, NY

Figure 10-15. Normal Doppler-derived data in various mechanical and bioprosthetic valves in the mitral position. In the mitral position, transthoracic Doppler echocardiography is an accurate and simple screening tool for prosthetic valve dysfunction. In general (see chart for exact values), a prosthetic transmitral early diastolic (E wave) peak velocity of less than 1.9 m/s, a mean transmitral gradient of less than 5 m/s, and a pressure half-time of less than 130 ms are markers of normal prosthetic mitral valve function. (*Adapted from* Barbetseas and Zoghbi [11].)

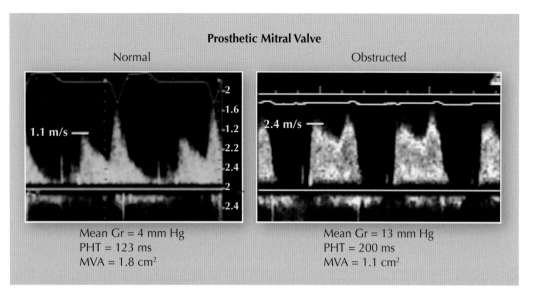

Prosthetic Mitral Valve

Normal

1.1 m/s

Mean Gr = 4 mm Hg
PHT = 123 ms
MVA = 1.8 cm²

Obstructed

2.4 m/s

Mean Gr = 13 mm Hg
PHT = 200 ms
MVA = 1.1 cm²

Figure 10-16. Normal and abnormal transmitral Doppler in mechanical prosthetic mitral valves. In the normal tracing (*left panel*), the peak velocity across the mitral valve is 1.1 m/s, the mean gradient (Gr) is 4 mm Hg, the pressure half time (PHT) is 123 ms, and the valve area is 1.8 cm², which are all within normal limits for mechanical mitral prostheses. In the abnormal tracing (*right panel*), the peak velocity across the mitral valve is 2.4 m/s, the mean gradient is 13 mm Hg, the PHT is 200 ms, and the valve area is 1.1 cm², which are all indicative of mitral prosthetic obstruction. MVA—mitral valve area. (*From* Barbetseas and Zoghbi [11]; with permission.)

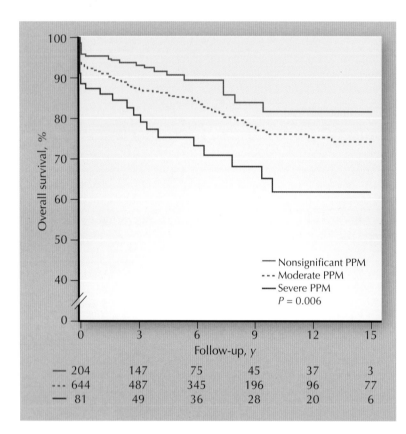

— Nonsignificant PPM
--- Moderate PPM
— Severe PPM
P = 0.006

— 204	147	75	45	37	3
--- 644	487	345	196	96	77
— 81	49	36	28	20	6

Figure 10-17. The concept of prosthesis-patient–mismatch (PPM) (*see* Fig. 10-13) also applies to mitral prosthetic valves. Analogous to the concept with prosthetic aortic valves, a prosthetic mitral valve area indexed to body surface area can be used to quantify mitral PPM. Mitral PPM can be classified as not clinically significant if greater than 1.2 cm²/m², as moderate if greater than 0.9 and less than 1.2 cm²/m², and as severe if less than 0.9 cm²/m² [16]. The presence of mitral valve PPM also affects patient survival, as shown in the figure. In 929 consecutive patients with mitral valve replacement, studied by Magne *et al.* [16], patients with severe PPM had a 6-year survival of 74.5%, which was significantly less than for patients with moderate PPM (84.1%) and for patients with nonsignificant PPM (90.2%, P = 0.002 for comparison). Twelve-year survival was also significantly lower in patients with severe PPM. Therefore, mitral prosthetic valves require appropriate sizing in relation to patient body surface area in order to optimize patient outcome. (*Adapted from* Magne *et al.* [16].)

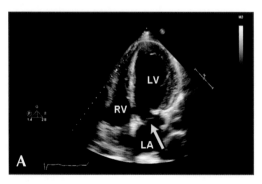

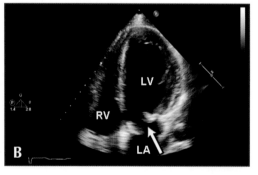

Figure 10-18. An example of mitral-prosthesis–patient mismatch (PPM). This 22-year-old patient who had refused systemic anticoagulation had a bioprosthetic mitral valve replacement 6 years prior for cleft mitral valve. Transthoracic echocardiography (ordered for exertional dyspnea) revealed a bioprosthetic valve in the mitral position, which was well seated despite

being inserted on an angle with respect to the long axis of the LV (**A**). The bioprosthetic mitral leaflets are seen in the closed position during early systole (**A**, *yellow arrow*) and appear thin and normal. Normal opening of the bioprosthetic mitral leaflets during diastole is shown (**B**, *white arrow*).

Continued on the next page

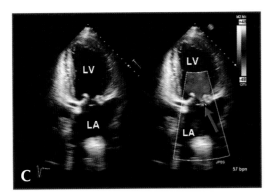
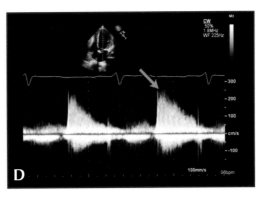

Figure 10-18. *(Continued)* Color Doppler reveals only trace mitral regurgitation (**C**, *red arrow*); it should be noted that significant left atrial shadowing by the mitral prosthesis is not normally encountered with bioprosthetic valves, and thus adequate detection of mitral regurgitation can often be made by transthoracic echocardiography. At a heart rate of 56 bpm, an elevated peak early mitral velocity (2.5 m/s) (*blue arrow*) can be seen, with a pressure half time of 193 ms, a mean mitral gradient of 11.8 mm Hg, and a time velocity integral (TVI) of 79.7 cm (**D**). As described in Figure 10-12, given an LV outflow tract (LVOT) diameter of 2.0 cm, and LVOT TVI of 26.3 cm, the calculated mitral bioprosthetic valve effective orifice area was 1.03 cm^2, qualifying as moderate PPM. LA—left atrium.

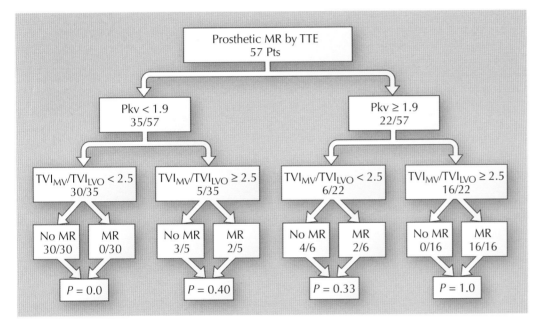

Figure 10-19. Use of the peak transmitral velocity on transthoracic echocardiography (TTE) in the detection of significant mechanical prosthetic mitral regurgitation (MR). Prosthetic valves are inherently mildly stenotic, resulting in elevated transvalvular peak velocities when compared with native valves (*see* Fig. 10-15). However, when significant prosthetic MR is present, a further increase in peak transmitral velocity occurs due to higher transvalvular flow. For mechanical prostheses, a peak velocity (Pkv) of transmitral flow in early diastole (E velocity) greater than 1.9 can indicate significant (greater than moderate) prosthetic MR in the absence of prosthetic valve stenosis. Furthermore, in significant MR, velocity and time velocity integral (TVI) in the LV outflow tract (LVOT) are decreased, but are increased through the prosthesis. Thus, the ratio of the mitral valve time velocity integral (TVI_{MV}) to the (TVI_{LVOT}) of more than 2.5 has been demonstrated to be a screening index for significant mechanical prosthetic mitral regurgitation [17]. Compared to peak velocity, the TVI ratio is less dependent on cardiac output. Pictured in the figure is an algorithm utilizing, first, the peak transmitral velocity, and second, the TVI_{MV}/ TVI_{LVOT} ratio in detecting significant prosthetic mitral regurgitation. (*From* Olmos *et al.* [17]; with permission.)

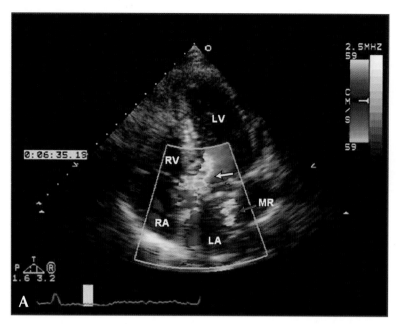

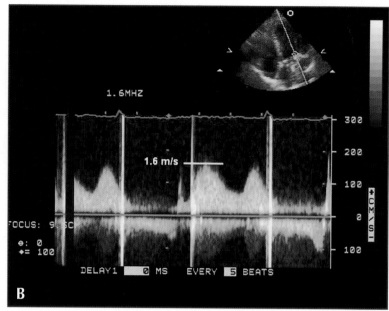

Figure 10-20. Transthoracic echocardiography in the detection of prosthetic mitral regurgitation. This 76-year-old woman with a history of mechanical prosthetic valve insertion for mitral regurgitation (MR) 8 years prior underwent echocardiography for routine monitoring of prosthetic valve function. Color Doppler imaging revealed prosthetic mitral regurgitation (**A**, *red arrow*), which is visualized in the left atrium (LA) during ventricular systole. In this case, therefore, although artifact interfered with clear LA visualization, color Doppler evidence of MR could nonetheless be detected. The aliased velocity of ejected blood through the aortic outflow tract (**A**, *yellow arrow*) is also shown. Continuous wave Doppler interrogation of the prosthetic mitral valve (**B**) revealed a peak transmitral velocity of 1.6 m/s and a mean gradient of 4.7 mm Hg, both within normal limits. These Doppler characteristics suggest a degree of prosthetic MR of less than moderate (*see* Fig. 10-19). LA—left atrium; RA—right atrium.

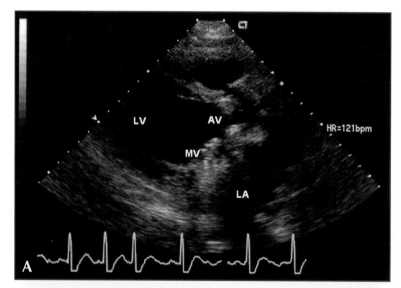

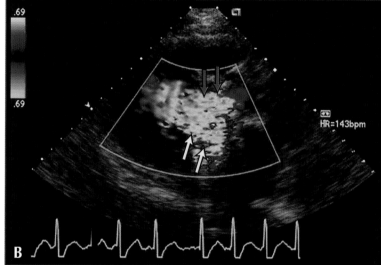

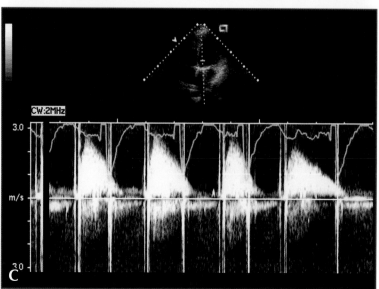

Figure 10-21. Transthoracic echocardiography (TTE) demonstrating aortic and mitral prosthetic valves with prosthetic aortic regurgitation and elevated transmitral velocities in atrial fibrillation. This 44-year-old man with a history of rheumatic heart disease underwent aortic and mitral valve replacement with mechanical prostheses 6 years prior. He presented with fatigue, fever, chills, and shortness of breath and underwent TTE. This revealed a relatively normal two-dimensional echocardiographic appearance of mechanical aortic (AV) and mitral valve (MV) prostheses (**A**). However, on color Doppler imaging (**B**), there was evidence of significant aortic regurgitation (*red arrows*) and high transmitral flow velocity (*yellow arrows*); note the confluence of mitral inflow and aortic regurgitation color jets, both occurring during diastole. Continuous wave Doppler interrogation of the mitral valve (**C**) revealed elevated transmitral velocities of approximately 2.5 m/s, taking into consideration variations in velocity due to atrial fibrillation. This patient underwent transesophageal echocardiography, revealing prosthetic mitral valve endocarditis with dehiscence of the valve and a moderate to severe periprosthetic leak (*see* Fig. 10-31). He also had moderate aortic regurgitation due to endocarditic involvement of the mechanical aortic valve. LA—left atrium.

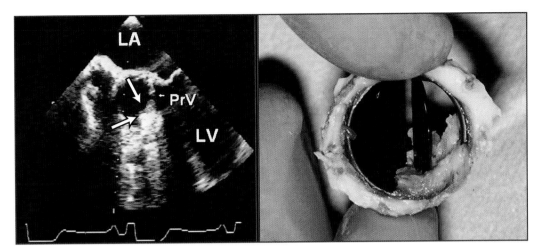

Figure 10-22. Mechanical bileaflet prosthesis with pannus formation. Transesophageal echocardiographic view of the mechanical aortic prosthesis at 0° rotation in the midesophagus. Note the considerable thickening visualized in the aortic prosthesis (*left panel, arrows*). The same valve is displayed after explantation, revealing the characteristic appearance of pannus formation with one of the mechanical leaflets stuck in the open position (*right panel*).

Pannus is a recognized cause of prosthetic valve dysfunction; the precise cause and subsequent prevention remain unknown. In mechanical bileaflet valves in the aortic position, pannus appears to originate in the neointima and periannular regions [18]. The structure of the pannus consists of myofibroblasts and an extracellular matrix, including collagen fiber. Identification of various growth factors on immunohistochemical staining suggests that pannus formation after prosthetic valve replacement may be associated with a process of periannular tissue healing via the expression of transforming growth factor-beta [18]. LA—left atrium; PrV—prosthetic valve.

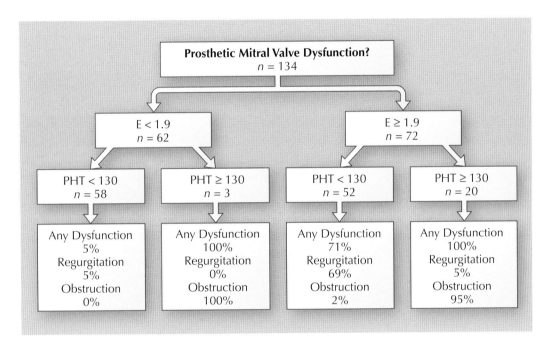

Figure 10-23. Use of peak transmitral diastolic velocity and pressure half time (PHT) by continuous wave Doppler in the detection of mechanical prosthetic mitral valve dysfunction. Similar to the detection of significant prosthetic mitral regurgitation (*see* Fig. 10-19), an elevated peak transmitral velocity in early diastole (E velocity) by continuous wave Doppler is suggestive of mitral valve obstruction. Thus, a peak E velocity more than 1.9 m/s can be used in order to detect mechanical prosthetic mitral valve dysfunction (regurgitation or obstruction). In obstruction, the PHT of the mitral valve prosthesis is prolonged (> 130 ms), whereas in regurgitation, it is not [19]. Thus, an algorithm combining an E more than 1.9 m/s, with PHT less than 130 ms can be used in transthoracic echocardiography to detect prosthetic MV dysfunction, then to differentiate its cause (regurgitation or obstruction). E—mitral early diastolic peak velocity. (*From* Fernandes *et al.* [19]; with permission.)

Normal Doppler Values with Various Types of Tricuspid Valve Prostheses

Valve Type	Peak Velocity, m/s Mean ± SD	Mean Gradient, mm Hg Mean ± SD	Pressure Half-Time, m/s Mean ± SD
Caged Ball			
Starr Edwards*	1.3 ± 0.2	3 ± 0.8	144 ± 46
Tilting disk			
Bjork-Shiley†	1.3	2.2	144
Bileaflet			
St. Jude Medical‡	1.2 ± 0.3	2.7 ± 1.1	108 ± 32
Heterograft	1.3 ± 0.2	3.0 ± 1.0	146 ± 39

*Edwards Lifesciences, Irvine, CA
†Pfizer, Inc., New York, NY
‡St. Jude Inc., St. Paul, MN

Figure 10-24. Normal Doppler-derived data in various mechanical and bioprosthetic valves in the tricuspid position. The same variables used in the assessment of mitral prostheses may be used in the assessment of tricuspid prostheses, although the velocity and mean gradient values are somewhat lower, owing to the larger size of tricuspid prostheses relative to mitral prostheses (see Fig. 10-15). In general, a peak velocity of early diastolic filling of less than 1.5 m/s and a mean gradient of less than 3 mm Hg are considered within normal limits (see chart for exact values). Although bioprosthetic valves were traditionally thought to be superior to mechanical ones in the tricuspid position due to the worry of thrombotic-related complications in the right side of the heart [20], more recent evidence has suggested that there may be no difference in early mortality, midterm mortality, or re-replacement rates between the two types of valves [21]. In addition, bioprosthetic valves in the tricuspid position may be particularly prone to pannus formation [22]. (Adapted from Connolly et al. [23].)

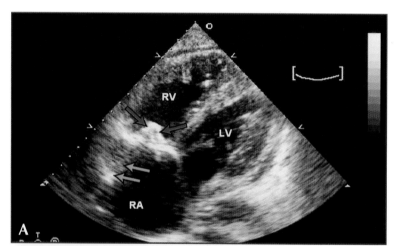

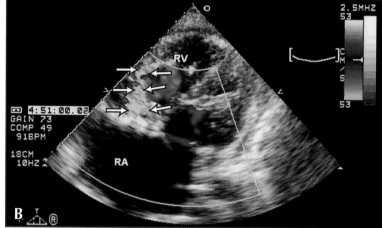

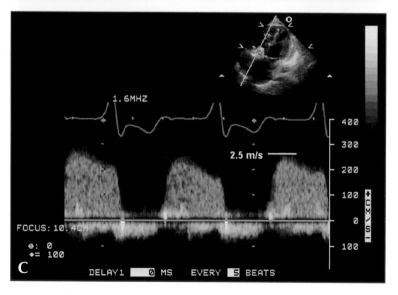

Figure 10-25. Mechanical prosthetic tricuspid valve (TV) with severe prosthetic TV stenosis. This 38-year-old patient with mechanical prosthetic tricuspid and pulmonic valves presented with increasing shortness of breath and fatigue. Transthoracic echocardiography in an oblique apical view (**A**) revealed a mechanical prosthetic tricuspid valve (red arrows) with reverberation artifact generated by the prosthesis (blue arrows), as well as RV dilatation. Color Doppler during diastole (**B**) showed a turbulent TV inflow jet (arrows) extending into the RV. Continuous wave Doppler interrogation (**C**) revealed an elevated peak tricuspid inflow velocity of 2.5 m/s with a mean gradient of 16 mm Hg, suggesting severe prosthetic TV stenosis. This patient had a history of noncompliance with warfarin (Coumadin; Bristol-Myers Squibb, Princeton, NJ). RA—right atrium.

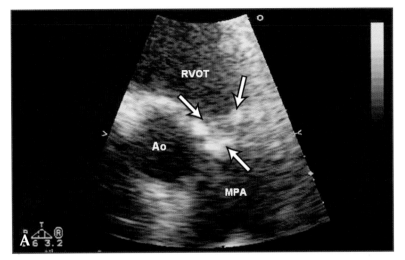

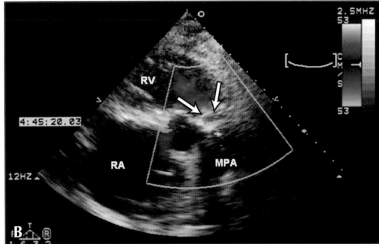

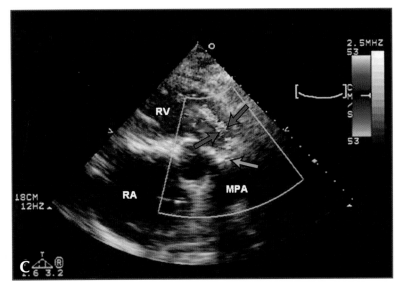

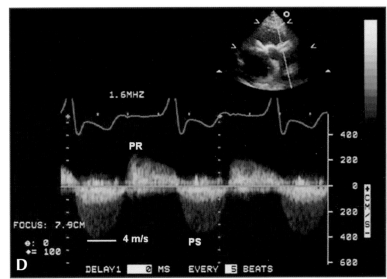

Figure 10-26. Prosthetic pulmonic valve with moderate prosthetic pulmonic stenosis (PS) and moderate pulmonic regurgitation (PR). The transthoracic echocardiogram on the same patient as in Figure 10-25 revealed a prosthetic valve in the pulmonic position (**A**, *arrows*) in the basal short-axis view. The aortic root (Ao) is seen to the left of the pulmonic prosthesis, and the bifurcation of the main pulmonary artery (MPA) is visualized inferior to the pulmonic valve. Color Doppler imaging (**B**) during systole revealed flow convergence (*arrows*) on the RV side of the prosthesis as blood passes through the prosthet-ic valve into the MPA. Color Doppler during diastole (**C**) revealed prosthetic PR (*red arrows*) into the RV outflow tract with flow convergence seen this time on the MPA side of the prosthesis (*blue arrow*). Continuous wave Doppler inter-rogation (**D**) of the PS jet revealed a peak velocity of 4 m/s during systole, indi-cating a peak gradient of 64 mm Hg. In diastole, the PR spectral envelope across the prosthetic pulmonic valve is visualized with an intermediate deceleration time and spectral density. These Doppler features suggest moderate prosthetic PS and PR. RA—right atrium; RVOT—RV outflow tract.

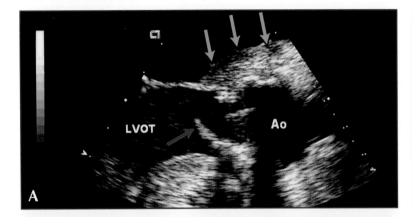

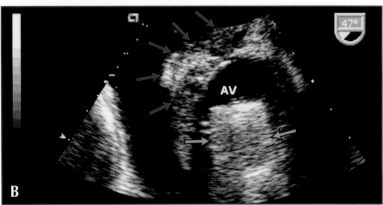

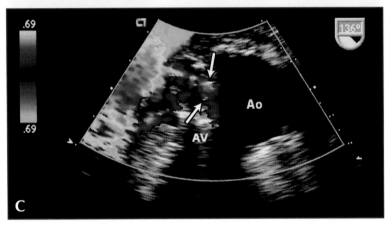

Figure 10-27. Mechanical aortic prosthesis with endocarditis complicated by aortic root abscess. This 56-year-old woman underwent prosthetic aortic valve (AV) placement 22 years prior with a single leaflet mechanical prosthesis for a bicuspid AV. She presented with a 3-week history of fever, anorexia, weight loss, and shortness of breath. Four out of four blood culture bottles on admission grew *Staphylococcus aureus*. Transthoracic echocardiography suggested a mass on the prosthetic AV, and transesophageal echocardiography (TEE) was performed. TEE long-axis view (**A**) revealed a vegetation (*red arrow*) on the LV outflow tract (LVOT) side of the prosthetic AV with marked thickening (*blue arrows*) along the posterior aortic root, suggestive of valvular abscess. The vegetation extended along the posterior aortic root and along the anterior

wall of the left atrium. Zoomed short-axis view on TEE (**B**) confirmed the presence of aortic root thickening strongly suggesting abscess (*red arrows*). Note the appearance of the monoleaflet mechanical prosthetic AV in short-axis view with characteristic reverberation artifact (*blue arrows*). On color Doppler imaging (**C**), only mild aortic insufficiency (*arrows*) was visualized without presence of a fistula involving the abscess. At surgery, this patient had prosthetic AV endocarditis, with the prosthesis on the verge of total dehiscence, being surrounded by abscess. She underwent successful AV replacement with a homograft and aortic root reconstruction and fully recovered.

Prosthetic valve endocarditis (PVE) is a serious condition with considerable morbidity and mortality and occurs at a rate of approximately 0.45% per year [24]. PVE can be divided into early (nosocomial) and late (community acquired) cases. As the microbiologic causes differ between early and late PVE, the cut off between early and late is generally regarded as 1 year [25]. For early PVE, staphylococci and HACEK (*Haemophilus, Actinobacillus, Cardiobacterium, Eikenella,* and *Kingella* species) organisms are common, whereas in late PVE, staphylococci, streptococci, and enterococci are common. Duration of intravenous antibiotic treatment of PVE is generally 4 to 6 weeks, longer than that for native valve endocarditis [25]. Surgical intervention is necessary in many cases of PVE and especially for complicated cases (abscess, paravalvular leak, fistulae, large vegetations, resistant organisms), although some uncomplicated cases may be treated with antibiotics alone [24,26]. Given the serious nature of PVE, with an in-hospital mortality of 20% to 30% [27,28], antibiotic prophylaxis in patients with prosthetic valves prior to dental or surgical procedures is of great importance. Ao—aorta.

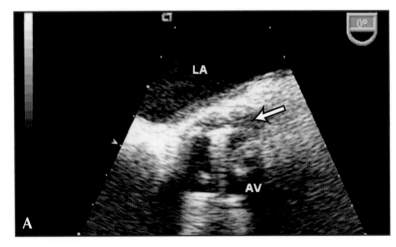

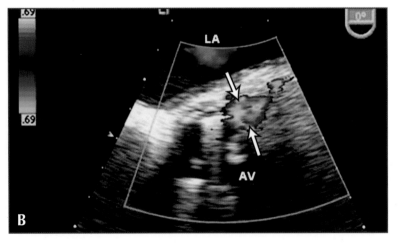

Figure 10-28. Bioprosthetic aortic valve (AV) with perivalvular abscess and leak. This 73-year-old patient underwent bioprosthetic aortic valve insertion 5 years prior for degenerative aortic stenosis. He presented with a 2-week history of fevers and weakness. Transesophageal echocardiography (TEE) short-axis images (**A**) revealed a bioprosthetic AV with an area of echolucency in the postero-

lateral aortic root (*arrow*), indicative of a cavity. Color Doppler imaging (**B**) in the same view revealed evidence of color flow into the cavity (*arrows*), whereas color M-mode imaging in the area of the cavity (**C**) revealed evidence of "to and fro" flow (*arrows*) between the aortic root and the cavity.

Continued on the next page

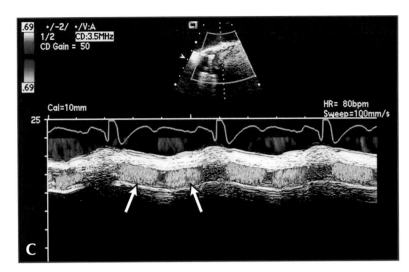

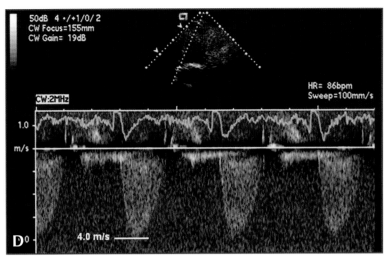

Figure 10-28. (*Continued*) Continuous wave Doppler on transthoracic imaging (**D**) showed an elevated peak velocity (4 m/s) across the aortic valve, resulting in a peak gradient of 64 mm Hg due to obstruction related to endocarditis (*see* Fig. 10-9). Thus, this patient had bioprosthetic endocarditis complicated by abscess formation with fistula formation from the aortic root into the abscess.

Periannular complications in prosthetic valve endocarditis (PVE) include abscess, pseudoaneurysm, and fistula formation [28]. These complications of PVE are readily identified by TEE with an accuracy of more than 95%. Periannular complications are more common in aortic PVE than mitral PVE, and tend to occur within 6 months of surgery [28]. Although surgical treatment (along with antibiotic therapy) is recommended for PVE with periannular complications, the in-hospital mortality remains high at approximately 38% [28]. LA—left atrium.

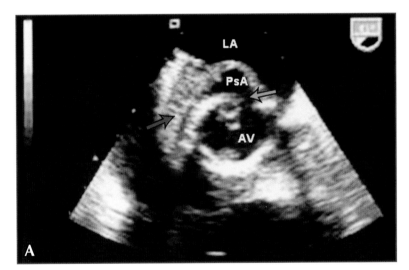

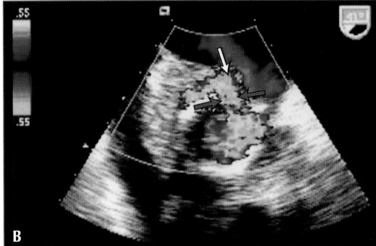

Figure 10-29. Prosthetic aortic valve (AV) endocarditis complicated by abscess and pseudoaneurysm (PsA) formation. On transesophageal echocardiographic (TEE) imaging in the basal short-axis view (**A**), an echolucent space is visualized in the superior aortic root, communicating (*blue arrow*) with the aortic annulus, suggestive of PsA formation. Note the aortic root thickening (*red arrow*), suggesting abscess formation. On color Doppler imaging during diastole (**B**), flow is seen exiting the PsA (*yellow arrow*) into the LV outflow (*red arrows*). The turbulent appearance of the diastolic flow suggested communication with the aortic root, which was confirmed at surgery.

Pseudoaneurysms of the mitral aortic intervalvular fibrosa are relatively uncommon and generally occur as complications of endocarditis,

valve surgery, or chest trauma [29]. Their importance is underscored by the complications of rupture, which may lead to cardiac tamponade and severe regurgitation. PsAs occur when infection or trauma causes dehiscence, creating a cavity between the medial wall of the left atrium (LA) and the aorta, communicating with the LV outflow tract [30]. The majority of intervalvular PsAs involve endocarditis of prosthetic AVs. The diagnosis can be detected by transthoracic echocardiography (TTE) or aortography. However, TEE is a more accurate means of diagnosis and characterization [29] and complements TTE visualization. PsAs are dynamic, expanding during isovolumic contraction and early systole, and collapsing during diastole. Ao—aorta.

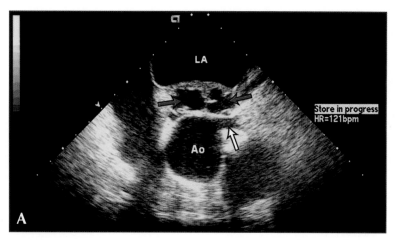

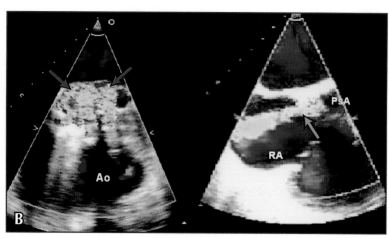

Figure 10-30. Prosthetic aortic valve endocarditis with pseudoaneurysm (PsA) formation and fistula formation into the right atrium (RA). This 62-year-old patient with a history of aortic valve replacement presented with fever, chills, and cough. Transthoracic echocardiography (TTE) was performed in order to evaluate prosthetic valve function due to persistent shortness of breath. TTE revealed significant thickening in the area of the aortic root, suggesting abscess formation. Transesophageal echocardiography (TEE) in the basal short-axis view (**A**) demonstrated two side-by-side echolucent spaces (*red arrows*) superior to the posterior aortic root. Note the clear visualization of the left main coronary artery (*white arrow*) and its bifurcation. Color Doppler imaging in the short-axis view during diastole (**B**, *left image*) revealed turbulent color (*red arrows*) filling these spaces, representing flow from the aortic root into the PsA during diastole. In the long-axis view during systole (**B**, *right image*) color flow can be visualized exiting the PsA (*blue arrow*) and entering the RA (fistula formation). In real-time imaging, pulsatility was observed as blood entered the PsA during diastole and exited during systole (*see* Fig. 10-29). Ao—aorta.

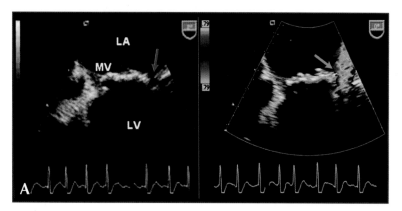

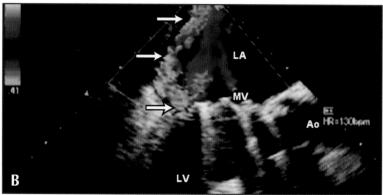

Figure 10-31. Mechanical prosthetic mitral valve (MV) endocarditis with paravalvular leak. This 44-year-old patient underwent aortic and mitral valve replacement with a mechanical bileaflet prosthesis 6 years prior for rheumatic valve disease. He presented with a 2-week history of sweats, chills, nausea, and dyspnea. Blood culture on admission grew *Streptococcus viridans* in two out of three sets. Transthoracic echocardiography revealed high transmitral prosthetic gradients with evidence of significant prosthetic mitral regurgitation (*see* Fig. 10-21). Two-dimensional transesophageal echocardiography (**A**, *left image*) revealed an echolucent area in the posterolateral mitral annulus (*red arrow*), suggestive of prosthetic dehiscence. Color Doppler imaging (**A**, *right panel*) revealed periprosthetic mitral regurgitation (*blue arrow*) through this echolucent space. An eccentric mitral regurgitation jet (**B**) is seen coursing along the posterior left atrium (LA) (*arrows*) and was graded as moderately severe. Thus, this patient had prosthetic mitral valve endocarditis complicated by annular abscess with dehiscence and significant periprosthetic mitral regurgitation. Ao—aorta; LA—left atrium.

Prosthetic Valve Thrombosis

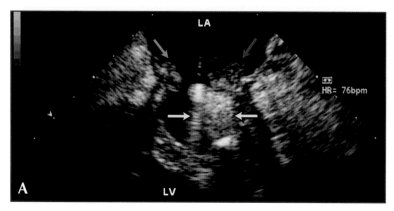

Figure 10-32. Mechanical mitral valve thrombosis. This 55-year-old woman with a history of mechanical valve insertion 3 years prior presented with shortness of breath and fatigue. Transthoracic echocardiography revealed an elevated transmitral gradient, thus transesophageal echocardiography (TEE) was performed. Long-axis view on TEE (**A**) revealed a bileaflet mechanical prosthesis in the mitral position with a large mass in the lateral aspect of the prosthesis (*red arrow*), and a smaller mass in the medial annulus (*blue arrow*). Note that the lateral leaflet does not open in diastole ("stuck leaflet") while the medial leaflet is open. Note also the intense reverberation artifact (*yellow arrows*) generated by the mechanical mitral prosthesis.

Continued on the next page

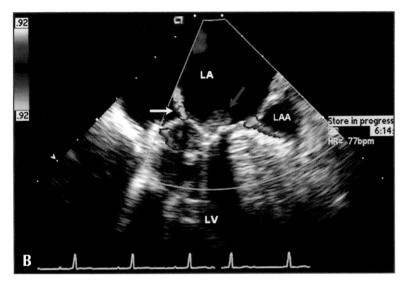

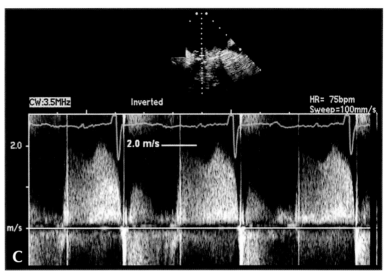

Figure 10-32. *(Continued)* Color Doppler imaging (**B**) revealed only mild central mitral regurgitation (*yellow arrow*). Note the appearance of the thrombus (*red arrow*) and the presence of color flow from the left atrium (LA) into the left atrial appendage (LAA), which had been previously surgically "closed." By continuous wave Doppler, the transmitral velocity was elevated at 2 m/s with an elevated mean gradient of 8 mm Hg (**C**). This patient underwent thrombolysis using streptokinase, with resolution of her symptoms and decrease of the transmitral velocity to 1.5 m/s, with a mean gradient of 3.8 mm Hg. She did not suffer any embolic complications.

Prosthetic valve thrombosis is a life-threatening condition that causes substantial morbidity and mortality, whether it occurs early or late after surgery [31]. Treatment options for prosthetic mechanical valve thrombosis include anticoagulation with heparin, thrombolysis, or surgical intervention. Although surgical intervention is an option for patients with valve thrombosis, espe-cially in those with very large clot burden, thrombolysis has increasingly been used to treat prosthetic valve thrombosis in patients without contraindications [32,33]. Some investigators have suggested thrombolysis as first-line therapy in patients without contraindications for mechanical valve thrombolysis [34]. There is also evidence that both repeated and slow rate infusions are more efficacious and may be associated with lower morbidity than bolus infusions [35]. After initial hemodynamic evaluation with transthoracic echocardiography, TEE is particularly useful for direct prosthesis visualization in order to differentiate the cause of valve obstruction, although fluoroscopy can be also be used [36]. When distinguishing thrombus from pannus formation as the cause of obstruction, pannus is more common in the aortic position, in patients with adequate anticoagulation, those with more than 1-month's duration of symptoms, and those with echodense (as opposed to soft) mass on the prosthesis by TEE [37].

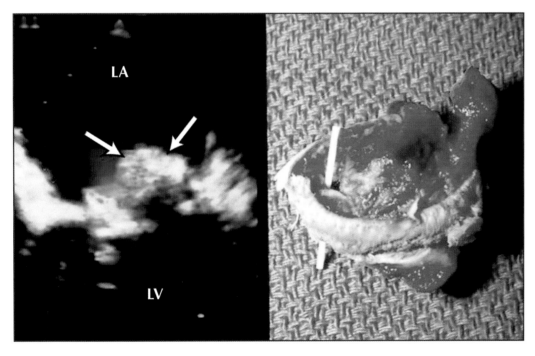

Figure 10-33. Pathologic correlation of mechanical mitral valve thrombosis findings at echocardiography. On transesophageal echocardiography (*left image*), soft tissue densities are visualized in the mitral prosthesis (*arrows*). At pathology after surgical resection, large thrombi are visualized. Note the bright red appearance of the thrombus and its extensive nature, involving nearly the entire prosthetic mitral valve orifice (*see* Fig. 10-32 for discussion of prosthetic valve thrombosis). LA—left atrium.

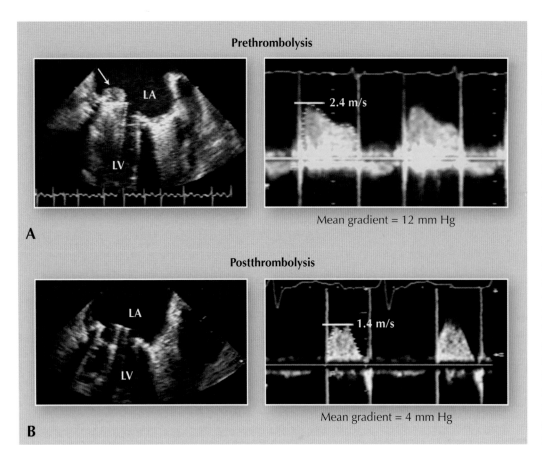

Prethrombolysis

LA

LV

2.4 m/s

Mean gradient = 12 mm Hg

A

Postthrombolysis

LA

LV

1.4 m/s

Mean gradient = 4 mm Hg

B

Figure 10-34. Pre- and post-thrombolysis echocardiographic Doppler of a thrombosed mechanical mitral valve. This patient, with a history of under-anticoagulation for her prosthetic mechanical mitral valve, presented with increasing dyspnea. Transesophageal echocardiography (TEE) revealed a mechanical bileaflet prosthetic mitral valve (**A**, *left*) with a large circular thrombus (*arrow*) on the left atrial (LA) side of the medial leaflet. As the frame is in diastole, note that only the lateral leaflet is open, the medial leaflet being "stuck" in the closed position by the thrombus. Continuous wave Doppler interrogation of the mitral prosthesis (**A**, *right*) reveals a peak velocity of 2.4 m/s with a mean gradient of 12 mm Hg, both indicative of valve obstruction (*see* Fig. 10-15 and 10-23). The patient was treated with intravenous streptokinase with marked relief of her dyspnea, and she had no complications. Repeat TEE of the mitral prosthesis (**B**, *left*) reveals no evidence of thrombus, with full opening of the prosthetic leaflets in diastole. Continuous wave Doppler (**B**, *right*) reveals a peak transmitral velocity of 1.4 m/s and a mean gradient of 4 mm Hg, both which are within normal limits for a mechanical mitral prosthesis.

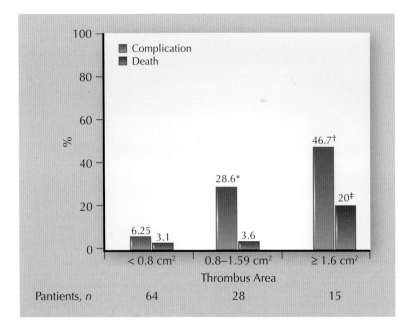

Figure 10-35. Role of transesophageal echocardiography (TEE) in prosthetic valve thrombolysis. In a multicenter study assessing the role of TEE in patient selection for thrombolysis, 107 patients with mechanical valve thrombosis (the majority mitral) were assessed [38]. Hemodynamic success was achieved in 85%, whereas complications were observed in 17.8% and death in 5.6%. Multivariate analysis demonstrated that TEE demonstration of thrombus area of more than 0.8 cm^2 and a history of stroke were independent predictors of complications after thrombolysis. The risk of complications was incremental to increasing thrombus size. Thus, TEE can help risk stratify individuals with prosthetic valve thrombosis and help select patients for thrombolysis. *P—0.003; †P—0.0001; ‡P—0.016. (*Adapted from* Tong *et al.* [38].)

New Directions in Prosthetic Valves

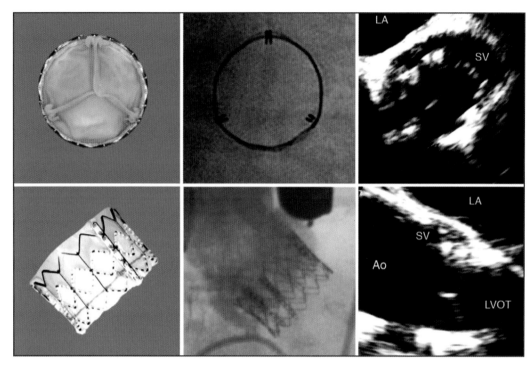

were of high surgical risk, Webb *et al.* [39] performed transcatheter implantation of a balloon expandable aortic valve stent. Valve implantation was successful in 86% of patients, with intraprocedural mortality of 2%. Mortality at 30 days was 12%, with improving outcomes associated with ongoing procedural experience. The figures (*Top and bottom, left panel*) shows a photograph of the balloon-expandable stent from the aortic aspect showing leaflets in the closed position (*Top, left panel*) and from the side showing the fabric sealing cuff (*Bottom, left panel*). Fluoroscopic images of the implanted and fully expanded valve are shown from the aortic aspect (*Top, middle panel*), and the aortic angiogram (*Bottom, middle panel*) shows the valve securely fixed in the annulus. During transesophageal echocardiography (*Top and Bottom, right panels*), short-axis (*Top, right panel*) and long-axis (*Bottom, right panel*) view shows the orientation of the implanted aortic valve relative to adjacent cardiac structures [39]. Ao—aorta; LA—left atrium; LVOT—LV outflow tract; SV—sinus of Valsalva. (*From* Webb et al. [39]; with permission.)

Figure 10-36. Percutaneous valve implantation in the aortic position. Given that open thoracic surgery is necessary for standard prosthetic valve implantation, there has been an interest in percutaneous valve deployment in the aortic and pulmonic positions. In selected patients with severe aortic stenosis whom

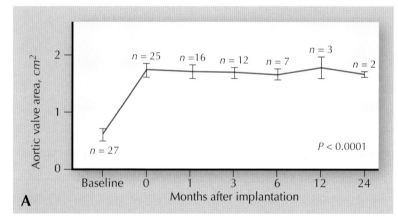

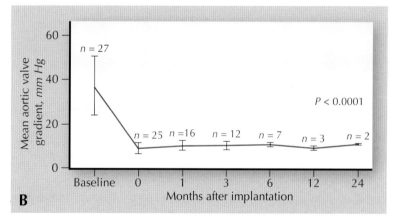

Figure 10-37. Improvement in aortic valve area and mean aortic valve gradient after percutaneous aortic valve implantation. Cribier *et al.* [40] developed an equine pericardium valve in a balloon expandable, stainless steel stent and tested its implantation in 36 patients with severe comorbidities and New York Heart Association (NYHA) class IV who were formally turned down for surgical aortic valve replacement. Twenty-seven patients (75%) were implanted successfully, with improvement in valve area (0.60 ± 0.11 cm^2 to 1.70 ± 0.10 cm^2) (**A**) and transvalvular gradient (37 ± 13 mm Hg to 9 ± 2 mm Hg, [**B**] $P <$

0.0001 for both comparisons). Postprocedural paravalvular aortic regurgitation was grade 0 to 1/4 in 10 patients, grade 2/4 in 12 patients, and grade 3/4 in 5 patients. Improvement in LV ejection fraction (EF) ($45 \pm 18\%$ to $53 \pm 14\%$, $P = 0.02$) was most pronounced in patients with EF less than 50% ($35 \pm 10\%$ to $50 \pm 16\%$, $P < 0.0001$), while 30-day major adverse events after successful implantation were 26% [40]. Thus, this study revealed that percutaneous valve replacement may be an option in selected patients who are too ill for open surgical aortic valve replacement. (*Adapted from* Cribier et al. [40].)

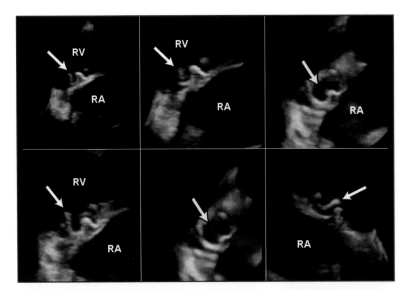

Figure 10-38. Three-dimensional transthoracic echocardiography (TTE) of a normally functioning bioprosthetic valve in the tricuspid position. Three-dimensional TTE can improve spatial resolution and in certain cases can provide anatomically correct and very detailed pictures of cardiac structures, at times mitigating the need for transesophageal echocardiography (TEE). In the case of bioprosthetic valves, if good transthoracic acoustic windows are present, exquisite imaging can be achieved, as depicted in the figure. The three struts of the bioprosthetic tricuspid valve can be well seen (*white arrows*), within which the thin, pliable, normal appearing bioprosthetic leaflets (*yellow arrows*) can be visualized. One of the advantages of three-dimensional echocardiography is that, from one full-volume capture (usually six to eight cardiac beats during breath hold), multiple cuts and orientations of the bioprosthetic valve can be obtained. However, for mechanical prostheses, acoustic shadowing can still pose a significant problem for three-dimensional TTE; in such cases, three-dimensional TEE can be used for optimal visualization (*see* Fig. 10-39). RA—right atrium.

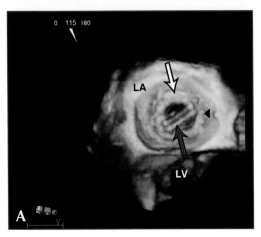
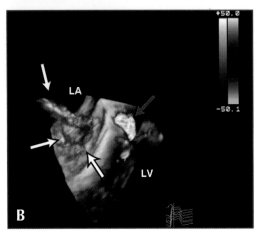

Figure 10-39. Three-dimensional transesophageal echocardiography (TEE) of a bileaflet mechanical mitral valve. Mechanical prosthetic valves in the atrioventricular position cause intense shadowing of the atria during transthoracic echocardiography and of the ventricles during TEE (*see* Fig. 10-4). The mechanical mitral valve (MV) is imaged from the atrial aspect (**A**); thus the reverberation artifact is confined to the ventricular side, allowing clear visualization of the mechanical mitral leaflets (*red arrow*), which are open during diastole. Note the clear visualization of the prosthetic MV ring (*white arrow*) and the suture points (*black arrowhead*). The regurgitant jets of the mechanical MV are well visualized (**B**), coursing into the left atrium. Three physiologic ("washing jets," *see* Fig. 10-6C) are seen (*white arrows*), which are normal for a bileaflet mechanical valve. Note color Doppler evidence of flow out the LV outflow tract (*red arrow*). LA—left atrium.

References

1. Vongpatanasin W, Hillis LD, Lange RA: Prosthetic heart valves. *N Engl J Med* 1996, 335:407–416.

2. Rahimtoola SH: Choice of prosthetic heart valve for adult patients. *J Am Coll Cardiol* 2003, 41:893–904.

3. Ikonomidis JS, Kratz JM, Crumbley AJ III, *et al.*: Twenty-year experience with the St. Jude mechanical valve prosthesis. *J Thorac Cardiovasc Surg* 2003, 126:2022–2031.

4. Butchart EG, Li HH, Payne N, *et al.*: Twenty years' experience with the Medtronic Hall valve. *J Thorac Cardiovasc Surg* 2001, 121:1090–1100.

5. Rizzoli G, Bottio T, Thiene G, *et al.*: Long-term durability of the Hancock II porcine bioprosthesis. *J Thorac Cardiovasc Surg* 2003, 126:66–74.

6. Rao V, Christakis GT, Sever J, *et al.*: A novel comparison of stentless versus stented valves in the small aortic root. *J Thorac Cardiovasc Surg* 1999, 117:431–436.

7. Yun KL, Sintek CF, Fletcher AD, *et al.*: Aortic valve replacement with the freestyle stentless bioprosthesis: five-year experience. *Circulation* 1999, 100(19 Suppl):II17–II23.

8. Hammermeister K, Sethi G, Henderson WG, *et al.*: Outcomes 15 years after valve replacement with a mechanical versus a bioprosthetic valve: final report of the Veterans Affairs randomized trial. *J Am Coll Cardiol* 2000, 36:1152–1158.

9. Davis EA, Greene PS, Cameron DE, *et al.*: Bioprosthetic versus mechanical prostheses for aortic valve replacement in the elderly. *Circulation* 1996, 94(9 Suppl): II121–II125.

10. Girard SE, Miller FA Jr, Orszulak TA, *et al.*: Reoperation for prosthetic aortic valve obstruction in the era of echocardiography: trends in diagnostic testing and comparison with surgical findings. *J Am Coll Cardiol* 2001, 37:579–584.

11. Barbetseas J, Zoghbi WA: Evaluation of prosthetic valve function and associated complications. *Cardiol Clin* 1998, 16:505–530.

12. Chafizadeh ER, Zoghbi WA: Doppler echocardiographic assessment of the St. Jude Medical prosthetic valve in the aortic position using the continuity equation. *Circulation* 1991, 83:213–223.

13. Pibarot P, Dumesnil JG: Hemodynamic and clinical impact of patient-prosthesis mismatch in the aortic valve position and its prevention. *J Am Coll Cardiol* 2000, 36:1131–1141.

14. Pibarot P, Dumesnil JG, Jobin J, *et al.*: Usefulness of the indexed effective orifice area at rest in predicting an increase in gradient during maximum exercise in patients with a bioprosthesis in the aortic valve position. *Am J Cardiol* 1999, 83:542–546.

15. Tasca G, Mhagna Z, Perotti S, *et al.*: Impact of prosthesis-patient mismatch on cardiac events and midterm mortality after aortic valve replacement in patients with pure aortic stenosis. *Circulation* 2006, 113:570–576. [Published erratum appears in *Circulation* 2006, 113:e288.]

16. Magne J, Mathieu P, Dumesnil JG, *et al.*: Impact of prosthesis-patient mismatch on survival after mitral valve replacement. *Circulation* 2007, 115:1417–1425.

17. Olmos L, Salazar G, Barbetseas J, *et al.*: Usefulness of transthoracic echocardiography in detecting significant prosthetic mitral valve regurgitation. *Am J Cardiol* 1999, 83:199–205.

18. Teshima H, Hayashida N, Yano H, *et al.*: Obstruction of St. Jude medical valves in the aortic position: histology and immunohistochemistry of pannus. *J Thorac Cardiovasc Surg* 2003, 126:401–407.

19. Fernandes V, Olmos L, Nagueh SF, *et al.*: Peak early diastolic velocity rather than pressure half-time is the best index of mechanical prosthetic valve function. *Am J Cardiol* 2002, 89:704–710.

20. Dalrymple-Hay MJ, Leung Y, Ohri SK, *et al.*: Tricuspid valve replacement: bioprostheses are preferable. *J Heart Valve Dis* 1999, 8:644–648.

21. Kaplan M, Kut MS, Demirtas MM, *et al.*: Prosthetic replacement of tricuspid valve: bioprosthetic or mechanical? *Ann Thorac Surg* 2002, 73:467–473.

22. Nakano K, Ishibashi-Ueda H, Kobayashi J, *et al.*: Tricuspid valve replacement with bioprostheses: long-term results and causes of valve dysfunction. *Ann Thorac Surg* 2001, 71:105–109.

23. Connolly HM, Miller FA Jr, Taylor CL, *et al.*: Doppler hemodynamic profiles of 82 clinically and echocardiographically normal tricuspid valve prostheses. *Circulation* 1993, 88:2722–2727.

24. Akowuah EF, Davies W, Oliver S, *et al.*: Prosthetic valve endocarditis: early and late outcome following medical or surgical treatment. *Heart* 2003, 89:269–272.

25. Piper C, Korfer R, Horstkotte D: Prosthetic valve endocarditis. *Heart* 2001, 85:590–593.

26. Tornos P: Management of prosthetic valve endocarditis: a clinical challenge. *Heart* 2003, 89:245–246.

27. Tornos P, Almirante B, Olona M, *et al.*: Clinical outcome and long-term prognosis of late prosthetic valve endocarditis: a 20-year experience. *Clin Infect Dis* 1997, 24:381–386.

28. San Roman JA, Vilacosta I, Sarria C, *et al.*: Clinical course, microbiologic profile, and diagnosis of periannular complications in prosthetic valve endocarditis. *Am J Cardiol* 1999, 83:1075–1079.

29. Afridi I, Apostolidou MA, Saad RM, *et al.*: Pseudoaneurysms of the mitral-aortic intervalvular fibrosa: dynamic characterization using transesophageal echocardiographic and Doppler techniques. *J Am Coll Cardiol* 1995, 25:137–145.

30. Karalis DG, Bansal RC, Hauck AJ, *et al.*: Transesophageal echocardiographic recognition of subaortic complications in aortic valve endocarditis. Clinical and surgical implications. *Circulation* 1992, 86:353–362.

31. Laplace G, Lafitte S, Labeque JN, *et al.*: Clinical significance of early thrombosis after prosthetic mitral valve replacement: a postoperative monocentric study of 680 patients. *J Am Coll Cardiol* 2004, 43:1283–1290.

32. Roudaut R, Lafitte S, Roudaut MF, *et al.*: Fibrinolysis of mechanical prosthetic valve thrombosis: a single-center study of 127 cases. *J Am Coll Cardiol* 2003, 41:653–658.

33. Shapira Y, Herz I, Vaturi M, *et al.*: Thrombolysis is an effective and safe therapy in stuck bileaflet mitral valves in the absence of high risk thrombi. *J Am Coll Cardiol* 2000, 35:1874–1880.

34. Silber H, Khan SS, Matloff JM, *et al.*: The St. Jude valve. Thrombolysis as the first line of therapy for cardiac valve thrombosis. *Circulation* 1993, 87:30–37.

35. Ozkan M, Kaymaz C, Kirma C, *et al.*: Intravenous thrombolytic treatment of mechanical prosthetic valve thrombosis: a study using serial transesophageal echocardiography. *J Am Coll Cardiol* 2000, 35:1881–1889.

36. Montorsi P, De Bernardi F, Muratori M, *et al.*: Role of cine-fluoroscopy, transthoracic, and transesophageal echocardiography in patients with suspected prosthetic heart valve thrombosis. *Am J Cardiol* 2000, 85:58–64.

37. Barbetseas J, Nagueh SF, Pitsavos C, *et al.*: Differentiating thrombus from pannus formation in obstructed mechanical prosthetic valves: an evaluation of clinical, transthoracic and transesophageal echocardiographic parameters. *J Am Coll Cardiol* 1998, 32:1410–1417.

38. Tong AT, Roudaut R, Ozkan M, *et al.*: Transesophageal echocardiography improves risk assessment of thrombolysis of prosthetic valve thrombosis: results of the international PRO-TEE registry. *J Am Coll Cardiol* 2004, 43:77–84.

39. Webb JG, Pasupati S, Humphries K, *et al.*: Percutaneous transarterial aortic valve replacement in selected high-risk patients with aortic stenosis. *Circulation* 2007, 116:755–763.

40. Cribier A, Eltchaninoff H, Tron C, *et al.*: Treatment of calcific aortic stenosis with the percutaneous heart valve: mid-term follow-up from the initial feasibility studies: the French experience. *J Am Coll Cardiol* 2006, 47:1214–1223.

Echocardiographic Assessment of the Tricuspid and Pulmonic Valves

Linda D. Gillam

Although the tricuspid and pulmonic valves are structurally similar to the mitral and aortic valves, they rarely undergo the chronic degenerative changes that affect their left-sided counterparts. Moreover, they are less likely to be affected by acquired diseases, such as endocarditis and the rheumatic process. The pulmonic valve is particularly immune. This is generally attributed to the relative protection afforded by the lower right-sided pressures. Congenital abnormalities such as Ebstein's anomaly and pulmonary stenosis are frequently encountered in the adult, and when the physiologic disturbance is mild it may have been undetected in childhood. The most common form of tricuspid dysfunction is functional (*ie*, when leaflet architecture is normal, but RV dysfunction and remodeling prevent normal valve closure). This condition accounts for most surgical procedures performed on the tricuspid valve. Echocardiography plays a unique role in the assessment of the tricuspid and pulmonic valves. However, their evaluation is often suboptimal because imaging protocols may overlook the views that best display pulmonic and tricuspid anatomy and function. The images selected for this chapter include the disorders that most commonly affect the tricuspid and pulmonic valves and illustrate the views that can be used to image them most effectively.

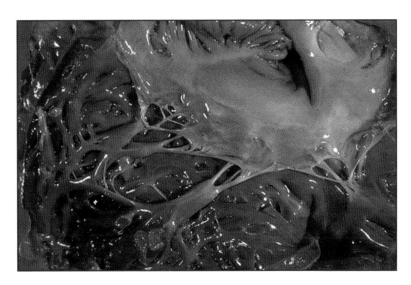

Figure 11-1. An autopsy specimen of a normal tricuspid valve is shown. The annulus is larger than that of the mitral valve, and it is more apically positioned. Note the relative sizes of the three leaflets: the anterior leaflet is largest, with an attachment that extends from the infundibulum to the inferoposterior wall. The posterior leaflet is the smallest, and it extends along the diaphragmatic surface as the septal leaflet attaches to the muscular and membranous septum with an irregular array of chordae. The papillary muscles are variable in number, size, and position.

Views for Assessing the Tricuspid Valve

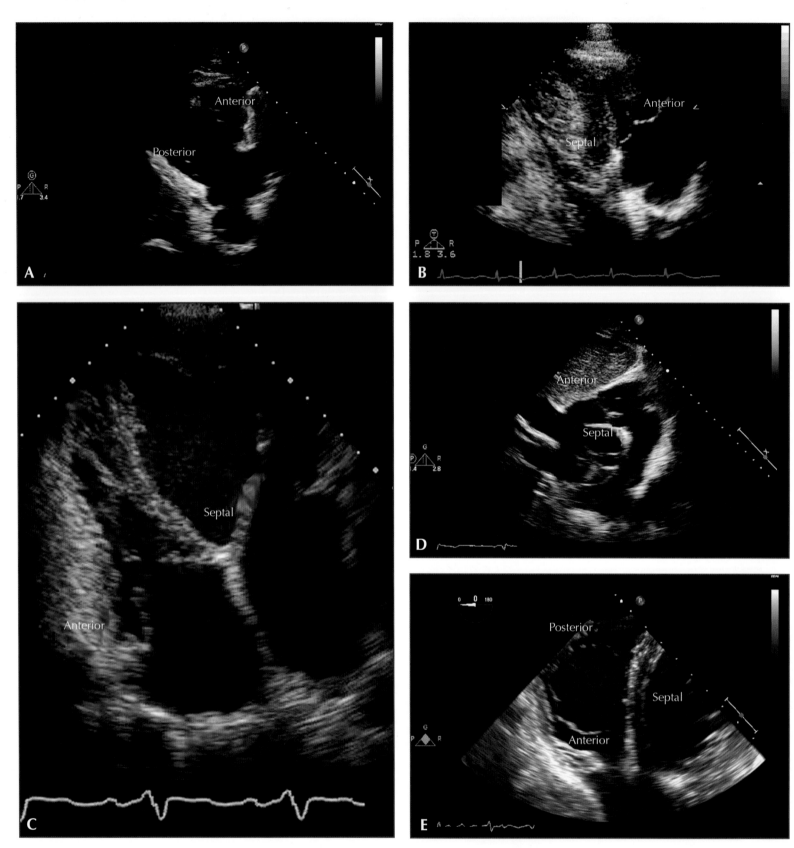

Figure 11-2. The standard two-dimensional echocardiographic views for imaging the tricuspid valve are shown. **A**, RV inflow tract view. When obtained properly, this view displays the diaphragmatic and anterior walls of the RV and the anterior and posterior leaflets of the tricuspid valve. This is a key view for visualizing the posterior leaflet. **B**, A nonstandard but common variant of this view is recognizable by the visualization of Tri interventricular septum and adjacent LV cavity. This view displays the anterior and septal leaflets. **C**, This apical four-chamber view demonstrates the anterior and septal leaflets. A similar view may be obtained from the subcostal window and from the midesophageal four-chamber transesophageal echocardiographic view. **D**, Subcostal short-axis view at the level of the great vessels is shown. This view displays the anterior and septal leaflets. A similar may be obtained parasternally. **E**, The short-axis transesophageal echocardiographic transgastric view is the only view that shows all leaflets simultaneously. It may be possible to obtain a comparable view using the parasternal short-axis view, particularly if the RV is dilated.

Abnormalities of the Tricuspid Valve

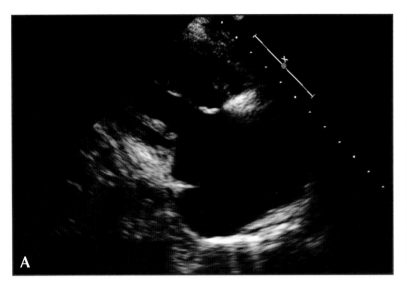

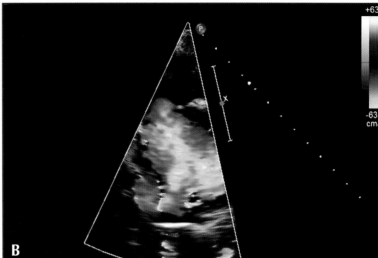

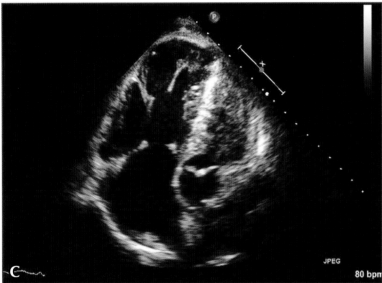

Figure 11-3. Right ventricular inflow tract views (**A** and **B**) demonstrate the typical features of carcinoid heart disease. The leaflets are thickened, retracted, and immobilized, creating a large regurgitant orifice. As a result, there is unrestricted tricuspid regurgitation, and the color regurgitant jet may appear relatively monochromic. In the apical five-chamber view of the same patient (**C**), the classic "drum stick" appearance of the leaflets is evident. The valvopathy occurs when serotonin and its metabolite 5 hydroxytryptophan secreted by carcinoid tumors causes an inflammatory reaction in the valves. Because the active metabolite is inactivated in the lungs, left-sided involvement occurs only when there is an intracardiac shunt or pulmonary metastases.

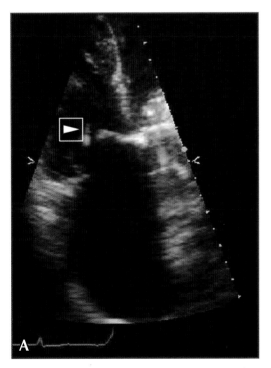

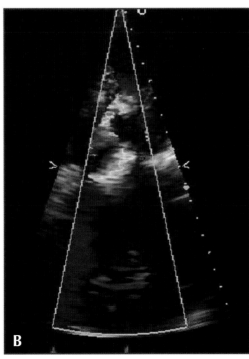

Figure 11-4. **A**, An apical four-chamber view demonstrates rheumatic tricuspid disease. A pathognomonic finding is diastolic leaflet doming (*arrowhead*) seen involving the septal leaflet. This occurs because the belly of the leaflet may remain mobile as the tip is restricted. Rheumatic tricuspid disease is generally accompanied by rheumatic mitral disease. It may be distinguished from carcinoid disease (where mitral involvement is rare) by the presence of commissural fusion and chordal thickening. **B**, In this diastolic frame, color flow demonstrates proximal flow convergence, a marker of stenosis. This patient also had moderate to severe tricuspid regurgitation.

Continued on the next page

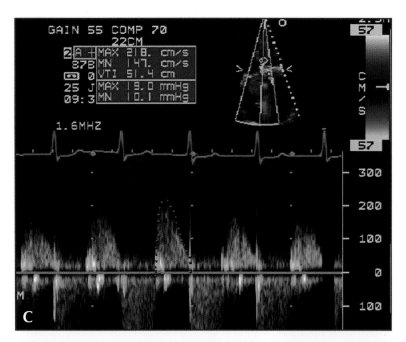

Figure 11-4. *(Continued)* **C**, Spectral Doppler can be used to derive transvalvular gradients.

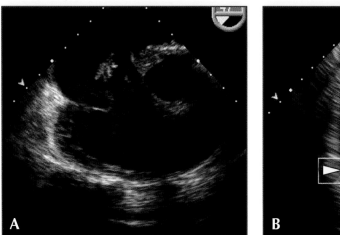

Figure 11-5. Tricuspid valve endocarditis is shown. Transesophageal midesophageal (**A**) and transgastric (**B**) echocardiograms demonstrate a large irregular vegetation (**B**, *arrowhead*) attached to the anterior leaflet of the tricuspid valve. The chordal attachments have been disrupted, and there is severe tricuspid regurgitation. Tricuspid endocarditis is typically a disease of intravenous drug abusers or the immuno-compromised. In approximately 50% of cases, the causative organism is *Staphylococcus aureus*.

Figure 11-6. The apical four-chamber view shows a flail septal leaflet. Flail tricuspid leaflet may be caused by trauma (*eg*, acceleration-deceleration injury) or endocarditis, and it is a recognized complication of RV biopsy. Spontaneous chordal rupture or RV papillary muscle rupture is extremely rare. The regurgitant jets are typically eccentric.

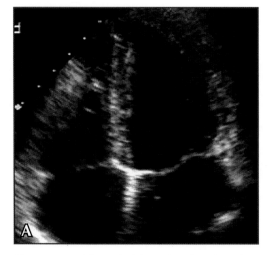
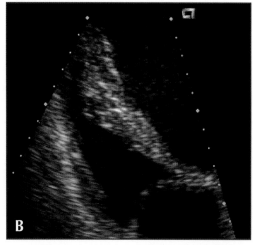
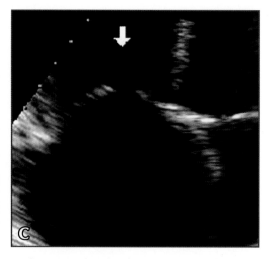

Figure 11-7. The apical four-chamber view shows normal closure pattern (**A**) and the apically tethered pattern (**B**) that is typical of functional tricuspid regurgitation. In extreme cases, there is complete failure of leaflet coaptation with a visible regurgitant orifice (**C,** *arrow*), and severe regurgitation occurs. Functional tricuspid regurgitation is the most common abnormality of the tricuspid valve and may be encountered as a consequence of either primary (myopathy, infarction) or secondary (pulmonary vascular disease, left-sided heart disease) RV dysfunction. The pathophysiology is likely analogous to that reported for the mitral valve with an imbalance between closure and tethering forces. Factors promoting tethering include annular dilation and geometric remodeling of the RV. Impaired RV systolic function (whether primary or secondary) reduces closure forces.

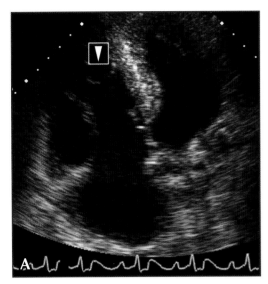
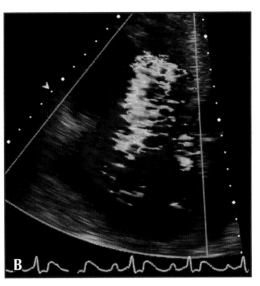

Figure 11-8. An apical four-chamber view of Ebstein's anomaly is shown. This most common congenital anomaly of the tricuspid valve is associated with apical displacement (**A**, *arrow*) of the septal, posterior, and (less commonly) the anterior leaflets. As is the case here, septal tissue may be immobilized by an arcade-like attachment along the interventricular septum. In this case, the septal leaflet becomes mobile only at the midventricular level. The anterior leaflet is large and sail-like. Tricuspid regurgitation and interatrial shunts are common. The apically displaced origin of the tricuspid regurgitant jet is shown (**B**). Although severe cases present with cyanosis in infancy, patients with milder forms may remain asymptomatic until late adulthood.

Figure 11-9. A four-chamber view demonstrates tricuspid atresia. The tricuspid valve is absent (*arrow*), and the RV is hypoplastic. There is a large atrial septal defect, which directs systemic venous return to the left side of the heart. Not shown is a small RV outflow tract and normal pulmonary valve. A Waterston shunt (also not shown) connects the ascending aorta to the main pulmonary artery.

Pulmonary Valve

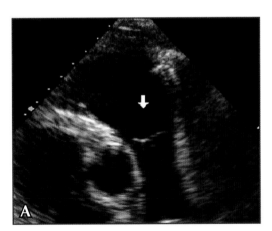
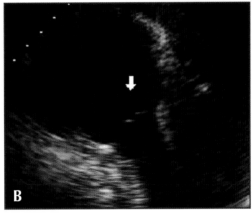
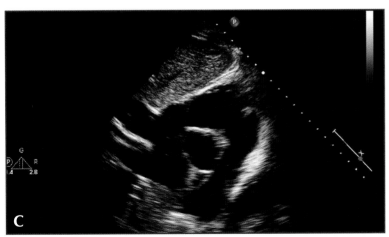
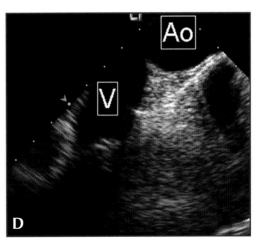

Figure 11-10. Although the pulmonic valve has three cusps (right, left, and anterior), it is rare to see all three in a single short two-dimensional echocardiographic image. Long-axis images of the valve (*arrow*) may be obtained transthoracically using basal parasternal (**A**), steeply anteriorly angulated apical (**B**) with the valve indicated (*arrow*), and subcostal (**C**) windows. Comparable views may be obtained with transesophageal echocardiography (TEE). TEE offers a unique view of the valve using a high esophageal window rotated slightly from that used to image the aortic arch (**D**). Ao—aorta; V—valve.

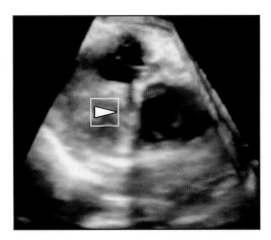

Figure 11-11. Three-dimensional echo-cardiographic views of the pulmonic valve (*arrowhead*) derived from midesophagheal. A systolic frame showing all 3 cusps is shown. Three-dimensional echocardiography can display all 3 cusps simultaneously.

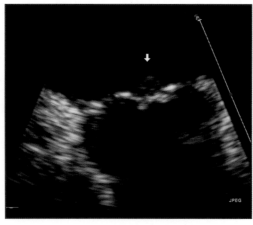

Figure 11-12. The parasternal image demonstrates a pulmonic valve vegetation (*arrow*). Pulmonic valve endocarditis is rare, but may accompany tricuspid valve or endocarditis or occur in the setting of congenital heart disease involving the pulmonic valve and/or pulmonary artery. In this case, the organism was *Staphylococcus aureus*.

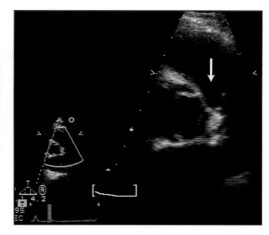

Figure 11-13. The parasternal systolic image of congenital valvular pulmonic stenosis is shown. The imaging hallmark is systolic doming of the valve (*arrow*). In real time, the valve has a jump rope appearance because the restricted tip projects into the pulmonary artery (PA) as the belly of the cusp is mobile. Color Doppler demonstrates turbulent flow, and spectral Doppler can be used to measure transvalvular gradients. In such patients, it is important to remember that RV systolic pressure (as estimated from the tricuspid regurgitant jet) will not equal PA systolic pressure. Instead, RV systolic pressure (RVSP) = PA systolic pressure + transvalvular gradient. Failure to recognize pulmonic stenosis may result in the misdiagnosis of pulmonary hypertension.

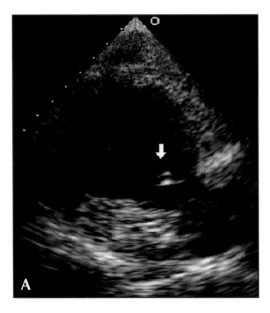

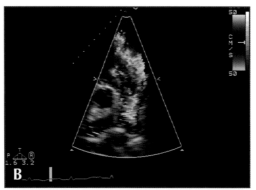

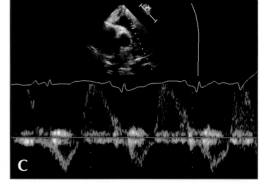

Figure 11-14. Postvalvotomy pulmonic valve with unrestricted pulmonic regurgitation is shown. **A,** A parasternal short-axis view of a congenitally stenotic pulmonic valve following valvuloplasty is depicted. Visualized cusp is thickened (*arrow*). In some cases, irregularly mobile fragments may be seen. **B,** Color flow mapping shows unrestricted regurgitation. When pulmonary artery pressure is normal, the flow may not have the typical mosaic pattern of high-velocity jets, and the severity of the regurgitation may be underestimated. **C,** Spectral Doppler shows a laminar regurgitant signal.

Suggested Reading

Attenhofer Jost CH, Connolly HM, Dearani J, et al.: Ebstein's anomaly. *Circulation* 2007, 115:277–285.

Bashore TM, Cabell C, Fowler V Jr: Update on infective endocarditis. *Curr Probl Cardiol* 2006, 31:274–352.

Gibson TC, Foale RA, Guyer DE, Weyman AE: Clinical significance of incomplete tricuspid valve closure seen on two-dimensional echocardiography. *J Am Coll Cardiol* 1984, 4:1052–1057.

Guyer DE, Gillam LD, Foale RA, et al.: Comparison of the echocardiographic and hemodynamic diagnosis of rheumatic tricuspid stenosis. *J Am Coll Cardiol* 2008, 3:1135–1144.

Moller JE, Pellikka PA, Bernheim AM, et al.: Prognosis of carcinoid heart disease: analysis of 200 cases over two decades. *Circulation* 2005, 112:3320–3327.

Pothineni KR, Duncan K, Yelamanchili P, et al.: Live/real time three-dimensional transthoracic echocardiographic assessment of tricuspid valve pathology: incremental value over the two-dimensional technique. *Echocardiography* 2007, 24:541–552.

Shah PM, Raney AA: Tricuspid valve disease. *Curr Probl Cardiol* 2008, 33:47–84.

Singh SK, Tang GH, Maganti MD, et al.: Midterm outcomes of tricuspid valve repair versus replacement for organic tricuspid disease. *Ann Thorac Surg* 2006, 82:1735–1741.

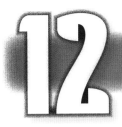

12 Myocardial Infarction

Kaitlyn My-Tu Lam, Kibar Yared, David McCarty, and Michael H. Picard

Echocardiography has many roles during and after myocardial infarction. These roles include diagnosis, quantifying prognosis, and assessment of complications. Identification of regional LV wall motion abnormalities and regional LV dysfunction can accelerate the diagnosis of acute myocardial infarction, especially when other findings are confusing. Such circumstances include chest pain in a patient with left bundle branch block on ECG, a patient whose biomarkers are mildly elevated in the presence of renal failure, or other entities that may alter creatine phosphokinase or troponin. It is important to keep in mind that other causes may present similar to acute myocardial infarction. Echocardiography can recognize such disease processes responsible for presentation. Global LV function, as measured by LV ejection fraction; size and location of infarction, as measured by wall motion score index, and inducible ischemia, as quantified on stress testing, have all been demonstrated to have prognostic value after myocardial infarction. Echocardiographic techniques have the ability to quantify each of these measures of prognosis. Echocardiography is valuable in assessing complications that may arise after myocardial infarction, ranging from recurrent chest pain, due to recurrent ischemia, to cardiogenic shock, due to a mechanical complication. Direct visualization of cardiac structure and function by transthoracic or transesophageal echocardiography enable rapid identification of the etiology of these complications, resulting in triage to optimum therapy. Lastly, new technologies, such as three-dimensional echocardiography and strain rate imaging, enhance display and quantitation of LV function by echocardiography. The goal of this chapter is to demonstrate the wide range of applications of echocardiography in myocardial infarction.

Echocardiographic Diagnosis of Myocardial Infarction

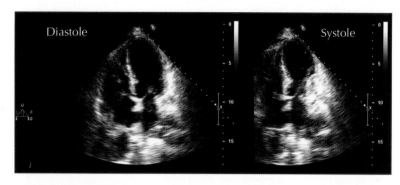

Figure 12-1. Regional LV wall motion abnormality on echocardiography is the hallmark of coronary artery disease and myocardial infarction. It is one of the earliest signs of myocardial ischemia and infarction and serves as a key component in the latest definition of both acute and prior myocardial infarction [1]. During ischemia and infarction, there is decreased thickening of the myocardium and reduced inward motion of the endocardial wall. Shown here is a transthoracic echocardiographic apical four-chamber view with regional wall motion abnormality during anterior myocardial infarction (diastole and systole). The extent of dysfunction involves the apical portion of the LV.

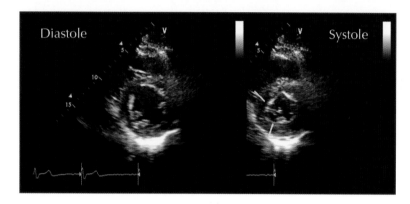

Figure 12-2. Diastolic and systolic frames from a transthoracic echocardiographic parasternal short axis view at mid-LV level demonstrate the circumferential extent of regional wall motion abnormality during inferior myocardial infarction (*between yellow lines*). The inferior septum and inferior wall are involved.

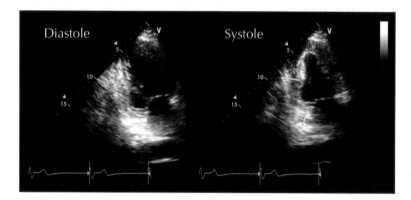

Figure 12-3. Transthoracic echocardiographic apical two-chamber view (from the same patient as Figure 12-2) demonstrates the longitudinal extent of regional wall motion abnormality after inferior myocardial infarction (*between yellow lines*).

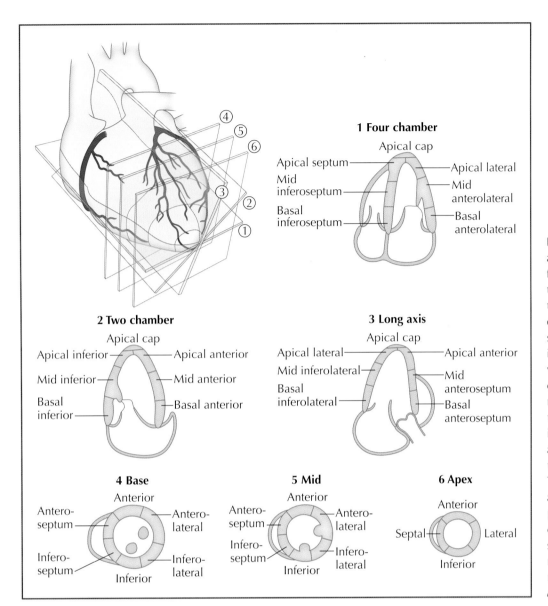

1 Four chamber

Apical cap

Apical septum — — Apical lateral

Mid inferoseptum — — Mid anterolateral

Basal inferoseptum — — Basal anterolateral

2 Two chamber

Apical cap

Apical inferior — — Apical anterior

Mid inferior — — Mid anterior

Basal inferior — — Basal anterior

3 Long axis

Apical cap

Apical lateral — — Apical anterior

Mid inferolateral — — Mid anteroseptum

Basal inferolateral — — Basal anteroseptum

4 Base

Anterior

Antero-septum — — Antero-lateral

Infero-septum — — Infero-lateral

Inferior

5 Mid

Anterior

Antero-septum — — Antero-lateral

Infero-septum — — Infero-lateral

Inferior

6 Apex

Anterior

Septal — — Lateral

Inferior

Figure 12-4. The standardized nomenclature and segmentation of the LV that is applicable for all the tomographic cardiac imaging modalities is shown here [2]. This differs slightly from the typical 16-segment model previously used in echocardiography due to the addition of a 17th segment, an apical cap. This 17-segment model is ideal for myocardial perfusion assessment and when comparing echocardiographic findings with other imaging modalities. The 16-segment model remains appropriate for wall motion quantitation and display because the apical cap does not include a full thickness of the myocardium [3]. In addition, assessment of motion and thickening of this 17th segment is difficult in clinical practice. The degree of wall motion in each LV segment is assessed visually in multiple views and by comparing it with other segments [4]. Segments are described as normal, hyperkinetic (enhanced systolic motion), hypokinetic (reduced systolic motion), akinetic (no systolic motion), and dyskinetic (paradoxical systolic motion). (*From* Lang *et al.* [3]; with permission.)

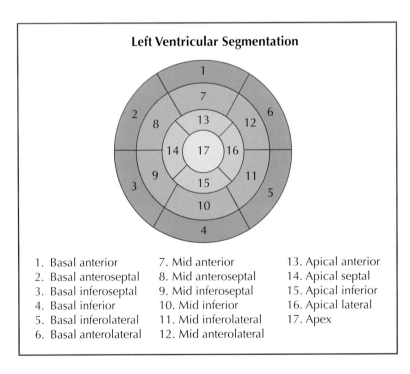

Left Ventricular Segmentation

1. Basal anterior
2. Basal anteroseptal
3. Basal inferoseptal
4. Basal inferior
5. Basal inferolateral
6. Basal anterolateral
7. Mid anterior
8. Mid anteroseptal
9. Mid inferoseptal
10. Mid inferior
11. Mid inferolateral
12. Mid anterolateral
13. Apical anterior
14. Apical septal
15. Apical inferior
16. Apical lateral
17. Apex

Figure 12-5. The myocardial segmental function can be displayed in a polar or "bulls-eye" diagram, as shown here. The degree of dysfunction can be displayed in each segment, or a wall motion score can be quantified by assigning a number to each segment based on its function (normal = 1, hypokinetic = 2, akinetic = 3, dyskinetic = 4). The points in each segment are summed and a wall motion score index is then calculated as the mean score per segment. (*Adapted from* American Society of Nuclear Cardiology [5].)

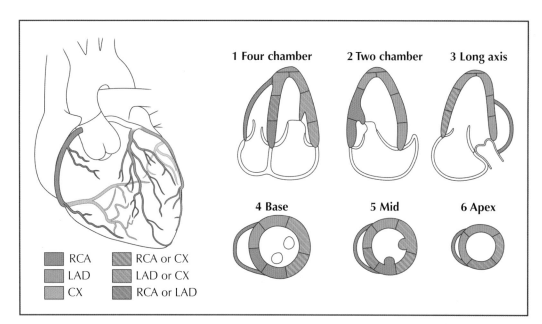

Figure 12-6. There is variability in the coronary arterial blood supply to the myocardium. However, this illustration shows the most common assignment of the LV segments to the artery that most often provides its blood supply. RCA – right coronary artery; LAD – left descending coronary artery; CX – circumflex coronary artery. (*From* Lang *et al.* [3]; with permission.)

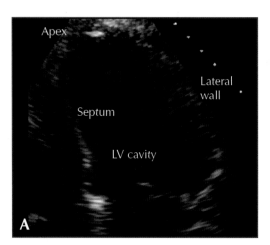 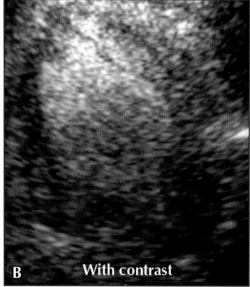

Figure 12-7. Complete LV endocardial border delineation is critical for the assessment of regional and global LV function in the setting of myocardial infarction. When images are not optimal (more than two endocardial segments not visualized), echocardiographic contrast agents can be used.

Echocardiographic contrast agents consist of a gas enclosed by a liquid, which can scatter sound strongly, and travel like red blood cells. Contrast-enhanced echocardiographic images are highly accurate in detecting regional wall abnormalities when compared with other cardiac imaging modalities and reduce interobserver variability for detection of wall motion abnormalities [6]. Contrast echocardiography can accurately identify LV thrombi after infarction and distinguish these from normal trabeculations [7]. Unenhanced (**A**) and contrast-enhanced (**B**) transthoracic apical echocardiographic images are shown here from a 78-year-old man who presented with syncope, elevated cardiac enzymes, but no chest pain. Echocardiography demonstrates LV dilatation with diffuse hypokinesia with regional variation and estimated ejection fraction of 26%. The images after contrast injection show improved endocardial definition and no evidence of LV thrombus (**B**).

Echocardiography to Assess Sequelae and Complications of Myocardial Infarction

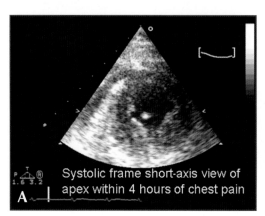 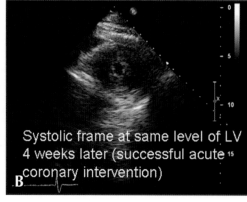

Figure 12-8. In an acute myocardial infarction (MI), reperfusion of the infarct-related artery (when performed within hours of the symptom onset) can result in the recovery of myocardial function [8]. This is demonstrated in these images from a 62-year-old man, who presented with his first acute anterior MI and received stenting of the mid-left anterior descending artery within 4 hours of symptom onset (**A**). The follow-up echo images are from 4 weeks later (**B**) and show resolution of the regional dysfunction.

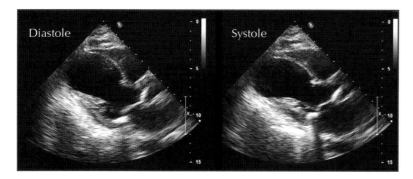

Figure 12-9. When early reperfusion is unsuccessful or not attempted in anterior myocardial infarction, then adverse remodeling in the form of infarct expansion can occur within hours of presentation. This early process is considered "functional" infarct expansion, and refers to the early process prior to the permanent structural changes of aneurysm formation [9].

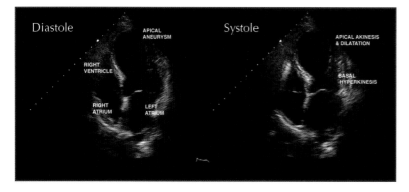

Figure 12-10. The functional expansion eventually becomes an aneurysm as the infarcted area undergoes further expansion and thinning. The wall of the aneurysm consists of all the layers of the myocardium; however, fibrous tissue replaces the necrotic muscle over time. The walls of the aneurysm are typically less than 7 mm thick in diastole, yet can be highly reflective on the ultrasound image due to increased fibrosis and calcification. An aneurysm is defined by the presence of distortion of the ventricular cavity shape in diastole. The walls of the aneurysm exhibit akinetic or dyskinetic motion in systole. True aneurysms characteristically have a wide neck, which is comparable to the maximal width of aneurysmal cavity. Nearly 90% of all aneurysms involve the cardiac apex and anterior wall. Apical aneurysms are frequently associated with LV thrombus. Ventricular aneurysms may contribute to cardiac decompensation, recurrent arrhythmia, and systemic emboli. Spontaneous rupture is rare and late rupture almost never occurs. Aneurysm formation after acute coronary syndrome is associated with higher mortality rates and subsequent clinical events [10,11].

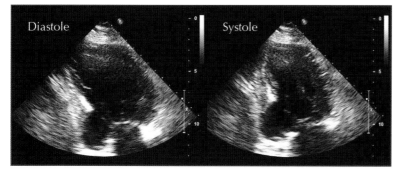

Figure 12-11. The same pathologic process can involve the inferior wall, although this is less common than the apical aneurysm. When aneurysms involve the inferior wall, the normal position of the posteromedial papillary muscle is often displaced, resulting in significant mitral regurgitation [12].

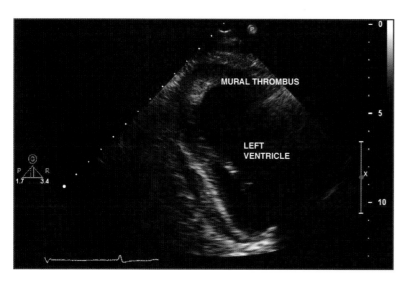

Figure 12-12. LV thrombus is a common complication of myocardial infarction. It has decreased in frequency since the introduction of reperfusion therapy. The reported incidence varies between 5% and 60%, depending on infarct size, location, and treatment [13,14]. Mural thrombi appear as focal echo-producing masses adjacent to the normal endocardial contour of the ventricle in regions of dyskinesis or akinesis. They may be fixed, pedunculated, mobile, or may have a fixed base with mobile filaments extending from the surface. They can have a speckled appearance and when organized may contain areas that are brighter or more reflective than the surrounding myocardium. Confirmation of thrombus requires its visualization on at least two views. Thrombi can generally be detected on echocardiography 6 to 10 days after acute infarction; however, delayed formation may occur with LV remodeling and worsening function. Detection within 48 hours is associated with poorer prognosis [15]. Mural thrombi are more common with anterior infarctions, larger infarctions, impaired LV function, and aneurysm formation. Thrombi are a potential source of arterial embolic events and studies report increased events with thrombi that are mobile, protrude into ventricular cavity, or are adjacent to zones of hyperkinetic wall motion [16].

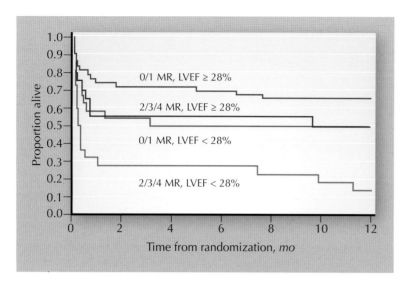

Figure 12-13. Cardiogenic shock is a major cause of death in patients admitted with acute myocardial infarction. A wide range of cardiac structural and functional abnormalities exist in patients who present with acute cardiogenic shock. LV failure is the cause of shock in more than 75% of all cases of cardiogenic shock, but other causes include ventricular septal rupture, acute mitral regurgitation (MR) from papillary muscle rupture, RV infarction, and cardiac tamponade [17]. Although echocardiography is commonly used in diagnosis and management of myocardial infarction and shock, the prognostic value of echocardiography early in the course of cardiogenic shock has only recently been demonstrated. Both short- and long-term mortality rates are independently associated with LV ejection fraction and severity of mitral regurgitation assessed by echocardiography at admission in patients with cardiogenic shock [18]. LVEF—LV ejection fraction; mo—months. (*From* Picard *et al.* [18]; with permission.)

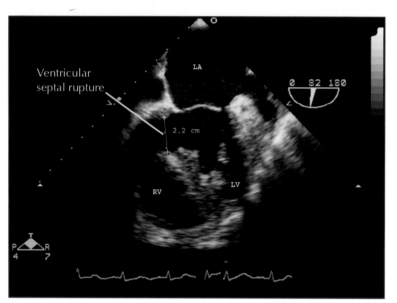

Figure 12-14. Rupture of the ventricular septum is a mechanical complication that can follow myocardial infarction and result in cardiogenic shock. In the era before reperfusion therapy, septal rupture was found in up to 3% of acute myocardial infarctions, but now the incidence has decreased to less than 1% [19,20]. Ventricular septal rupture occurs more frequently with anterior rather than other types of acute myocardial infarction. Risk factors include advanced age, female sex, lack of collateral coronary circulation, and hypertension [21]. In the absence of coronary reperfusion, septal rupture generally occurs within the first week after infarction. The median time from the onset of symptoms of acute myocardial infarction to rupture is generally 24 hours or less in patients who have received thrombolysis [19]. Typical patients present with chest pain, shortness of breath, and hypotension with a harsh holosystolic murmur with or without a palpable thrill at the left lower sternal border. Pulmonary edema, biventricular failure, and cardiogenic shock ensue. The transesophageal echocardiographic image shown is from an 82-year-old man who presented with acute-onset shortness of breath and biventricular failure. It demonstrates a 2.2-cm inferobasal ventricular septal defect (*green line*). There is also evidence of RV dilation and diffuse hypokinesis. LA—left atrium

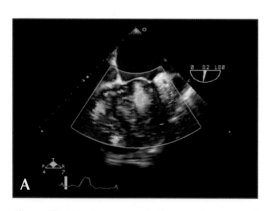
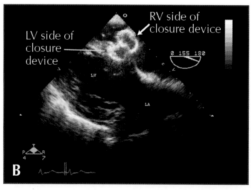

Figure 12-15. Acute ventricular septal rupture after myocardial infarction results in a left-to-right shunt, with increased pulmonary blood flow and volume overload of both ventricles and the left atrium. With ongoing shunting, RV and LV systolic function deteriorates, and forward flow diminishes. This leads to compensatory systemic vasoconstriction and increased systemic vascular resistance, which increases the magnitude of the left-to-right shunt. The degree of shunting is determined by the size of the defect, the ratio of pulmonary to systemic vascular resistance, and LV and RV function. As the LV fails and the systolic pressure declines, left-to-right shunting decreases. In anterior myocardial infarctions, the septal rupture tends to be apical, whereas in inferior infarctions, the septal defect is more basal and larger, resulting in a poorer prognosis. Immediate stabilization with intra-aortic balloon pump and urgent surgical repair results in improved survival compared with balloon pump and medical management, or later surgery [20]. **A,** Color Doppler flow through a large inferoseptal defect. **B,** Transesophageal echocardiographic image after successful percutaneous transcatheter device closure.

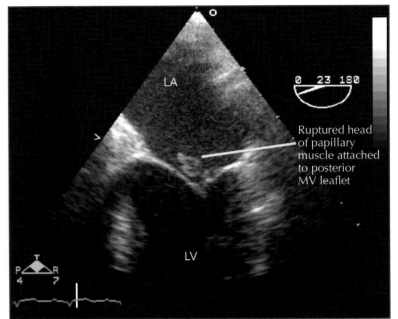

Figure 12-16. Acute papillary muscle rupture complicates about 1% of transmural myocardial infarctions. Patients present with acute pulmonary edema and cardiogenic shock [22,23]. The associated myocardial infarction is often small, with patients dying from LV volume overload from severe acute mitral regurgitation (MR) rather than primary pump failure. The condition more commonly complicates inferior myocardial infarction with involvement of the posteromedial papillary muscle because this muscle receives blood from a single coronary artery, typically the posterior descending coronary artery. The anterolateral papillary muscle is less commonly involved, as it receives a dual blood supply from the left anterior descending and left circumflex coronary artery systems. Following initial stabilization with an intra-aortic balloon pump, surgery is the treatment of choice. Images from a transesophageal echocardiogram demonstrate the free portion of the ruptured posteromedial papillary muscle prolapsing into the left atrium. Hyperdynamic LV function is often associated with acute, severe mitral regurgitation. MV—mitral valve.

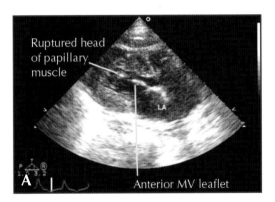
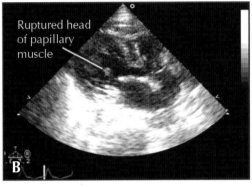
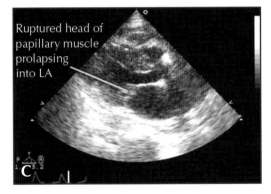
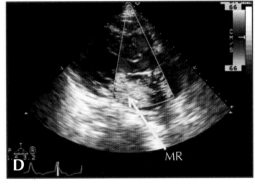

Figure 12-17. A common echocardiographic finding in acute papillary muscle rupture, complicating myocardial infarction (MI), is the presence of acute, severe mitral regurgitation (MR) and shock in a patient with a small MI and increased LV ejection fraction. In these transthoracic echocardiographic images from a patient with cardiogenic shock, the series of images from diastole through systole demonstrate the mobile portion of the ruptured papillary muscle. Color Doppler confirms the severe MR. MV—mitral valve.

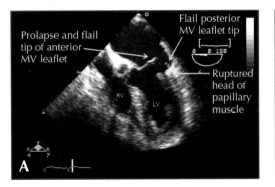
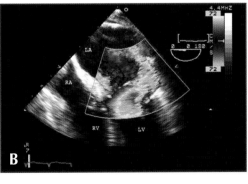

moves into the left atrium; for a prolapsed leaflet, the coaptation of leaflets remains present, but other portions of the leaflet are displaced into the left atrium. This transesophageal image shows prolapse and flail of both leaflets following rupture of the anterolateral papillary muscle in a 72-year-old woman with lateral myocardial infarction and shock (**A**). The accompanying color Doppler image shows the severe mitral regurgitation (wide vena contracta) directed away from the anterior leaflet of the mitral valve into the left atrium (**B**).

Figure 12-18. Rupture of the papillary muscle from myocardial infarction may be partial or complete. The spectrum of mitral valve (MV) dysfunction can range from flail of one or both leaflets, to flail of a portion of one leaflet, to prolapse of a leaflet. When a leaflet is flail, the tip has lost its support and

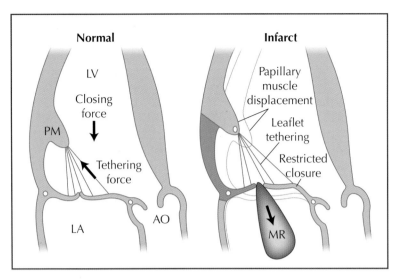

Figure 12-19. Ischemic mitral regurgitation (MR) frequently follows myocardial infarction and may accompany either extensive infarction with generalized LV dilation, or localized infarction of the inferior wall. In the setting of myocardial ischemia or infarction, several of the forces that control mitral valve closure will be affected. These include papillary muscle (PM) position, mitral valve closure position as controlled by chordal tension, and closing forces from ventricular systolic pressure development [24]. (*From* Levine *et al.* [24]; with permission.) AO—aorta; LA—left atrium.

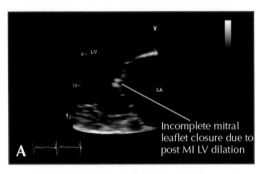

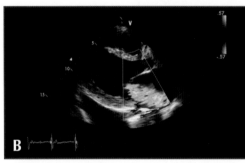

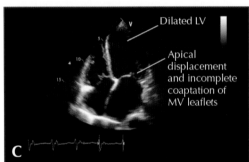

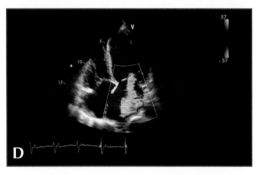

Figure 12-20. Functional mitral regurgitation (occurring in the presence of anatomically normal mitral leaflets) occurs in up to 25% of patients following acute myocardial infarction (MI) and confers an adverse prognosis [25,26]. In the transthoracic echocardiographic images shown here, LV remodeling after large anterior MI has led to global LV dilation and dilation of the mitral annulus (**C**). The LV dilation resulted in displacement of the papillary muscles away from the mitral annulus, leading to apical leaflet tethering in systole, inadequate coaptation (**A**), and severe mitral regurgitation (**B** and **D**). Coexistent ventricular dysfunction additionally reduces the closing force acting on the leaflets, which would oppose tethering and exacerbate the degree of regurgitation [24]. MV—mitral valve.

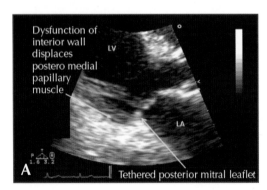

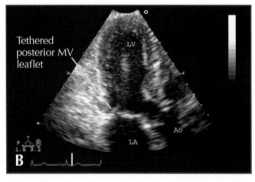

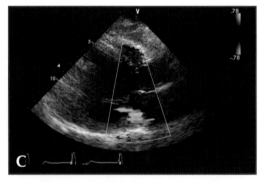

Figure 12-21. Inferior myocardial infarction, by itself, can result in ischemic mitral regurgitation. In this setting, displacement of the posteromedial papillary muscle occurs; the chordae tendineae from this papillary muscle are pulled away from the mitral valve, resulting in tethering of the posterior mitral valve leaflet, and reduction of its motion and ability to coapt with the anterior leaflet normally (**A**). Because the posterior mitral leaflet closing position is moved apically, yet the anterior mitral leaflet's tip closing position is unchanged, the anterior leaflet will appear to prolapse relative to the posterior leaflet (**B**). The jet of mitral regurgitation will be directed posteriorly (**C**) [24].

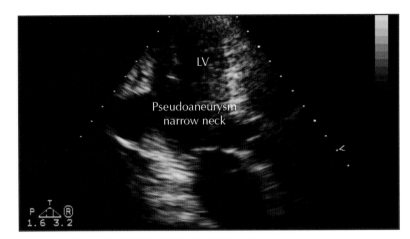

Figure 12-22. Pseudoaneurysm (false aneurysm) of the LV forms when extravasated blood from rupturing of the ventricular free wall is contained by localized pericardial adhesions, or hematoma. It is most commonly associated with inferior myocardial infarction and has a high rate of rupture and mortality [27,28]. Symptoms that are frequently reported include chest pain, syncope, arrhythmia, systemic embolism, or clinical features of tamponade. Some patients are asymptomatic. Echocardiography can usually distinguish pseudoaneurysm from true aneurysm by the appearance of the connection between the aneurysm and ventricular cavity. Pseudoaneurysms have a narrow neck communication that causes an abrupt interruption in ventricular contour. Doppler color flow mapping will demonstrate bidirectional flow between the pseudoaneurysm and ventricular cavity. Because of its high mortality rate in patients, surgical repair is the recommended management.

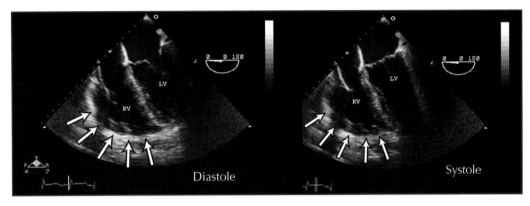

Figure 12-23. Clinically evident RV infarction occurs in less than 3% of all myocardial infarctions and is most often associated with inferior infarction. It typically occurs with occlusion of the right coronary artery proximal to its acute marginal branches; however, it may occur with occlusion of the left circumflex artery in a left-dominant coronary circulation [29]. Echocardiographic findings include RV dilation, wall motion abnormalities of the diaphragmatic or free walls, and abnormal interventricular septal motion [30]. Tricuspid annular dilation can cause significant tricuspid regurgitation. The short-axis view has been shown to be useful in identifying hemodynamically important RV infarction [31]. Interatrial septal bowing toward the left atrium, indicative of increased right atrial to left atrial pressure gradient, is an important prognostic marker in RV infarction. Patients with this finding have more hypotension and heart block and have a higher mortality rate than patients without it [32]. The images shown are from a 51-year-old man who developed cardiogenic shock in the setting of acute inferior myocardial infarction. Transesophageal echocardiogram revealed relatively preserved LV function, but profound RV systolic dysfunction and dilation, consistent with RV myocardial infarction. In addition to percutaneous intervention to the occluded right coronary artery, the patient was treated with fluids.

Echocardiography in the Differential Diagnosis of Myocardial Infarction

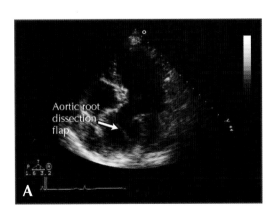
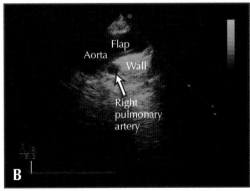

Figure 12-24. The clinical presentation of aortic dissection can mimic an acute coronary syndrome; however, the echocardiographic features are different. Dissections are characterized on echocardiography by the presence of an intimal flap, which is seen as a linear echo that exhibits low amplitude but high-frequency motion within the aortic lumen. In contrast, artifacts typically exhibit high-amplitude but low-frequency motion, similar to the motion of surrounding structures. Transesophageal echocardiography has a high sensitivity (99%) and specificity (98%) for detecting dissections and their complications [33]. The transthoracic echocardiographic images shown are from a 42-year-old woman who presents with sudden onset of tearing substernal chest pain radiating to her jaw. Her parents had early-onset coronary artery disease, and her brother had aortic repair surgery. The ECG showed sinus rhythm with nonspecific ST-segment and T-wave changes. Transthoracic echocardiography showed markedly dilated aortic root and ascending aorta (52 mm at sinus of Valsalva), moderate aortic insufficiency, and type 1 aortic dissection. The images displayed show the dissection flap in the aortic root on the apical five-chamber view (**A**) and in the ascending aorta and aortic arch on the suprasternal notch view (**B**).

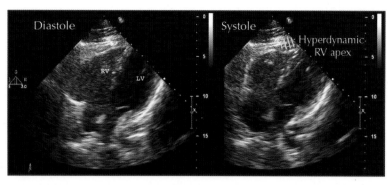

Figure 12-25. The presentation of acute pulmonary embolus can mimic acute myocardial infarction. The echocardiographic findings of pulmonary emboli depend on the hemodynamic consequences of the embolic event. If there is compromising of the pulmonary vasculature and increased pulmonary vascular afterload, signs of RV strain may be apparent. They include RV enlargement and systolic dysfunction, abnormal septal motion, tricuspid and pulmonary regurgitation, pulmonary hypertension, and pulmonary artery dilatation. RV wall motion abnormality, sparing the apex, has a high specificity (94%) for the diagnosis of acute pulmonary embolism [34]. However, a normal echocardiogram is common, especially when the emboli are small, and therefore does not exclude the diagnosis of pulmonary embolus. The images shown are from a 34-year-old woman with 2 days of chest pain and dyspnea. She used oral contraceptive pills, and had recently taken a long airplane flight. The ECG shows Q wave in lead III and T-wave inversion in V1-6. Biomarkers were mildly elevated. Chest CT showed right pulmonary artery embolus. The echocardiogram shows RV dilation with hyperdynamic RV apical motion (*yellow lines*) in association with hypokinesis of other wall segments. The shape of the interventricular septum (diastolic interventricular septal flattening) was consistent with RV volume overload.

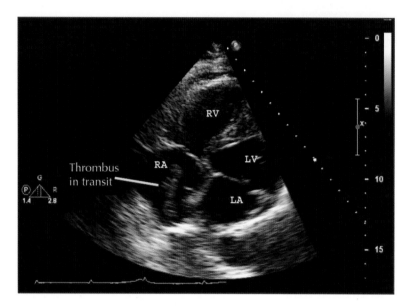

Figure 12-26. Echocardiography can differentiate myocardial infarction from pulmonary embolus when thrombus in transit is documented in the vena cavae, right atrium, RV, or pulmonary artery. This transthoracic echocardiogram is from a 65-year-old woman 10 days after hip replacement surgery who complained of chest pain and severe shortness of breathe. The ECG and CXR were normal. Her troponin and D-dimer biomarkers were both elevated. Her echocardiogram showed a long, serpentine, mobile mass, prolapsing through the tricuspid valve, RV dilation, and RV hypokinesis. LA—left atrium; RA—right atrium.

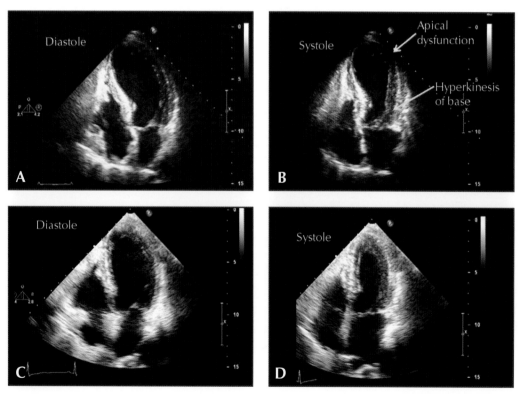

Figure 12-27. Stress-induced or "Tako-tsubo" cardiomyopathy mimics myocardial infarction in having similar symptoms, ECG changes, biomarker alterations, and echocardiographic wall motion abnormalities. The major difference is that epicardial coronary arteries are normal. This cardiomyopathy is characterized by transient dysfunction of the LV apex and compensatory hyperkinesis of the basal segments. In severe cases, LV outflow tract obstruction from the basal hyperkinesis, and resultant severe mitral regurgitation, can contribute to hemodynamic compromise. Acute complications include arrythmias, pulmonary edema, cardiogenic shock, thrombus formation, and stroke. This disease predominantly affects postmenopausal women and is typically triggered by an intense emotional or physical stress [35]. It is hypothesized that the disorder is caused by microvascular dysfunction from a surge in catecholamine output [36]. Patients who recover from the acute episode usually have normalization of their function by 1 month; however, recurrent episodes may occur. The images are from a 69-year-old woman who presented with substernal chest heaviness after intense emotional stress. Her ECG showed ST elevation in the anterior leads and her cardiac enzymes were elevated. Immediate coronary angiography showed no obstructive epicardial coronary artery disease. Initial transthoracic echocardiogram showed classic changes (**A** and **B**), which completely resolved within 1 month (**C** and **D**).

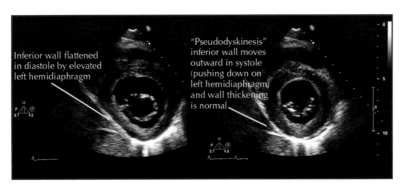

Figure 12-28. Wall motion abnormalities as a result of coronary artery disease can be mimicked when extracardiac structures distort the normal LV wall position in diastole; then the wall moves outward in systole as opposed to the

normal inward motion. In this situation, the systolic wall thickening is normal because the myocardium is normal. This motion has been termed "pseudodyskinesis" [37]. Pseudodyskinesis can be recognized by a characteristic flattening of the inferior wall at end diastole followed by its becoming round at end systole. Conversely, patients with a true inferior myocardial infarction have a normally round inferior wall contour at end diastole, with akinesis or outward bulging of that wall in systole [38]. This paradoxical wall motion abnormality has been reported in patients with liver disease. It has also been noted with other processes that cause elevation of the left hemidiaphragm, including volume loss of the left chest [38]. The left hemidiaphragm abuts and can compress the inferior wall of the LV. Diastolic and systolic images of the short axis of the LV at midventricular level demonstrate pseudodyskinesis with flattening of the inferior wall in diastole (*yellow line*), outward motion in systole causing rounding of the wall (*yellow line*), and normal systolic wall thickening.

New Echocardiographic Technologies: Applications in Myocardial Infarction

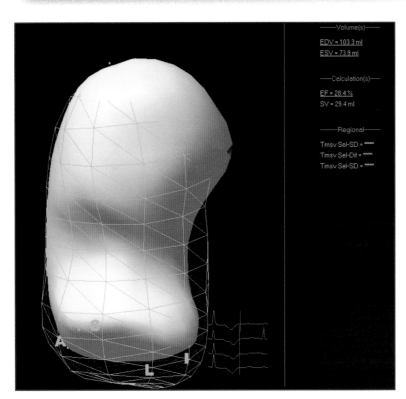

Figure 12-29. Three-dimensional echocardiography is now feasible with the use of matrix array transducers, which obtain a volume of ultrasound data. This three-dimensional ultrasound data set can then be cropped to yield various images of the heart. The endocardial borders of the LV can then be manually or automatically detected throughout the cardiac cycle to yield displays and measures of cardiac shape, volume, and function [39]. In this figure, the three-dimensional display of the LV in diastole (*white wire frame*) and systole (*yellow solid*) are superimposed to reveal a large, inferoapical aneurysm. A—anterior mitral valve annulus; EDV–end-diastolic volume; ESV–end-systolic volume; EF–ejection fraction; I—interior mitral valve annulus; L—lateral mitral valve annulus; S—septal mitral valve annulus; SV—stroke volume.

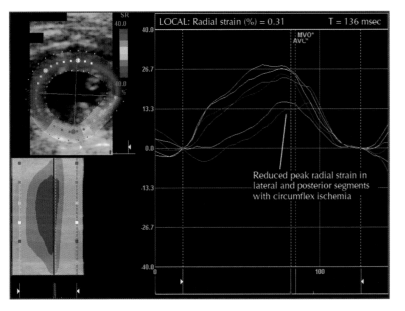

Figure 12-30. Myocardial strain or deformation can be quantified on echocardiography by Doppler and two-dimensional speckle or feature tracking techniques. This offers a quantitative method to assess regional function [40,41]. In short-axis image planes, the change in location of individual speckles can be tracked and compared with baseline in order to quantify radial and circumferential strain. In this illustration, radial strain is displayed in an experimental model of circumflex coronary artery territory ischemia. Although anterior, septal, and inferior segments (*red, yellow*, and *blue*) exhibit normal systolic thickening and radial strain, the lateral and posterior segments (*green* and *purple*) show a reduction in the degree of radial strain (thickening) due to myocardial ischemia. AVC—aortic valve closure; MVO—mitral valve opening.

References

1. Thygesen K, Alpert JS, White HD: Universal definition of myocardial infarction. *Eur Heart J* 2007, 28:2525–2538.

2. Cerqueira MD, Weissman NJ, Dilsizian V, *et al.*: Standardized myocardial segmentation and nomenclature for tomographic imaging of the heart: a statement for healthcare professionals from the Cardiac Imaging Committee of the Council on Clinical Cardiology of the American Heart Association. *Circulation* 2002, 105:539–542.

3. Lang RM, Bierig M, Devereux RB, *et al.*: Recommendations for chamber quantification: a report from the American Society of Echocardiography's Guidelines and Standards Committee and the Chamber Quantification Writing Group, developed in conjunction with the European Association of Echocardiography, a branch of the European Society of Cardiology. *J Am Soc Echocardiogr* 2005, 18:1440–1463.

4. Mann DL, Gillam LD, Weyman AE: Cross-sectional echocardiographic assessment of regional left ventricular performance and myocardial perfusion. *Prog Cardiovasc Dis* 1986, 29:1–52.

5. American Society of Nuclear Cardiology: Imagining guidelines for nuclear cardiology procedures, part 2. *J Nucl Cardiol* 1999, 6:G47–G84.

6. Hoffman R, von Bardeleben S, Kasprzak J, *et al.*: Analysis of regional left ventricular function by cineventriculography, cardiac magnetic resonance imaging and unenhanced and contrast-enhanced echocardiography: a multicenter comparison of methods. *J Am Coll Cardiol* 2007, 47:121–128.

7. Mansencal N, Nasr IA, Pilliere R, *et al.*: Usefulness of contrast echocardiography for assessment of left ventricular thrombus after acute myocardial infarction. *Am J Cardiol* 2007, 99:1667–1670.

8. Davidoff R, Picard MH, Force T, *et al.*: Spatial and temporal variability in the pattern of recovery of ventricular geometry and function after acute occlusion and reperfusion. *Am Heart J* 1994, 127:1231–1241.

9. Picard MH, Wilkins GT, Ray PA, Weyman AE: Natural history of left ventricular size and function after acute myocardial infarction: assessment and prediction by echocardiographic endocardial surface mapping. *Circulation* 1990, 82:484–494.

10. Visser CA, Kan G, Meltzer RS, *et al.*: Incidence, timing and prognostic value of left ventricular aneurysm formation after myocardial infarction: a prospective, serial echocardiographic study of 158 patients. *Am J Cardiol* 1986, 57:729–732.

11. Meizlish JL, Berger HJ, Plankey M, *et al.*: Functional left ventricular aneurysm formation after acute anterior transmural myocardial infarction: incidence, natural history, and prognostic implications. *N Engl J Med* 1984, 311:1001–1006.

12. Levine RA, Hung J: Ischemic mitral regurgitation, the dynamic lesson: clues to the cure. *J Am Coll Cardiol* 2003, 42:1929–1932.

13. Nayak D, Aronow WS, Sukhija R, *et al.*: Comparison of frequency of left ventricular thrombi in patients with anterior wall versus non-anterior wall acute myocardial infarction treated with antithrombotic and antiplatelet therapy with or without coronary revascularization. *Am J Cardiol* 1999, 83:529–530.

14. Chiarella F, Santoro E, Domenicucci S, *et al.*: Predischarge two-dimensional echocardiographic evaluation of left ventricular thrombosis after acute myocardial infarction in the GISSI-3 study. *Am J Cardiol* 1998, 81:822–827.

15. Domenicucci S, Chiarella F, Bellotti P, *et al.*: Early appearance of left ventricular thrombi after anterior myocardial infarction: a marker of higher in-hospital mortality in patients not treated with antithrombotic drugs. *Eur Heart J* 1990, 11:51–58.

16. Jugdutt BI, Sivaram CA: Prospective two-dimensional echocardiographic evaluation of left ventricular thrombus and embolism after acute myocardial infarction. *J Am Coll Cardiol* 1989, 13:554–564.

17. Menon V, Hochman JS: Management of cardiogenic shock complicating acute myocardial infarction. *Heart* 2002, 88:531–537.

18. Picard MH, Davidoff R, Sleeper LA, *et al.*: Echocardiographic predictors of survival and response to early revascularization in cardiogenic shock. *Circulation* 2003, 107:279–284.

19. Birnbaum Y, Fishbein MC, Blanche C, Seigel RJ: Ventricular septal rupture after myocardial infarction. *N Engl J Med* 2002, 347:1426–1432.

20. Crenshaw BS, Granger CB, Birnbaum Y, *et al.*: Risk factors, angiographic patterns, and outcomes in patients with ventricular septal defect complicating acute myocardial infarction. *Circulation* 2000, 101:27–32.

21. Antman E: ST-Elevation myocardial infarction: management. In *Braunwald's Heart Disease: A Textbook of Cardiovascular Medicine*, edn 7. Edited by Braunwald E, Zipes DP, Libby P, Bonow R. Philadelphia: Elsevier Saunders; 2005:1167–1226.

22. Barbour DJ, Roberts WC: Rupture of a left ventricular papillary muscle during acute myocardial infarction: analysis of 22 necropsy patients. *J Am Coll Cardiol* 1986, 8:558–565.

23. Nishimura RA, Schaff HV, Shub C, *et al.*: Papillary muscle rupture complicating acute myocardial infarction: analysis of 17 patients. *Am J Cardiol* 1983, 51:373–377.

24. Levine RA, Schwammenthal E: Ischemic mitral regurgitation on the threshold of a solution: from paradoxes to unifying concepts. *Circulation* 2005, 112:745–758.

25. Lamas GA, Mitchell GF, Flaker GC, *et al.*: Clinical significance of mitral regurgitation after acute myocardial infarction. Survival and Ventricular Enlargement Investigators. *Circulation* 1997, 96:827–833.

26. Grigioni F, Enriquez-Sarano M, Zehr KJ, *et al.*: Ischemic mitral regurgitation: long-term outcome and prognostic implications with quantitative Doppler assessment. *Circulation* 2001, 103:1759–1764.

27. Frances C, Romero A, Grady D: Left ventricular pseudoaneurysm. *J Am Coll Cardiol* 1998, 32:557–561.

28. Yeo TC, Malouf JF, Oh JK, Seward JB: Clinical profile and outcome in 52 patients with cardiac pseudoaneurysm. *Ann Intern Med* 1998, 128:299–305.

29. Andersen HR, Falk E, Nielsen D: Right ventricular infarction: frequency, size and topography in coronary heart disease: a prospective study comprising 107 consecutive autopsies from a coronary care unit. *J Am Coll Cardiol* 1987, 10:1223–1232.

30. D'Arcy B, Nanda NC: Two-dimensional echocardiographic features of right ventricular infarction. *Circulation* 1982, 65:167–173.

31. Bellamy GR, Rasmussen HH, Nasser FN, *et al.*: Value of two-dimensional echocardiography, electrocardiography, and clinical signs in detecting right ventricular infarction. *Am Heart J* 1986, 112:304–309.

32. Lopez-Sendon J, Lopez de Sa E, Roldan I, *et al.*: Inversion of the normal interatrial septum convexity in acute myocardial infarction: incidence, clinical relevance and prognostic significance. *J Am Coll Cardiol* 1990, 15:801–805.

33. Erbel R, Engberding R, Daniel W, *et al.*: Echocardiography in diagnosis of aortic dissection. *Lancet* 1989, 1:457–461.

34. McConnell MV, Solomon SD, Rayan ME, *et al.*: Regional right ventricular dysfunction detected by echocardiography in acute pulmonary embolus. *Am J Cardiol* 1996, 78:469–473.

35. Tsuchihashi K, Ueshima K, Uchida T, *et al.*: Transient left ventricular apical ballooning without coronary artery stenosis: a novel heart syndrome mimicking acute myocardial infarction. Angina Pectoris-Myocardial Infarction Investigations in Japan. *J Am Coll Cardiol* 2001, 38:11–18.

36. Gianni M, Dentali F, Grandi AM, *et al.*: Apical ballooning syndrome or takotsubo cardiomyopathy: a systematic review. *Eur Heart J* 2006, 27:1523–1529.

37. Yosefy C, Levine RA, Picard MH, *et al.*: Pseudodyskinesis of the inferior left ventricular wall: recognizing an echocardiographic mimic of myocardial infarction. *J Am Soc Echocardiogr* 2007, 20:1374–1379.

38. Vennalaganti PR, Ostfeld RJ, Malhotra D, *et al.*: Pseudodyskinesis: a novel mechanism for abnormal motion of the heart's diaphragmatic wall. *J Am Soc Echocardiogr* 2006, 19:1294.

39. Corsi C, Lang RM, Veronesi F, *et al.*: Volumetric quantification of global and regional left ventricular function from real-time three-dimensional echocardiographic images. *Circulation* 2005, 112:1161–1170.

40. Yip G, Abraham T, Belohlavek M, Khandheria BK: Clinical applications of strain rate imaging. *J Am Soc Echocardiogr* 2003, 16:1334–1342.

41. Sutherland GR, Di Salvo G, Claus P, *et al.*: Strain and strain rate imaging: a new clinical approach to quantifying regional myocardial function. *J Am Soc Echocardiogr* 2004, 17:788–802.

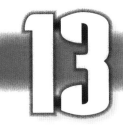

13

Hypertrophic Cardiomyopathy

Carolyn Y. Ho and Barry J. Maron

Over the past 35 years, echocardiographic imaging has played a fundamental role in our understanding of the clinical diagnosis and pathophysiology of hypertrophic cardiomyopathy (HCM). Echocardiography has provided key insights into natural history and has refined management of this complex and heterogeneous disease. In this chapter, we will illustrate specific areas in which echocardiographic findings have direct implications for patient care by integrating representative images with clinical data and pathologic observations.

The power of echocardiographic imaging is particularly well suited to studying the considerable morphologic diversity, varied patterns of LV hypertrophy, dynamic remodeling, and complex perturbations of cardiac function associated with HCM. To demonstrate this principle, we have used the expanse of technical evolution in echocardiography from M-mode, two-dimensional, and Doppler imaging.

The specific practical and clinical applications of echocardiography to HCM will be demonstrated by presentations relevant to diagnosis and recognition of morphologic variants, the spectrum and evolution of phenotypic expression, mechanisms of dynamic LV outflow tract obstruction, assessment of diastolic function, as well as clinical management, including risk stratification for sudden death and the evaluation of the consequences of invasive therapeutic interventions (surgical septal myectomy and alcohol septal ablation).

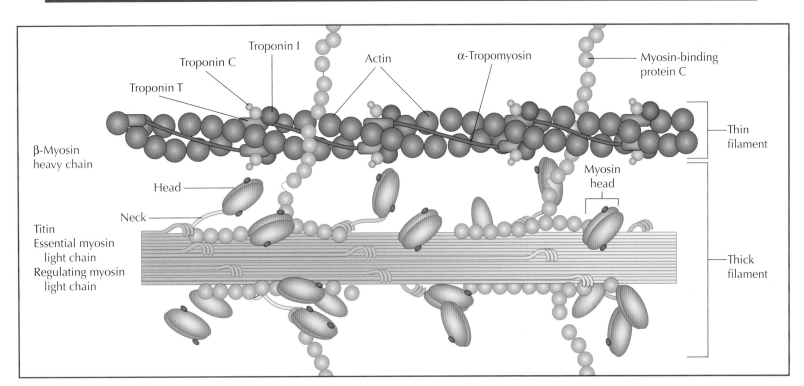

Figure 13-1. Hypertrophic cardiomyopathy (HCM) is caused by mutations in sarcomere genes. The sarcomere is the functional unit of contraction of the myocyte and the molecular motor of the heart. Force is generated by cyclical cross-bridge formation between actin and β-myosin heavy chain, which leads to interdigitation of the thick and thin filaments during the power stroke. This motor is powered by the hydrolysis of ATP and coordinated by carefully orchestrated fluxes in intracellular Ca^{2+} concentration. HCM is a disease of the sarcomere that is caused by dominantly acting mutations in contractile proteins. Over 600 mutations have been identified in 11 different components of the sarcomere apparatus. Mutations in the cardiac isoforms of β-myosin heavy chain, myosin binding protein C, and troponin T are the most common. Together, they account for over 80% of cases where a mutation has been identified [1,2]. (*From* Nabel [3]; with permission.)

Left Ventricular Morphology in Hypertrophic Cardiomyopathy

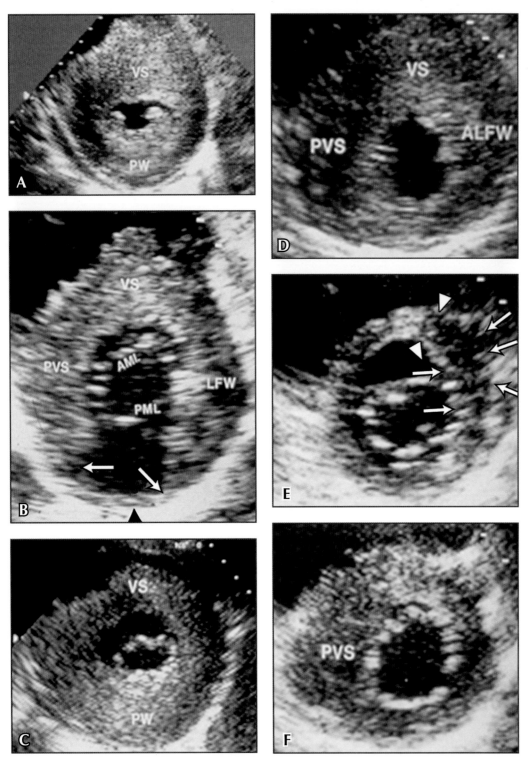

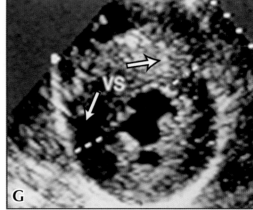

Figure 13-2. There is marked heterogeneity in the pattern and extent of LV hypertrophy in hypertrophic cardiomyopathy (HCM). The vast majority of patients with HCM demonstrate asymmetric LV hypertrophy; however, virtually every pattern of wall thickening has been reported, which is shown in the diastolic still frame parasternal short-axis images. No direct correlation between the distribution of LV hypertrophy and clinical outcomes has been demonstrated. Wall thickening is diffuse, involving substantial portions of the ventricular septum (VS) and anterolateral free wall (ALFW) (**A**, **B**, and **D**). At the papillary muscle level, all segments of the LV wall are hypertrophied, including the posterior wall (PW); however, the pattern of thickening is asymmetric, with massive hypertrophy of the anterior portion of the ventricular septum (50 mm) (**A**). Hypertrophy is diffuse, involving three segments of the LV, but sparing the basal posterior wall (< 10 mm) (**B**, *arrows*). Marked asymmetric hypertrophy in a distinct pattern from that seen previous (**A**, **B**, and **D**) is shown, in which thickening of the posterior wall is predominant and the ventricular septum is of nearly normal thickness (**C**). Prominent diffuse hypertrophy is shown (**D**). Hypertrophy, predominantly of the lateral free wall (**E**, *arrows*) and only a small portion of the contiguous anterior septum, is shown (**E**, *arrowheads*). Hypertrophy predominantly of the posterior ventricular septum (PVS) and, to a lesser extent, the contiguous portion of the anterior septum is shown (**F**). Thickening of the anterior and posterior septum to a similar degree (**G**, *arrows*) but with sparing of the free wall is shown. Calibration marks are 1 cm. AML—anterior mitral leaflet; LFW—LV free wall; PML—posterior mitral leaflet; PVS—posterior/inferior ventricular septum.

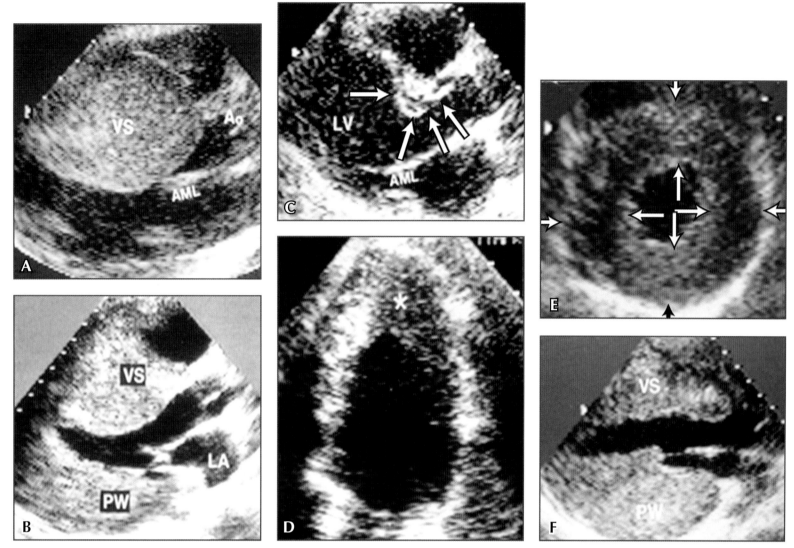

Figure 13-3. Additional morpohologic patterns of hypertrophic cardiomyopathy (HCM), shown in a composite of diastolic parasternal still frame images. Massive asymmetric septal hypertrophy is shown, with ventricular septum (VS) thickness greater than 50 mm (**A**). Septal hypertrophy with more prominent distal portion involvement is shown (**B**). Hypertrophy is confined to the proximal septum just below the aortic valve (**C**, *arrows*).

Hypertrophy is localized to the LV apex (**D**, *asterisk*) (*ie*, apical HCM). Relatively mild hypertrophy in a concentric pattern showing similar or identical thicknesses within each segment is shown (**E**, *paired arrows*). Inverted pattern with posterior free wall (PW), which is thicker (40 mm) than the anterior ventricular septum (VS) (**F**). Calibration marks are 1 cm. AML—anterior mitral valve leaflet; LA—left atrium.

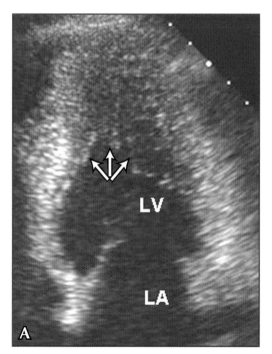

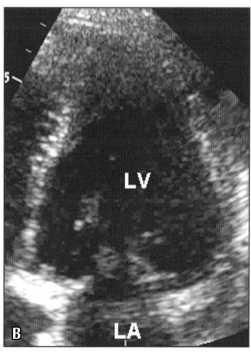

Figure 13-4. Apical hypertrophy is a well-described morphologic variant of hypertrophic cardiomyopathy (HCM), in which hypertrophy is confined to the distal portion of the LV chamber below the level of the papillary muscles (**A**, *arrows*). Apical HCM is always a nonobstructive form of the disease. If visualization of the distal LV is suboptimal, administration of echocardiographic contrast can assist in the detection of apical hypertrophy (**B** and **C**). There is poor visualization of the LV apex prior to contrast administration (**B**).

Continued on the next page

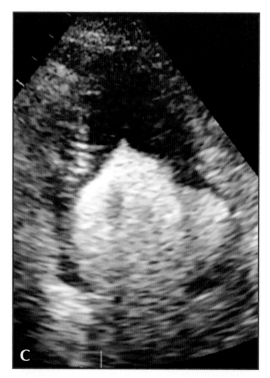

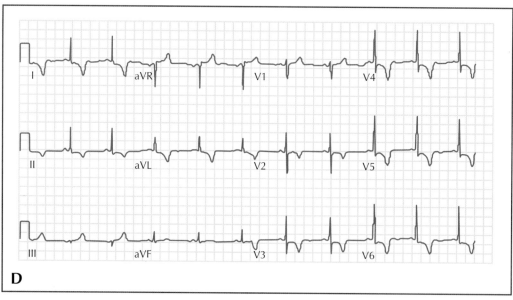

Figure 13-4. *(Continued)* The typical spade-shaped LV cavity is apparent with the administration of echocardiographic contrast, indicative of apical wall thickening (**C**). Apical HCM is often associated with giant negative T waves on ECG, present in the lateral precordial leads (**D**).

Apical HCM was first reported in Japan [4], and the prevalence of this variant is higher in Japanese patients than in those of Western descent (13%–25% vs 1%–2%) [5]. Although early reports suggested a more benign prognosis for this morphologic form, a spectrum of clinical outcomes is now recognized [6]. No particular genetic mutations have been associated with apical HCM and are often varied within family morphology [7]. AVS—anterior ventricular septum; LA—left atrium.

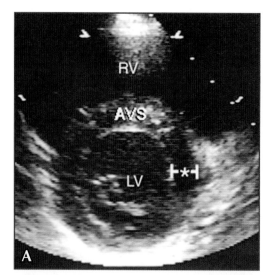

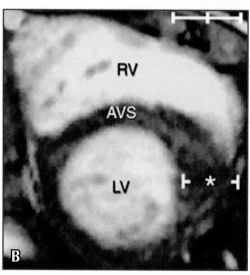

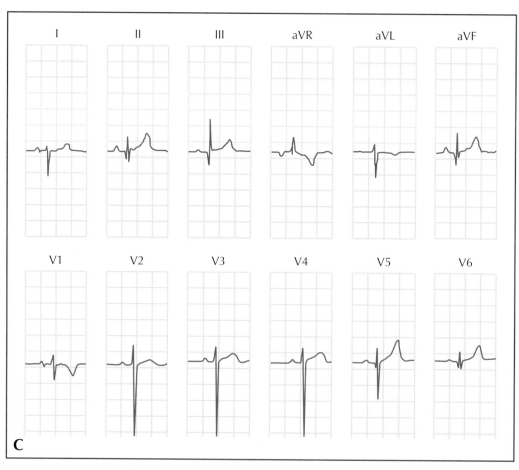

Figure 13-5. Echocardiography's capabilities are limited when determining LV morphology. The images are taken from a 13-year-old boy. Both he and his identical twin have nonobstructive hypertrophic cardiomyopathy (HCM). The two-dimensional parasternal short-axis echocardiographic image (**A**) suggests normal wall thickness; however, the anterolateral freewall (*asterisk*) is not well visualized because of beam spread and limited lateral resolution. Accurate measurement of lateral wall thickness is difficult.

Continued on the next page

Figure 13-5. *(Continued)* A cardiac MRI image from the same cross-sectional plane as the echocardiogram is diagnostic of HCM, demonstrating segmental hypertrophy confined to the anterolateral LV free wall (20 mm) and a small portion of the contiguous anterior septum (**B**, *asterisk*). The ECG is distinctly abnormal, showing Q waves in inferior leads II, III, aVF, and V6, as well as deep S waves in the right precordial leads (**C**). There is also diminished R wave voltage in the lateral precordial leads [8]. AVS—anterior ventricular septum.

Left Ventricular Outflow Obstruction in Hypertrophic Cardiomyopathy

A highly visible feature of HCM is obstruction and mechanical impedance to LV outflow. Subaortic gradients and associated mitral regurgitation are present in the majority of patients and significantly contribute to symptoms of exercise intolerance and heart failure. Echocardiography can evaluate the mechanism of obstruction and, with Doppler interrogation, precisely determine the magnitude of the gradient.

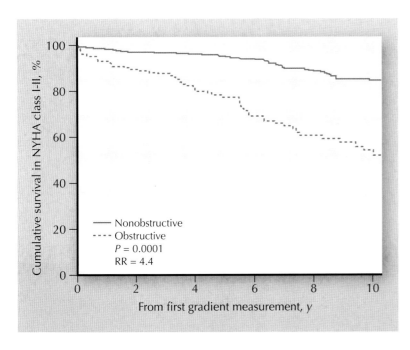

Figure 13-6. Impact of outflow obstruction ($\geq$ 30 mm Hg) on progression to severe heart failure related symptoms and death in 1101 hypertrophic cariomyopathy (HCM) patients. In this large retrospective cohort study, the presence of LV outflow obstruction (gradient $\geq$ 30 mm Hg) over long periods predicted adverse outcomes. The probability of progression to severe heart failure (New York Heart Association class III or IV) or death from heart failure or stroke among 224 patients with LV outflow tract obstruction and 770 patients without obstruction is shown in this Kaplan-Meier survival curve. Patients with obstruction were more likely to progress to severe symptoms of heart failure and heart-failure–related death with a relative risk (RR) in excess of 4 [9].

Obstruction at rest occurs in about 25% of patients, but the propensity to develop obstruction is more common and may be missed without careful and systematic evaluation incorporating provocative maneuvers. Exercise provides the most physiologic and clinically relevant provocation. A variety of factors predispose to the development of obstruction, including anatomic and functional abnormalities common to HCM. Septal hypertrophy, developmentally small LV outflow tract, hyperdynamic LV function, and elongated mitral leaflets all contribute to promoting drag effect, which results in systolic anterior motion of the mitral valve and mitral septal contact, the predominant mechanism by which LV outflow tract obstruction occurs in HCM.

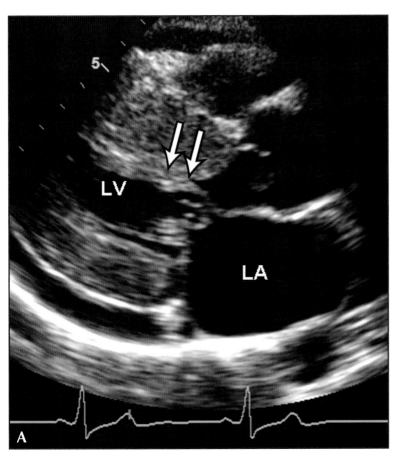

Figure 13-7. LV outflow obstruction and mechanisms of systolic anterior motion (SAM) is shown. Typical SAM of the mitral apparatus is shown in these midsystolic still frame parasternal long-axis (**A**) and apical four-chamber (**B**) images. The point at which the anterior mitral leaflet makes septal contact (**A** and **B**, *arrows*) creating LV outflow tract obstruction is shown. The mitral leaflets are elongated and flexible, with the tip of the anterior mitral leaflet making localized septal contact; this is typical in younger patients (as shown here). Older patients with SAM may have leaflets of normal length situated in a particularly small LV outflow tract, in which septal contact is affected by mild SAM and posterior motion of the septum.

Continued on the next page

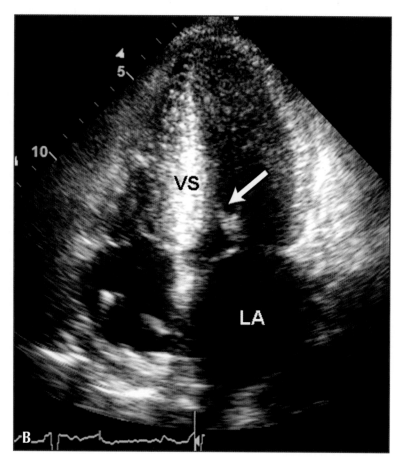

Figure 13-7. *(Continued)* Proposed mechanisms for SAM include Venturi effect or drag forces (the more likely of the two). The Venturi effect theory proposes that the hypertrophied basal septum creates a local low pressure region in the outflow tract that acts to pull the mitral valve anteriorly. The drag effect theory emphasizes the importance of anterior displacement of the mitral apparatus, which exposes more leaflet surface area to blood flow in the LV outflow tract. The hypertrophied proximal septum redirects blood flow posteriorly and laterally, creating a pressure gradient between the LV cavity and outflow tract, which pushes the underside of the mitral leaflets towards the septum and creates a self-amplifying loop where longer durations of SAM septal contact lead to further increases in the gradient [10]. LA—left atrium; VS—ventricular septum.

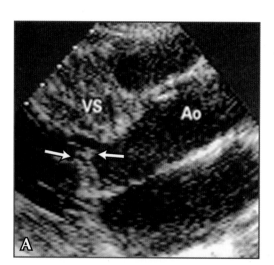 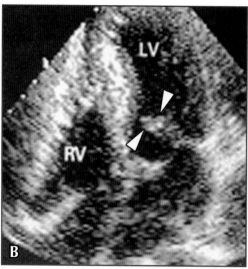 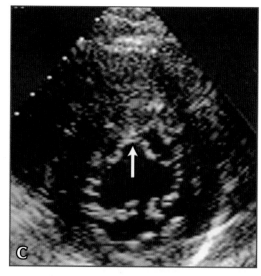

Figure 13-8. These still frame images illustrate typical systolic anterior motion (SAM) with an acutely angled bend formed by the anterior mitral leaflet as it makes septal contact. This produces mechanical impedance to LV outflow as well as mitral regurgitation (MR). A parasternal long-axis view (**A**) shows typical SAM, in which the anterior mitral leaflet (*arrows*) bends acutely and becomes virtually perpendicular to the LV outflow tract in systole, resulting in localized septal contact and obstruction to flow. An apical four-chamber view (**B**) demonstrates the same acutely angled conformation of SAM. A parasternal short-axis image (**C**) demonstrates that the typical anterior motion of the mitral valve occurs in the center of the anterior leaflet (*arrow*).

Continued on the next page

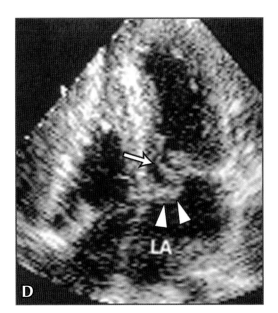

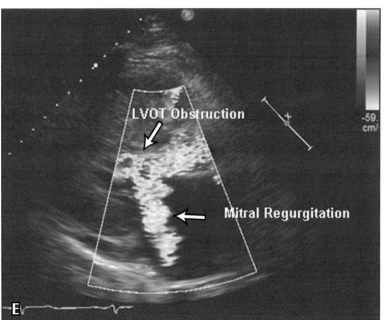

Figure 13-8. (Continued) An apical four-chamber view (**D**) shows greatly elongated mitral leaflets, particularly the anterior leaflet (AML), producing LV outflow obstruction from SAM (*arrow*), as well as systolic prolapse into the left atrium (*arrowheads*) due to deformation of the enlarged valve in the small LV cavity (mitral valve prolapse is not due to myxomatous degeneration). MR is usually mild to moderate in degree, and is invariably associated with SAM due to leaflet malcoaptation as the mitral valve moves towards and contacts the septum in midsystole (**E**). Because of the anterior displacement of the mitral apparatus, MR caused by SAM is directed posteriorly. MR that is more centrally or anteriorly directed suggests intrinsic mitral valve disease (*eg*, myxomatous changes with mitral valve prolapse, anomalous chordal structures, or abnormal papillary muscles) and should trigger careful scrutiny of valvular morphology and function. Ao—aorta; LA—left atrium; VS—ventricular septum.

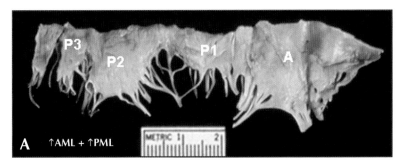

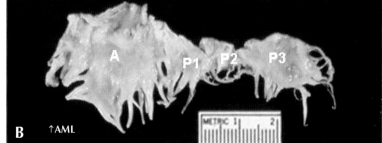

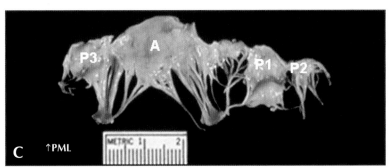

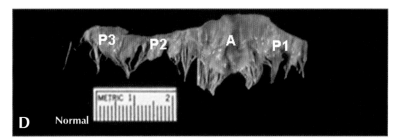

Figure 13-9. Diverse structural abnormalities of the mitral valve are seen in hypertrophic cardiomyopathy (HCM) and likely represent a primary manifestation of the underlying cardiomyopathy [11]. These photographs show pathologic mitral valve specimens from three patients with obstructive HCM compared with a normal control patient without cardiovascular disease. Valves have been opened with the circumference displayed in a horizontal orientation, exposing the atrial surface. Variations in valvular size and structure are demonstrated. **A**, A 31-year-old patient with large valve (22 cm^2), in which both the anterior (A) and posterior (P) mitral leaflets are greatly elongated and increased in area. **B**, A 29-year-old patient with large valve (18 cm^2) primarily due to elongation and enlargement of the anterior leaflet. **C**, A 60-year-old patient with segmental elongation and increased area confined to a lateral scallop of the posterior mitral leaflet, which has virtually the same length as the normal size anterior leaflet. **D**, A normal mitral valve from a patient without cardiovascular disease. Valve area is normal (11 cm^2), and leaflets are of normal length and thickness. AML—anterior mitral leaflet; PML—posterior mitral leaflet.

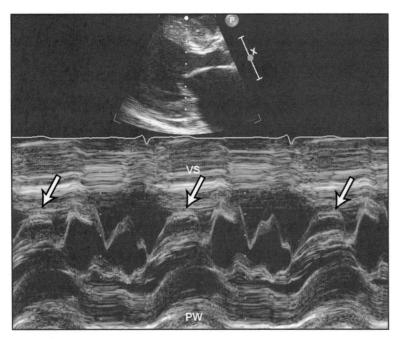

Figure 13-10. M-mode representation of systolic anterior motion (SAM). The anterior motion of the mitral valve and septal contact in midsystole is indicated (*arrows*). The degree and duration of SAM septal contact relate directly to the magnitude of the outflow gradient [12]. The prolonged contact shown in this figure is most consistent with an outflow tract gradient of more than 75 mm Hg. PW—posterior wall; VS—ventricular septum.

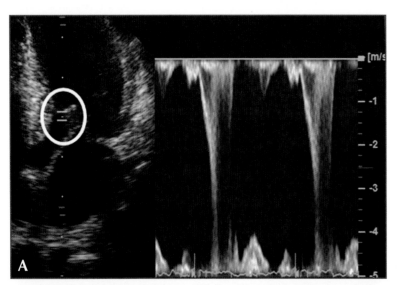

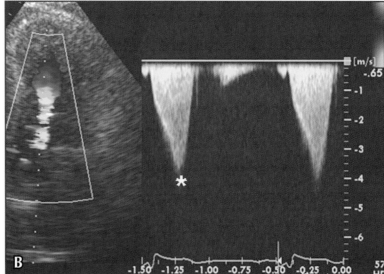

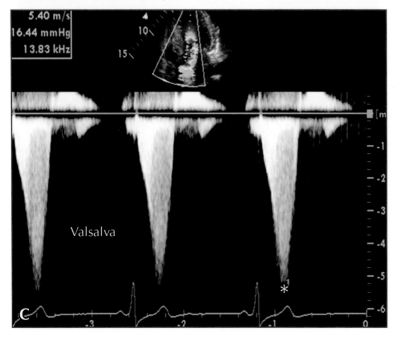

Figure 13-11. The intraventricular pressure gradient between the LV cavity and the outflow tract, produced by systolic anterior motion (SAM), can be localized and quantified by pulse and continuous wave Doppler. Interrogation starts with pulse wave Doppler in the mid LV cavity, advancing the sample volume (**A**, *circle*) to the outflow tract in order to identify the site of flow velocity acceleration (typically at the site of maximal SAM-septal contact). Continuous wave Doppler identifies the peak instantaneous outflow gradient of 4.1 m/s (**B**, *asterisk*) with the modified Bernoulli equation peak LV outflow tract (LVOT) gradient of 68 mm Hg at rest is predicted. The peak velocity (**C**, *asterisk*) increases to 5.4 m/s (peak instantaneous gradient 116 mm Hg) with Valsalva maneuver. Obstruction in hypertrophic cardiomyopathy is dynamic and is highly influenced by loading conditions; therefore, echocardiographic estimation of the magnitude of obstruction should be performed at rest and with provocative maneuvers. Gradients are accentuated by maneuvers that decrease preload (ie, strain phase of Valsalva maneuver, volume depletion, and tachycardia), decrease afterload, or increase contractility. It is critical to distinguish the Doppler signal from the LVOT from the jet of mitral regurgitation (MR).

Continued on the next page

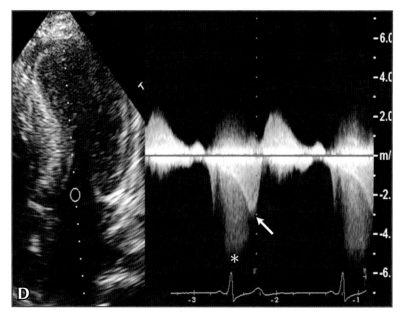

Figure 13-11. (*Continued*) The MR waveform has a more symmetric parabolic shape and begins at the onset of systole (during isovolumic contraction, at the onset of the QRS complex on an echocardiogram) with an abrupt increase in peak velocity (5.5 m/s) (**D**, *asterisk*). Of note, the later peaking midsystolic signal from the LV outflow tract is evident, embedded within the MR signal (3.1 m/s) (**D**, *arrow*). Guidance with two-dimensional and color flow Doppler imaging can usually separate the signals from these two jets.

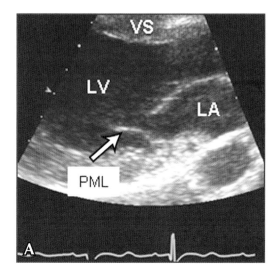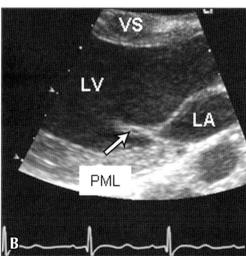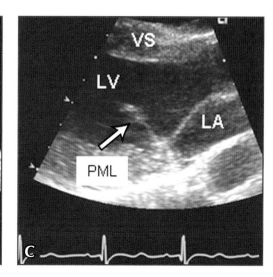

Figure 13-12. These sequential still frame long-axis images show systolic anterior motion (SAM) due to anterior motion of the posterior mitral leaflet (PML) towards the ventricular septum, from late diastole (**A**) to early systole (**B**), and to midsystole (**C**). Although the anterior mitral leaflet is responsible for septal contact in the vast majority of cases, a greatly elongated posterior leaflet alone produces septal contact (*arrows*) in ~5% to 10% of obstructive patients. In this unusual situation, the PML is both displaced distally and is longer or of equal length to the anterior leaflet. As a consequence, the anterior leaflet coapts near the base of the posterior leaflet (rather than distally at the tips), leaving a residual portion of the posterior leaflet to move into the outflow tract and make contact with the septum [13]. LA—left atrium; VS—ventricular septum.

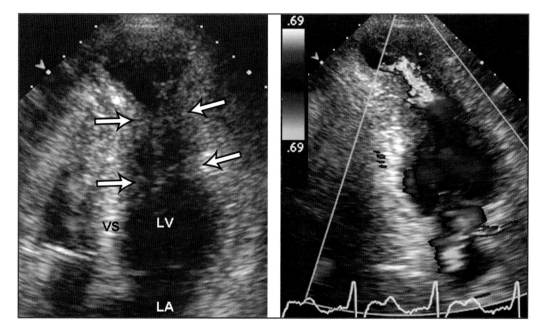

Figure 13-13. Apical aneurysm formation in hypertrophic cardiomyopathy (HCM). Apical four-chamber images showing a large LV apical aneurysm with (*right panel*) and without (*left panel*) color flow due to muscular midcavity narrowing and obstruction (*left panel, arrows*). Apical aneurysms in HCM are of varying size and are not related to concomitant atherosclerotic coronary disease. Development of these aneurysms may be associated with sudden death, progressive heart failure, and thromboembolic complications. LA—left atrium; VS—ventricular septum.

Remodeling of the Phenotype of Hypertrophic Cardiomyopathy

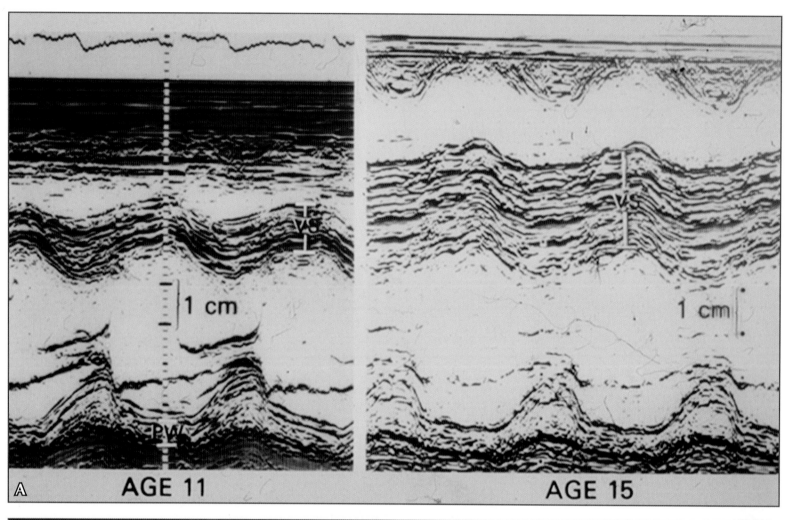

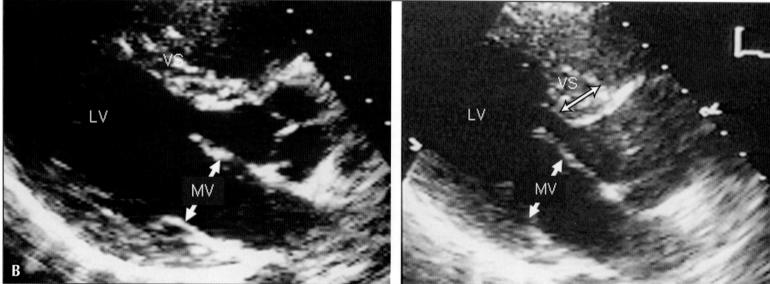

Figure 13-14. Progression of LV hypertrophy over time. Spontaneous development of marked hypertrophy in the basal anterior ventricular septum (VS) during adolescence in a hypertrophic cardiomyopathic (HCM) family member is shown (**A**). M-mode echocardiograms obtained at the same cross-sectional level in a girl with a family history of HCM. At 11 years of age, the anterior VS thickness was at the upper limit of normal (10 mm) (**A**, *left panel*). At 15 years of age, there is a marked increase in septal thickness to 33 mm (**A**, *right panel*). Phenotypic development delayed to adulthood in a patient with familial HCM is also shown (**B**). An initial echocardiogram was performed on a 29-year-old man, and a pathogenic myosin binding protein C mutation was identified in his family (**B**, *left panel*). A parasternal long-axis view at end-diastole shows normal thickness of the VS and elongated mitral valve (MV) leaflets. The patient was found to carry the causal gene mutation, but was asymptomatic at this time. Follow-up echocardiography 6 years later (at 35 years of age) revealed phenotypic progression (**B**, *right panel*). The long-axis view demonstrates greatly elongated MV leaflets, as well as hypertrophy of the anterior basal septum, which bulges prominently into the LV outflow tract [14].

Continued on the next page

Figure 13-14. *(Continued)* The penetrance (*ie*, the clinical expression of a gene mutation) of LV hypertrophy in HCM is dependent on age. Phenotypic conversion most commonly occurs during adolescence in association with the pubertal growth spurt. Wall thickness and echocardiographic studies may be normal during childhood but can increase abruptly over a short period.

This underscores the need for longitudinal clinical and echocardiographic evaluation of all family members at risk for HCM. If genetic testing results are available, this serial follow-up can be focused solely on family members who have inherited the causal sarcomere mutation [15]. Family members who do not carry the gene mutation are not at risk for developing HCM.

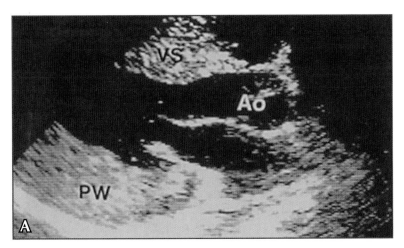

Figure 13-15. Serial echocardiography identifies evolution to the end-stage phenotype of hypertrophic cardiomyopathy (HCM). **A**, At 16 years of age, this patient had typical features of HCM with marked LV hypertrophy (ventricular septum and posterior free wall measure 32 mm), small LV cavity (end-diastolic dimension 38 mm), and an ejection fraction of 70%, when asymptomatic. **B**, At 23 years of age (7 years later), he presented with New York Heart Association (NYHA) functional class II heart failure symptoms. Repeat echocardiography demonstrated development of the end-stage phenotype with regression of LV wall thickness, LV dilatation (end-diastolic dimension 70 mm), and reduced ejection fraction (30%).

The end-stage phenotype of HCM is characterized by a heterogeneous pattern of cardiac remodeling with transition from the typical hypertrophied, nondilated, and hyperdynamic state to one of systolic dysfunction and often restrictive physiology, LV wall thinning, and cavity dilatation (**A** and **B**). Approximately 2% of HCM patients are affected over a broad age range (14–74 years), with about one half presenting by 40 years of age [16]. Recognition of end stage HCM depends on the presence of diminished LV ejection fraction (< 50%); only ~50% of patients show associated LV cavity enlargement or regression in wall thickness. Clinical course is variable and unpredictable, but generally unfavorable. Cardiac transplantation is the only definitive option when heart failure becomes refractory to medical therapy. Ao—aorta; LA—left atrium; PW—posterior wall; VS—ventricular septum.

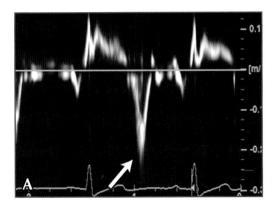 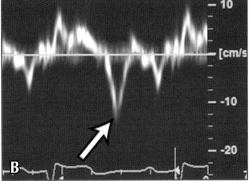 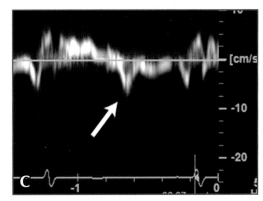

Figure 13-16. Impaired LV relaxation is present prior to the development of LV hypertrophy (LVH) in relatives with sarcomere gene mutations. Tissue Doppler imaging (TDI) studies on genotyped hypertrophic cardiomyopathy (HCM) family members have demonstrated that individuals with sarcomere gene mutations may have impaired LV relaxation early in life prior to the development of LVH [17,18]. A healthy 23-year-old family member who does not carry the causal myosin heavy chain (*MYH7*) gene mutation has a normal, brisk E' velocity of 22 cm/s (**A**, *arrow*), indicating normal LV relaxation. An asymptomatic and active 23-year-old female relative who carries the *MYH7* mutation, but does not have LVH or other echocardiographic features of HCM, nonetheless shows mild reduction in E' velocity to 10.5 cm/s, indicative of subtly impaired LV relaxation (**B**). Lastly, a 24-year-old female relative carries the *MYH7* mutation and has overt HCM with LVH (**C**). TDI demonstrates a striking reduction in E' velocity (6 cm/s), indicating a marked impairment in LV relaxation. The two-dimensional echocardiographic images obtained at the same examination are shown in Figure 13-17.

These studies imply that diastolic abnormalities are a primary manifestation of the underlying sarcomere mutation, rather than simply a secondary consequence of LV hypertrophy, myocardial fibrosis, and myocyte disarray, characteristic of overt HCM. Although the models are not fully characterized, studies on genetically engineered animal models of HCM have suggested that the mechanisms of diastolic dysfunction involve decreased rates of actin-myosin cross-bridge detachment (slowed actin-myosin dissociation kinetics), and decreased rates of calcium reuptake into the sarcoplasmic reticulum [19,20].

Although diastolic dysfunction is commonly regarded as an important pathophysiologic abnormality in clinically overt HCM, to date no consistent relationship has been demonstrated between transmitral Doppler flow patterns and the extent of LVH, the presence or absence of obstruction, LV end-diastolic pressure, heart-failure–related symptoms, or exercise capacity [21–24]. The ratio of the early transmitral flow velocity and TDI annular velocity (E/E') has been examined as a surrogate for left-sided heart filling pressures [25]; however, a recent study demonstrated only a modest correlation between the E/E' ratio and directly measured left atrial pressure in patients with HCM, suggesting that this method may not reliably estimate intracardiac filling pressures in this patient population [26].

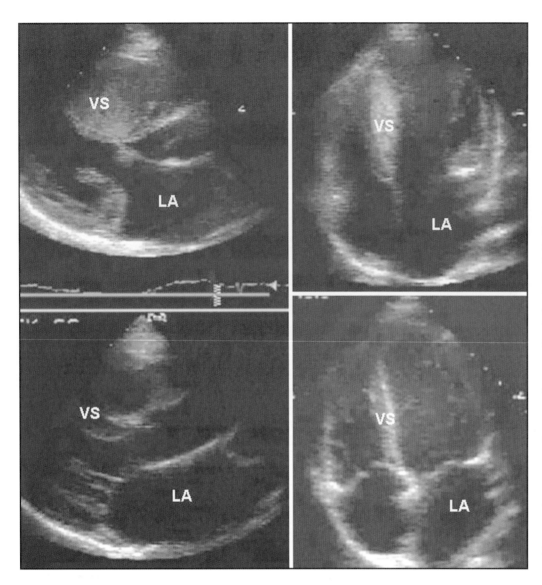

Figure 13-17. Recognition of preclinical hypertrophic cardiomyopathy (HCM) requires genetic studies in families. Parasternal long-axis and apical four-chamber images from a 24-year-old woman with overt HCM are shown (*top panels*). She has marked asymmetric septal hypertrophy with severe systolic anterior motion, causing LV outflow tract obstruction. Genetic testing identified a myosin heavy chain (*MYH7*) gene mutation as the etiology of HCM in her family. Parasternal long-axis and apical four-chamber images from her 23-year-old cousin show a normal standard echocardiographic examination, without LV hypertrophy or other diagnostic features of HCM (*bottom panels*). Genetic testing revealed that she also carries the causal *MYH7* mutation, illustrating the inability of echocardiography alone to identify preclinical gene mutation carriers without LV hypertrophy who are destined to develop HCM. As shown in Figure 13-13B, a subtle reduction in myocardial relaxation velocity (E′) by tissue Doppler interrogation is frequently, but not invariably, seen in young preclinical gene mutation carriers. LA—left atrium; VS—ventricular septum.

Echocardiography in the Differential Diagnosis of Hypertrophic Cardiomyopathy

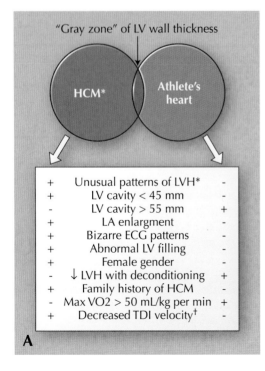

A

Figure 13-18. Athlete's heart versus hypertrophic cardiomyopathy (HCM) is depicted. Clinical features and noninvasive testing, including echocardiography, can aid in distinguishing HCM from the benign, physiologic hypertrophy associated with intense athletic training (**A**). Although most athletes have normal or only mildly increased LV wall thickness, ~2% of elite athletes have LV wall thickness of 13 mm or more and fall into an ambiguous morphologic "gray zone" between physiological hypertrophy and HCM. Although this uncertainty cannot be definitively resolved clinically in all athletes, careful and integrative analysis using these criteria and potentially genetic testing may clarify this diagnostic dilemma in most individuals [27,28]. *LV hypertrophy (LVH), in which asymmetry is prominent, the anterior ventricular septum is spared, or the region of predominant thickening involves the posterior septum or LV free wall. †Both systolic and diastolic myocardial velocities may be reduced in asymptomatic, active patients with HCM, but not in athletes (in one study, S′ = 8.8 vs 10.6 cm/s; E′ = 11.7 vs 18.9 cm/s; HCM vs athletes) [29].

Continued on the next page

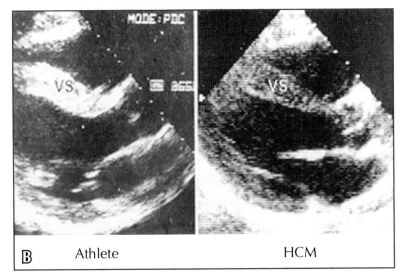

B Athlete   HCM

Figure 13-18. *(Continued)* These parasternal long-axis images (**B**) demonstrate the difficulty in discriminating between an athlete's heart and HCM by LV wall thickness alone. Both the athlete (*left panel*) and patient with HCM (*right panel*) have similar LV morphology and comparable degrees of LVH (maximal wall thickness in both cases ~16 mm). Incorporation of clues from other clinical features, as described above, can aid in resolving the differential diagnosis. Making this distinction between HCM and an athlete's heart is crucial because HCM is an important and lifelong genetic disease, in which consequences could be adversely modified by continued involvement in competitive athletics. Moreover, there are significant implications to the individual's family associated with a diagnosis of HCM. TDI—tissue Doppler imaging; VO$_2$—maximal oxygen consumption; VS—ventricular septum.

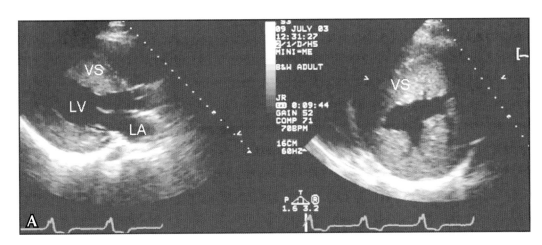

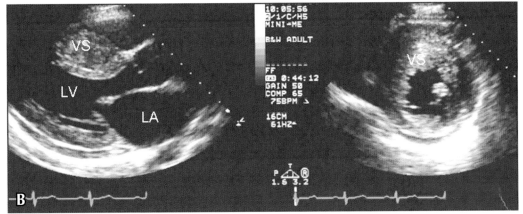

Figure 13-19. Phenocopies that mimic the clinical presentation of hypertrophic cardiomyopathy (HCM) are shown. Parasternal images from an 18-year-old man with a *LAMP2* mutation causing Danon disease, a storage disease that clinically mimics HCM due to a sarcomere gene mutation, are shown (**A**). There is marked diffuse LV hypertrophy (LVH) with a maximal LV septal wall thickness of 35 mm. In contrast, the parasternal images from a 20-year-old man (**B**) with a mutation in myosin heavy chain, also showing marked, diffuse LVH, with a maximal wall thickness of 30 mm, are shown. These discrete disease entities (HCM and metabolic cardiomyopathies) are usually indistinguishable by standard cardiac imaging, and they underscore the limitations of echocardiography in differentiating sarcomeric HCM from its phenocopies.

Genetic studies of families and sporadic cases of unexplained LVH with conduction abnormalities (*eg*, progressive atrioventricular block, atrial fibrillation, and ventricular pre-excitation) have identified a distinct category of genetic cardiac hypertrophy that is caused by mutations in the *PRKAG2* gene, encoding the γ2 regulatory subunit of AMP-activated protein kinase, as well as mutations in the X-linked lysosome-associated membrane protein (*LAMP2*) gene. Mutations in these genes may be present in a significant minority of individuals who carry a clinical diagnosis of HCM, particularly if combined features of LVH and pre-excitation are present [30]. LA—left atrium; VS—ventricular septum.

Echocardiography in the Clinical Management of Hypertrophic Cardiomyopathy

In addition to basic diagnostic considerations (*ie*, screening family members for evidence of disease and identifying the presence and measuring the magnitude of outflow obstruction), echocardiography plays an important role in the management of HCM as part of risk assessment for sudden cardiac death and assessing response to treatment.

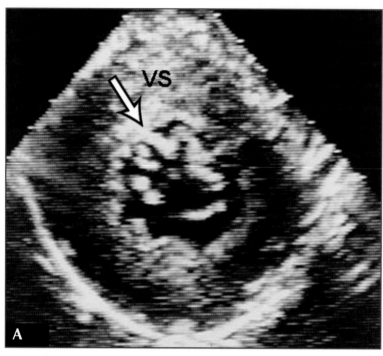

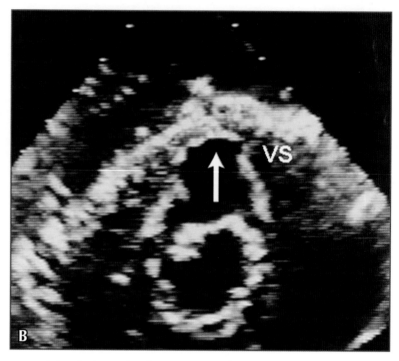

Figure 13-20. Surgical septal myectomy is shown. In preoperative, the parasternal short-axis view (**A**) shows marked hypertrophy of the ventricular septum (VS) with systolic anterior motion (SAM) of the anterior mitral leaflet (*arrow*), causing severe outflow tract obstruction and mitral regurgitation. After myectomy (postoperative), the parasternal short-axis view shows a myectomy "notch" (**B**, *arrow*) representing the portion of the upper septum that was resected, thereby increasing the cross sectional area of the LV outflow tract and eliminating SAM and obstruction. Furthermore, elimination of SAM and normalization of mitral valve coaptation abolishes mitral regurgitation. Long-term outcomes following myectomy are excellent, with improvement of symptoms, exercise capacity, and overall prognosis, including survival, as compared with nonoperated patients who have not had surgery for obstruction [31].

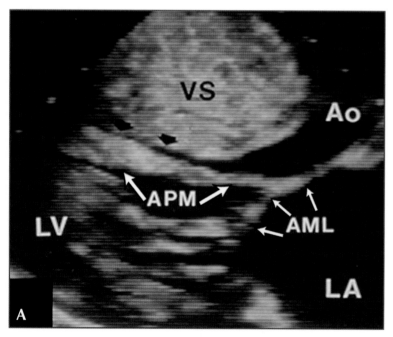

Figure 13-21. Anatomic variant of hypertrophic cardiomyopathy (HCM) amenable only to surgical myectomy is shown. In this preoperative echocardiogram (**A**), the parasternal long-axis image of this morphologic variant of HCM shows that the hypertrophied anterolateral papillary muscle (APM) inserts directly into the anterior mitral leaflet (AML). This produces mid cavity obstruction (*arrowheads*) due to muscular apposition with the ventricular septum (VS). This anomaly may be difficult to recognize with standard transthoracic echocardiography, but is defined more easily by transesophageal and/or intraoperative imaging. In the surgical treatment of obstruction, this anomalous papillary muscle must be addressed to fully attend to outflow obstruction.

Continued on the next page

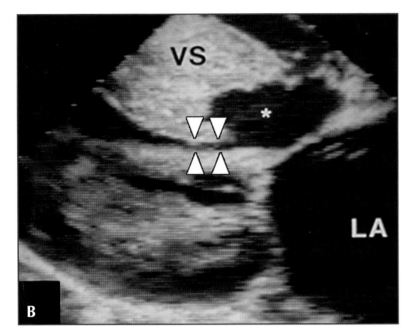

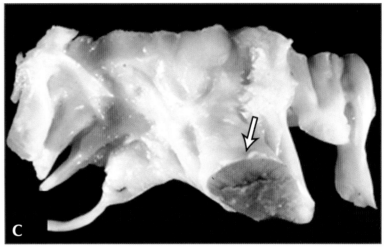

Figure 13-21. *(Continued)* In postoperative echocardiography, the parasternal long-axis image after standard surgical myectomy (Morrow procedure) (**B**) shows that the resection does not extend sufficiently distal, allowing muscular obstruction due to anomalous papillary muscle to persist (*arrowheads*), despite enlargement of the proximal LV outflow tract (*asterisk*). This underscores the necessity for a more extended myectomy

resection, beyond the point of muscular apposition, in such patients. Furthermore, alcohol septal ablation would likely not be effective in this anatomic setting. In a pathologic specimen, the excised mitral valve shows a massively hypertrophied and anomalous papillary muscle (**C**), which inserts directly into the anterior mitral leaflet without the interposition of chordae tendineae (*arrow*). Ao—aorta.

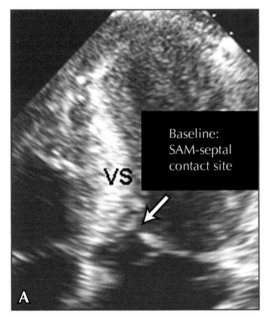
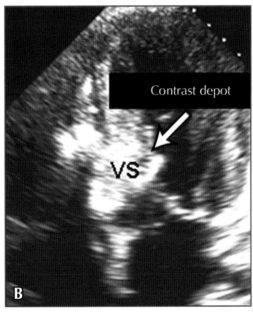
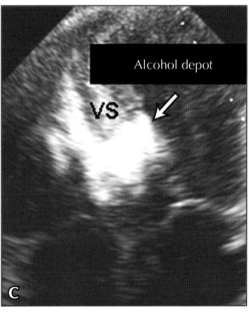

Figure 13-22. Alcohol septal ablation is the deliberate and controlled creation of a septal myocardial infarction. Ethanol (100%) is injected into a septal perforator coronary artery, which results in transmural scar formation and thinning of the proximal septum, thereby decreasing systolic anterior motion (SAM) and outflow tract obstruction. Although alcohol ablation has been associated with improvement in symptoms, exercise tolerance, and oxygen consumption, long-term results are not yet available. During the procedure, contrast echocardiography guidance plays an important role in determining patient suitability, targeting the appropriate septal perforator branch for injection, and reducing the likelihood of potential complications [32,33]. A baseline apical four-chamber view identifies the area of maximal SAM septal contact

to target for ablation (**A**, *arrow*). Intracoronary injection of echocardiographic contrast verifies that the selected septal perforator branch supplies the target area of the ventricular septum (VS) at the site of maximal SAM septal contact. The contrast agent highlights the region supplied by the injected septal branch with an echogenic signal created by the accumulation of contrast within the myocardium (**B**, *arrow*). This delineates the site of potential ablation and determines whether infarction size will be excessive or involve the RV or other unintended structures. Alcohol is then instilled into the selected septal perforator branch, targeting the same region of the septum, as highlighted by the intracoronary contrast and seen as an intensely echobright signal from the alcohol collection within the myocardium (**C**, *arrow*).

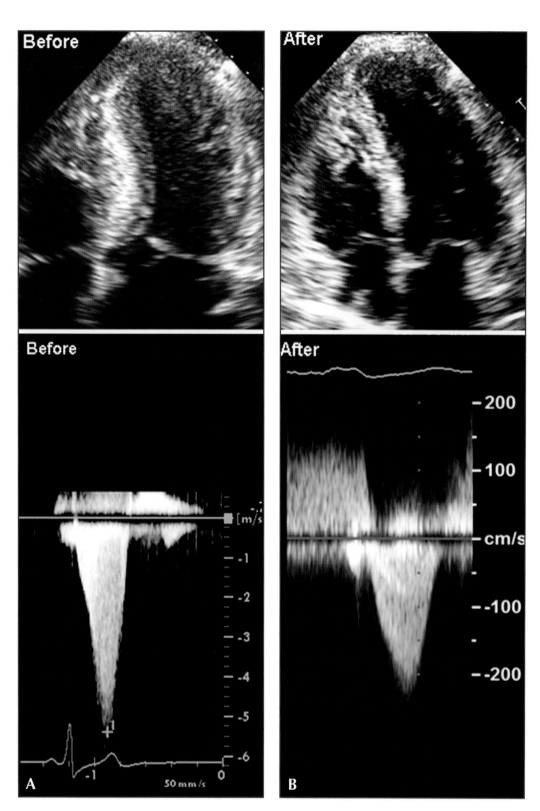

Figure 3-23. Hemodynamic effects of successful alcohol septal ablation are shown. Mid systolic apical four-chamber view (before ablation) (**A**) demonstrates severe systolic anterior motion (SAM) with prolonged septal contact, resulting in a resting gradient of 100 mm Hg. Two months after septal ablation (**B**), there is thinning of the proximal septum and amelioration of SAM. Resting gradient has decreased to 20 mm Hg.

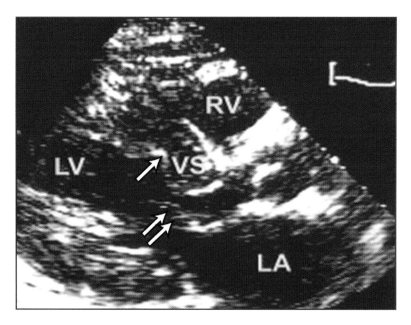

Figure 3-24. Failed alcohol septal ablation is shown. In this patient, septal perforator artery distribution was unfavorable, supplying a portion of the ventricular septum (VS) (*single arrow*) distal to the target location of systolic anterior motion septal contact (*double arrows*). Consequently, outflow obstruction and heart failure symptoms persisted following the procedure. LA—left atrium.

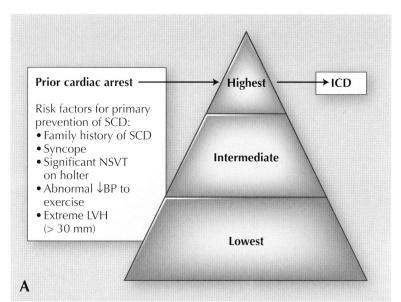

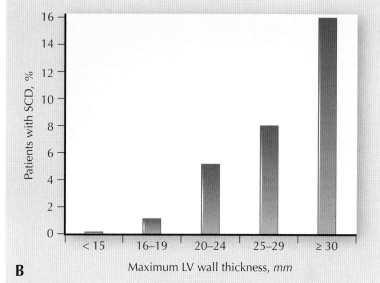

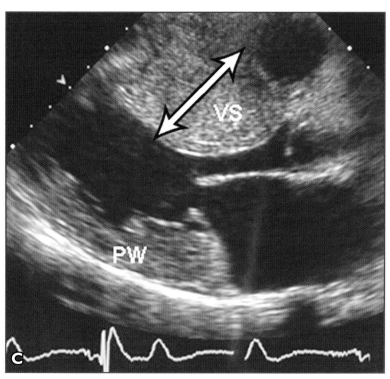

Figure 3-25. Echocardiography in the assessment of risk for sudden cardiac death in hypertrophic cardiomyopathy (HCM) is shown. **A**, HCM is associated with an increased risk of sudden cardiac death (SCD). Clinical predictors of increased risk include a family history of SCD, unexplained syncope, hypotensive blood pressure response to exercise, nonsustained ventricular tachycardia (NSVT) on ambulatory Holter monitoring, and extreme LV hypertrophy (LVH) (wall thickness ≥ 30 mm by echocardiography). In this regard, routine echocardiographic examination can identify high risk patients with extreme LVH who may be eligible for implantable cardiovertor defibrillator (ICD) therapy for primary prevention of SCD [34–36].

B, Young patients with extreme hypertrophy (maximal wall thickness ≥ 30 mm), even those with few or no symptoms, have increased long-term risk of SCD. In contrast, the majority of patients with mild hypertrophy appear to be at lower risk for SCD [36]. However, it is important to recognize that the positive predictive accuracy for a wall thickness of 30 mm or more is less than 20%, suggesting that interpretation of this parameter must be in the context of a thorough clinical assessment, including assessment of other risk factors such as family history of SCD, presence of arrhythmias, symptoms, and blood pressure response to exercise [37].

C, A parasternal long-axis view from a young asymptomatic patient with HCM demonstrating extreme LVH with a maximal septal wall thickness of 45 mm is shown (*arrows*). In HCM, the magnitude of hypertrophy shows a direct relationship with the risk of SCD. PW—posterior wall; VS—ventricular septum.

References

1. Maron BJ, Towbin JA, Thiene G, et al.: Contemporary definitions and classification of the cardiomyopathies: an American Heart Association Scientific Statement from the Council on Clinical Cardiology, Heart Failure and Transplantation Committee; Quality of Care and Outcomes Research and Functional Genomics and Translational Biology Interdisciplinary Working Groups; and Council on Epidemiology and Prevention. *Circulation* 2006, 113:1807–1816.

2. Ho CY, Seidman CE: A contemporary approach to hypertrophic cardiomyopathy. *Circulation* 2006, 113:e858–e862.

3. Nabel E: Cardiovascular disease. *N Engl J Med* 2003, 349:60–72.

4. Yamaguchi H, Ishimura T, Nishiyama S, et al.: Hypertrophic nonobstructive cardiomyopathy with giant negative T waves (apical hypertrophy): ventriculographic and echocardiographic features in 30 patients. *Am J Cardiol* 1979, 44:401–412.

5. Kitaoka H, Doi Y, Casey SA, et al.: Comparison of prevalence of apical hypertrophic cardiomyopathy in Japan and the United States. *Am J Cardiol* 2003, 92:1183–1186.

6. Eriksson MJ, Sonnenberg B, Woo A, et al.: Long-term outcome in patients with apical hypertrophic cardiomyopathy. *J Am Coll Cardiol* 2002, 39:638–645.

7. Arad M, Penas-Lado M, Monserrat L, et al.: Gene mutations in apical hypertrophic cardiomyopathy. *Circulation* 2005, 112:2805–2811.

8. Rickers C, Wilke NM, Jerosch-Herold M, et al.: Utility of cardiac magnetic resonance imaging in the diagnosis of hypertrophic cardiomyopathy. *Circulation* 2005, 112:855–861.

9. Maron MS, Olivotto I, Betocchi S, et al.: Effect of left ventricular outflow tract obstruction on clinical outcome in hypertrophic cardiomyopathy. *N Engl J Med* 2003, 348:295–303.

10. Sherrid MV, Gunsburg DZ, Moldenhauer S, Pearle G: Systolic anterior motion begins at low left ventricular outflow tract velocity in obstructive hypertrophic cardiomyopathy. *J Am Coll Cardiol* 2000, 36:1344–1354.

11. Klues HG, Maron BJ, Dollar AL, Roberts WC: Diversity of structural mitral valve alterations in hypertrophic cardiomyopathy. *Circulation* 1992, 85:1651–1660.

12. Spirito P, Maron BJ: Significance of left ventricular outflow tract cross-sectional area in hypertrophic cardiomyopathy: a two-dimensional echocardiographic assessment. *Circulation* 1983, 67:1100–1108.

13. Klues HG, Roberts WC, Maron BJ: Morphological determinants of echocardiographic patterns of mitral valve systolic anterior motion in obstructive hypertrophic cardiomyopathy. *Circulation* 1993, 87:1570–1579.

14. Maron BJ, Niimura H, Casey SA, et al.: Development of left ventricular hypertrophy in adults in hypertrophic cardiomyopathy caused by cardiac myosin-binding protein C gene mutations. *J Am Coll Cardiol* 2001, 38:315–321.

15. Maron BJ, Seidman JG, Seidman CE: Proposal for contemporary screening strategies in families with hypertrophic cardiomyopathy. *J Am Coll Cardiol* 2004, 44:2125–2132.

16. Harris KM, Spirito P, Maron MS, et al.: Prevalence, clinical profile, and significance of left ventricular remodeling in the end-stage phase of hypertrophic cardiomyopathy. *Circulation* 2006, 114:216–225.

17. Nagueh SF, Bachinski LL, Meyer D, et al.: Tissue Doppler imaging consistently detects myocardial abnormalities in patients with hypertrophic cardiomyopathy and provides a novel means for an early diagnosis before and independently of hypertrophy. *Circulation* 2001, 104:128–130.

18. Ho CY, Sweitzer NK, McDonough B, et al.: Assessment of diastolic function with Doppler tissue imaging to predict genotype in preclinical hypertrophic cardiomyopathy. *Circulation* 2002, 105:2992–2997.

19. Gao WD, Perez NG, Seidman CE, et al.: Altered cardiac excitation-contraction coupling in mutant mice with familial hypertrophic cardiomyopathy. *J Clin Invest* 1999, 103:661–666.

20. Spindler M, Saupe KW, Christe ME, et al.: Diastolic dysfunction and altered energetics in the alphaMHC403/+ mouse model of familial hypertrophic cardiomyopathy. *J Clin Invest* 1998, 101:1775–1783.

21. Briguori C, Betocchi S, Losi MA, et al.: Noninvasive evaluation of left ventricular diastolic function in hypertrophic cardiomyopathy. *Am J Cardiol* 1998, 81:180–187.

22. Nihoyannopoulos P, Karatasakis G, Frenneaux M, et al.: Diastolic function in hypertrophic cardiomyopathy: relation to exercise capacity. *J Am Coll Cardiol* 1992, 19:536–540.

23. Nishimura RA, Appleton CP, Redfield MM, et al.: Noninvasive Doppler echocardiographic evaluation of left ventricular filling pressures in patients with cardiomyopathies: a simultaneous Doppler echocardiographic and cardiac catheterization study. *J Am Coll Cardiol* 1996, 28:1226–1233.

24. Spirito P, Maron BJ: Relation between extent of left ventricular hypertrophy and diastolic filling abnormalities in hypertrophic cardiomyopathy. *J Am Coll Cardiol* 1990, 15:808–813.

25. Nagueh SF, Lakkis NM, Middleton KJ, et al.: Doppler estimation of left ventricular filling pressures in patients with hypertrophic cardiomyopathy. *Circulation* 1999, 99:254–261.

26. Geske JB, Sorajja P, Nishimura RA, Ommen SR: Evaluation of left ventricular filling pressures by Doppler echocardiography in patients with hypertrophic cardiomyopathy: correlation with direct left atrial pressure measurement at cardiac catheterization. *Circulation* 2007, 116:2702–2708.

27. Maron BJ: Distinguishing hypertrophic cardiomyopathy from athlete's heart: a clinical problem of increasing magnitude and significance. *Heart* 2005, 91:1380–1382.

28. Maron BJ, Pelliccia A, Spirito P: Cardiac disease in young trained athletes: insights into methods for distinguishing athlete's heart from structural heart disease, with particular emphasis on hypertrophic cardiomyopathy. *Circulation* 1995, 91:1596–1601.

29. Cardim N, Oliveira AG, Longo S, et al.: Doppler tissue imaging: regional myocardial function in hypertrophic cardiomyopathy and in athlete's heart. *J Am Soc Echocardiogr* 2003, 16:223–232.

30. Arad M, Maron BJ, Gorham JM, et al.: Glycogen storage diseases presenting as hypertrophic cardiomyopathy. *N Engl J Med* 2005, 352:362–372.

31. Ommen SR, Maron BJ, Olivotto I, et al.: Long-term effects of surgical septal myectomy on survival in patients with obstructive hypertrophic cardiomyopathy. *J Am Coll Cardiol* 2005, 46:470–476.

32. Faber L, Ziemssen P, Seggewiss H: Targeting percutaneous transluminal septal ablation for hypertrophic obstructive cardiomyopathy by intraprocedural echocardiographic monitoring. *J Am Soc Echocardiogr* 2000, 13:1074–1079.

33. Shamim W, Yousufuddin M, Wang D, et al.: Nonsurgical reduction of the interventricular septum in patients with hypertrophic cardiomyopathy. *N Engl J Med* 2002, 347:1326–1333.

34. Maron BJ, Shen WK, Link MS, et al.: Efficacy of implantable cardioverter-defibrillators for the prevention of sudden death in patients with hypertrophic cardiomyopathy. *N Engl J Med* 2000, 342:365–373.

35. McKenna WJ, Behr ER: Hypertrophic cardiomyopathy: management, risk stratification, and prevention of sudden death. *Heart* 2002, 87:169–176.

36. Spirito P, Bellone P, Harris KM, et al.: Magnitude of left ventricular hypertrophy and risk of sudden death in hypertrophic cardiomyopathy. *N Engl J Med* 2000, 342:1778–1785.

37. Elliott PM, Gimeno Blanes JR, Mahon NG, et al.: Relation between severity of left-ventricular hypertrophy and prognosis in patients with hypertrophic cardiomyopathy. *Lancet* 2001, 357:420–424.

Dilated and Restrictive/Infiltrative Cardiomyopathies

Rodney H. Falk

The American Heart Association (AHA) and the European Society of Cardiology (ESC) have recently and independently published documents that define and reclassify the cardiomyopathies [1,2]. Both classifications stress, in their respective definitions, the central role of a disorder of cardiac muscle that is not due to congenital, coronary, or valvular disease and is not secondary to hypertension. The European guidelines define cardiomyopathy as "a myocardial disorder, in which the heart muscle is structurally and functionally abnormal, in the absence of coronary artery disease, hypertension, valvular disease and congenital heart disease sufficient to cause the observed myocardial abnormality" [2]. The AHA definition states that "cardiomyopathies are a heterogeneous group of diseases of the myocardium associated with mechanical and/or electrical dysfunction that usually (but not invariably) exhibit inappropriate ventricular hypertrophy or dilatation and are due to a variety of causes that frequently are genetic. Cardiomyopathies either are confined to the heart, or are part of a generalized systemic disorder, often leading to cardiovascular death of progressive heart failure-related disability" [1]. Although not formally part of the definition, the AHA scientific statement stresses that "it is also important to specify those disease entities that have not been included as cardiomyopathies in the present contemporary classification. These include pathological myocardial processes and dysfunction that are a direct consequence of cardiovascular abnormalities, such as those which occur with valvular heart disease, systemic hypertension, congenital heart disease, and atherosclerotic cardiac disease producing ischemic myocardial damage secondary to impairment in coronary flow." Concern is raised about the classification of cardiomyopathies as hypertrophic, dilated, or restrictive, not only because this classification

mixes a morphologic hypertrophic or dilated with a functional designation, namely "restrictive," but also because a single disease may fall into more than one category. The suggestion is therefore made that this classification of "dilated-hypertrophic-restrictive" should probably be abandoned [1].

From an echocardiographic standpoint, there is still some value in retaining these categories. Echocardiographically, a fairly precise assessment of LV cavity size, wall thickness, and systolic and diastolic function can be made. This allows for the distinction between diseases that predominantly cause wall thickening, such as hypertrophic cardiomyopathy and infiltrative cardiomyopathy and cardiac disorders that tend to result in ventricular dilation with associated systolic dysfunction. The echocardiographic assessment of cardiac disease, particularly among patients manifesting a dilated LV with systolic dysfunction, cannot easily distinguish a specific diagnosis among the multiple etiologies that may be responsible for the dysfunction. However, echocardiographic appearances are extremely helpful in defining the severity of dysfunction and for pointing the clinician in a specific direction. As will be apparent in the upcoming examples, it is feasible to have a dilated LV with a restrictive pathophysiology; however, the potential etiology of this finding is entirely different from a similar Doppler appearance in a patient with a normal-sized LV and preserved LV ejection fraction. Thus, from an echocardiographic standpoint there remains a value in this classification, with the caveat that it is primarily descriptive. Despite limitations of this classification, pointed out in both the AHA and ESC position papers, both continue to use it nonetheless in their updated classifications. The new US and European classifications of cardiomyopathies are shown in this chapter (*see* Figs. 14-1 and 14-2).

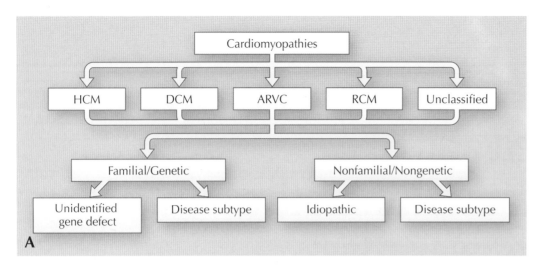

A

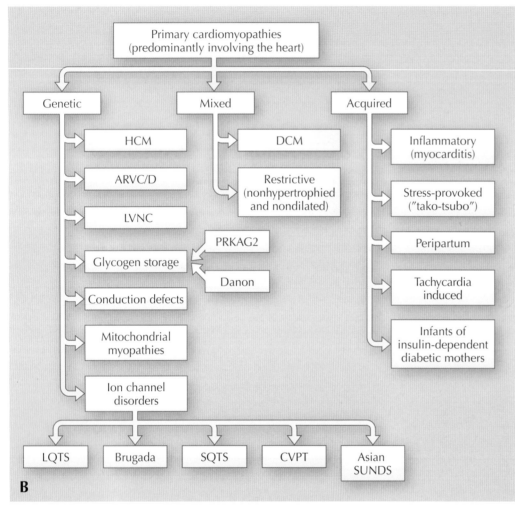

B

Figure 14-1. A, Summary of European Society of Cardiology (ESC) proposed classification system of cardiomyopathies. ARVC—arrhythmogenic right ventricular cardiomyopathy; DCM—dilated cardiomyopathy; HCM—hypertrophic cardiomyopathy; RCM—restrictive cardiomyopathy. (*From* Elliott *et al.* [2]; with permission.) **B,** American Heart Association (AHA) proposed classification of cardiomyopathies. CVPT—catecholamine-induced polymorphic ventricular tachycardia; SUNDS—sudden unexpected nocturnal death syndrome. (*Adapted from* Maron *et al.* [1].)

Examples of Different Diseases That Cause Cardiomyopathies

	HCM	DCM	ARVC	RCM	Unclassified
Familial	Familial, unknown gene	Familial, unknown gene	Familial, unknown gene	Familial, unknown gene	LV noncompaction
	Sarcomeric protein mutations	Sarcomeric protein mutations (see HCM)	Intercalated disk protein mutations	Sarcomeric protein mutations	Barth syndrome
	β Myosin heavy chain	Z-band	Plakoglobin	Troponin I 9RCM ± HCM)	Lamin A/C
	Cardiac myosin binding protein C	Muscle LIM protein	Desmoplakin	Essential light chain of myosin	ZASP
	Cardiac troponin I	TCAP	Plakophilin 2	Familial amyloidosis	α-Dystrobrevin
	Troponin-T	Cytoskeletal genes	Desmoglein 2	Transthyretin	
	α-Tropomyosin	Dystrophin	Desmocollin 2	(RCM + nephropathy)	
	Essential myosin light chain	Desmin	Cardiac ryanodine receptor (RyR2)	Apolipoprotein	
	Regulatory myosin light chain	Metavinculin	Transforming growth factor - β3	(RCM + nephropathy)	
	Cardiac actin	Sarcoglycan complex		Desminopathy	
	α-Myosin heavy chain	CRYAB		Pseudoxanthoma elasticum	
	Titin	Epicardin		Hemochromatosis	
	Troponin C	Nuclear membrane		Anderson-Fabry disease	
	Muscle LIM protein	Lamin A/C		Glycogen storage disease	
	Glycogen storage diseases (eg, Pompe; PRKAG2, Forbes, Danon)	Emerin			
	Lysosomal storage diseases (eg, Anderson-Fabry, Hurler's)	Mildly dilated CM			
	Disorders of fatty acid metabolism	Intercalated disc protein mutations (see ARVC)			
	Carnitine deficiency	Mitochondrial cytopathy			
	Phosphorylase B kinase deficiency				
	Mitochondrial cytopathies				
	Syndromic HCM				
	Noonan's syndrome				
	LEOPARD syndrome				
	Friedreich's ataxia				
	Beckwith-Wiedemann syndrome				
	Swyer's syndrome				
	Other				
	Phospholamban promoter				
	Familial amyloid				
Nonfamilial	Obesity	Myocarditis (infective/toxic/immune)	Inflammation	Amyloidosis	Takotsubo cardio-myopathy
	Infants of diabetic mothers	Kawaski disease		Scleroderma	
	Athletic training	Eosinophilic (Churg Strauss syndrome)		Endomyocardial fibrosis	
	Amyloid (prealbumin)	Viral persistence		Hypereosinophilic syndrome	
		Drugs		Idiopathic	
		Pregnancy		Chromosomal cause	
		Endocrine		Drugs (serotonin, methysergide, ergotamine, mercurial agents, busulfan)	
		Nutritional: thiamine, carnitine, selenium, hypophosphatemia, hypocalcemia		Carcinoid heart disease	
		Alcohol		Metastatic cancers	
		Tachycardiomyopathy		Radiation	
				Drugs (anthracyclines)	

Figure 14-2. Examples of the diseases causing cardiomyopathy, classified according to the European Society of Cardiology (ESC) criteria. Diseases causing dilated and restrictive cardiomyopathy are highlighted. ARVC—arrhythmogenic right ventricular cardiomyopathy; CRYAB—alpha-B-crystallin; DCM—dilated cardiomyopathy; HCM—hypertrophic cardiomyopathy; LVNC—LV noncompaction; LQTS—Long QT Syndrome; RCM—restrictive cardiomyopathy; SQTS—Short QT Syndrome; TCAP—titin cap protein. (*From* Elliott *et al.* [2]; with permission.)

Dilated Cardiomyopathy

Dilated cardiomyopathy is defined by the AHA Working Group as "ventricular chamber enlargement and systolic dysfunction with normal wall thickness" [1] and by the ESC as "the presence of LV dilatation and LV systolic dysfunction in the absence of abnormal loading conditions (such as hypertension or valve disease), or of coronary artery disease sufficient to cause global systolic impairment" [2]. It has long been recognized that although the severity of LV dysfunction is related to prognosis, it correlates poorly with the presence or severity of symptoms [3]. In contrast, symptoms in cardiomyopathy relate well to LV filling pressure, which in turn can be evaluated by Doppler echocardiography [4]. Thus, although dilated cardiomyopathy is always associated with systolic dysfunction, it is the diastolic function that drives symptoms. The following images illustrate some of the features of dilated cardiomyopathy.

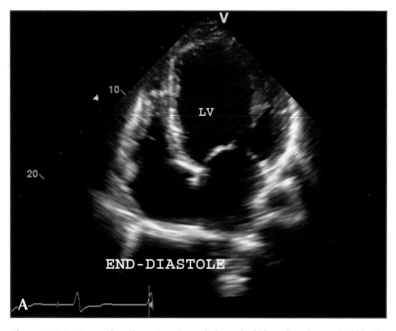
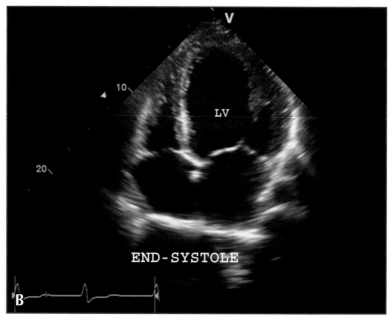

Figure 14-3. Four-chamber view in end-diastole (**A**) and end-systole (**B**) of a patient with a dilated cardiomyopathy and a severely reduced LV ejection fraction. In this patient, the RV was normal in size, and the atria are only minimally dilated.

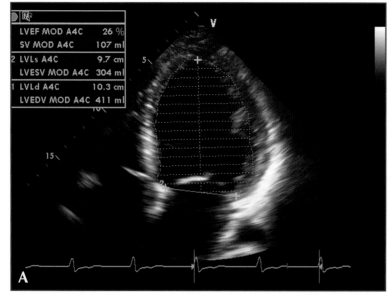
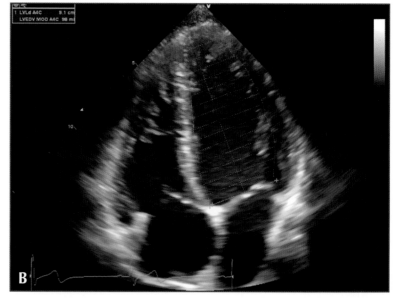

Figure 14-4. End-diastolic volume measurement in the four-chamber view (A4C). In the patient illustrated on the left, the calculated LV ejection fraction (LVEF), using the Simpson rule of disks, is 26% (**A**). Note that the calculated LV volumes are markedly increased (411 mL in diastole and 304 mL in systole). Thus, even with a severely reduced ejection fraction, the stroke volume (SV) at rest was normal, resulting in a normal cardiac output. In addition to the marked dilation of the ventricle in severe dilated cardiomyopathy, the shape of the ventricle alters, becoming more spherical. The "sphericity index" is calculated as the ratio of the length of the ventricle measured in the apical long axis to the width of the widest point [5–7]. A normal sphericity index is greater than 1.6. In the *left-hand panel* (**A**), the sphericity index of the ventricle is calculated as 1.2, which is markedly abnormal and indicative of pathologic remodeling. In the *right panel* (**B**), a normal ventricle is illustrated with a calculated LV end-diastolic volume of 98 mL and a sphericity index of 2.1. LVEDV—LV end-diastolic volume; LVESV—LV end-systolic volume; LVLd—LV long-axis length in end-diastole; LVLs—LV long-axis length in end-systole.

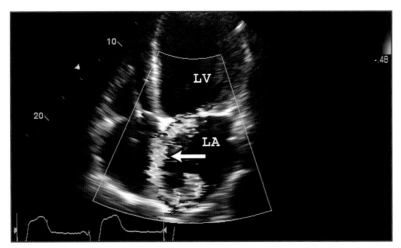

Figure 14-5. Ventricular remodeling in dilated cardiomyopathy results in apical and lateral displacement of the papillary muscles and dilation of the mitral annulus, predisposing to mitral regurgitation (MR) [5,8]. This patient had a mitral valve repair, which initially improved his secondary MR. This later recurred, a phenomenon related to ongoing ventricular remodeling in the severely dilated LV [9,10]. Note also the pacing/implantable cardioverter-defibrillator wire going through the tricuspid valve. Biventricular pacing in this patient did not improve the LV ejection fraction or his MR. It has been suggested that (as in this case) patients with a dilated cardiomyopathy and a severely dilated LV, defined as an LV end-diastolic dimension of more than 75 mm, have a relatively poor response to resynchronization therapy [10]. The *arrow* points to the eccentric MR jet. LA—left atrium.

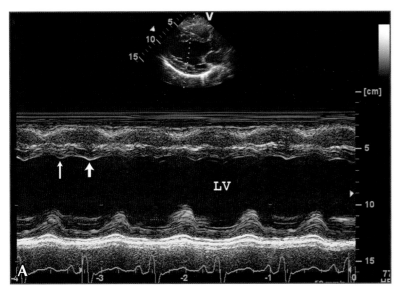

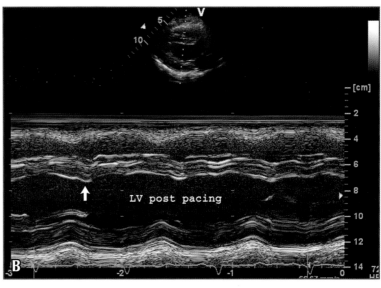

Figure 14-6. Intraventricular conduction delay, typified by left bundle branch block, can result in a significant reduction of ejection fraction and/or cardiac output [11]. M-mode of the LV before (**A**) and after (**B**) biventricular pacing in a patient presenting with heart failure. Note the paradoxical septal motion characterized by an initial brief downward motion (**A**, *narrow arrow*), followed by motion toward LV cavity during diastole (**A**, *broad arrow*). This is normalized by biventricular pacing, with systolic septal motion toward the LV cavity (**B**, *arrow*). In addition to improved synergy, the LV size has decreased after biventricular pacing.

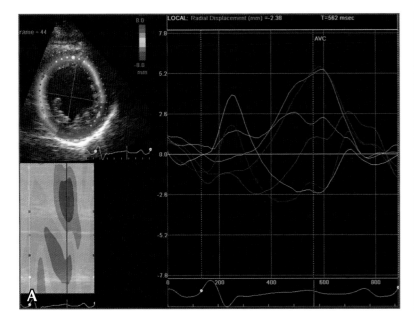

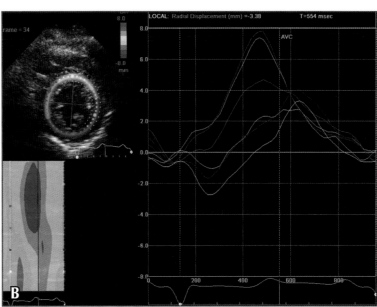

Figure 14-7. The same patient as in Figure 14-6, demonstrating improvement of dyssynergy by the technique of speckle tracking [12–14]. The prepacing image is shown (*left*). The onset of systole is characterized by a brief positive deflection of the ventricular septum (*yellow and red lines on graph*) followed by a paradoxical negative (outward) deflection throughout the remainder of systole. Following pacing (**B**), dyssynchrony is improved (but not fully normalized), and all segments move concordantly during systole and diastole.

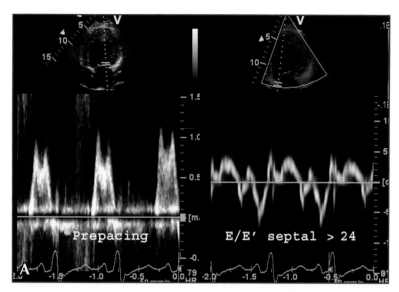

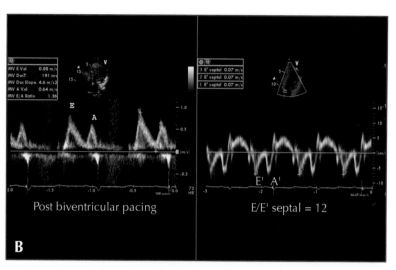

Figure 14-8. A, Transmitral Doppler and tissue Doppler prior to resynchronization therapy shows a pattern of decreased LV compliance (pseudonormalization of transmitral Doppler flow pattern). Transmitral E/A ratio is more than 1.0, but the tissue Doppler shows a marked reversal of E'/A'. E/E' ratio is 24, indicative of elevated LV end-diastolic pressure [15]. **B**, Following biventricular pacing, the transmitral E/A is normal, with normalization of E'/A' and a lower E/E' ratio, indicative of the improvement in diastolic function and decrease in LV filling pressure. MV—mitral valve.

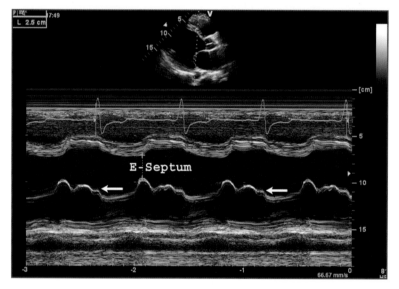

Figure 14-9. In a diseased ventricle, when ventricular end-diastolic pressure is elevated, mitral valve (MV) closure may be interrupted by an abnormal elevation of left atrial pressure, causing it to briefly reopen. This results in an M-mode appearance of an additional notch on the MV known as an A-C notch (also referred to as a B-bump [*horizontal arrow*]) [16,17]. Note also the increased E point septal separation, suggestive of a low stroke volume [18,19].

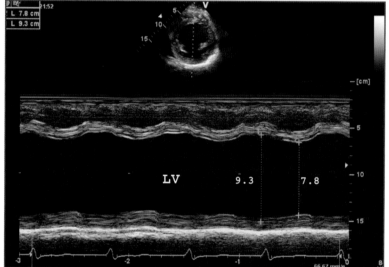

Figure 14-10. M-mode from a patient with a severely dilated LV due to a dilated cardiomyopathy. Although the LV wall thickness (10 mm) is within normal limits for a normal sized LV, it represents eccentric LV hypertrophy in this markedly dilated ventricle. Using the Devereaux formula, LV mass (in grams) = $0.8\{1.04[([LVEDD + IVSd + PWd]^3 - LVEDD^3)]\} + 0.6$ the calculated LV mass is markedly increased at 532 g or 260 g/m^2, with a normal range in men of 49 to 115 g/m^2. LVEDD—LV end-diastolic dimension; PWd—posterior wall thickness in diastole; IVSd—interventricular septal thickness in diastole [20].

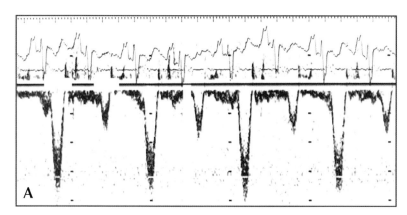

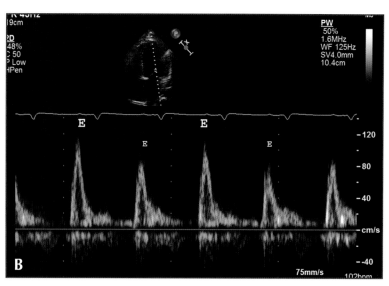

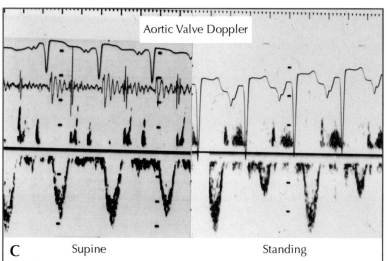

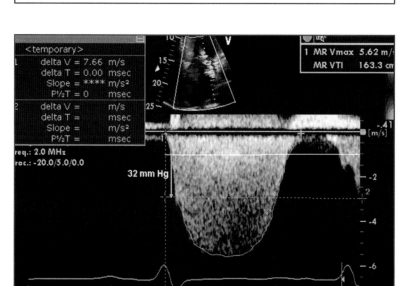

Figure 14-11. Doppler manifestation of pulsus alternans due to severe LV dysfunction in dilated cardiomyopathy. Aortic Doppler alternans is shown (**A**); in another patient, alternans of the mitral inflow Doppler tracing is demonstrated (**B**) [21]. Pulsus alternans is usually associated with a severely reduced LV ejection fraction and tends to occur at the heart rates of 100 bpm or more. It is an intermittent phenomenon and, in susceptible patients, may be precipitated by standing [22] (**C**).

Figure 14-12. Example of calculation of "isovolumic" dP/dt (rate of rise of LV pressure) using the mitral regurgitation (MR) jet. The time taken for the LV pressure to rise by 32 mm Hg is derived from the rate of rise of the MR Doppler signal between a velocity of 1 m/s (representing an LV to left atrial pressure difference of 4 mm Hg by the Bernoulli equation) and 3 m/s (representing 36 mm Hg). At 3 m/s, the LV pressure is still below the aortic diastolic pressure (hence the dP/dt represents isovolumic contraction) [23]. A normal value is greater than 1100 mm Hg/s, and a value of less than 600 mm Hg/s has been shown to indicate a poorer chance of survival in a group of patients with a reduced LV ejection fraction [24]. In the example, which was taken from a patient with a dilated cardiomyopathy, ejection fraction of 35%–40%, and new onset of heart failure, the time taken for the pressure to rise 32 mm Hg was 20 ms, giving a calculated dP/dt of 1600 mm Hg/s, which is well within the normal range.

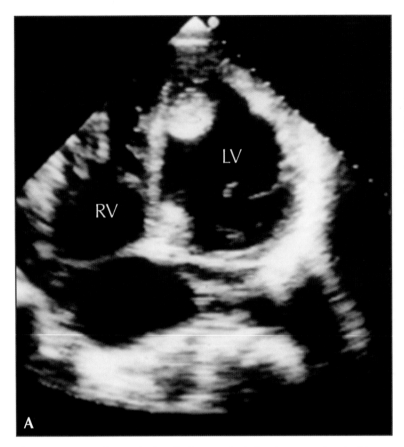

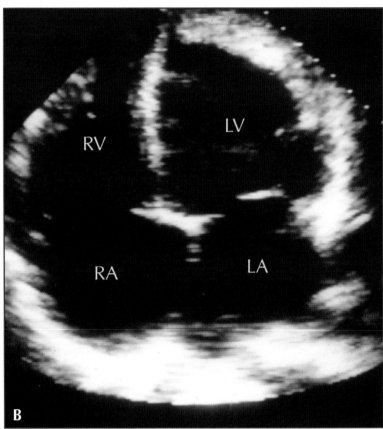

Figure 14-13. Left ventricular dilation, particularly when associated with low cardiac output, may result in thrombus formation in the LV cavity. In this example, recorded in a patient with an alcoholic cardiomyopathy and ejection fraction of approximately 10%, a very large "cannonball" thrombus is seen in the region of the apical septum. Despite the unusually large size of this thrombus, it was best visualized on this off-axis apical view of the LV (**A**) and is not appreciated on the standard four-chamber view (**B**). LA—left atrium; RA—right atrium.

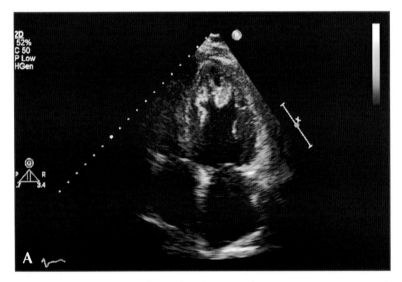

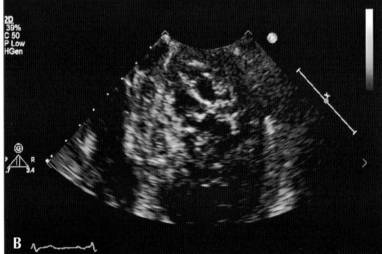

Figure 14-14. An unusual form of cardiomyopathy may occur in patients with the congenital abnormality of LV noncompaction [25]. This is characterized by prominent LV trabeculae and deep interventricular recesses. The myocardial wall may be thin; the epicardium is compacted, and the endocardium is often thickened. This may result in an appearance mimicking LV thrombus (**A**). An appearance of hypertrabeculation in the LV cavity (**B**) is typical of this condition. Although designated by the European Society of Cardiology as an "unclassified cardiomyopathy" [2], it may result in a dilated cardiomyopathy. In the example shown, the patient was asymptomatic with a normal ejection fraction, undergoing echocardiography because of an abnormal electrocardiogram. Although rare, the prevalence of noncompaction is not precisely known, in part because of differing definitions [2,26,27]. (*Courtesy of* Ravin Davidoff, MD.)

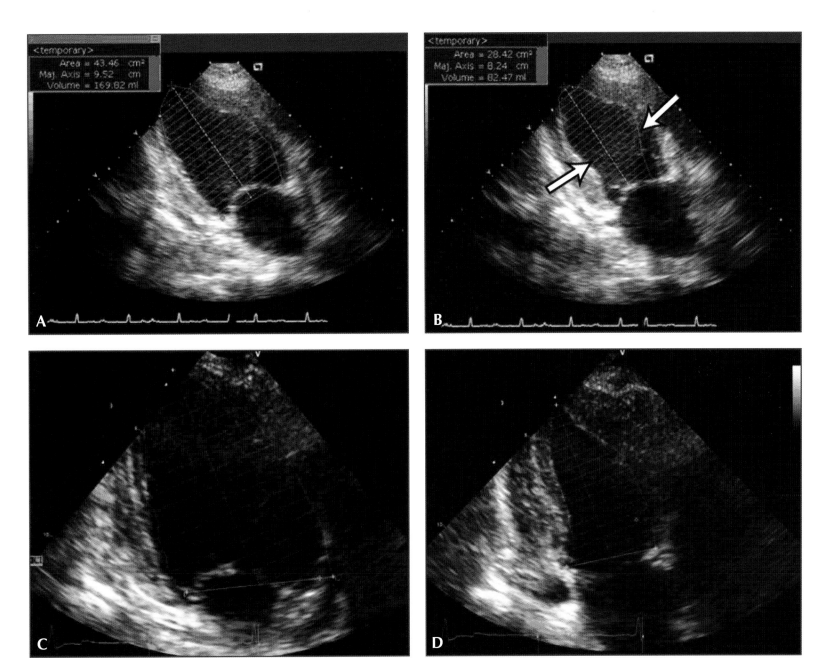

Figure 14-15. An acute, catecholamine-mediated cardiomyopathy may occur following severe emotional trauma. It is characterized by reversible and often severe regional LV dysfunction with electrocardiographic changes mimicking myocardial infarction. In the majority of cases, the LV apex is involved, resulting in dyskinesis or ballooning of the apical segments, giving rise to the term "apical ballooning syndrome" or Takotsubo cardiomyopathy (named for the shape of the LV, which resembles a narrow-necked Japanese octopus pot) [28]. However, other regions of the ventricle may be involved. This example is recorded from a 70-year-old woman with a newly diagnosed ascending aortic aneurysm, severe aortic regurgitation, and acute chest pain with ST segment elevation. End-diastolic frame in the apical two-chamber view is shown (**A**). The echocardiogram showed mid-anterior and apical-anterior wall akinesis and mid- and apical-inferior wall akinesis with a "hinge point" seen at end-systole (**B**, *arrows*). No aortic dissection was present, and coronary angiography revealed normal coronary arteries. No clear reason for the severe regional dysfunction could be found other than presumptive Takotsubo cardiomyopathy, and it was opted to postpone surgery for 2 months in order to reassess LV function. Two months later, her LV function was entirely normal at end-diastole (**C**) and end-systole (**D**), and she underwent an uncomplicated aortic root and valve replacement.

Restrictive/Infiltrative Cardiomyopathy

The term "restrictive cardiomyopathy" is imprecise, referring to a cardiomyopathy characterized by a nondilated nonhypertrophied LV, usually with relatively preserved LV ejection fraction, but with significant diastolic dysfunction. Although patients with restrictive cardiomyopathy frequently have restrictive pathophysiology, this is not always the case, and this hemodynamic profile can be seen in cardiomyopathy of any type. It is quite common in decompensated dilated cardiomyopathy, in which the Doppler pattern is often reversible following treatment (*see* Fig. 14-16). With the exception of "primary restrictive nonhypertrophied cardiomyopathy," the classification of many cardiomyopathies formerly described as "restrictive cardiomyopathy" has been virtually dropped from the AHA cardiomyopathy classification, primarily because of this imprecision of the terminology.

In contrast, restrictive cardiac pathophysiology secondary to systemic disorders (the most common of which is amyloidosis) is still classified as a restrictive cardiomyopathy by the European classification, with the AHA preferring to classify this and most other most types as a "secondary cardiomyopathy due to infiltrative disease." Amyloidosis is the most common disorder to cause a cardiomyopathy with a predominantly restrictive pathophysiology [29]. As the spectrum of cardiac amyloid involvement ranges from an asymptomatic stage to severe and rapidly progressive restrictive heart disease [30], the designation as an infiltrative cardiomyopathy appears to be more precise. The images reflect the spectrum of findings in patients with cardiac amyloidosis, and represent the nature of the infiltration, not only on the ventricles, but also on the oft neglected atria.

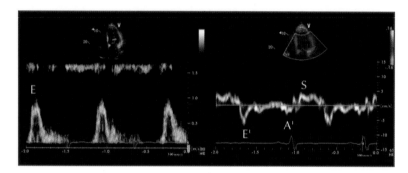

Figure 14-16. An example of restrictive mitral inflow, taken from a patient with a dilated cardiomyopathy and decompensated heart failure, demonstrating that restrictive pathophysiology is not necessarily an indicator of restrictive cardiomyopathy.

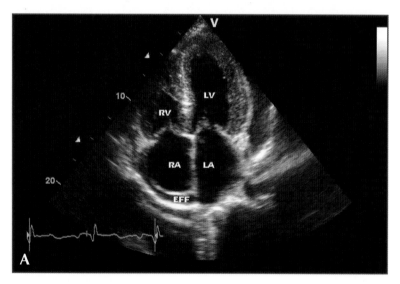

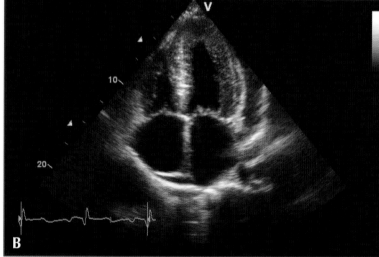

Figure 14-17. Apical four-chamber view in diastole (**A**) and systole (**B**) from a patient with light chain amyloidosis and rapidly progressive heart failure. The typical features of amyloid cardiomyopathy are seen. The LV walls are increased in thickness due to amyloid infiltration and the LV size is relatively small, giving a calculated LV end-diastolic volume of only 52 mL, an end-systolic volume of 26 mL, and a calculated LV ejection fraction (LVEF) of 50%, but a stroke volume of only 26 mL. The atria are dilated and differ minimally in size between systole and diastole, suggestive of atrial failure despite sinus rhythm. A small pericardial effusion (EFF) is present. LA—left atrium; RA—right atrium.

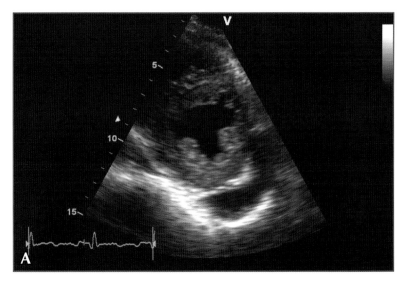
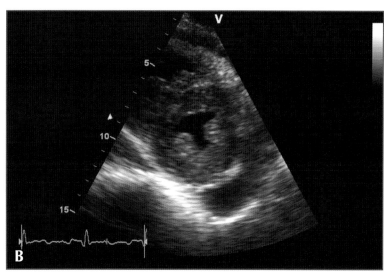

Figure 14-18. Same patient as in Figure 14-17. Parasternal short-axis views at the level of the papillary muscles in diastole (**A**) and systole (**B**), showing thick walls with a small cavity and a preserved LV ejection fraction. There is increased myocardial echogenicity; the papillary muscles are prominent due to infiltration, and a pericardial effusion is seen again.

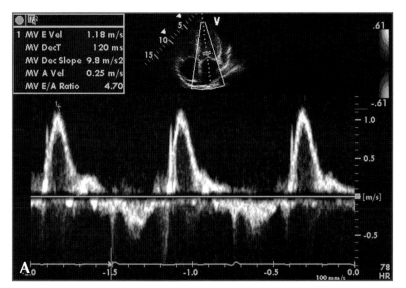
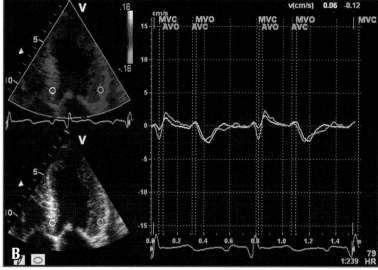

Figure 14-19. Same patient as in Figures 14-17 and 14-18, showing transmitral Doppler (**A**) with a deceleration time of the E wave of 120 ms, representing a restrictive filling pattern. The transmitral A wave is diminutive despite sinus rhythm, due to a combination of atrial failure and high LV filling pressure [31]. A tracing of tissue Doppler recorded from the basal septum and lateral wall in the apical four-chamber view is shown (**B**). In contrast to the relatively well preserved ejection fraction seen in Figures 14-17 and 14-18, there is severe impairment of longitudinal ventricular contraction, with a peak S' wave of less than 2.0 cm/s [32]. E' and A' are also markedly reduced, typical of restrictive pathophysiology. AVC—aortic valve closure; AVO—aortic valve opening; MV—mitral valve; MVC—mitral valve closure; MVO—mitral valve opening; Vel—velocity; DecT—deceleration time.

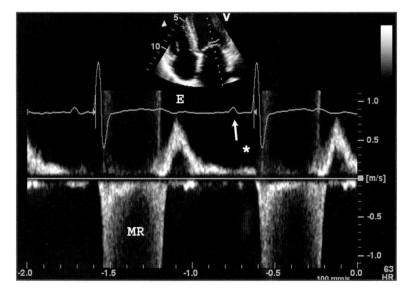

Figure 14-20. Transmitral Doppler from another patient with light chain amyloidosis showing a normal deceleration time of the mitral E wave, but with an absence of the A wave. The patient was in sinus rhythm (*arrow*), and the Doppler appearance is due to electromechanical dissociation of the atrium as a result of atrial amyloid infiltration. These patients are at high risk of atrial thrombus formation and thromboembolism [31,33]. Spectral Doppler of mitral regurgitation (MR) is also seen. Severe MR is rare and was only mild in this patient.

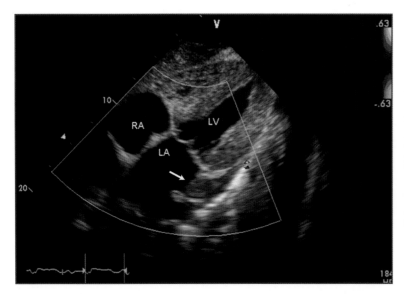

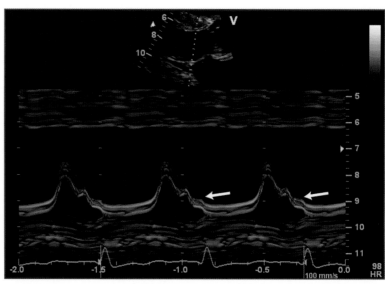

Figure 14-21. Subcostal four-chamber view in a patient with severe amyloid cardiomyopathy and sinus rhythm with absent A wave on transmitral and tissue Doppler. The left atrial appendage is well visualized and contains a round thrombus (*arrow*), which protrudes slightly into the cavity of the left atrium (LA). No atrial fibrillation had ever been documented in this patient. At autopsy, atrial thrombi are common in amyloid heart disease, even if no atrial arrhythmia had been present during life [33]. RA—right atrium.

Figure 14-22. M-mode of the mitral valve in a patient with severe amyloid cardiomyopathy. Note the AC notch (*arrows*) indicative of elevated LV end-diastolic pressure. The septum and posterior walls are thick and, despite a normal end-diastolic cavity size, there is an increased E-point septal separation consistent with low stroke volume and indicative that this echocardiographic sign is independent of LV dilation [19]. Compare this with Figure 14-9, which was recorded from a patient with dilated cardiomyopathy.

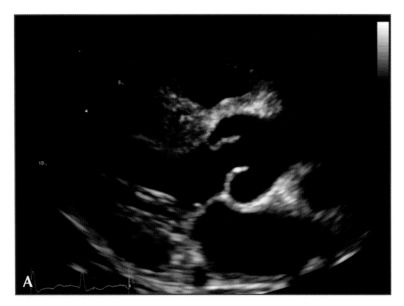

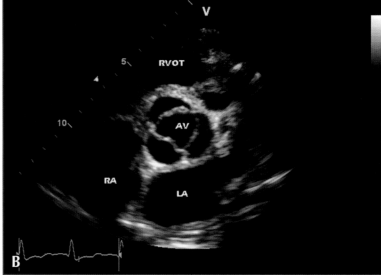

Figure 14-23. Maximum aortic valve opening in a patient with amyloid cardiomyopathy and low stroke volume. The aortic leaflets are infiltrated, but pliable. The reduced opening is a result of the low stroke volume and not a result of aortic stenosis. **A**, Parasternal long-axis view. **B**, Short-axis view.

There is a generalized increase in echogenicity, making it common to see three valves (aortic, pulmonary, and tricuspid) simultaneously in real time in the short-axis view at the level of the aortic valve (AV), an otherwise unusual finding. LA—left atrium; RA—right atrium; RVOT—RV outflow tract.

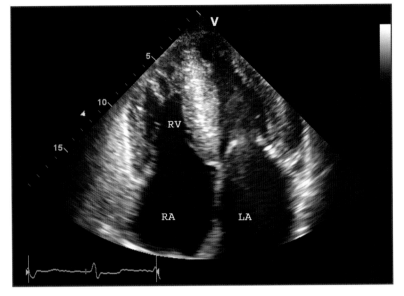

Figure 14-24. Four-chamber view of severe amyloid cardiomyopathy due to deposition of wild-type transthyretin (senile systemic amyloidosis), showing severe LV thickening with small cavity and marked biatrial enlargement. The image is obtained in mid-diastole and spontaneous echocardiographic contrast can be seen in the mid-left atrium (LA) through the mitral valve and into the LV (compare the "haziness" of the LA and LV cavity with that on the right side, where no spontaneous echo contrast was seen.) This is indicative of stasis of blood in both the LA and LV cavity. RA—right atrium.

References

1. Maron BJ, Towbin JA, Thiene G, *et al.*: Contemporary definitions and classification of the cardiomyopathies: an American Heart Association Scientific Statement from the Council on Clinical Cardiology, Heart Failure and Transplantation Committee; Quality of Care and Outcomes Research and Functional Genomics and Translational Biology Interdisciplinary Working Groups; and Council on Epidemiology and Prevention. *Circulation* 2006, 113:1807–1816.

2. Elliott P, Andersson B, Arbustini E, *et al.*: Classification of the cardiomyopathies: a position statement from the European Society of Cardiology working group on myocardial and pericardial diseases. *Eur Heart J* 2008, 29:270–276.

3. Franciosa JA, Park M, Levine TB: Lack of correlation between exercise capacity and indexes of resting left ventricular performance in heart failure. *Am J Cardiol* 1981, 47:33–39.

4. Parthenakis FI, Kanoupakis EM, Kochiadakis GE, *et al.*: Left ventricular diastolic filling pattern predicts cardiopulmonary determinants of functional capacity in patients with congestive heart failure. *Am Heart J* 2000, 140:338–344.

5. Kono T, Sabbah HN, Stein PD, *et al.*: Left ventricular shape as a determinant of functional mitral regurgitation in patients with severe heart failure secondary to either coronary artery disease or idiopathic dilated cardiomyopathy. *Am J Cardiol* 1991, 68:355–359.

6. Kono T, Sabbah HN, Rosman H, *et al.*: Left ventricular shape is the primary determinant of functional mitral regurgitation in heart failure. *J Am Coll Cardiol* 1992, 20:1594–1598.

7. Di Donato M, Dabic P, Castelvecchio S, *et al.*: Left ventricular geometry in normal and post-anterior myocardial infarction patients: sphericity index and 'new' conicity index comparisons. *Eur J Cardiothorac Surg* 2006, 29(Suppl 1):S225–S230.

8. Kono T, Sabbah HN, Rosman H, *et al.*: Mechanism of functional mitral regurgitation during acute myocardial ischemia. *J Am Coll Cardiol* 1992, 19:1101–1105.

9. Hung J, Papakostas L, Tahta SA, *et al.*: Mechanism of recurrent ischemic mitral regurgitation after annuloplasty: continued LV remodeling as a moving target. *Circulation* 2004, 110(11 Suppl 1):II85–II90.

10. Diaz-Infante E, Mont L, Leal J, *et al.*: Predictors of lack of response to resynchronization therapy. *Am J Cardiol* 2005, 95:1436–1440.

11. Toquero J, Geelen P, Goethals M, Brugada P: What is first, left bundle branch block or left ventricular dysfunction? *J Cardiovasc Electrophysiol* 2001, 12:1425–1428.

12. Teske AJ, De Boeck BW, Melman PG, *et al.*: Echocardiographic quantification of myocardial function using tissue deformation imaging, a guide to image acquisition and analysis using tissue Doppler and speckle tracking. *Cardiovasc Ultrasound* 2007, 5:27.

13. Sengupta PP, Krishnamoorthy VK, Korinek J, *et al.*: Left ventricular form and function revisited: applied translational science to cardiovascular ultrasound imaging. *J Am Soc Echocardiogr* 2007, 20:539–551.

14. Edvardsen T, Helle-Valle T, Smiseth OA: Systolic dysfunction in heart failure with normal ejection fraction: speckle-tracking echocardiography. *Prog Cardiovasc Dis* 2006, 49:207–214.

15. Ommen SR, Nishimura RA, Appleton CP, *et al.*: Clinical utility of Doppler echocardiography and tissue Doppler imaging in the estimation of left ventricular filling pressures: a comparative simultaneous Doppler-catheterization study. *Circulation* 2000, 102:1788–1794.

16. Konecke LL, Feigenbaum H, Chang S, *et al.*: Abnormal mitral valve motion in patients with elevated left ventricular diastolic pressures. *Circulation* 1973, 47:989–996.

17. Araujo AQ, Araujo AQ: Elucidating the B bump on the mitral valve M-mode echogram in patients with severe left ventricular systolic dysfunction. *Int J Cardiol* 2004, 95:7–12.

18. Silverstein JR, Laffely NH, Rifkin RD: Quantitative estimation of left ventricular ejection fraction from mitral valve E-point to septal separation and comparison to magnetic resonance imaging. *Am J Cardiol* 2006, 97:137–140.

19. Child JS, Krivokapich J, Perloff JK: Effect of left ventricular size on mitral E point to ventricular septal separation in assessment of cardiac performance. *Am Heart J* 1981, 101:797–805.

20. Devereux RB, Alonso DR, Lutas EM, *et al.*: Echocardiographic assessment of left ventricular hypertrophy: comparison to necropsy findings. *Am J Cardiol* 1986, 57:450–458.

21. Perk G, Tunick PA, Kronzon I: Systolic and diastolic pulsus alternans in severe heart failure. *J Am Soc Echocardiogr* 2007, 20:905.e5–905.e7.

22. Friedman B, Daily WM, Sheffield RS: Orthostatic factors in pulsus alternans. *Circulation* 1953, 8:864–873.

23. Bargiggia GS, Bertucci C, Recusani F, *et al.*: A new method for estimating left ventricular dP/dt by continuous wave Doppler-echocardiography. Validation studies at cardiac catheterization. *Circulation* 1989, 80:1287–1292.

24. Kolias TJ, Aaronson KD, Armstrong WF: Doppler-derived dP/dt and -dP/dt predict survival in congestive heart failure. *J Am Coll Cardiol* 2000, 36:1594–1599.

25. Stollberger C, Finsterer J: Left ventricular hypertrabeculation/noncompaction. *J Am Soc Echocardiogr* 2004, 17:91–100.

26. Kohli SK, Pantazis AA, Shah JS, *et al.*: Diagnosis of left-ventricular non-compaction in patients with left-ventricular systolic dysfunction: time for a reappraisal of diagnostic criteria? *Eur Heart J* 2008, 29:89–95.

27. Anderson RH: Ventricular non-compaction a frequently ignored finding? *Eur Heart J* 2008, 29:10–11.

28. Gianni M, Dentali F, Grandi AM, *et al.*: Apical ballooning syndrome or takotsubo cardiomyopathy: a systematic review. *Eur Heart J* 2006, 27:1523–1529.

29. Falk RH: Diagnosis and management of the cardiac amyloidoses. *Circulation* 2005, 112:2047–2060.

30. Klein AL, Hatle LK, Taliercio CP, *et al.*: Serial Doppler echocardiographic follow-up of left ventricular diastolic function in cardiac amyloidosis. *J Am Coll Cardiol* 1990, 16:1135–1141.

31. Dubrey S, Pollak A, Skinner M, Falk RH: Atrial thrombi occurring during sinus rhythm in cardiac amyloidosis: evidence for atrial electromechanical dissociation. *Br Heart J* 1995, 74:541–544.

32. Koyama J, Ray-Sequin PA, Falk RH: Longitudinal myocardial function assessed by tissue velocity, strain, and strain rate tissue Doppler echocardiography in patients with AL (primary) cardiac amyloidosis. *Circulation* 2003, 107:2446–2452.

33. Feng D, Edwards WD, Oh JK, *et al.*: Intracardiac thrombosis and embolism in patients with cardiac amyloidosis. *Circulation* 2007, 116:2420–2426.

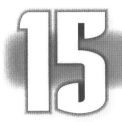

Pulmonary Embolism, Pulmonary Hypertension, and Diseases of the Right Ventricle

Judy R. Mangion and Scott D. Solomon

Echocardiography is being used more and more often in the setting of pulmonary embolism, pulmonary hypertension, and diseases of the RV. Although echocardiography is not recommended as a routine imaging test for diagnosis of pulmonary embolism, it is an outstanding tool in risk stratification and prognostication in patients with known pulmonary emboli; in the acute setting, it can serve an important role in identifying patients with RV systolic dysfunction who should be considered for thrombolysis or surgical embolectomy. With respect to isolated pulmonary hypertension, echocardiography provides an established noninvasive method for accurately quantifying pulmonary artery pressures and measuring the impact of pulmonary hypertension on RV systolic function. In many cases, echocardiography may be the first test to recognize the presence of pulmonary vascular disease, and the identification of pulmonary hypertension or RV dysfunction will often lead to further cardiopulmonary investigation.

Historically, the qualitative and quantitative assessment of diseases affecting the RV has lagged behind that of the LV; however, recent research has proven that diseases affecting the right side of the heart have the same clinical consequences and negative prognosis as similar diseases affecting the left side of the heart and therefore deserve equal attention.

This chapter will include examples of both transthoracic and transesophageal echocardiography in the setting of pulmonary embolism. Various echocardiographic features of cor pulmonale will also be presented. The need for quantitative assessment of regional RV systolic function, particularly in the setting of suspected RV myocardial infarction, will be emphasized, and tools for improving the visualization of the RV, including ultrasound contrast, will be demonstrated. The identification of volume and pressure overload of the RV with echocardiography will also be emphasized in various clinical scenarios. Finally, a classic case study of arrhythmogenic RV dysplasia will be presented.

Pulmonary Embolism

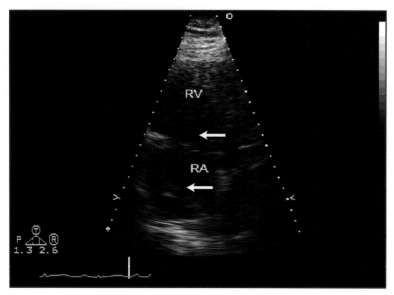

Figure 15-1. Pulmonary embolism, thrombus in transit. Apical four-chamber view, demonstrating large mobile thrombi (*arrows*) within a dilated and hypokinetic RA and RV, which is consistent with acute pulmonary emboli. The appearance of thrombus in transit has been described as similar to "sausage links." Because most pulmonary emboli originate from the deep veins in the legs, it is hypothesized that the valves within the deep veins create indentations in the thrombus, which contribute to the "sausage link" appearance.

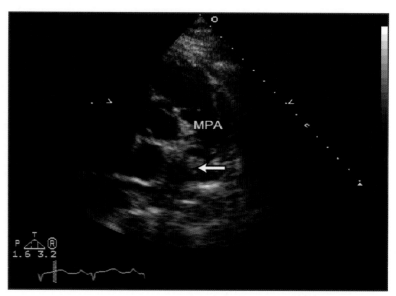

Figure 15-2. Pulmonary embolism, thrombus within the right pulmonary artery (*arrow*). Main pulmonary artery and bifurcation view. Although echocardiography is often used in the setting of pulmonary embolism, it is not recommended as a routine imaging test for the diagnosis of pulmonary embolism because most patients with pulmonary embolism will have a "normal" echo. In patients with known pulmonary emboli, or with strong clinical suspicion for pulmonary emboli, it is important to visualize the pulmonary artery and branches, as in this case example. MPA—main pulmonary artery.

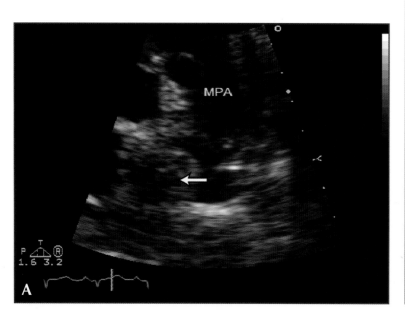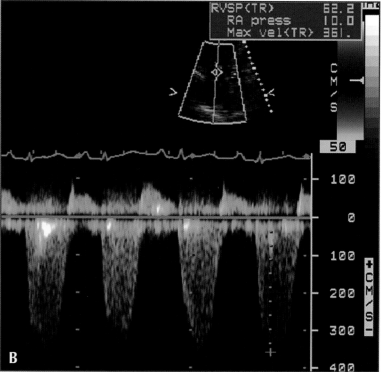

Figure 15-3. A, Pulmonary embolism, thrombus within the right pulmonary artery (*arrow*), magnified view. **B,** Continuous wave Doppler recording of the maximal velocity tricuspid regurgitant jet in a patient with acute pulmonary embolism, obtained from the apical four-chamber view. The simplified Bernoulli equation is used in order to calculate the peak pressure difference between the right atrium and RV (mm Hg pressure = $4V^2$, where V = the peak of tricuspid regurgitant jet in m/s) and the estimated right atrial pressure is added to estimate the pulmonary artery systolic pressure, which in this case is 62 mm Hg and is consistent with moderate pulmonary hypertension. Note that an acute massive pulmonary embolism can cause RV failure without causing substantial elevations in pulmonary artery pressure. When measuring pulmonary artery pressures noninvasively, it is important to ensure visualization of the complete tricuspid regurgitant envelope. Agitated saline or ultrasound contrast agents can be used to enhance the tricuspid regurgitant spectral Doppler tracing. MPA—main pulmonary artery.

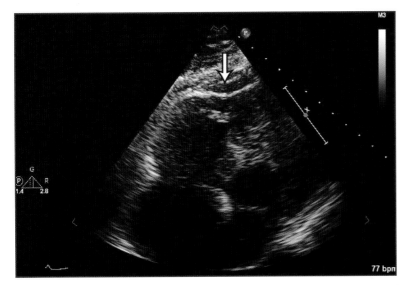

Figure 15-4. Apical four-chamber view, demonstrating RV dilatation, hypokinesis, as well as McConnell's sign (*arrow*), which are markers of acute pulmonary embolism. Echocardiography is an outstanding clinical tool in selecting patients with pulmonary embolism who may have a poor prognosis, with RV systolic dysfunction being the most powerful predictor of in-hospital death (six-fold increase). McConnell's sign refers to the presence of RV free wall segmental hypokinesis with sparing of the RV apex. This sign may be a helpful screening tool to distinguish acute pulmonary embolism from other etiologies of RV systolic dysfunction, and it has been estimated to have a sensitivity of 77%, specificity of 94%, and negative predictive value of 96%.

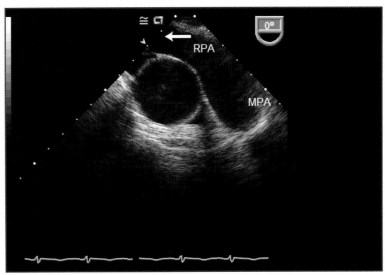

Figure 15-5. Pulmonary embolism, thrombus within the right pulmonary artery (RPA) (*arrow*) identified with transesophageal echocardiography. Main pulmonary artery (MPA) and bifurcation view. Direct visualization of pulmonary embolism may be achieved with transesophageal echocardiography if the embolus is large and centrally located.

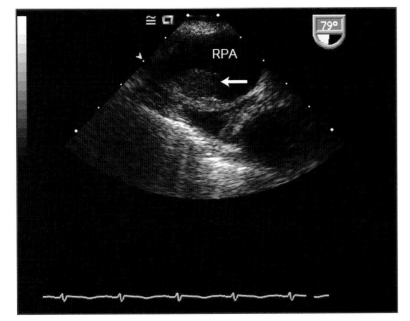

Figure 15-6. Pulmonary embolism, magnified transverse view of thrombus within the right pulmonary artery (RPA) (*arrow*), obtained with transesophageal echocardiography.

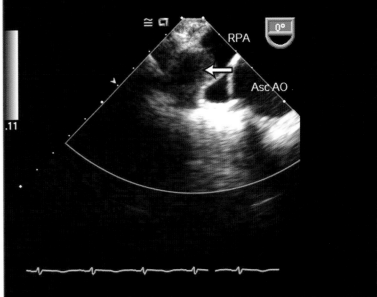

Figure 15-7. Pulmonary embolism, magnified view accentuated with tissue Doppler, demonstrating large thrombus within the right pulmonary artery (RPA) (*arrow*), visualized with transesophageal echo. AscAO—ascending aorta.

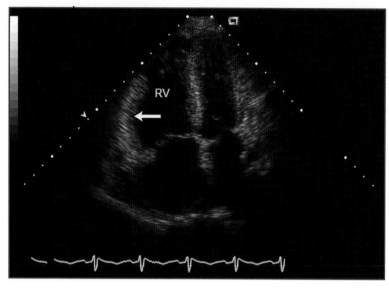

Figure 15-8. Severe pulmonary hypertension. Apical four-chamber view demonstrating severe RV dilatation with severe generalized RV systolic dysfunction. In addition, there is RV hypertrophy (*arrow*). RV hypertrophy is the response to RV pressure overload and it is defined echocardiographically as a free wall thickness of 6 mm or greater.

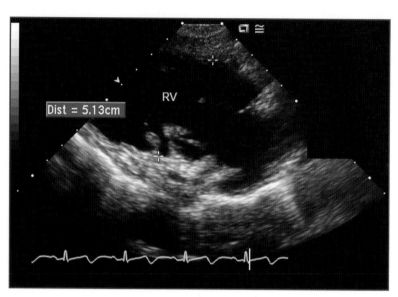

Figure 15-9. RV inflow view, demonstrating severe RV enlargement with severe generalized RV systolic dysfunction in a patient with severe pulmonary hypertension. This view is obtained from the parasternal long-transducer position with the transducer tilted downward. This should be a standard view for the assessment of RV size and systolic function.

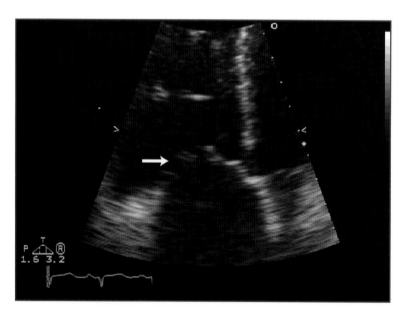

Figure 15-10. Apical four-chamber view of the RV and tricuspid valve, demonstrating apical displacement of the tricuspid valve closure pattern (*arrow*), which is often observed in the presence of RV dilatation and RV papillary muscle dysfunction. The tricuspid leaflets coapt in systole above the plane of the tricuspid annulus, so-called prayer pattern.

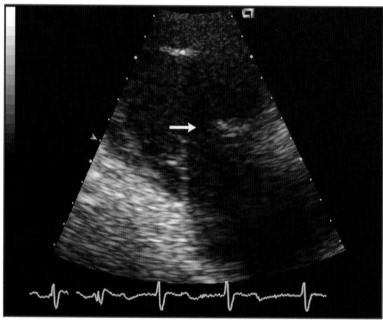

Figure 15-11. Apical four-chamber view of the RV and tricuspid valve in a patient with severe cor pulmonale. The RV and tricuspid valve annulus are markedly dilated and there is total lack of tricuspid leaflet coaptation in systole (*arrow*).

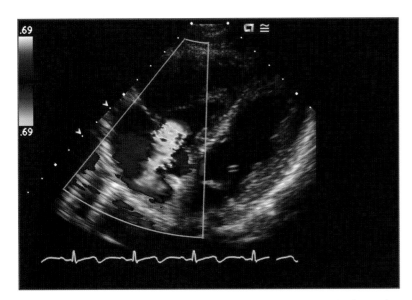

Figure 15-12. Apical four-chamber view of the RV and tricuspid valve with color Doppler in the same patient as Fig. 15-11, demonstrating resultant severe wide-open unrestricted tricuspid insufficiency. In this setting, the simplified Bernoulli equation often cannot accurately measure pulmonary artery systolic pressure because pressure in the right atrium is equivalent to pressure in the RV; therefore, there is no "pressure gradient."

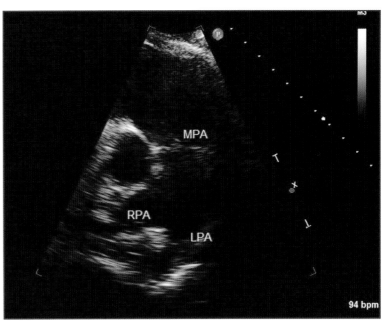

Figure 15-13. Main pulmonary artery (MPA) and bifurcation view, demonstrating severely dilated MPA and branches in a patient with severe pulmonary hypertension. LPA—left pulmonary artery; RPA—right pulmonary artery.

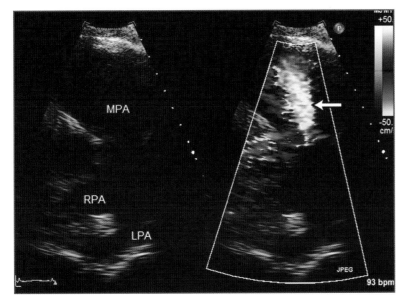

Figure 15-14. Main pulmonary artery (MPA) and bifurcation view with color Doppler interrogation of the pulmonic valve in the same patient as Fig. 15-13, demonstrating moderate pulmonic insufficiency (*arrow*). LPA—left pulmonary artery; RPA—right pulmonary artery.

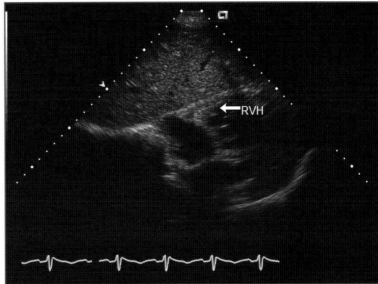

Figure 15-15. Subcostal four-chamber view in a patient with severe pulmonary hypertension demonstrating RV hypertrophy (RVH; *arrow*).

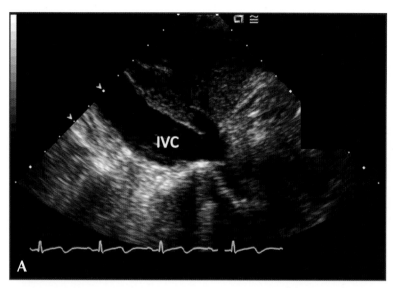

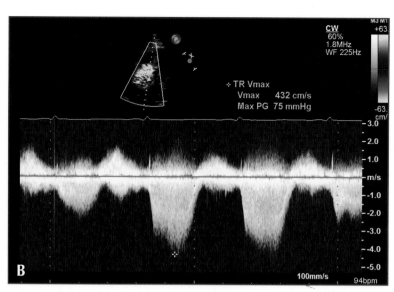

Figure 15-16. **A**, Subcostal view of the inferior vena cava (IVC) in a patient with severe cor pulmonale. The IVC is markedly dilated and plethoric and is indicative of an elevated right atrial pressure of at least 20 mm Hg. **B**, Continuous wave Doppler recording of the maximal velocity (V max) tricuspid regurgitant jet in a patient with severe pulmonary hypertension, obtained from the apical four-chamber view. The simplified Ber-noulli equation is used to calculate the peak pressure difference between the right atrium and the RV (mm Hg pressure = $4V^2$), and the estimated right atrial pressure is added in order to estimate the pulmonary artery systolic pressure, which in this case is estimated at (75 mm Hg + right atrial pressure) and is consistent with severe pulmonary hypertension.

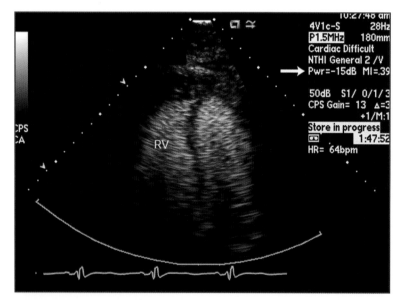

Figure 15-17. Apical four-chamber view of the RV, demonstrating enhanced opacification with an ultrasound contrast agent. Ultrasound contrast agents are an established tool for improving the assessment of regional wall motion. In using contrast for the RV, it is important to adjust machine settings to optimize the visualization of contrast. The power or mechanical index (MI) should always be low. In this example, the MI = 0.39 (*arrow*).

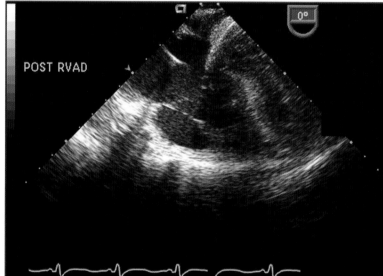

Figure 15-18. Midesophageal four-chamber view, transesophageal echocardiogram, in a patient who has had surgical removal of an RV assist device (RVAD). There is profound RV systolic dysfunction.

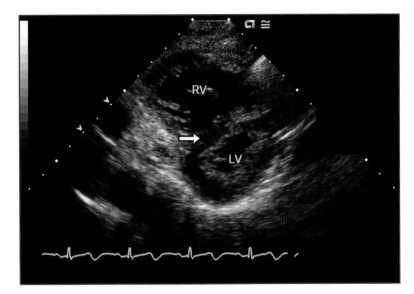

Figure 15-19. Parasternal short-axis view of the LV and RV, demonstrating flattening of the interventricular septum in systole (*arrow*), representing pressure overload of the RV, which is observed in severe pulmonary hypertension.

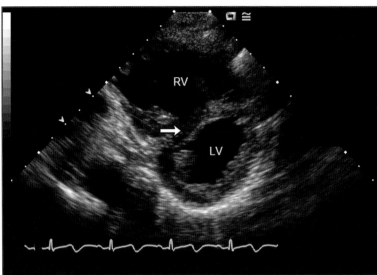

Figure 15-20. Parasternal short-axis view of the LV and RV, demonstrating flattening of the interventricular septum in diastole (*arrow*), representing volume overload of the RV, which in this patient was secondary to severe tricuspid insufficiency. Other causes of RV volume overload include anomalous pulmonary veins and intracardiac shunts.

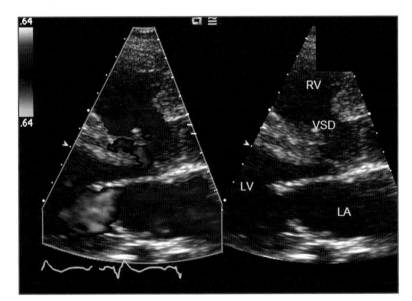

Figure 15-21. Parasternal long-axis view with color Doppler interrogation of the interventricular septum in a patient with congenital ventricular septal defect (VSD), patent ductus arteriosus, and resultant Eisenmenger's physiology. Congenital heart disease may cause secondary forms of pulmonary hypertension. When pulmonary vascular resistance exceeds systemic resistance, the left to right shunt is replaced by a right to left shunt (Eisenmenger's physiology) and the patient becomes cyanotic. LA—left atrium.

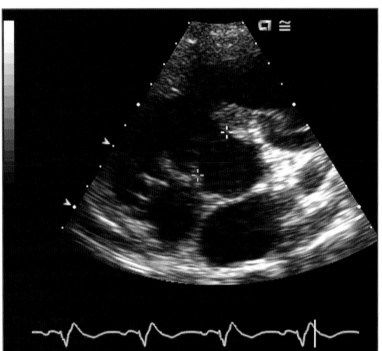

Figure 15-22. Parasternal short-axis view in the same patient as Figure 15-21 with large membranous ventricular septal defect (VSD), patent ductus arteriosus, and Eisenmenger's physiology. The VSD measures 2.2 cm.

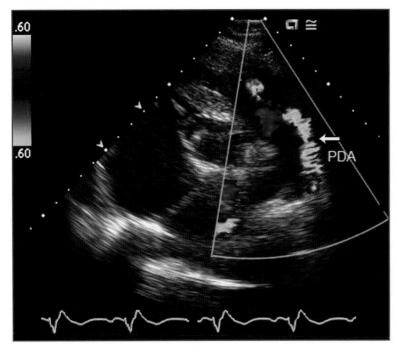

Figure 15-23. Parasternal short-axis view with color Doppler interrogation of the pulmonary artery branches in the same patient as in Figure 15-21, demonstrating the presence of a large patent ductus arteriosus (PDA) (*arrow*). The transmission of aortic pressure to the pulmonary tree over time results in severe pulmonary hypertension. When the pulmonary vascular resistance progresses to systemic levels, the left to right shunt will reverse (Eisenmenger's physiology).

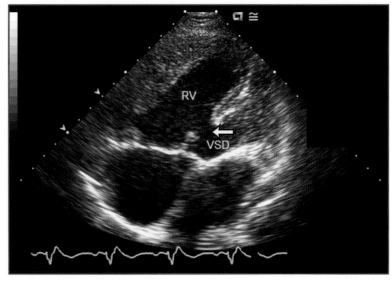

Figure 15-24. Apical four-chamber view in the same patient as in Figure 15-21 with ventricular septal defect (VSD), patent ductus arteriosus, and Eisenmenger's physiology. The large VSD is visualized well in this view (*arrow*). There is also marked RV hypertrophy.

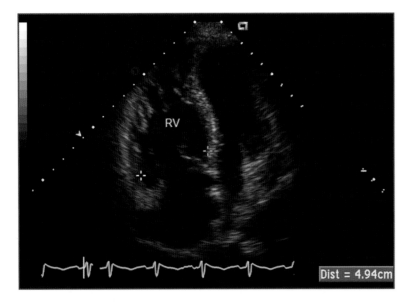

Dist = 4.94cm

Figure 15-25. Apical four-chamber view of the left and right heart demonstrating RV enlargement with preserved RV systolic function. The RV measures 4.9 cm. RV enlargement with normal systolic function should always prompt a careful assessment as to the etiology of RV volume overload. Common causes include atrial septal defects and anomalous pulmonary veins. Transesophageal echocardiography is recommended for further evaluation when the cause of RV volume overload is not obvious from transthoracic imaging.

Right Ventricular Infarction

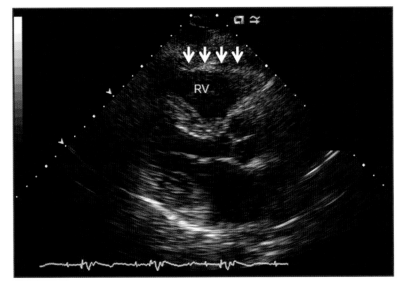

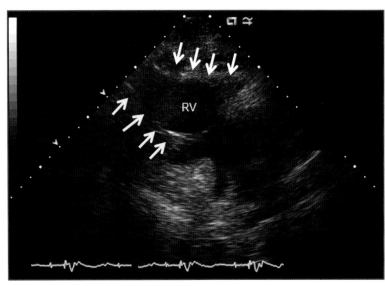

Figure 15-26. Parasternal long-axis view of the RV in a patient with suspected RV myocardial infarction. The echocardiographic assessment of RV systolic function, particularly in the setting of suspected RV infarction, requires visualization of the RV from multiple windows and a segmental approach to describing wall motion. In the parasternal long-axis view, the RV outflow tract is visualized (*arrows*) and contracts normally.

Figure 15-27. Parasternal RV inflow view in a patient with suspected RV myocardial infarction. In this view, the anterior wall (*white arrows*) and inferior wall (*yellow arrows*) of the RV are visualized. The inferior free wall of the RV is hypokinetic.

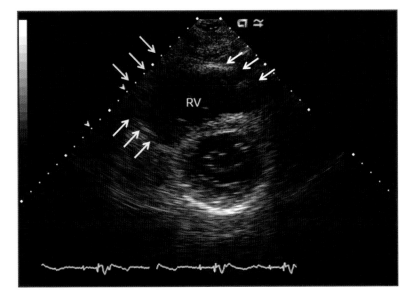

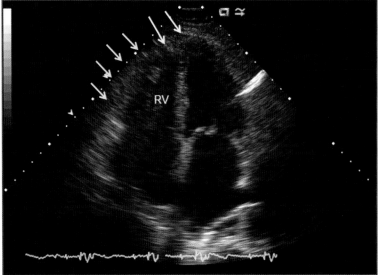

Figure 15-28. Parasternal short-axis view of the RV and LV in a patient with suspected RV myocardial infarction. The anterior wall (*white arrows*), lateral wall (*pink arrows*), and inferior wall (*yellow arrows*) of the RV are visualized. The lateral and inferior segments of the RV are hypokinetic.

Figure 15-29. Apical four-chamber view of the RV and LV in a patient with suspected RV myocardial infarction. The lateral free wall (*pink arrows*) and apex (*blue arrows*) of the RV are visualized. Both the lateral free wall and apex are hypokinetic.

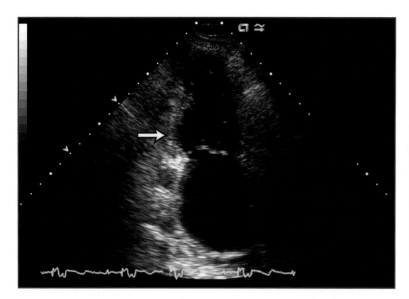

Figure 15-30. Apical two-chamber view of the LV in a patient with myocardial infarction with suspected RV involvement. The basal one half of the inferior wall of the LV is akinetic (*arrow*). This is consistent with right coronary artery infarction. The right coronary artery provides predominant flow to the RV, supplying the lateral wall through acute marginal branches. It also supplies the posterior wall and posterior interventricular septum through the posterior descending artery.

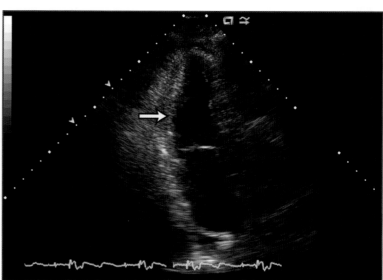

Figure 15-31. Apical three-chamber view of the LV in the same patient as Figure 15-23 with myocardial infarction and suspected RV involvement. The basal one half of the posterior wall of the LV is akinetic (*arrow*). This is also consistent with right coronary artery infarction.

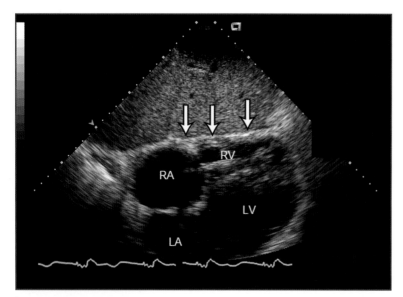

Figure 15-32. Subcostal four-chamber view of the RV in the same patient as Figure 15-23 with myocardial infarction and suspected RV involvement. The inferior surface of the RV is hypokinetic (*arrows*). LA—left atrium; RA—right atrium.

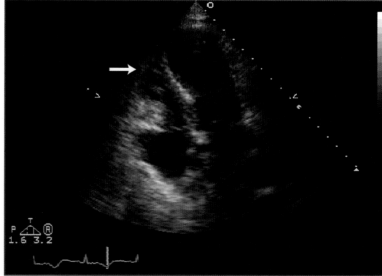

Figure 15-33. Apical four-chamber view of the RV, demonstrating severe RV apical hypokinesis (*arrow*). The etiology of the wall motion abnormality in this patient was believed to be either a left anterior descending coronary artery infarct or the Takotsubo syndrome, also known as stress-induced cardiomyopathy. The anterior wall and apex of the RV are supplied by the conus artery branch of the right coronary artery and by branches of the left anterior descending coronary artery.

Arrhythmogenic Right Ventricular Dysplasia

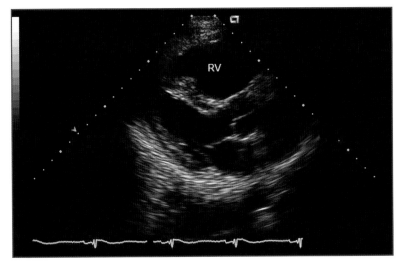

Figure 15-34. Parasternal long-axis view of the RV in a patient with ventricular tachycardia. The right RV is markedly dilated and severely hypokinetic. The myocardium appears thin, although focal RV aneurysm is not present. Findings are suggestive of arrhythmogenic RV dysplasia. In RV dysplasia, there is fatty tissue replacement of the myocardium. Echo criteria for the diagnosis include RV enlargement with diffuse or focal hypokinesis and thinning of the myocardium. Localized aneurysms are a hallmark, but are not always present. In some cases, the echo may be normal, and RV abnormalities may progress over time.

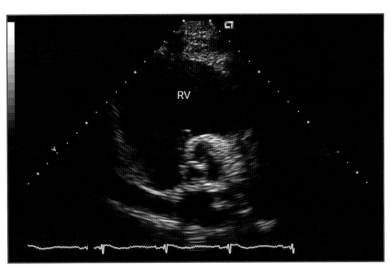

Figure 15-35. Parasternal short-axis view of the RV outflow tract in a patient with arrhythmogenic RV dysplasia. Again, the RV is dilated and hypokinetic. The myocardium appears thinned, although no focal RV aneurysm is identified. RV dysplasia is an important cause of sudden cardiac death, and it can be difficult to diagnose.

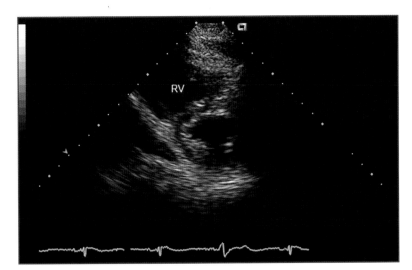

Figure 15-36. Parasternal short-axis view of the RV and LV in the same patient as Figure 15-34 and Figure 15-35. The RV is dilated and hypokinetic. There is thinning of the RV myocardium, suggestive of fatty infiltration; however, no discrete aneurysms are identified. LV systolic function is normal.

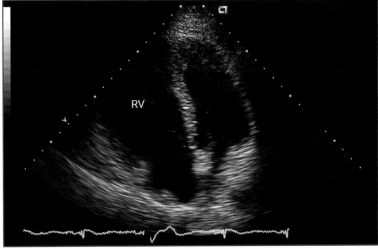

Figure 15-37. Apical four-chamber view of the RV and LV in the same patient as Figures 15-34, 15-35, and 15-36. Again, the RV is severely dilated and severely hypokinetic. The patient underwent electrophysiology testing and was noted to have inducible left bundle branch block morphology ventricular tachycardia, confirming arrhythmogenic RV dysplasia. An implantable cardiac defibrillator was placed.

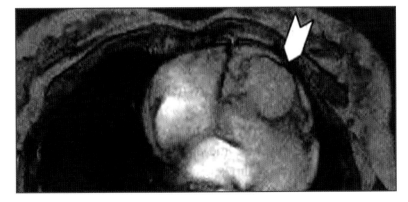

Figure 15-38. Cardiac MRI shows small focal aneurysm at the RV apex (*arrow*), consistent with arrhythmogenic RV dysplasia. Focal aneurysms of the RV in this disease are most commonly observed at the RV inflow, RV apex, and infundibulum or RV outflow area (triangle of dysplasia). The diagnosis should be considered in patients with ventricular tachycardia of left bundle branch morphology, T-wave inversions in leads V1–V3, late potentials on signal-average ECG, and family history of sudden cardiac death before age 35, or family history of arrhythmogenic RV dysplasia.

Suggested Reading

Burgess MI, Bright-Thomas RJ, Ray SG: Echocardiographic evaluation of right ventricular function. *Eur J Echocardiogr* 2002, 3:252–262.

de Groote P, Millaire A, Foucher-Hossein C, *et al.*: Right ventricular ejection fraction is an independent predictor of survival in patients with moderate heart failure. *J Am Coll Cardiol* 1998, 32:948–954.

Goldhaber SZ: Echocardiography in the management of pulmonary embolism. *Ann Intern Med* 2002, 136:691–700.

Kinch JW, Ryan TJ: Right ventricular infarction. *N Engl J Med* 1994, 330:1211–1217.

Solomon SD, ed: *Essential Echocardiography*. Totowa, NJ: Humana Press Inc; 2007.

Weyman A, ed: *Principles and Practice of Echocardiography*, edn 2. Philadelphia: Lea & Febiger; 1994.

Zornoff LA, Skali H, Pfeffer MA, *et al.*: Right ventricular dysfunction and risk of heart failure and mortality after myocardial infarction. *J Am Coll Cardiol* 2002, 39:1450–1455.

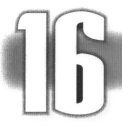

16

Pericardial Disease and Cardiac Masses

Gerard P. Aurigemma, Dennis A. Tighe,
Jae K. Oh, and Raul E. Espinoza

Echocardiography is the most important clinical tool in the diagnosis and management of the various pericardial diseases and cardiac masses that are initially diagnosed during routine echocardiography [1]. Distinguishing normal variants, benign degenerative changes, and even artifacts from cardiac tumors presents a challenge to even the most experienced echocardiographer. This chapter will review commonly encountered pericardial abnormalities and the most common cardiac tumors and will emphasize pathophysiologic principles when appropriate.

The pericardium consists of an outer sac (the fibrous pericardium) and an inner double-layered sac (the serous pericardium). The visceral layer of the serous pericardium, or epicardium, covers the heart and proximal great vessels. It is reflected to form the parietal pericardium, which lines the fibrous pericardium. Pericardial effusion, tamponade, pericardial cyst, and absent pericardium are readily recognized on two-dimensional echocardiography. The detection of pericardial effusion was greatly facilitated by echocardiography and was one of its initial clinical applications over 40 years ago [2]. Therapeutically, echocardiography also has a role in guiding safe pericardiocentesis [3,4]. Although constrictive pericarditis may escape diagnosis on clinical

grounds, or even with two-dimensional echocardiography alone, the characteristic respiratory variation in mitral inflow and hepatic vein Doppler velocities as well as tissue Doppler recording of mitral annulus velocity has added reliability and confidence to the noninvasive diagnosis of constrictive pericarditis [5,6] and enhanced our understanding of its pathophysiology. Although two-dimensional Doppler echocardiography (including tissue Doppler analysis [7]) can usually supply enough data to make the diagnosis of pericardial disease, transesophageal echocardiography (TEE) is a useful adjunct. TEE examinations supplement the findings of transthoracic echocardiography in providing measurements of pericardial thickness [8] and in detecting loculated pericardial effusion or other structural abnormalities of the pericardium; pulmonary vein Doppler recordings are also invaluable in the evaluation of diastolic function.

The various applications of echocardiography that are beneficial in the evaluation of pericardial diseases are illustrated in this chapter. In addition, we will review common cardiac mass lesions encountered in clinical practice. Primary cardiac tumors are rare; most (75%) are benign [9]. The most common cardiac tumors are myxomas, with the remaining divided among lipomas, papillary fibroelastomas, and rhabdomyomas.

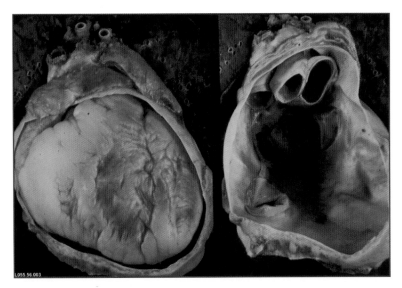

Figure 16-1. The pericardium provides mechanical protection for the heart as well as providing lubrication in order to reduce friction between the heart and surrounding structures. Note that the reflection of the pericardium in the cephalad portion of the heart means that the proximal portions of the great vessels are intrapericardial structures. This anatomic fact has clinical implications in a number of cardiac disorders, including acute proximal aortic dissection, which is a presenting sign of hemopericardium. The pericardium also has a significant hemodynamic impact on the atria and ventricles. The nondistensible pericardium limits acute distention of the heart. Ventricular volume is greater at any given ventricular filling pressure, with the pericardium removed as opposed to being intact (pericardial restraint). The pericardium also contributes to diastolic coupling between two ventricles—the distention of one ventricle alters the filling of the other, which is an effect that is important in the pathophysiology of cardiac tamponade and constrictive pericarditis. Ventricular interdependence becomes more marked at high ventricular filling pressures and greater ventricular volumes. Abnormalities of the pericardium can range from the pleuritic chest pain of pericarditis to marked heart failure and even death from tamponade or constriction. (*Courtesy of* William D. Edwards, MD.)

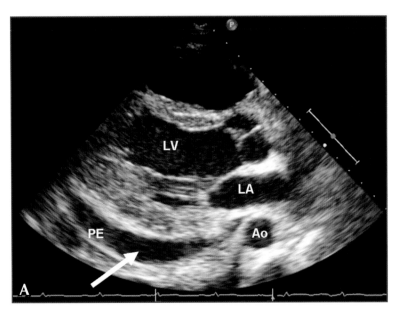

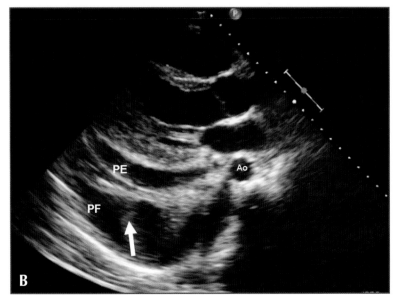

Figure 16-2. A parasternal long-axis view from the study of a patient with a pericardial effusion (PE) (**A**) located posterior to the LV is shown. Note that the pericardial fluid tracks between the left atrium (LA) and the descending thoracic aorta (Ao) (*arrow*). The same study is also shown at greater imaging depth (**B**). This image shows pleural fluid (PF) and lung parenchyma (**B**, *arrow*). It can be challenging to distinguish a pericardial from a pleural fluid collection. However, some clues that serve as indications include 1) pleural fluid, which is located predominantly posterior to the heart, rather than surrounding the heart, circumferentially; 2) pleural fluid, which will not track between the Ao and the LA, as is shown (**A**) for the pericardial effusion; 3) the presence of lung parenchyma, or atelectatic lung, will not be seen within a pericardial effusion.

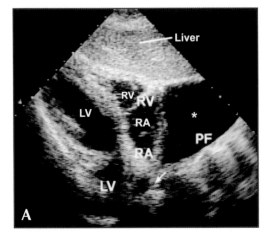

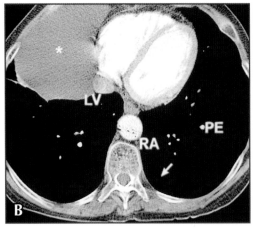

Figure 16-3. A pericardial cyst (*asterisk*) is shown as demonstrated by two-dimensional echocardiography and MRI. A pericardial cyst is a benign structural abnormality of the pericardium that is usually found incidentally on chest radiography in an asymptomatic person. Most frequently, it is located at the right costophrenic angle, but it can also be found at the left costophrenic angle, hilum, or superior mediastinum.

The differential diagnosis of the chest radiograph finding includes malignant tumor, cardiac chamber enlargement, and diaphragmatic hernia. A pericardial cyst appears as a cystic structure attached to the heart on cardiac imaging. Two-dimensional echocardiography (**A**), CT, or MRI (**B**) may be used to differentiate a pericardial cyst from a solid tumor. The subcostal view shows an echo-free space (**A**, *asterisk*) next to the right atrial (RA) wall, which is the most common location for pericardial cyst. A CT scan of the chest shows a large pericardial cyst (**B**, *asterisk*) from the same patient. The subcostal view is usually the most helpful in detecting a pericardial cyst (**A**). Contrast or color flow imaging shows no blood flow in the cystic structure (*asterisk*). Usually no treatment is necessary in asymptomatic patients. PE—pericardial effusion; PF—pleural fluid; RA—right atrium.

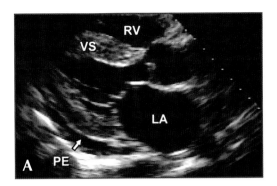

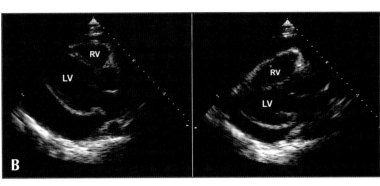

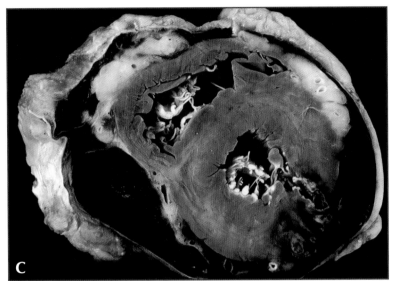

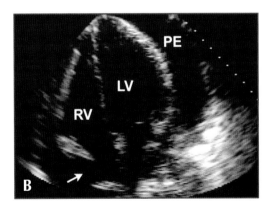

Figure 16-4. When the pericardial space contains fluid or unclotted blood, it is detected as an echo-free area (**A**). A smaller pericardial effusion (PE) may be detected as a loculated echo-free space that is visualized only during systole. When the amount of effusion is greater than 25 mL, an echo-free space persists throughout the cardiac cycle. As a PE increases in size, movement of the parietal pericardium decreases [10]. When the PE is massive, the heart may exhibit a swinging motion within the pericardial cavity (**B**), which is responsible for "electrical alternans." Conversely, cardiac tamponade can also occur with a small PE if it develops rapidly (*eg*, myocardial perforation after acute myocardial infarction or during pacemaker implantation) [11]. This image demonstrates a pathologic specimen with hemopericardium caused by myocardial perforation after a lateral wall myocardial infarction (**C**). In this situation, echocardiography may demonstrate clotted blood in the pericardium. A subcostal image of the clot (**D**, *short arrow*) and PE in a patient who had myocardial rupture soon after acute myocardial infarction is shown. LA—left atrium; VS—ventricular septum. (*Panel C courtesy of* William D. Edwards, MD.)

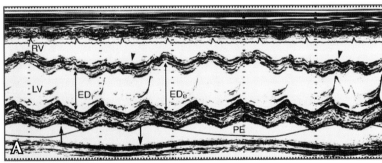

Figure 16-5. M-mode and two-dimensional echocardiographic signs of cardiac tamponade are shown. Early diastolic collapse of the RV, late diastolic right atrial (RA) inversion, abnormal ventricular septal motion, respiratory variation in ventricle chamber size, and plethora of the inferior vena cava with blunted respiratory changes are shown (**A**) [12,13]. In health, intrapericardial pressure is equal to intrathoracic pressure and is transmitted uniformly through the intrapericardial space. However, as pericardial fluid accumulates, changes in intrathoracic pressure become disassociated from intrapericardial pressure. With inspiration, pulmonary venous pressure falls more than LV diastolic pressure, giving a reduced transmitral pressure gradient. Concurrently, the constraining pericardial effusion prevents the RV from expanding in order to accommodate systemic venous return (*ie*, increased ventricular interdependence). As a result, the ventricular septum (VS) shifts leftward during inspiration. With expiration, the process reverses and the septum moves rightward. Increasing intrapericardial pressure also leads to diastolic compression of the RV and RA, as well as high systemic venous pressure, manifested as plethora of the inferior vena cava. The characteristic M-mode echocardiogram of cardiac tamponade is shown (**A**) [14,15]. Abnormal ventricular septal motion (**A**, *arrowheads*) is related to respiratory variation in ventricular filling and increased ventricular interdependence. LV end-diastolic dimension (EDi) decreases with inspiration (**A**, *upward arrow*) and increases with expiration (EDe) (**A**, *downward arrow*). A still frame image of an apical four-chamber view demonstrates late diastolic inversion of the RA (**B**, *arrow*).

Continued on the next page

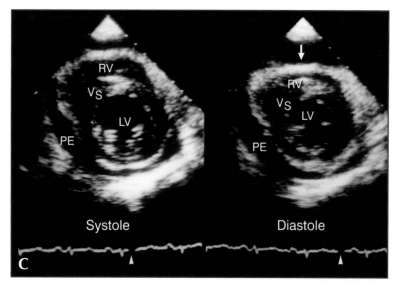

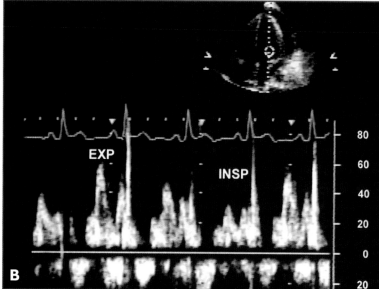

Figure 16-5. *(Continued)* However, RA diastolic inversion is not specific for tamponade, and it can be seen in patients without hemodynamic compromise. As the size of the pericardial effusion (PE) increases and hemodynamic compromise occurs, the duration of RA inversion also increases. Early diastolic collapse (**C**, *arrows*) of the RV is specific for tamponade. In early diastole, when RV pressure is lowest, intrapericardial pressure is higher than RV pressure, which causes early diastolic collapse or inversion of the RV. This finding is responsible for the blunted "y" descent on the jugular vein in cardiac tamponade.

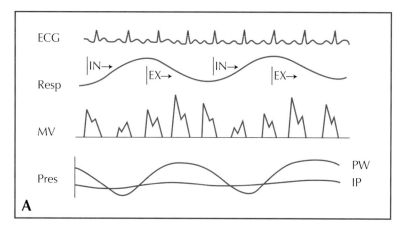

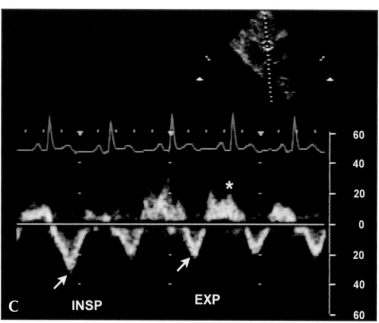

intrapericardial pressure falls substantially less than intrathoracic pressure. Therefore, the LV filling pressure gradient (from pulmonary wedge pressure to LV diastolic pressure) decreases with INSP. With the associated decreased transmitral pressure gradient, the mitral valve (MV) opening is delayed, which lengthens the isovolumic relaxation time (IVRT) and decreases mitral E velocity with INSP. In cardiac tamponade, the degree of ventricular filling depends on the other ventricle because of the relatively fixed cardiac volume (increased ventricular interdependence); thus, reciprocal changes occur in the right-sided heart chambers. With expiration (EXP), the transmitral pressure gradient increases and systemic venous return decreases. The IVRT shortens, mitral E velocity increases, and reversal of diastolic flow becomes more pronounced in the hepatic veins.

A schematic diagram of simultaneous ECG, respirometer (Resp), MV Doppler, and pressure (Pres) changes in intrapericardial (IP) and pulmonary capillary wedge (PW) is shown (**A**). IP pressure does not change much with respiration, whereas PW pressure decreases with INSP, which results in respiratory variation in LV filling and MV inflow Doppler velocity recording. Doppler mitral inflow velocities with respiratory variation are shown (**B**). Mitral E velocity is higher with EXP than with INSP. Pulsed-wave Doppler recording of the hepatic vein velocities is shown (**C**, *arrows*). Diastolic flow reversal increases (*asterisk*) with EXP.

Figure 16-6. Characteristic Doppler recordings from a patient with cardiac tamponade are shown. The Doppler features of pericardial tamponade are more sensitive than the two-dimensional echocardiographic findings. Normally, intrapericardial pressure (*ie*, left atrium [LA] and LV diastolic pressures) and intrathoracic pressure (*ie*, pulmonary capillary wedge pressure) fall to the same degree during inspiration (INSP); in cardiac tamponade, however,

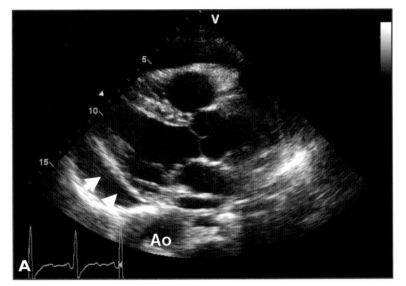

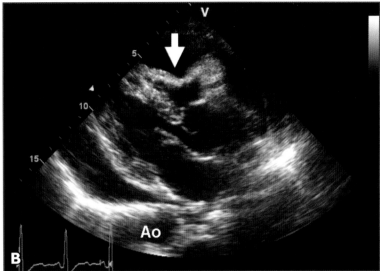

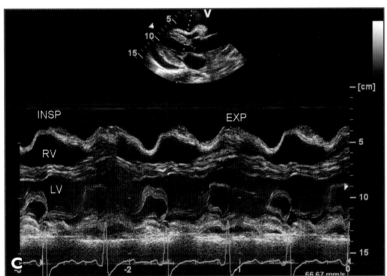

Figure 16-7. Two-dimensional and M-mode evidence of cardiac tamponade in a patient with metastatic lung cancer is shown. Other malignant tumors associated with pericardial effusion (PE) include lymphoma and breast cancer. Parasternal long-axis images (**A** and **B**) are shown, taken in isovolumic systole and mid diastole, respectively. There is a circumferential PE, which tracks between the left atrium (LA) and aorta (Ao) (**A**, *arrows*). In mid diastole, prior to atrial contraction, there is collapse of the RV free wall (**B**, *arrow*). This occurs because at this phase of the cardiac cycle, intrapericardial pressure exceeds RV diastolic pressure. An M-mode taken from the same study is also shown (**C**). This demonstrates the same features as the still frame two-dimensional images (**A** and **B**). In addition, this panel demonstrates respirophasic changes in the RV and LV chambers. Note that there are reciprocal changes in RV and LV dimensions, consistent with ventricular interaction; RV size is larger in inspiratory beats and smaller in expiratory beats, the converse is found for the LV. EXP—expiration; INSP—inspiration.

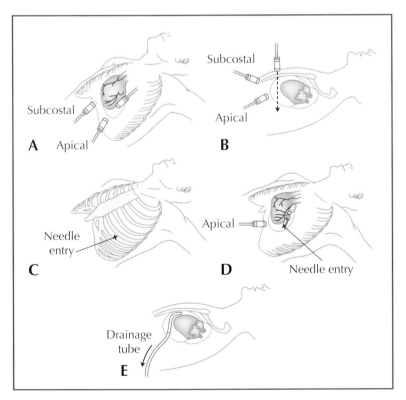

Figure 16-8. Schematics of two-dimensional echocardiography-guided peri-cardiocentesis are shown. The most effective treatment for cardiac tampon-ade is the removal of the pericardial fluid. Although pericardiocentesis is life saving, a blind percutaneous attempt has a high rate of complications, includ-ing pneumothorax, puncturing of the cardiac wall, or death. Two-dimensional echocardiography can guide pericardiocentesis by locating the optimal site of puncture (**A**, **B**, and **C**), determining the depth of the pericardial effusion (and the distance from the puncture site to the effusion), and by monitor-ing the results of the pericardiocentesis (**D** and **E**), usually from the subcostal view. At the Mayo Clinic, most pericardiocentesis procedures are performed by an echocardiographer with the guidance of two-dimensional echocar-diography [3,4]. The most common location of needle entry is para-apical (67%), followed by subcostal (19%). Unusual locations, such as left axillary or right parasternal area, are occasionally used depending on two-dimensional echocardiographic findings [4].

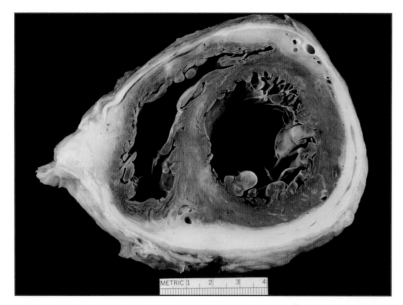

Figure 16-9. A pathology specimen of typical constrictive pericarditis is shown. Constrictive pericarditis is not a rare condition, but it can escape clinical detection if it is not being considered. The figure shows a thickened and fibrotic pericardium, which limits diastolic filling and can lead to heart failure despite normal or even supranormal ejection fraction (EF). Because constrictive pericarditis is potentially curable, it should be considered in patients with heart failure and normal EF, especially when there is a predisposing factor, such as pericarditis, prior cardiac surgery, or thoracic radiation. In fact, recent series of etiologies of constrictive pericarditis have shown that the leading causes were postsurgical (29%), idiopathic (26%), pericarditis (16%), and radiation (11%) [16,17]. In the authors' opinions, constrictive pericarditis should always be considered in patients with signs and symptoms of chronic liver disease, especially when ascites and peripheral edema coexist with elevated jugular venous pressure.

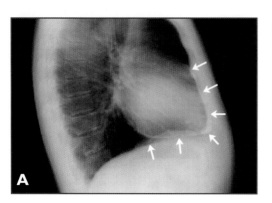
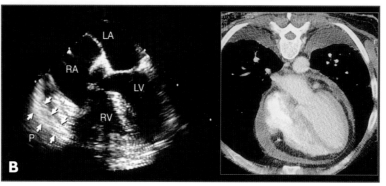

Figure 16-10. Typical chest radiograph, transesophageal echocardiography (TEE) (**A**), and CT/MRI findings (**B**) of constrictive pericarditis are shown. Pericardial calcification (**A**, *arrows*) on chest radiograph is helpful, but it is present in only 25% of cases [17]. It is best seen from the lateral view, where it is located in contiguity with the RV and across the diaphragmatic surface of the heart. Pericardial calcification reflects constrictive pericarditis of long duration and is associated with a higher surgical mortality. A thick pericardium is a usual finding in this condition, but pericardial thickness may be normal on imaging in up to 20% of cases. Thickness of the pericardium is often difficult to determine by transthoracic echocardiography, but TEE is usually reliable in measuring the pericardial thickness (**B**, *arrows*). Pericardial thickness measured by TEE has correlated well with measurements by CT [9]. Talreja *et al.* [18] observed that 18% of patients with surgically proven constriction had normal pericardial thickness on direct measurement of surgical specimens.

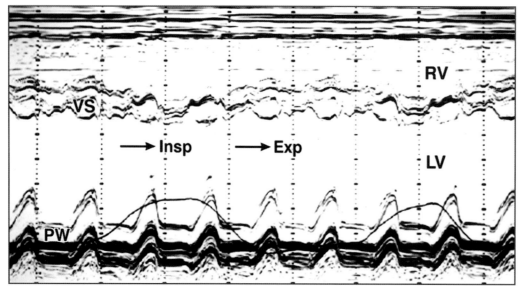

Figure 16-11. M-mode echocardiographic features of constrictive pericarditis include thickened pericardium, abnormal ventricular septal (VS) motion, flattening of the LV posterior wall (PW) during diastole, and respiratory variation in ventricular size. Explanations for these characteristic findings are related to dissociation between intrathoracic and intracardiac pressure, as well as exaggerated ventricular interdependence in diastolic filling. Restrictive cardiomyopathy, a condition in which the hemodynamic profile may be confused with constrictive pericarditis, does not feature extensive respiratory-related changes in ventricular filling [19–27].

A thickened or inflamed pericardium prevents full transmission of the intrathoracic pressure changes that occur with respiration to the pericardial and intracardiac cavities, creating respiratory variation in the left-sided filling pressure gradient (*ie*, the pressure difference between the pulmonary vein and the left atrium). With inspiration (Insp), intrathoracic pressure falls (3–5 mm Hg normally) and the pressure in other intrathoracic structures (pulmonary vein, pulmonary capillaries) falls to a similar degree. This inspiratory pressure change is not fully transmitted to the intrapericardial and intracardiac cavities. As a result, the driving pressure gradient for LV filling decreases immediately after Insp (Insp) and increases with expiration (Exp). This characteristic hemodynamic pattern is best illustrated by simultaneous pressure recordings from the LV and the pulmonary capillary wedge together with mitral inflow velocities (*see* Fig. 16-12). (*From* Oh *et al.* [10]; with permission.)

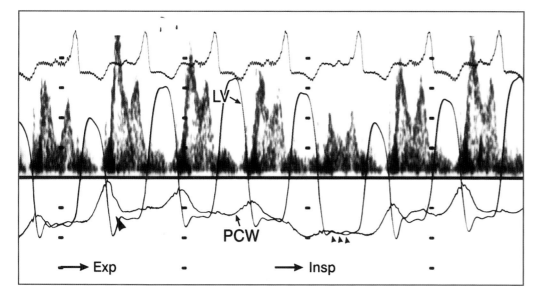

Figure 16-12. Simultaneous pressure recordings are shown from the LV and pulmonary capillary wedge (PCW) together with mitral inflow velocity on a Doppler echocardiogram. The onset of the respiratory phase is indicated. With the onset of expiration (Exp), PCW pressure increases much more than LV diastolic pressure, creating a large driving pressure gradient (*large arrowhead*). With inspiration (Insp), however, PCW decreases much more than LV diastolic pressure, with a very small driving pressure gradient (*three small arrowheads*). These respiratory changes in the LV filling gradient are well reflected by the changes in the mitral inflow velocities recorded on Doppler echocardiography. (*From* Oh *et al.* [10]; with permission.)

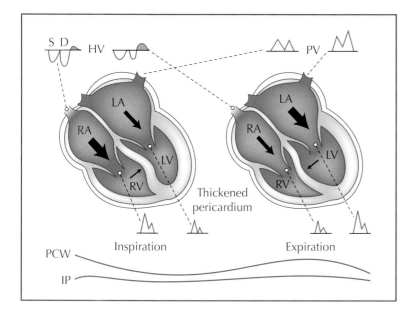

Figure 16-13. Schematic diagram of differential ventricular filling varying with respiration is shown. Pulmonary capillary wedge (PCW) pressure changes with respiration, whereas intrapericardial (IP) or LV diastolic pressure changes minimally with respiration. Diastolic filling (or distensibility) of the LV and RV rely on each other because the overall cardiac volume is relatively fixed within the thickened or noncompliant pericardium. Hence, reciprocal respiratory changes occur in the filling of the LV and RV. With inspiration, decreased LV filling allows increased filling in the RV. As a result, the ventricular septum shifts to the left, and tricuspid inflow E velocity and hepatic vein diastolic forward flow velocity increase. With expiration, LV filling increases, causing the ventricular septum to shift to the right, which limits RV filling. Tricuspid inflow decreases and hepatic vein diastolic forward flow decreases, with significant flow reversals during diastole. Diastolic forward flow velocity is usually higher than systolic forward flow velocity in the hepatic vein, which corresponds to the Y and X waves of systemic venous pressure, respectively. HV—hepatic vein; LA—left atrium; PV—pulmonary vein; RA—right atrium. (*Adapted from* Oh *et al.* [10].)

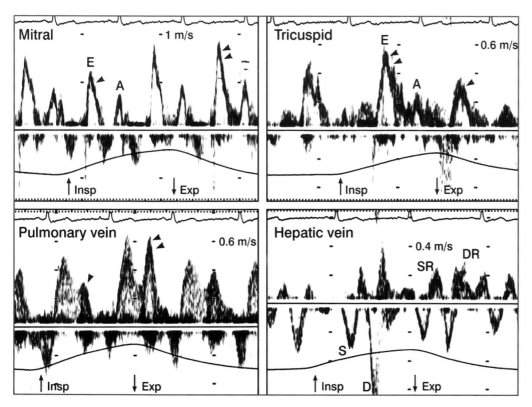

Figure 16-14. Typical respiratory variations of mitral, tricuspid, pulmonary vein, and hepatic vein Doppler velocity flow in constrictive pericarditis. Note the reciprocal relationship between peak transmitral and peak transtricuspid velocities. Exp—expiration; Insp—inspiration; DR—diastolic reversal; SR—systolic reversal. (*From* Oh *et al.* [10]; with permission.)

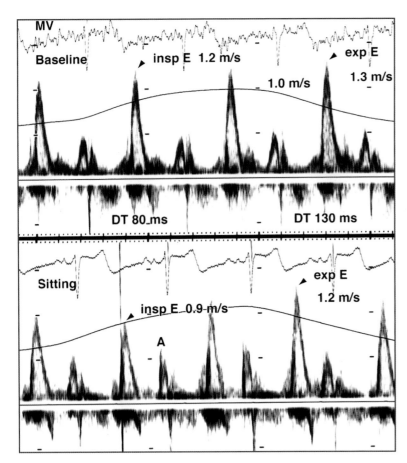

Figure 16-15. Atypical Doppler findings in constrictive pericarditis are shown. Optimally, a respiratory variation of 25% or greater in the mitral inflow E velocity and increased diastolic flow reversal with expiration (exp) in the hepatic veins should be demonstrated in order to establish the diagnosis of constrictive pericarditis [7]. Up to 30% of patients with constrictive pericarditis demonstrate less than 25% respiratory variation in mitral E velocity, however, because of mixed constriction and restriction, or marked increase of atrial pressures. If an attempt is made to decrease preloads (sitting position), a repeat mitral Doppler examination may unmask the expected respiratory variation [21]. Therefore, the lack of respiratory variation in mitral inflow does not necessarily exclude the diagnosis of constrictive pericarditis, especially when mitral inflow velocities demonstrate high filling pressure with restrictive features. A repeat examination of mitral inflow Doppler and hepatic vein Doppler should be performed in the sitting position to unmask the respiratory variation in mitral inflow velocities. DT—deceleration time; insp—inspiration; MV—mitral valve.

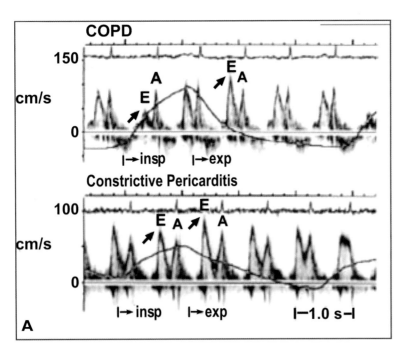

Figure 16-16. Transmitral (**A**) and superior vena cava (SVC) (**B**) spectral profiles in chronic obstructive pulmonary disease (COPD) (*upper*) and constrictive pericarditis (*lower*) are shown. It is important to recognize that acute RV dilatation from pulmonary embolism or RV infarction, pleural effusion, and COPD can also produce respirophasic changes in transmitral velocities. Once clinical and two-dimensional echocardiographic features are taken into account, however, most of these conditions do not present a significant diagnostic problem in the interpretation of the Doppler data. Patients with COPD, however, may have signs and symptoms of right-sided heart failure similar to those of constrictive pericarditis.

Several features of the Doppler echocardiographic examination can be used to distinguish COPD from constrictive pericarditis. For one, in COPD, transmitral velocities are not usually "restrictive" because the LV filling pressure is not increased (**B**, *upper figure*). Secondly, in COPD, the highest mitral

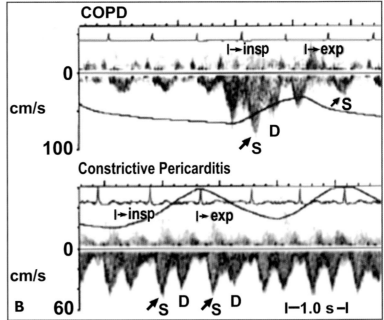

E velocity occurs toward the end of expiration (exp), but in constrictive pericarditis, it occurs immediately after the onset of exp. This difference may not be helpful, however, when the patient is tachypneic, or if gating problems exist between the respirometer and the real time Doppler recording. Third, the Doppler finding that most reliably distinguishes between these two entities is flow velocity in the SVC. In chronic obstructive lung disease, SVC flow is markedly increased with inspiration (insp) because the underlying mechanism for respiratory variation in COPD is an exaggerated decrease in intrathoracic pressure with insp. This greater negative pressure enhances blood flow to the right atrium from the SVC. In constrictive pericarditis, by contrast, SVC systolic flow velocities do not change significantly with respiration, with a difference in systolic forward flow velocity between insp and exp usually less than 20 cm per second. These differences are illustrated (**B**). (*From Boonyaratavej et al.* [28]; with permission.)

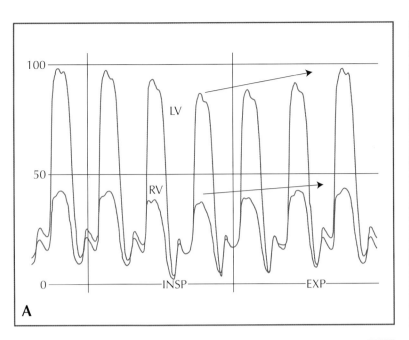

A

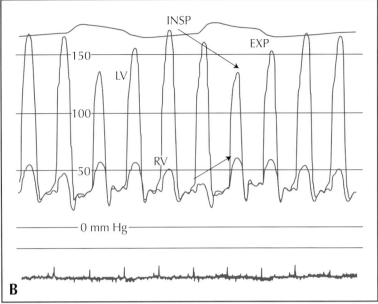

B

ℂ Diagnostic Criteria For Constrictive Pericarditis Using Noninvasive Doppler Hemodynamics or Invasive Cardiac Catheterization

Criterion	Constriction	Restriction
LVEDP-RVEDP, *mm Hg*	5 or less	> 5
RVSP, *mm HG*	< 50	> 50
RVEDP/RVSP	0.33 or greater	< 0.3

Figure 16-17. Invasive hemodynamic diagnostic criteria for distinguishing constrictive pericarditis from restrictive cardiomyopathy (RCM) are shown (**A** and **B**) and summarized (**C**). Despite the significant difference in the pathophysiologic mechanisms, there is significant overlap in hemodynamic parameters between these two entities. Increased atrial pressures, equalization of end-diastolic pressures (EDP), and dip-and-plateau or "square root"

sign of the ventricular diastolic pressure recording have traditionally been considered hemodynamic features typical of constrictive pericarditis. Almost identical hemodynamic pressure tracings can be obtained in patients with RCM. Therefore, in addition to these hemodynamic features, respiratory variation in ventricular filling and increased ventricular interdependence should be demonstrated in order to diagnose constrictive pericarditis, whether invasively or noninvasively [20,29]. The dissociation between intrathoracic and intracardiac pressure changes with inspiration (INSP) is seen in simultaneous recordings of LV and pulmonary capillary wedge pressures (*see* Fig. 16-12). Ventricular interdependence is also observed in simultaneous recordings of LV and RV pressures. **A**, With INSP, which induces less filling of the LV, LV peak systolic pressure decreases; the opposite changes occur in the RV so that RV peak systolic pressure (SP) increases with INSP. **B**, Ejection time also varies with respiration in opposite directions in LV and RV. This discordant pressure change between the LV and RV in constrictive pericarditis does not occur in RCM, in which changes in LV and RV systolic pressures with respiration are concordant. EXP—expiration.

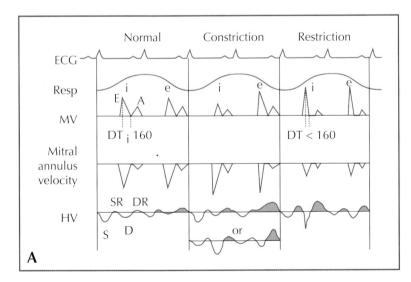

A

Figure 16-18. A, Summary of Doppler findings in constrictive pericarditis and restrictive cardiomyopathy. In restrictive cardiomyopathy, the mitral inflow velocity rarely shows respiratory variation (unless the patient also has chronic obstructive lung disease), although the velocity profile appears similar to that of constrictive pericarditis, with increased E velocity, an E/A ratio usually greater than 2.0, and a short deceleration time (DT) usually less than 160 ms. Hepatic vein systolic flow reversals are more prominent with inspiration in restrictive cardiomyopathy, although it is not unusual to see significant diastolic flow reversals in the hepatic vein during inspiration and expiration in patients with advanced constrictive pericarditis (the two possible patterns are shown) or with combined constrictive pericarditis and restrictive cardiomyopathy. Therefore, invasively or noninvasively, the differentiation between these two entities is based on the respiratory patterns of ventricular filling. Septal mitral annular velocity by tissue Doppler imaging is of enormous help in making this distinction; mitral annular velocity is markedly decreased in restrictive cardiomyopathy because myocardial relaxation is reduced in myocardial diseases, whereas it is well preserved or even augmented in constrictive pericarditis because the longitudinal motion of the heart is the main mechanism of its diastolic filling. HV—hepatic vein; DR—diastolic reversal; MV—mitral valve; SR—systolic reversal.

Continued on the next page

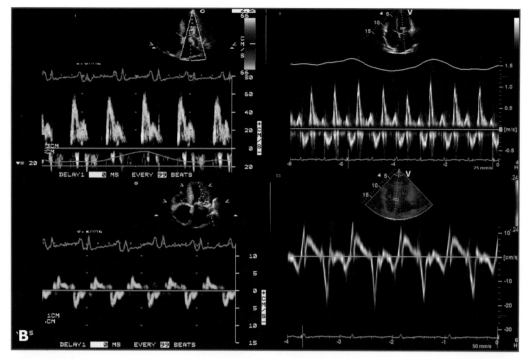

Figure 16-18. (Continued) **B**, Clinical examples are given to reinforce the principles outlined in the schematic diagram (**A**). In restrictive cardiomyopathy (biopsy-proven amyloidosis) (*left panel*) and in surgically confirmed constrictive pericarditis (*right panel*), the transmitral flow patterns look similar; E/A ratio is elevated, and the deceleration time is short. However, in contrast to constrictive pericarditis, in restrictive cardiomyopathy, there is minimal respirophasic variation in transmitral E wave. The other crucial distinguishing feature is the tissue Doppler spectra. In restrictive cardiomyopathy, the peak tissue Doppler E wave is low (> 5 cm/s). By contrast, in constrictive pericarditis, because of the critical role played by longitudinal lengthening in generating LV filling, the tissue Doppler E velocity is orders of magnitude higher.

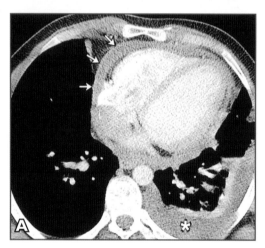

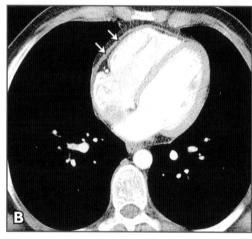

Figure 16-19. Transient (or effuso-constrictive) pericarditis showing resolution of thick pericardium over a 1-week period with steroid treatment. Approximately 7% to 10% of patients with acute pericarditis have a transient constrictive phase. These patients usually have a moderate pericardial effusion, and, as the pericardial effusion disappears, the pericardium remains inflamed, thickened, and noncompliant, resulting in constrictive hemodynamics. The patient presents with dyspnea, peripheral edema, increased jugular venous pressure, and, sometimes, ascites, as in patients with chronic constrictive pericarditis. This transient constrictive phase may last 2 to 3 months before it gradually resolves spontaneously or with treatment with anti-inflammatory agents. When hemodynamics and findings typical of constriction develop in patients with acute pericarditis, initial treatment is indomethacin for 2 to 3 weeks, and if there is no response, steroids may be administered for 1 to 2 months (60 mg daily × 1 week, then tapered over 6 to 8 weeks) after being certain that pericarditis is not caused by bacterial infection, including tuberculosis. Constrictive hemodynamics can be diagnosed readily with Doppler echocardiography (**A**); resolution of constrictive physiology can be documented clinically and by follow-up echocardiography (**B**) [30–32]. Effuso-constrictive pericarditis [30–32] may be a form of transient constrictive pericarditis that may resolve without pericardiectomy.

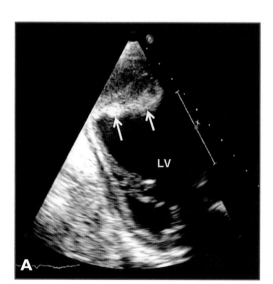

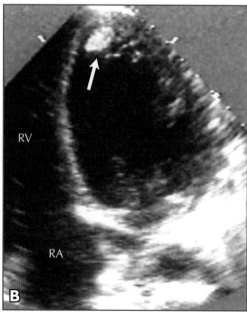

Figure 16-20. Left ventricular apical thrombus is shown. An apical two-chamber image shows a large layered LV apical thrombus (**A**, *arrows*) occupying the distal one-third of the LV. A more discrete LV apical thrombus is also shown (**B**, *arrow*). As compared with the previous findings (**A**), this thrombus protrudes into the cavity and exhibits greater echodensity. The latter finding is suggestive of greater duration. A thrombus that protrudes into the cavity or is mobile represents a relatively high-risk situation for peripheral embolization. Laminated (layered) thrombus is much less likely to result in peripheral embolization. Factors that predispose to LV thrombus development include a recent myocardial infarction (especially a large infarction involving the apex), LV aneurysm, and a dilated cardiomyopathy. Although the examples shown (**A** and **B**) are difficult to miss, small thrombi can be easily missed. RA—right atrium.

Continued on the next page

Figure 16-20. *(Continued)* Use of a high-frequency transducer with coned-down apical views, the apical short-axis view, or other off-axis/tangential views may be required to image these thrombi. The use of echocardiographic contrast agents may improve detection of thrombi in cases where the image quality is poor. The differential diagnosis of LV apical thrombus includes apical hypertrophic cardiomyopathy, prominent trabeculations and/or false tendons, LV noncompaction, endocardial fibroelastosis, and the hypereosinophilic syndrome.

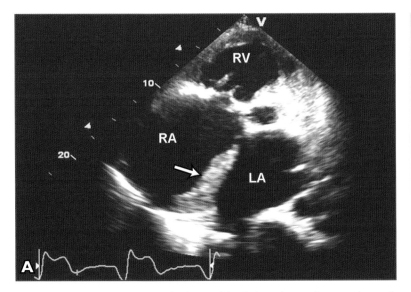

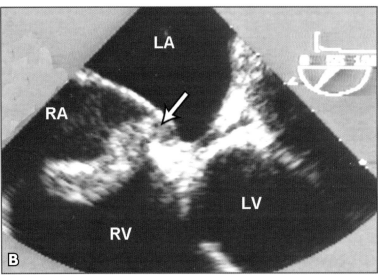

Figure 16-21. Two examples of right atrial (RA) thrombi are shown. A layered thrombus (**A**, *arrow*) along the RA aspect of the interatrial septum is observed in this off-axis apical view. Both the left atrium (LA) and the RA are dilated, and a prosthetic tricuspid valve is in place. The genesis of the thrombus was most likely related to stagnant RA blood flow in this patient with rheumatic heart disease, atrial fibrillation, and a subtherapuetic international normalized ratio. A thrombus in transit is also seen within the RA (**B**). The thrombus is seen passing through a patent foramen ovale (**B**, *arrow*). This patient suffered both a pulmonary embolism and an embolism to the left arm. Note that the RA and the RV are dilated, and the interatrial septum bows from right to left in this TEE view, suggesting that elevated right-sided heart pressures were present. Although thrombus within the right atrial appendage can be observed among patients with atrial fibrillation, its incidence is much less common when compared with the occurrence of thrombus within the left atrial appendage.

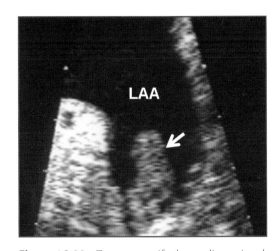

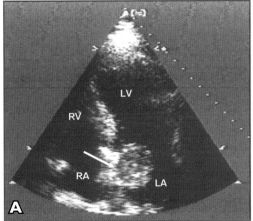

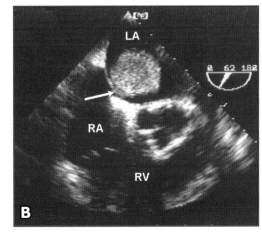

Figure 16-22. Zoom-magnified two-dimensional transesophageal echocardiographic (TEE) view shows a thrombus within the body of the left atrial appendage [LAA] (*arrow*). Thrombus within the LAA can be found in conditions characterized by stagnant blood flow. The clinical conditions most commonly associated include atrial fibrillation, atrial flutter, and mitral stenosis. Spontaneous echo contrast material ("smoke") may also be observed. Thrombus within the LAA should not be confused with the presence of pectinate muscles, which are normal anatomic structures seen in the LAA. Pectinate muscles are most reliably observed in the vertical TEE views as multiple, linear, erect structures. The LAA has more than one lobe in 80% of individuals; thus, careful scanning in multiple planes is required to exclude the presence of an LAA thrombus.

Figure 16-23. A mass protruding into the left atrial (LA) cavity with attachment in the region of the fossa ovalis (**A**, *arrow*) is shown. The mass was somewhat mobile on real time imaging, but did not obstruct mitral inflow. The transesophageal echocardiogram of the same patient is also shown (**B**). The region of the fossa ovalis (*arrow*) where the mass is demonstrated to have a broad-based attachment is shown. Histologic evaluation confirmed this mass to be a myxoma. Primary cardiac tumors are rare (autopsy incidence 0.017%–0.33%). Among the primary cardiac tumors, myxoma is the most common type. Cardiac myxomas most commonly occur within the LA, originating near the region of the fossa ovalis, although they may originate from any endocardial surface and from the cardiac valves. Presentation can include manifestations of constitutional symptoms, peripheral embolic phenomena, or they can be secondary to an obstruction of mitral inflow. In the present era, many cases are diagnosed with routine echocardiography performed for other indications. Although thrombus is always a diagnostic concern, the echocardiographic appearance of the mass in this case is typical for that of an LA myxoma. The treatment of choice is surgical excision. Follow-up echocardiography should be obtained annually for several years following removal of the mass to evaluate for potential recurrence. RA—right atrium.

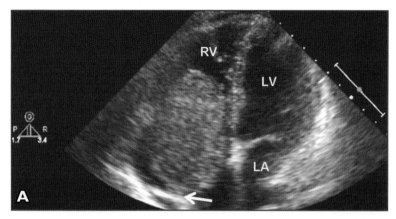

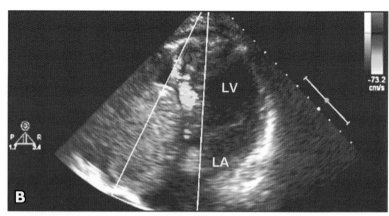

Figure 16-24. A large mass (**A**, *arrow*) that attaches to the superior wall of the right atrium (RA) and extends into the RV is shown. The mass was mobile on real time imaging. Color flow Doppler demonstrates that diastolic inflow into the RV has a turbulent pattern as it processes around the large mass (**B**). On physical examination, the patient had an early diastolic sound, consistent with a "tumor plop," as well as a holosystolic murmur consistent with tricuspid regurgitation. A large myxoma was found and removed in surgery. The RA is the second most common location for occurrence of a cardiac myxoma. LA—left atrium.

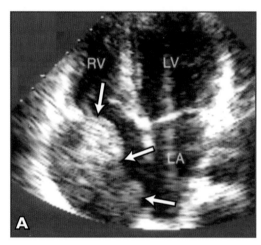

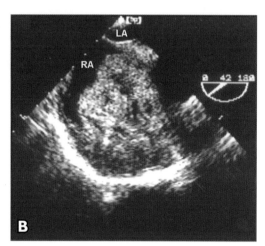

Figure 16-25. An image from the apical four-chamber plane demonstrates a large inhomogeneous mass (**A**, *arrows*) occupying the majority of the right atrial (RA) cavity. A diffuse attachment to the lateral atrial wall is present. Compared with the right atrial myxoma shown (*see* Fig. 16-24), this mass was not mobile. The transesophageal echocardiogram of the same patient is also shown (**B**). A large inhomogeneous mass occupies the majority of the RA cavity and is broadly attached to the free wall. A pericardial effusion was not observed. Histology showed this mass to be a hemangiosarcoma.

Primary cardiac tumors are significantly less common than are tumors that have metastasized to the heart (secondary tumors) [9]. Among the primary cardiac tumors, the incidence of malignant tumors is much less compared with benign tumors. The most common primary malignant cardiac tumors are the sarcomas, such as hemangiosarcoma, fibrosarcoma, and rhabdomyosarcoma. At the time of diagnosis, the sarcomas tend to be large and often have metastasized distantly. Other malignant primary cardiac tumors include mesothelioma, cardiac lymphoma, and malignant teratoma. LA—left atrium.

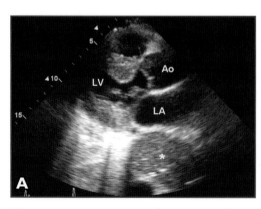

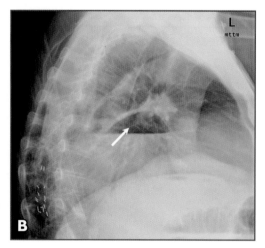

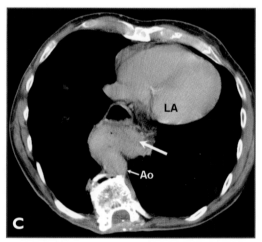

Figure 16-26. An image in the parasternal long-axis view shows an apparent mass lesion (**A**, *asterisk*) located posterior to the left atrium (LA). The lateral chest x-ray of the same patient is also shown (**B**). An air fluid level within the chest (**B**, *arrow*) is observed, suggesting the presence of a hiatal hernia. A noncontrast enhanced CT scan of the same patient shows a large hiatal hernia (**C**, *large arrow*) adjacent to the LA and descending thoracic aorta (Ao). With transthoracic echocardiography, the administration of a carbonated beverage can produce a contrast effect within the hiatal hernia, and it can be used as a diagnostic maneuver to demonstrate its true nature as a "pseudomass."

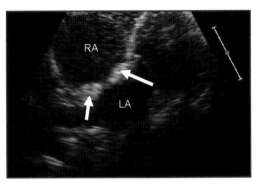
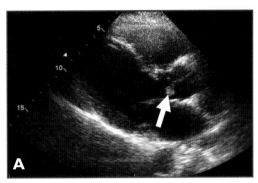
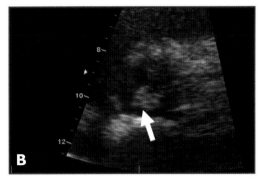

Figure 16-27. Lipomatous hypertrophy of the interatrial septum, depicted from a subcostal view. Fatty infiltration of the interatrial septum results in a marked thickening and increased echogenicity of the inferior and superior portions of the septum. A characteristic sparing of the region of the fossa ovalis ("dumb-bell appearance") is observed (*arrows*). This condition is more commonly found among elderly women and has been associated with an increased incidence of atrial arrhythmia by some investigators. Most investigators, however, believe that this condition is benign, and it is not associated with any significant clinical manifestations. LA—left atrium; RA—right atrium.

Figure 16-28. Parasternal long- (**A**) and short-axis (**B**) images taken from the study of a 67-year-old man found to have a papillary fibroelastoma on echocardiography. These images (*arrows*) demonstrate that this tumor is found on the noncoronary cusp of the aortic valve, as is shown (**B**). The echocardiographic appearance is typically a round echogenic mass, which may be sessile or minimally mobile. Papillary fibroelastomas may or may not be pedunculated, are generally found on left-sided cardiac valves, and are more commonly on the aortic valve than the mitral valve. However, these tumors may be found anywhere in the heart [33]. As is the case here, a papillary fibroelastoma is found incidentally. When encountered in the course of an evaluation for a cardiac source of cerebral embolism, surgical excision is considered, especially if the fibroelastoma exceeds 1 cm in diameter.

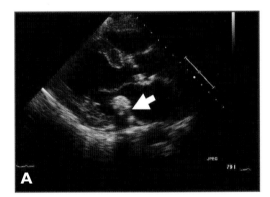
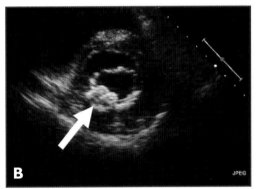
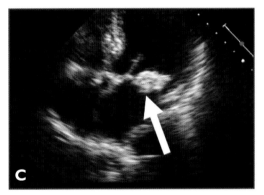

Figure 16-29. Parasternal long-axis (**A**), short-axis (**B**), and apical four-chamber views (**C**) taken from the study of an 86-year-old woman are shown. These images show the typical appearance of caseous calcification of the mitral annulus. (*arrows*) This entity is typically rounded, echodense, and immobile, and it is usually located primarily on the posterior aspect of the mitral annulus. There may be areas of central lucency. Pathologically, caseous calcification is a solid mass, containing toothpaste-like white material, hence the sobriquet "toothpaste tumor." The central areas of lucency represent liquefaction necrosis. The true prevalence of this entity is unknown, although Harpaz *et al.* [34] estimate that it is found in 0.63% of autopsies of patients with mitral annular calcification. There do not appear to be specific symptoms associated with caseous calcification of the mitral annulus, nor is therapy required. However, it is important to recognize it so that it is not confused with a cardiac tumor or an abscess complicating infective endocarditis.

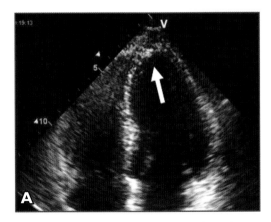
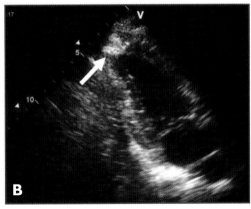
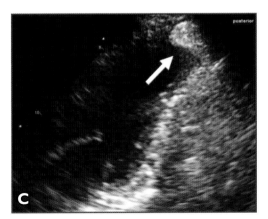

Figure 16-30. These images are taken from the two-dimensional echocardiography and MRI study of an asymptomatic 44-year-old man. Apical views demonstrate a round echo-dense mass located at the apex (*arrows*). This mass was relatively difficult to discern on the apical four-chamber view (**A**), and it was better seen on the apical two-chamber view in the extreme inferior portion of the apex (**B**). An additional off-axis view (**C**) was necessary for optimal visualization. Cardiac MRI was also performed, and showed a solitary, well-defined, spherical mass arising from the endocardial surface of the apex (*arrow*).

Continued on the next page

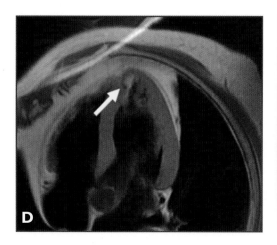

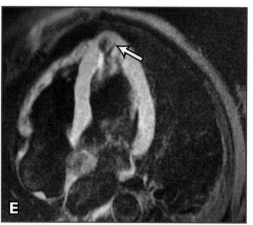

Figure 16-30. (*Continued*) On T1-weighted fast spin-echo MRI, the mass was hyperintense (**D**). On T1-weighted fast spin-echo with fat suppression sequence, the mass appeared hypointense (**E**, *arrow*), suggestive of lipoma. Cardiac lipomas account for 10% of all cardiac tumors. They are well encapsulated and are generally composed of mature fat cells. Solitary cardiac lipomas are much less frequently encountered than lipomatous hypertrophy of the interatrial septum, and can be found anywhere in the heart. As is the case here, cardiac lipomas are generally incidental findings and in most cases require no treatment or surgical intervention [35].

References

1. Little WC, Freeman GL: Pericardial disease. *Circulation* 2006, 113:1622–1632.

2. Feigenbaum H, Waldhausen JA, Hyde LP: Ultrasound diagnosis of pericardial effusion. *JAMA* 1965, 191:711–714.

3. Callahan JA, Seward JB, Tajik AJ: Cardiac tamponade: pericardiocentesis directed by two-dimensional echocardiography. *Mayo Clin Proc* 1985, 60:344–347.

4. Tsang TS, Enriquez-Sarano M, Freeman WK, *et al.*: Consecutive 1127 therapeutic echocardiographically guided pericardiocenteses: clinical profile, practice patterns, and outcomes spanning 21 years. *Mayo Clin Proc* 2002, 77:429–436.

5. Hatle LK, Appleton CP, Popp RL: Differentiation of constrictive pericarditis and restrictive cardiomyopathy by Doppler echocardiography. *Circulation* 1989, 79:357–370.

6. Oh JK, Hatle LK, Seward JB, *et al.*: Diagnostic role of Doppler echocardiography in constrictive pericarditis. *J Am Coll Cardiol* 1994, 23:154–162.

7. Garcia MJ, Rodriguez L, Ares M, *et al.*: Differentiation of constrictive pericarditis from restrictive cardiomyopathy: assessment of left ventricular diastolic velocities in longitudinal axis by Doppler tissue imaging. *J Am Coll Cardiol* 1996, 27:108–114.

8. Ling LH, Oh JK, Tei C, *et al.*: Pericardial thickness measured with transesophageal echocardiography: feasibility and potential clinical usefulness. *J Am Coll Cardiol* 1997, 29:1317–1323.

9. Burke A, Virmani R: Tumors of the heart and great vessels. In: *Atlas of Tumor Pathology*, 3rd series. Edited by Rosai J and Sobin LH. Washington, DC: Armed Forces Institute of Pathology; 1996:80–86.

10. Oh JK, Seward JB, Tajik AJ: *The Echo Manual*, edn 2. Baltimore: Lippincott Williams & Wilkins; 1999.

11. Spodick DH: Acute cardiac tamponade. *N Engl J Med* 2003, 349:684–690.

12. Gillam LD, Guyer DE, Gibson TC, *et al.*: Hydrodynamic compression of the right atrium: a new echocardiographic sign of cardiac tamponade. *Circulation* 1983, 68:294–301.

13. Armstrong WF, Schilt BF, Helper DJ, *et al.*: Diastolic collapse of the right ventricle with cardiac tamponade: an echocardiographic study. *Circulation* 1982, 65:1491–1496.

14. Burstow DJ, Oh JK, Bailey KR, *et al.*: Cardiac tamponade: characteristic Doppler observations. *Mayo Clin Proc* 1989, 64:312–324.

15. Appleton CP, Hatle LK, Popp RL: Cardiac tamponade and pericardial effusion: respiratory variation in transvalvular flow velocities studied by Doppler echocardiography. *J Am Coll Cardiol* 1988, 11:1020–1030.

16. Ling LH, Oh JK, Schaff HV, *et al.*: Constrictive pericarditis in the modern era: evolving clinical spectrum and impact on outcome after pericardiectomy. *Circulation* 1999, 100:1380–1386.

17. Ling LH, Oh JK, Breen JF, *et al.*: Calcific constrictive pericarditis: is it still with us? *Ann Intern Med* 2000, 132:444–450. [Published erratum appears in *Ann Intern Med* 2000, 133:659.]

18. Talreja DR, Edwards WD, Danielson GK, *et al.*: Constrictive pericarditis in 26 patients with histologically normal pericardial thickness. *Circulation* 2003, 108:1852–1857.

19. Vaitkus PT, Kussmaul WG: Constrictive pericarditis versus restrictive cardiomyopathy: a reappraisal and update of diagnostic criteria. *Am Heart J* 1991, 122:1431–1441.

20. Hurrell DG, Nishimura RA, Higano ST, *et al.*: Value of dynamic respiratory changes in left and right ventricular pressures for the diagnosis of constrictive pericarditis. *Circulation* 1996, 93:2007–2013.

21. Oh JK, Tajik AJ, Appleton CP, *et al.*: Preload reduction to unmask the characteristic Doppler features of constrictive pericarditis: a new observation. *Circulation* 1997, 95:796–799.

22. Talreja DR, Nishimura RA, Oh JK, Holmes DR: Constrictive pericarditis in the modern era: novel criteria for diagnosis in the cardiac catheterization laboratory. *J Am Coll Cardiol* 2008, 51:315–319.

23. Sohn DW, Kim YJ, Kim HS, *et al.*: Unique features of early diastolic mitral annulus velocity in constrictive pericarditis. *J Am Soc Echocardiogr* 2004, 17:222–226.

24. Ha JW, Oh JK, Ommen SR, *et al.*: Diagnostic value of mitral annular velocity for constrictive pericarditis in the absence of respiratory variation in mitral inflow velocity. *J Am Soc Echocardiogr* 2002, 15:1468–1471.

25. Rajagopalan N, Garcia MJ, Rodriguez L, *et al.*: Comparison of new Doppler echocardiographic methods to differentiate constrictive pericardial heart disease and restrictive cardiomyopathy. *Am J Cardiol* 2001, 87:86–94.

26. Ha JW, Ommen SR, Tajik AJ, *et al.*: Differentiation of constrictive pericarditis from restrictive cardiomyopathy using mitral annular velocity by tissue Doppler echocardiography. *Am J Cardiol* 2004, 94:316–319.

27. Ha JW, Oh JK, Ling LH, *et al.*: Annulus paradoxus: transmitral flow velocity to mitral annular velocity ratio is inversely proportional to pulmonary capillary wedge pressure in patients with constrictive pericarditis. *Circulation* 2002, 106:976–978.

28. Boonyaratavej S, Oh JK, Tajik AJ, *et al.*: Comparison of mitral inflow and superior vena cava Doppler velocities in chronic obstructive pulmonary disease and pericarditis. *J Am Coll Cardiol* 1998, 32:2043–2048.

29. Wu LA, Nishimura RA: Images in clinical medicine: pulsus paradoxus. *N Engl J Med* 2003, 349:666.

30. Haley JH, Tajik AJ, Danielson GK, *et al.*: Transient constrictive pericarditis: causes and natural history. *J Am Coll Cardiol* 2004, 43:271–275.

31. Hancock EW: A clearer view of effusive-constrictive pericarditis. *N Engl J Med* 2004, 350:435–437.

32. Sagrista-Sauleda J, Angel J, Sanchez A, *et al.*: Effusive-constrictive pericarditis. *N Engl J Med* 2004, 350:469–475.

33. Klarich KW, Enriquez-Sarano M, Gura GM, *et al.*: Papillary fibroelastoma: echocardiographic characteristics for diagnosis and pathologic correlation. *J Am Coll Cardiol* 1997, 30:784–790.

34. Harpaz D, Auerbach I, Vered Z, *et al.*: Caseous calcification of the mitral annulus: a neglected, unrecognized diagnosis. *J Am Soc Echocardiogr* 2001, 14:825–831.

35. Ganame J, Wright J, Bogaert J: Cardiac lipoma diagnosed by cardiac magnetic resonance imaging. *Eur J Heart* 2008, 29:697.

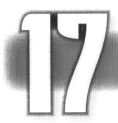

Echocardiographic Assessment of the Left Atrium and Evaluation for Cardiac Source of Embolus

Fay Y. Lin and Jorge R. Kizer

Cardiac ultrasound provides accurate assessment of the left atrium (LA) [1]. It is the cornerstone for evaluation of suspected cardiogenic and aortogenic cerebral infarction, permitting identification of structural variants or abnormalities that can serve as substrates for embolism [2]. LA dilatation is the morphophysiologic expression of abnormal LV function [3]. The full spectrum of pathological processes affecting the LV have (as a common consequence) impairment of myocardial relaxation and an increase in ventricular stiffness [3]. The resulting increase in LV filling pressure is transmitted to the LA, which undergoes compensatory enlargement in order to normalize wall tension [3]. LA size can offer a window into the severity and duration of vascular, myocardial, or valvular disease processes, with effects on the LV [4]. Beyond acting as a marker for ventricular and vascular disease, LA dilatation has direct pathogenetic implications, resulting in stasis and dysrhythmias, which foster thrombosis within its walls [4]. Echocardiographic LA size [4,5] (particularly when determined volumetrically [6,7]) has been shown to provide powerful prognostic information for incident coronary and cerebral vascular events, heart failure, and dysrhythmias in individuals with and without clinically overt cardiovascular disease.

The cerebral circulation receives almost 15% of cardiac output, supplying an organ that is extraordinarily sensitive to ischemia [2]. Embolism of cardiac or aortic origin is most often clinically manifest in the brain, where its most negative consequences can occur [2]. Out of the nearly 90% of strokes that are ischemic in nature, approximately 20% are the result of high-risk cardiac or aortic abnormalities [2]. Another 30% of strokes have no definable etiology; however, these strokes frequently have embolic features, suggesting that they may have a cardiac or aortic cause [2]. Thus, the heart and aorta may be involved in the pathogenesis of as many as half of all ischemic strokes.

Various cardiac, pulmonary vascular, and proximal aortic abnormalities, are associated with stroke. They may be grouped into high-risk and moderate or uncertain risk sources of embolism (*see* Fig. 17-5) based on the magnitude of their associations and the quality of evidence in support thereof [2]. For some cardiac sources of embolism, high-quality transthoracic echocardiography is sufficient for evaluation [2]. For others, particularly abnormalities of the interatrial septum and aortic atheroma, transesophageal echocardiography (TEE) is necessary for diagnosis (*see* Fig. 17-5). The yield of TEE is highest in patients without clinical evidence of cardiovascular disease, as well as younger adults with stroke [8].

Careful attention should be paid to the following components in the standard evaluation of TEE in patients with stroke of undetermined etiology: 1) left-sided (and, in the presence of intracardiac shunting, right-sided) cardiac valves, with close-up imaging in multiple planes; 2) LA and left atrial appendage size and function, thrombus or smoke; 3) close-up evaluation of the interatrial septum in multiple planes, both with two-dimensional and color Doppler imaging; 4) agitated saline or contrast injection in order to assess for right to left shunting, with satisfactory opacification at rest and with provocative maneuvers (*eg*, Valsalva, coughing); leftward bowing of the septum is important to confirm a favorable (right to left) transseptal gradient with provocative maneuvers; 5) atheromatous disease of the aortic root, ascending aorta, and aortic arch.

The evidence base for secondary stroke prevention with cardiogenic or aortogenic stroke is mostly observational, with the exception of atrial fibrillation [2]. In general, stroke in association with high-risk cardiac findings mandates anticoagulation, with the exception of tumors and infective endocarditis, for which surgical resection or appropriate antibiotic therapy is indicated [2]. By contrast, there is less (and often insufficient evidence) to guide therapy for stroke patients with moderate or uncertain risk findings [2]. In both settings, treatment needs to be individualized and informed by the balance between risk of embolic recurrence and major (specifically intracerebral) hemorrhage [2].

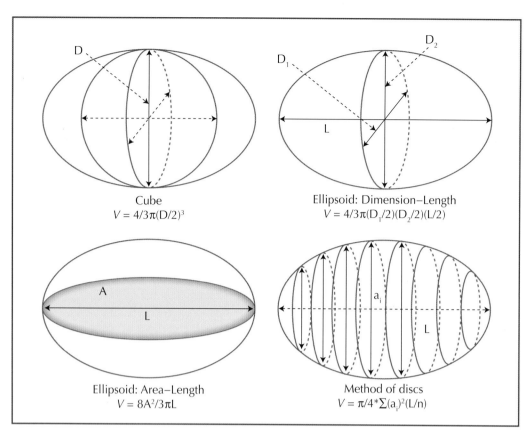

Cube
$$V = 4/3\pi(D/2)^3$$

Ellipsoid: Dimension–Length
$$V = 4/3\pi(D_1/2)(D_2/2)(L/2)$$

Ellipsoid: Area–Length
$$V = 8A^2/3\pi L$$

Method of discs
$$V = \pi/4 * \Sigma(a_i)^2(L/n)$$

Figure 17-1. Measurement of the anteroposterior diameter of the left atrium (LA) in parasternal views has been the standard in transthoracic echocardiography. However, this one-dimensional measurement does not accurately reflect the magnitude of LA dilatation because enlargement along an anteroposterior axis is constrained by the sternum anteriorly and the spine posteriorly, such that greater degrees of dilatation become increasingly asymmetric along the mediolateral and inferosuperior planes [1]. Volumetric echocardiographic determinations of LA volume are preferable because they compare well with cine CT and MRI, and they have superior prognostic ability when compared to linear LA dimension [1].

Although the cube model (where D = anteroposterior diameter) offers a simple approach to volume determination, accurate quantification is best achieved by the ellipsoid model and Simpson's method of discs [1]. LA volume, modeled as a prolate ellipse, can be calculated using the biplane dimension length formula (where medio-lateral and inferosuperior diameters can be substituted for D_1 and D_2); however, more reliable estimation of minor-axis dimensions of the LA can be achieved by tracing long-axis areas along the entire LA border and applying the biplane area-length formula [1]. Alternatively, LA volume can be computed as the sum of the volumes of stacked oval discs using Simpson's rule.

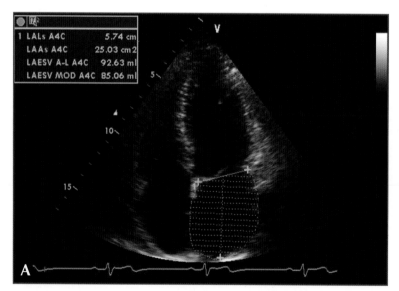

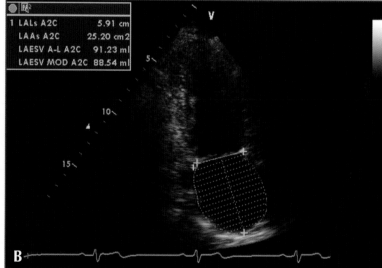

Figure 17-2. Determination of left atrial (LA) volume by transthoracic echocardiography, based on the area-length ellipsoid approach and the method of discs. Planimetry of the LA from orthogonal four-chamber (**A**) and two-chamber (**B**) apical views is performed, taking care to exclude the pulmonary veins and left atrial appendage and using the plane of the mitral annulus as the inferior margin [1]. Online software packages can provide areas and volumes based on single plane determinations as shown, or computations involving orthogonal planes. Single plane approaches to the area length method and Simpson's rule achieve reasonable accuracy; however, biplane approaches make fewer assumptions [1]. The latter approach is favored because available studies have predominantly used the biplane method. Normal LA volume indexed to body surface area using either method in community-based studies is 22 ± 6 mL/m² [1]. A2C—apical two-chamber; A4C—apical four-chamber; LAA—left atrial appendage; LAESV—left atrial end-systolic volume.

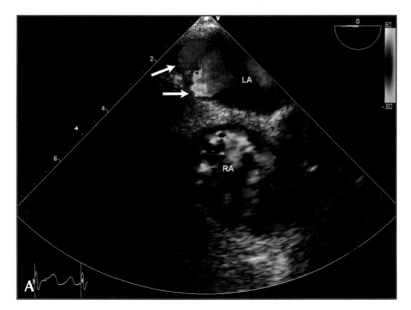

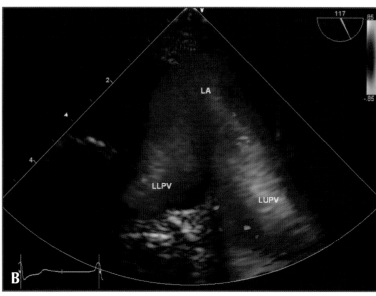

Figure 17-3. Identification of all four pulmonary veins permits visualization of invading lung carcinoma or pulmonary veins thrombus. It may also allow detection of pulmonary vein stenosis, following an invasive electrophysiologic ablation procedure, and it provides reassurance against the presence of partially anomalous pulmonary venous connection, a condition most commonly associated with the presence of atrial septal defect. Pulmonary veins may be imaged both in transverse and longitudinal planes by transesophageal echocardiography. **A,** Color Doppler evaluation of the right-sided pulmonary veins in the transverse plane (*arrows*); right lower (*upper arrow*); and right upper (*lower arrow*) pulmonary veins. **B,** Color Doppler evaluation of the left sided pulmonary veins in the longitudinal plane. LA—left atrium; LLPV—left lower pulmonary vein; LUPV—left upper pulmonary vein; RA—right atrium.

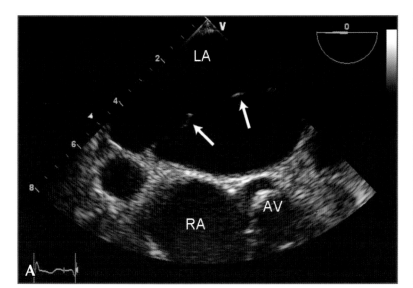

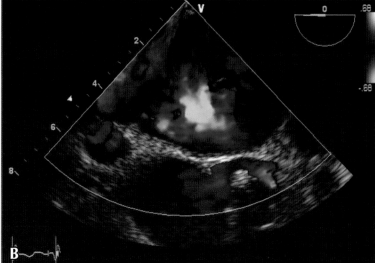

Figure 17-4. A 59-year-old woman with type 2 diabetes mellitus and hypertension is referred for transesophageal echocardiography because of transient ischemic attack. A linear structure separating the superior aspect from the inferior aspect of the left atrium (LA) (*arrows*) is appreciated on midesophageal views in the transverse (**A** and **B**) and longitudinal (**C**) planes, consistent with cor triatriatum. This rare congenital anomaly is characterized by persistence of a fibrous or fibromuscular membrane that separates the LA into proximal (accessory) and distal (true) chambers, which, when obstructive, mimics mitral stenosis, leading to the development of pulmonary hypertension and right-sided heart failure [9]. When the openings in the membrane are nonobstructive as demonstrated by color Doppler in this patient (**B**), isolated cor triatriatum may remain clinically silent throughout the patient's life [9]. Either LA chamber may communicate with the right atrium (RA) through a patent foramen ovale or atrial septal defect [9], but no interatrial shunting, or other cardiac sources of embolism were identified in this patient. AV—aortic valve; SVC—superior vena cava.

Proximal Sources of Embolism*

High Risk		Medium or Uncertain Risk
Cyanotic congenital heart disease	**Primary cardiac tumors**	**Interatrial septal abnormalities**
Atrial dysrhythmias	Myxoma	Patent foramen ovale†
Atrial fibrillation	Papillary fibroelastoma	Atrial septal defect
Sick sinus syndrome	Malignant tumors	Atrial septal aneurysm
Atrial flutter†	**Metastatic tumors to the heart**	**Pulmonary arteriovenous malformation**
Left atrial/LAA thrombus	**Vegetations**	**Spontaneous echo contrast ("smoke")†**
Atrial dysrhythimias	Infective endocarditis	**Mitral valve prolapse**
Mitral valve stenosis	Nonbacterial thrombotic (marantic) endocarditis	**Valvular calcification**
LV thrombus	**Prosthetic cardiac valve**	Mitral annular calcification
Acute myocardial infarction	**Complex aortic atheroma†**	Aortic valve sclerosis/stenosis
Dilated cardiomyopathy		**Valvular strands†**

Figure 17-5. Proximal sources of embolism. (*Adapted from* Doufekias *et al.* [2].) *High-quality transthoracic echocardiography (TTE) is considered sufficient for evaluation if positive, obviating the need for transesophageal echocardiography (TEE) in some patients. However, if TTE is negative, TEE can provide additional diagnostic yield, particularly for vegetations and atrial septal defect [2]. †TEE is required for diagnosis. LAA—left atrial appendage.

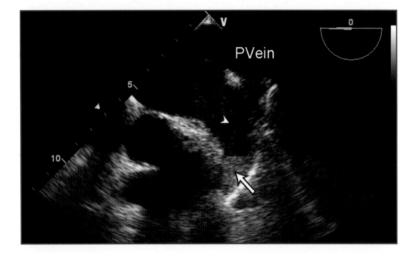

Figure 17-6. Echodense thrombus (*arrow*) fills the apex of the left atrial appendage (LAA) in a patient with atrial fibrillation (AF); midesophageal view, transverse plane, transesophageal echocardiography. Spontaneous echo contrast or "smoke" (*arrowhead*) is noted in the appendage proximal to the apical thrombus. AF is the preeminent cardioembolic condition, and it is the principal cause of stroke in individuals aged 75 or older [10]. Embolization of LAA thrombus accounts for approximately two-thirds of AF-associated strokes [10]. Dense smoke reflects rouleaux formation, determined by stasis, fibrinogen concentration, and hematocrit level [11], and it is a harbinger of thrombosis and thromboembolism [12]. Management of LAA thrombus consists of anticoagulation with warfarin, aiming for a target international normalized ratio level of 2.0 to 3.0, with documentation of thrombus resolution at follow up [13]. PVein—pulmonary vein.

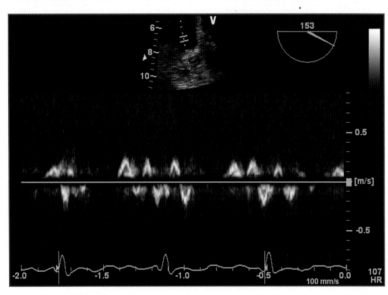

Figure 17-7. Pulsed-wave Doppler interrogation of the left atrial appendage (LAA) during transesophageal echocardiography in a patient with atrial fibrillation. Both filling and emptying velocities are reduced (peak 23 cm/s), consistent with impaired contractile function of the appendage. Reduced LAA flow velocities with lack of visible fibrillatory contractions on two-dimensional imaging were defined in a cross-sectional study as less than 25 cm/s and were found to be more commonly associated with "smoke" as opposed to higher velocities [14]. In a longitudinal study, peak LAA emptying velocity less than 20 cm/s was associated with prevalence of dense smoke and thrombus in the LAA, as well as incidence of thromboembolic events [12].

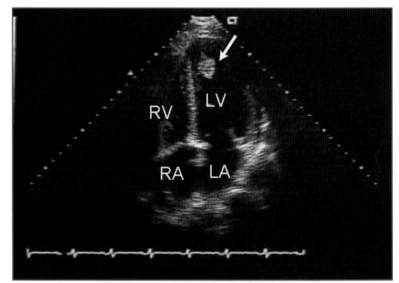

Figure 17-8. Apical four-chamber view transthoracic echocardiography (TTE) demonstrating a mobile, globular echodensity (*arrow*) adherent to the apical septum in a patient with nonischemic cardiomyopathy, consistent with thrombus (*arrow*). Like LA thrombus, LV thrombus is associated with structural heart disease. Both ischemic and nonischemic cardiomyopathies constitute substrates for thrombus formation, the risk of which is directly proportional to reduction in global LV ejection fraction [15–17]. Acute myocardial infarction is a major predisposing condition, particularly in an anterior location [18], although the incidence of LV thrombosis in the contemporary setting of primary percutaneous coronary intervention has declined to 10% of anterior ST elevation myocardial infarctions [19]. Treatment of LV thrombus involves anticoagulation for a minimum of 3 months, with documentation of thrombus resolution by serial TTEs [2]. RA—right atrium.

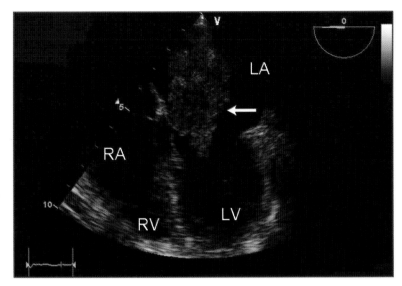

Figure 17-9. A 17-year-old woman presented with bilateral cerebellar and occipital strokes. Transesophageal echocardiography (midesophageal view, transverse plane) reveals a large mass (*arrow*) adherent to the interatrial septum and with multiple frond-like extensions, which is seen to prolapse across the mitral valve in diastole. Surgical resection showed a friable tumor, confirmed histopathologically to be a villous myxoma. Myxomas are the most common primary cardiac tumor, and may be polypoid or villous in nature [20]. They occur most frequently in the left atrium (LA), where they are attached to the limbus of the fossa ovalis [20]. As a result, these tumors often become clinically manifest through systemic embolism, for which surgical removal is indicated [2,20]. RA—right atrium.

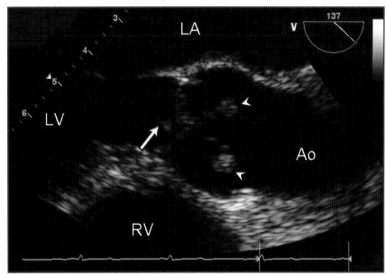

Figure 17-10. Multiple papillary fibroelastomas found incidentally in a 53-year-old woman with lone atrial fibrillation (AF) undergoing transesophageal echocardiography prior to pulmonary vein ablation. Round homogeneous echodensities attached by a stalk are seen on the aortic side of the leaflets (*arrowheads*) on a midesophageal view, longitudinal plane. Also noted are linear strands on the ventricular side of the leaflets, consistent with Lambl's excrescences (*arrow*). Papillary fibroelastoma is the second most common primary cardiac tumor, principally found on left-sided valvular surfaces (aortic greater than mitral) [21]. These tumors are usually single, but may be multiple, and are generally well circumscribed and often pedunculated [21]. Surgical resection is advocated for large mobile tumors, especially those greater than 1 cm in diameter, because of the risk of embolism [2,8]. Ao—aorta; LA—left atrium; RA—right atrium.

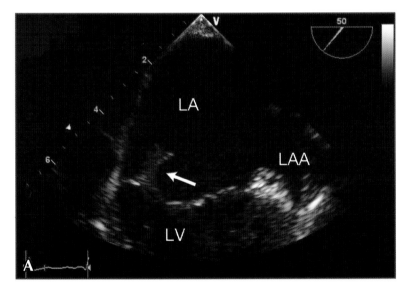

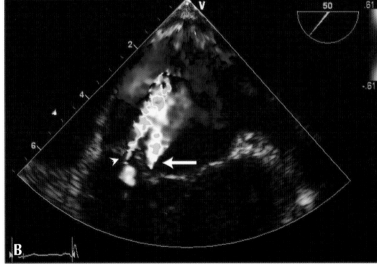

Figure 17-11. Transesophageal echocardiography in a 55-year-old man with multiple cerebral infarcts and *Staphylococcus aureus* bacteremia reveals an echodensity with mobile extensions on the anterior mitral valve leaflet (*arrow*, **A**), consistent with vegetation. There is echocardiographic dropout of the anterior leaflet in the region of the vegetation through which color flow is demonstrated (*arrowhead*, **B**), consistent with leaflet perforation and mild to moderate mitral regurgitation; a second jet of commissural mild to moderate mitral regurgitation (*arrow*, **B**) is also visualized.

Mitral valve vegetations are more commonly associated with clinical embolism than aortic valve vegetations [22]. Vegetation size, especially a dimension greater than 10 mm, is a major determinant of propensity for embolization, as is mobility [23]. Both large size and high mobility characterize the vegetation shown. When severe, valvular regurgitation from leaflet destruction, heart failure, recurrent embolism despite antibiotics, and infection by certain pathogens, calls for consideration of valve replacement [24]. LA—left atrium; LAA—left atrial appendage.

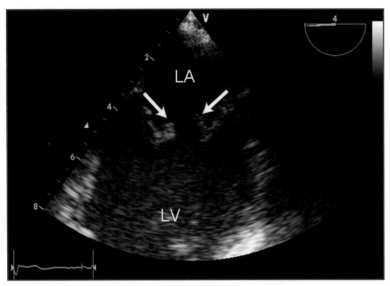

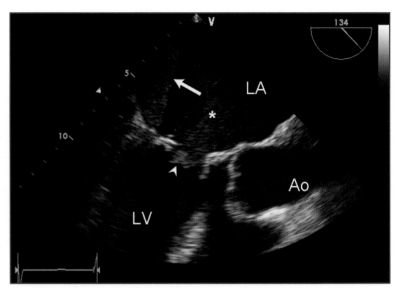

Figure 17-12. Globular echodensities (*arrows*) are visualized on the anterior and posterior mitral leaflets during transesophageal echocardiograph (midesophageal view, transverse plane) in a 36-year-old woman with systemic lupus erythematosus (SLE) and positive antiphospholipid antibodies who suffered a right temporoparietal stroke. There were no clinical signs of infection and multiple blood cultures were negative. Findings are consistent with nonbacterial thrombotic (marantic) endocarditis. Aseptic vegetations, composed of platelet fibrin aggregates, which deposit on damaged valvular endothelium, occur in the setting of neoplastic disease, as well as chronic inflammatory (or of infectious) processes [25], which SLE with associated antiphospholipid syndrome is an exemplar. Systemic anticoagulation is indicated, and specifically in the case of nonbacterial thrombotic endocarditis associated with malignancy, unfractionated or low molecular weight heparin is recommended [26].

Figure 17-13. A 70-year-old man with history of prior mitral valve replacement presents with bilateral occipital infarcts. Transesophageal echocardiography (midesophageal view, longitudinal plane) shows thrombosis of a posterior bioprosthetic leaflet (*arrowhead*) resulting in severe mitral stenosis with left atrial (LA) stasis (spontaneous echocardiographic contrast, *asterisk*) and formation of mural thrombus (*arrow*). Systemic embolization complicates both biologic and mechanical valvular prostheses, with incidence ranging from 1% to 4% per year [26]. Eighty percent of clinical thromboemboli associated with prosthetic valves involve the cerebral circulation. The risk of cerebral embolism is higher in the mitral position (2%–3.5% per year) than the aortic position (1%–2% per year), and it is increased in the setting of atrial fibrillation [26]. Ao—aorta.

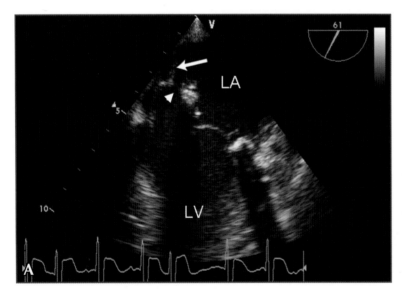

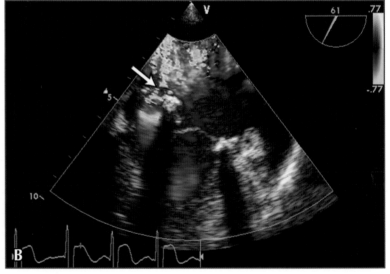

Figure 17-14. A 72-year-old man with a history of mitral valve replacement presents with fever, a right homonymous hemianopsia, and left-sided hemisensory loss. MRI of the brain reveals left-occipital and right-thalamic infarcts. Transesophageal echocardiograph (midesophageal view, transverse plane), shows a mobile echodensity on the mitral annulus (**A**, *arrow*), consistent with vegetation. An area of echocardiographic dropout beyond the sewing ring is also apparent (**A**, *arrowhead*), through which there is

a jet of moderate paravalvular mitral regurgitation (**B**, *arrow*). Rocking motion of the bioprosthesis also was appreciated, consistent with partial dehiscence from prosthetic valve endocarditis. Prosthetic heart valves offer a potential nidus for infection, which, like native valve endocarditis, may also manifest through cerebral embolism. Of note, although the patient was in AF, there was no evidence of LAA thrombus. (*Courtesy of* Daniel Krauser, MD). LA—left atrium.

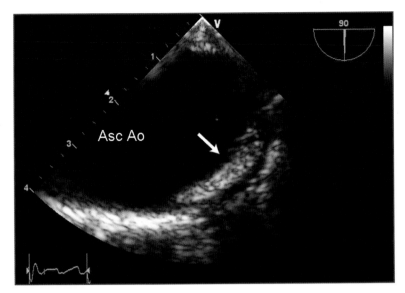

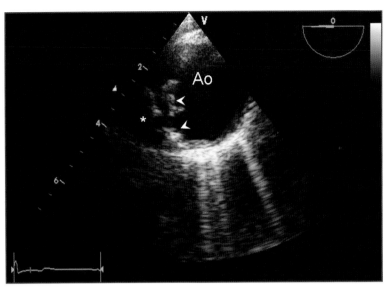

Figure 17-15. Upper esophageal view of the distal aortic arch, demonstrating the presence of sessile plaque protruding 4 mm into the lumen (*arrow*), consistent with complex aortic atheroma. Although some studies have failed to reveal an association between complex aortic atheroma and stroke in the general population [27], the presence of protruding aortic plaque greater of 4 mm or more in thickness has been shown to markedly increase the risk of stroke recurrence [28]. Complex aortic atheroma not only serves as a marker for atherosclerotic disease, but also acts as a direct emboligenic substrate through atherothromboembolism [29]. In the absence of mobile components, professional society guidelines generally favor antiplatelet therapy in addition to aggressive atherosclerosis risk factor modification for this condition [2]. AscAo—ascending aorta.

Figure 17-16. Upper esophageal view of the aortic (Ao) arch in a patient with cardiac catheterization complicated by stroke reveals the presence of prominent atheromatous plaque (*asterisk*) with large mobile echodensities on its surface (*arrowheads*). Cardiac catheterization carries a small but definite risk of stroke in part through disruption of the atheromatous plaque surface and resulting thrombogenesis [30]. Complex aortic atheroma with mobile components may also be detected in stroke patients who have not had endovascular instrumentation, reflecting erosion or ulceration of vulnerable atheromatous plaque and subsequent thromboembolization. Short-term anticoagulation may be considered for secondary stroke prevention in such settings [2].

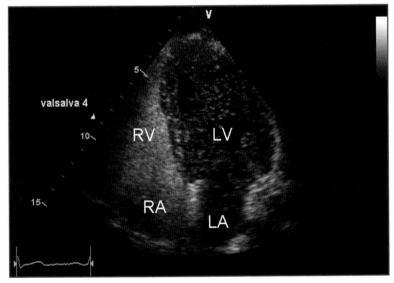

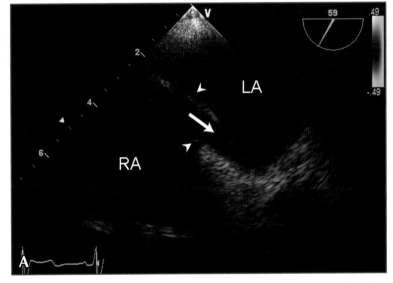

Figure 17-17. Apical four-chamber view transthoracic echocardiograph (TTE) illustrating passage of numerous microbubbles from the right to left side of the heart during the release phase of the Valsalva maneuver, consistent with the presence of an interatrial shunt. Injection of agitated saline or contrast agents that are filtered by the lungs is essential for the evaluation of right to left interatrial shunts, and should involve maneuvers to increase right atrial pressure (*eg*, Valsalva, coughing) [8]. The advent of second harmonic imaging has improved the sensitivity of TTE with agitated saline injection for right to left interatrial shunts, which can be complementary to transesophageal echocardiography where sedation and esophageal intubation may interfere with adequate performance of provocative (right atrial pressure-raising maneuvers) [2]. LA—left atrium; RA—right atrium.

Figure 17-18. **A**, Transesophageal echocardiograph (TEE) (midesophageal view, longitudinal plane) showing a large patent foramen ovale (*arrow*) with maximal separation between the primum and secundum septa (*arrowheads*) of 0.6 cm. Bidirectional flow was present, consistent with an incompetent septum primum valve.

Continued on the next page

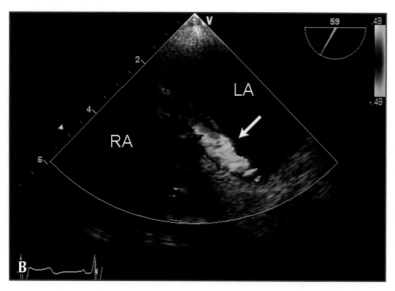

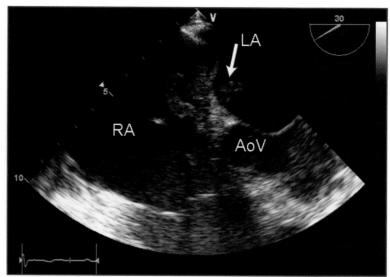

Figure 17-18. *(Continued)* **B,** Demonstration of right to left interatrial flow by color Doppler *(arrow)*. Patent foramen ovale is associated with ischemic stroke, especially in younger adults without an alternative stroke etiology [8]. The presumptive mechanism is paradoxical embolism, but such a diagnosis requires demonstration of venous thrombosis, which is detected in a minority of patients using duplex sonography of the lower extremities [8]. However, magnetic resonance venography of the pelvis and distal lower extremity venography suggest that a proportion of patients with unexplained arterial embolism and patent foramen ovale have thrombosis of the pelvic [31] or calf veins [32] as the underlying mechanism. LA—left atrium; RA—right atrium.

Figure 17-19. A 46-year-old woman was found to have acute cerebral infarcts in multiple vascular distributions after an episode of loss of consciousness. Transesophageal echocardiography (midesophageal view, transverse plane) shows an oblong branching echodensity *(arrow)* trapped in a patent foramen ovale, consistent with "thrombus-in-transit." Right-sided chamber dilatation with moderate pulmonary hypertension led to performance of CT of the chest, which revealed pulmonary embolism. The present case is a rare instance of "thrombus-in-transit" in a patient with brain embolism and patent foramen ovale, which proves the cause of the stroke to be paradoxical embolism. Barring contraindications, prompt thoracotomy for thrombectomy and closure of patent foramen ovale appears to be the most sensible approach towards preventing potentially catastrophic systemic embolism, although anticoagulation is required for a minimum of 6 to 12 months in the setting of idiopathic venous thromboembolism [33]. *(Adapted from* Doufekias *et al.* [2].) AoV—aortic valve; LA—left atrium; RA—right atrium.

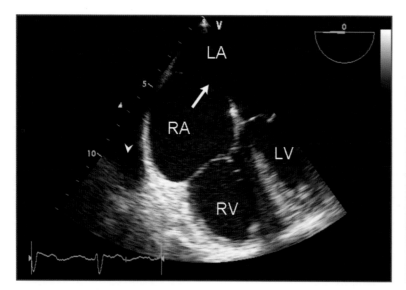

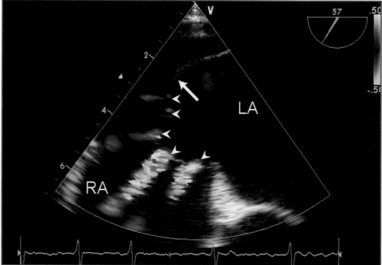

Figure 17-20. Distal esophageal transesophageal echocardiography showing a large ostium secundum atrial septal defect *(arrow)* with a maximal diameter of 3.1 cm. A pleural effusion is also seen *(arrowhead)*. An atrial septal defect provides a conduit for paradoxical embolization, although this condition that is much less common in the general population than patent foramen ovale, needs to be considered in the patient with cryptogenic brain embolism [34]. In the presence of venous thrombosis, intermediate term anticoagulation is indicated [33], but surgical or percutaenous closure is warranted in the patient with ischemic stroke and suspected paradoxical embolism [35]. LA—left atrium; RA—right atrium.

Figure 17-21. Distal esophageal transesophageal echocardiography demonstrates a prominent atrial septal aneurysm *(arrow)* with multiple fenestrations *(arrowheads)* *(ie,* small ostium secundum defects). Color Doppler demonstrates left to right flow across the multiple defects. An atrial septal aneurysm results from redundancy of the interatrial septum with exaggerated deviation from the midline originally defined as 15 mm or more [36] and subsequently, in populations with stroke, as greater than or equal to 11 mm [37]. Atrial septal aneurysms are associated with interatrial shunts in 50% to 90% of cases, which is thought to explain in large measure their relation to ischemic stroke [8]. They have also been linked to atrial fibrillation, as in the present case, providing another potential mechanism for the observed association with stroke [8]. In the latter case, anticoagulation is warranted for secondary stroke prevention [13]. *(Courtesy of* Daniel Krauser, MD). LA—left atrium; RA—right atrium.

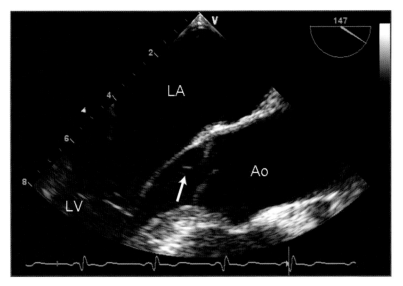

Figure 17-22. Transesophageal echocardiography (TEE) midesophageal view, longitudinal plane, shows a linear strand (*arrow*) on the ventricular side of the aortic (Ao) valve leaflets, consistent with a Lambl's excrescence. Lambl's excrescences are believed to result from valvular wear and tear, whereby fibrin is deposited serially and covered by a single layer of endothelial cells [38]. Although case-control studies suggested an association between valvular strands and stroke [38], valvular strands are common findings in left-sided heart valves and subsequent longitudinal studies have failed to confirm a relation [39–41]. Moreover, a TEE substudy of a randomized controlled trial comparing aspirin versus warfarin for secondary stroke prevention found no difference in stroke recurrence and death in patients with valvular strands assigned to aspirin versus warfarin [41]. Thus, these findings do not require therapy beyond standard antiplatelet treatment for secondary stroke prevention [2]. LA—left atrium.

References

1. Lang RM, Bierig M, Devereux RB, *et al.*: Recommendations for chamber quantification: a report from the American Society of Echocardiography's Guidelines and Standards Committee and the Chamber Quantification Writing Group, developed in conjunction with the European Association of Echocardiography, a branch of the European Society of Cardiology. *J Am Soc Echocardiogr* 2005, 18:1440–1463.

2. Doufekias E, Segal AZ, Kizer JR: Cardiogenic and aortogenic brain embolism. *J Am Coll Cardiol* 2008 (in press).

3. Abhayaratna WP, Seward JB, Appleton CP, *et al.*: Left atrial size: physiologic determinants and clinical applications. *J Am Coll Cardiol* 2006, 47:2357–2363.

4. Kizer JR, Bella JN, Palmieri V, *et al.*: Left atrial diameter as an independent predictor of first clinical cardiovascular events in middle-aged and elderly adults: the Strong Heart Study (SHS). *Am Heart J* 2006, 151:412–418.

5. Vaziri SM, Larson MG, Benjamin EJ, Levy D: Echocardiographic predictors of non-rheumatic atrial fibrillation. *Circulation* 1994, 89:724–730.

6. Tsang TS, Abhayaratna WP, Barnes ME, *et al.*: Prediction of cardiovascular outcomes with left atrial size: is volume superior to area or diameter? *J Am Coll Cardiol* 2006, 47:1018–1023.

7. Moller JE, Hillis GS, Oh JK, *et al.*: Left atrial volume: a powerful predictor of survival after acute myocardial infarction. *Circulation* 2003, 107:2207–2212.

8. Kizer JR, Devereux RB: Clinical practice: patent foramen ovale in young adults with unexplained stroke. *N Engl J Med* 2005, 353:2361–2372. [Published erratum appears in *N Engl J Med* 2006, 354:2401.]

9. Perloff JK, ed: Congenital obstruction to left atrial flow: cor triatriatum. In *The Clinical Recognition of Congenital Heart Disease.* Philadelphia: W.B. Saunders; 1994:178–185.

10. Hart RG, Halperin JL: Atrial fibrillation and stroke: concepts and controversies. *Stroke* 2001, 32:803–808.

11. Rastegar R, Harnick DJ, Weidemann P, *et al.*: Spontaneous echo contrast video-density is flow-related and is dependent on the relative concentrations of fibrinogen and red blood cells. *J Am Coll Cardiol* 2003, 41:603–610.

12. Transesophageal echocardiographic correlates of thromboembolism in high-risk patients with nonvalvular atrial fibrillation. The Stroke Prevention in Atrial Fibrillation Investigators Committee on Echocardiography. *Ann Intern Med* 1998, 28:639–647.

13. Fuster V, Ryden LE, Cannom DS, *et al.*: ACC/AHA/ESC 2006 Guidelines for the Management of Patients with Atrial Fibrillation: a report of the American College of Cardiology/American Heart Association Task Force on Practice Guidelines and the European Society of Cardiology Committee for Practice Guidelines (Writing Committee to Revise the 2001 Guidelines for the Management of Patients With Atrial Fibrillation): developed in collaboration with the European Heart Rhythm Association and the Heart Rhythm Society. *Circulation* 2006, 114:e257–e354. [Published erratum appears in *Circulation* 2007, 116:e138.]

14. Mugge A, Kuhn H, Nikutta P, *et al.*: Assessment of left atrial appendage function by biplane transesophgeal echocardiography in patients with nonrheumatic atrial fibrillation: identification of a subgroup of patients at increased embolic risk. *J Am Coll Cardiol* 1994, 23:599–607.

15. Dries DL, Rosenberg YD, Waclawiw MA, Domanski MJ: Ejection fraction and risk of thromboembolic events in patients with systolic dysfunction and sinus rhythm: evidence for gender differences in the studies of left ventricular dysfunction trials. *J Am Coll Cardiol* 1997, 29:1074–1080.

16. Loh E, Sutton MS, Wun CC, *et al.*: Ventricular dysfunction and the risk of stroke after myocardial infarction. *N Engl J Med* 1997, 336:251–257.

17. Freudenberger RS, Hellkamp AS, Halperin JL, *et al.*: Risk of thromboembolism in heart failure: an analysis from the Sudden Cardiac Death in Heart Failure Trial (SCD-HeFT). *Circulation* 2007, 115:2637–2641.

18. Chiarella F, Santoro E, Domenicucci S, *et al.*: Predischarge two-dimensional echocardiographic evaluation of left ventricular thrombosis after acute myocardial infarction in the GISSI-3 study. *Am J Cardiol* 1998, 81:822–827.

19. Kalra A, Jang IK: Prevalence of early left ventricular thrombus after primary coronary intervention for acute myocardial infarction. *J Thromb Thrombolysis* 2000, 10:133–136.

20. Reynen K: Cardiac myxomas. *N Engl J Med* 1995, 333:1610–1617.

21. Gowda RM, Khan IA, Nair CK, *et al.*: Cardiac papillary fibroelastoma: a comprehensive analysis of 725 cases. *Am Heart J* 2003, 146:404–410.

22. Cabell CH, Pond KK, Peterson GE, *et al.*: The risk of stroke and death in patients with aortic and mitral valve endocarditis. *Am Heart J* 2001, 142:75-80.

23. Di Salvo G, Habib G, Pergola V, *et al.*: Echocardiography predicts embolic events in infective endocarditis. *J Am Coll Cardiol* 2001, 37:1069–1076.

24. Mylonakis E, Calderwood SB: Infective endocarditis in adults. *N Engl J Med* 2001, 345:1318–1330.

25. Reisner SA, Brenner B, Haim N, *et al.*: Echocardiography in nonbacterial thrombotic endocarditis: from autopsy to clinical entity. *J Am Soc Echocardiogr* 2000, 13:876–881.

26. Salem DN, Stein PD, Al-Ahmad A, *et al.*: Antithrombotic therapy in valvular heart disease: native and prosthetic: the Seventh ACCP Conference on Antithrombotic and Thrombolytic Therapy. *Chest* 2004, 126:457S–482S.

27. Meissner I, Khandheria BK, Sheps SG, *et al.*: Atherosclerosis of the aorta: risk factor, risk marker, or innocent bystander? A prospective population-based transesophageal echocardiography study. *J Am Coll Cardiol* 2004, 44:1018–1024.

28. Atherosclerotic disease of the aortic arch as a risk factor for recurrent ischemic stroke. The French Study of Aortic Plaques in Stroke Group. *N Engl J Med* 1996, 334:1216–1221.

29. Rundek T, Di Tullio MR, Sciacca RR, *et al.*: Association between large aortic arch atheromas and high-intensity transient signals in elderly stroke patients. *Stroke* 1999, 30:2683–2686.

30. Segal AZ, Abernethy WB, Palacios IF, *et al.*: Stroke as a complication of cardiac catheterization: risk factors and clinical features. *Neurology* 2001, 56:975–977.

31. Cramer SC, Rordorf G, Maki JH, *et al.*: Increased pelvic vein thrombi in cryptogenic stroke. Results of the Paradoxical Emboli From Large Veins in Ischemic Stroke (PELVIS) Study. *Stroke* 2004, 35:46–50.

32. Stollberger C, Slany J, Schuster I, *et al.*: The prevalence of deep venous thrombosis in patients with suspected paradoxical embolism. *Ann Intern Med* 1993, 119:461–465. [Published erratum appears in *Ann Intern Med* 1994, 120:347.]

33. Buller HR, Agnelli G, Hull RD, *et al.*: Antithrombotic therapy for venous thrombo-embolic disease: the Seventh ACCP Conference on Antithrombotic and Thrombolytic Therapy. *Chest* 2004, 126(3 Suppl):401S–428S. [Published erratum appears in *Chest* 2005, 127:416.]

34. Harvey JR, Teague SM, Anderson JL, *et al.*: Clinically silent atrial septal defects with evidence for cerebral embolization. *Ann Intern Med* 1986, 105:695–697.

35. Therrien J, Webb G: Clinical update on adults with congenital heart disease. *Lancet* 2003, 362:1305–1313.

36. Hanley PC, Tajik AJ, Hynes JK, *et al.*: Diagnosis and classification of atrial septal aneurysm by two-dimensional echocardiography: report of 80 consecutive cases. *J Am Coll Cardiol* 1985, 6:1370–1382.

37. Mas JL, Arquizan C, Lamy C, *et al.*: Recurrent cerebrovascular events associated with patent foramen ovale, atrial septal aneurysm, or both. *N Engl J Med* 2001, 345:1740–1746.

38. Voros S, Nanda NC, Thakur AC, *et al.*: Lambl's excrescences (valvular strands). *Echocardiography* 1999, 16:399–414.

39. Roldan CA, Shively BK, Crawford MH: Valve excrescences: prevalence, evolution and risk for cardioembolism. *J Am Coll Cardiol* 1997, 30:1308–1314.

40. Cohen A, Tzourio C, Chauvel C, *et al.*: Mitral valve strands and the risk of ischemic stroke in elderly patients. *Stroke* 1997, 28:1574–1578.

41. Homma S, Di Tullio MR, Sciacca RR, *et al.*: Effect of aspirin and warfarin therapy in stroke patients with valvular strands. *Stroke* 2004, 35:1436–1442.

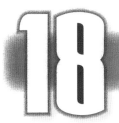

Three-Dimensional Echocardiography and Hand-Carried Cardiac Ultrasound

Victor Mor-Avi, Kirk T. Spencer, Lissa Sugeng, and Roberto M. Lang

From the time that ultrasound imaging first provided insight into the human heart, our diagnostic capabilities have exponentially increased as a result of the growing knowledge and developing technology. This chapter focuses on two exciting and recent developments in echocardiography: real-time three-dimensional imaging and hand-carried imaging systems. Although they are continuing their meteoric rise, these tools currently provide valuable clinical information that empowers us with new levels of confidence in the diagnosis of heart disease and is steadily winning the trust of cardiologists worldwide.

Three-Dimensional Echocardiography

The potential for three-dimensional imaging to overcome the limitations of two-dimensional imaging became obvious in the early 1980s when the initial results of off-line three-dimensional reconstructions from serial multiplane acquisition were reported [1,2]. Such acquisition required electrocardiogram gating and relied on the assumption that all planes would be acquired during the same respiratory phase to ensure for each plane to have an identical shape and position of the ventricle within the chest. Over the past decade, a different approach was pursued in order to eliminate the need for tedious multiplane acquisition and time consuming three-dimensional reconstruction. This approach is based on real-time volumetric imaging by using transducers that contain arrays of piezoelectric elements capable of scanning pyramidal volumes, rather than single-plane sectors. In the early 1990s, a dedicated system, based on the use of a sparse array transducer with parallel processing, allowed real-time three-dimensional ultrasound imaging of the heart for the first time [3]. Despite the relatively low spatial and temporal resolution, this system allowed fast acquisition of pyramidal datasets during a single breath hold without the need for off-line reconstruction.

This system was then used to demonstrate the additional benefits of this modality in multiple clinical scenarios, thus providing the basis for the development of smaller transthoracic matrix phased-array transducers with larger numbers of crystals and faster scanners. These newer systems are based on modern digital processing and improved image formation algorithms in order to allow higher spatial and temporal resolution for real-time volumetric imaging and have since become commercially available. Their increasing availability gave rise to growing research efforts geared towards embracing this new technology. More recently, novel electronic circuitry, with advanced miniaturized beam forming technology that accommodates thousands of elements, was developed to fit into the tip of a transesophageal transducer. This fully sampled matrix array transesophageal probe allows real-time three-dimensional acquisition and online display of unique three-dimensional views of unparalleled quality for optimal visualization of cardiac structures [4].

The usefulness of three-dimensional echocardiography has been demonstrated in several areas, including 1) direct evaluation of cardiac chamber volumes and mass without the need for geometric modeling and the detrimental effects of foreshortened views; 2) direct three-dimensional assessment of regional LV wall motion and quantification of systolic asynchrony to guide ventricular resynchronization therapy; 3) volumetric imaging and quantification of myocardial perfusion; 4) unique realistic views of cardiac valves, and 5) three-dimensional color Doppler imaging with volumetric evaluation of regurgitant lesions and shunts.

Although quantification of LV size and function relied on tedious, manual, or at best semiautomated tracing of endocardial boundaries in multiple planes in earlier three-dimensional studies, today it is based on almost fully automated frame-by-frame detection of the three-dimensional endocardial surface from real-time three-dimensional datasets. Almost all studies that have directly compared the accuracy of three-dimensional measurements of LV volumes and ejection fraction (EF) have demonstrated the superiority of the three-dimensional approach over the two-dimensional methodology, which was shown to consistently underestimate LV volumes. This superiority was demonstrated in both accuracy and reproducibility when compared with independent reference techniques, such as radionuclide ventriculography and MRI [5–8]. The use of real-time three-dimensional imaging in combination with contrast enhancement has been shown to improve the visualization of the endocardial surface in patients with poor acoustic windows [9]. Measurements of LV mass rely not only on endocardial but also on epicardial visualization, which is known to be even more challenging because of the difficulties in identifying the epicardial border. The use of three-dimensional imaging has led to significant improvements in the accuracy and reproducibility of three-dimensional estimates of LV mass compared with their traditional M-mode and two-dimensional counterparts. Quantification of LV volumes, EF, and mass using real-time three-dimensional echocardiography is gaining widespread popularity because of its accuracy and ease of use [8], and it is poised to be routinely used in daily clinical practice.

Volumetric imaging differs substantially from two-dimensional imaging, and it is thus extremely appealing because three-dimensional datasets contain complete dynamic information on LV chamber contraction and filling, from which any ventricular wall can be viewed in any plane and allow more accurate interpretation of regional wall motion. Several studies have explored the potential of quantitative evaluation of regional LV function based on segmental analysis of the dynamic three-dimensional endocardial surface for objective detection of wall motion abnormalities [10,11]. A clinically useful by-product of the three-dimensional quantification of regional LV wall motion is the ability to quantify the temporal aspects of regional endocardial systolic contraction, which have been used for objective serial diagnosis of LV systolic asynchrony in order to guide resynchronization therapy [12–14] and to assess its benefits.

The ability of conventional contrast-enhanced echocardiographic imaging to provide accurate information on the extent and severity of perfusion abnormalities is also limited by its two-dimensional nature. Despite the obvious appeal of the three-dimensional imaging in this context, its use in humans has not been explored until recently. Real-time three-dimensional echocardiography offers an opportunity for online volumetric imaging of the entire heart during a single contrast maneuver. The feasibility of volumetric perfusion imaging was recently tested in experimental animals in conjunction with a new technique for volumetric quantification of myocardial perfusion from contrast-enhanced real-time three-dimensional echocardiographic datasets, as well as in patients undergoing percutaneous coronary interventions [15,16].

Most studies using three-dimensional echocardiography in the context of valvular heart disease have focused on the evaluation of the mitral valve. A variety of mitral valve abnormalities have been demonstrated by three-dimensional reconstructions using gated

transesophageal acquisition. These studies have played a crucial role in describing and quantifying the geometry of the mitral annulus, leaflet surface, tethering distances, and tenting volumes [17]. These studies have also defined and quantified the relationship between the mitral apparatus and the position of the papillary muscles, thus providing insight into the pathophysiology of mitral regurgitation.

The development of matrix array transducers has enabled real-time volumetric imaging of the mitral valve from the transthoracic approach [18], and more recently from the transesophageal approach, with an exquisite level of detail. The use of transthoracic real-time three-dimensional echocardiography in the evaluation of mitral stenosis, mitral valve prolapse, mitral valve perforation, and mitral valve dehiscence and accuracy of mitral valve area measurements has been previously established [19–21]. The main advantage of three-dimensional echocardiography is its ability to achieve a perpendicular en face cut plane of the mitral valve orifice, which enables accurate mitral valve orifice measurements.

Characterization of the mitral valve apparatus using three-dimensional echocardiography has shed new light into the pathophysiology of mitral regurgitation in patients with nonischemic and ischemic cardiomyopathy. It has been recognized that changes in mitral annular size may not be the sole cause of ischemic or dilated mitral regurgitation, and that the presence of mitral regurgitation in these patients is predominantly a disease of the remodeled myocardium rather than secondary to valvular pathology.

The collective experience in visualizing aortic valve disease is more limited when compared with the mitral valve. The challenges with the three-dimensional imaging of the aortic valve are related to the fact that aortic leaflets are thinner and frequently present with heavy calcification, both of which are responsible for drop out artifacts. In patients with aortic stenosis, planimetry of the aortic valve from transesophageal images is more accurate with three-dimensional than with two-dimensional imaging [22]. Transthoracic three-dimensional echocardiography has also resulted in improved visualization of bicuspid aortic valves, aortic vegetations, prosthetic aortic valve regurgitation, and subaortic pathology.

Three-dimensional color flow imaging did not come to fruition until gated transesophageal echocardiography (TEE) methods and computer software allowed reconstruction of three-dimensional color flow jets superimposed on the reconstructed gray scale data. With the ability to combine three-dimensional color flow with gray scale information, it became possible to improve the detection of the origin and direction of regurgitant jets, measure regurgitant orifice areas, as well as improve the identification of the origin of valvular and paravalvular regurgitation and the detection of multiple jets [23,24]. Volumetric color flow imaging has overcome some of its initial limitations and proved useful in estimating regurgitant volumes, stroke volumes, and cardiac output together with the delineation of valve regurgitation.

The recent addition of the transesophageal matrix array transducer provides unique three-dimensional views of cardiac anatomy in real time, including the mitral valve, interatrial septum, left atrial appendage, pulmonic veins, and the LV. The exceptional quality of the images of the mitral valve reported by several investigators suggests that this modality will become the "gold standard" for preoperative planning of mitral valve surgery and guidance of percutaneous interventions. This transducer also provides unparalleled views of both bioprosthetic and mechanical valve components, including leaflets, rings, and struts. The significant improvements in three-dimensional image quality with this probe have also enabled parallel development of three-dimensional volumetric quantification techniques.

Future advances in transducer and computer technology will allow wider angle acquisition and color flow imaging to be completed in a single cardiac cycle, which will shorten data acquisition and eliminate stitching artifacts. Transducers will have a smaller footprint with higher spatial and temporal resolution. In addition, transducers limited to two-dimensional imaging will be gradually phased out and replaced by new probes that will be versatile in their capability of imaging in different modes, including two-dimensional, three-dimensional, and color and tissue Doppler, just like the recently developed matrix TEE probe. With these multitasking transducers, it may be possible to significantly reduce the number of steps required to complete an echocardiographic examination, and thus reduce the time of the test. We also anticipate that improved quantification of all cardiac chambers, including flow dynamics, will be performed on the imaging system in an increasingly automated fashion, which will gradually eliminate the need for off-line analysis. This is of crucial importance in intervention settings, such as the catheterization laboratory and the operating department, where immediate visual and quantitative feedback is important. For the purposes of interpretation and storage, it is vital that the three-dimensional datasets are incorporated into digital information systems with full rendering and quantification capabilities.

In summary, we anticipate that (similar to transthoracic real-time three-dimensional imaging, which is being continuously integrated into the routine echocardiographic examination), transesophageal real-time three-dimensional imaging will become routine in the operating department and as a guiding tool for different percutaneous procedures in the coming years. Currently, there is sufficient evidence that three-dimensional imaging is superior to traditional two-dimensional echocardiography and should be routinely used in two clinic scenarios: quantification of LV volume and EF, and quantification of the mitral valve orifice area in mitral stenosis. Future clinical applications of this technology are also likely to include stress testing with real-time volumetric or simultaneous multiplane imaging from a single transducer position. Overall, the large number of recent publications on real-time three-dimensional echocardiographic imaging reflects the rapidly growing body of knowledge necessary for widely accepting and incorporating this methodology into the arsenal of clinic cardiac imaging [25]. In some instances, the scientific evidence seems strong enough to endorse the use of three-dimensional echocardiography as a new standard in the clinical evaluation of the heart.

Hand-Carried Cardiac Ultrasound

The evolution of ultrasound machines over the last decade has focused on improved performance, enhanced analysis, and the incorporation of new technologies. This has augmented the diagnostic capabilities of cardiac ultrasound, but it has also driven up the cost of echocardiographic platforms substantially. Several ultrasound manufacturers have recently developed devices that are small enough to be carried easily and used at the patient's bedside. Although these devices have become commercially available only recently, Roelandt et al. [26] introduced real-time bedside imaging using a hand-held ultrasound scanner as early as 1978.

Investigators have begun working with these small platforms, and many have been coining their own terminology for this technology. The American Society of Echocardiography Task Force on New Technology has suggested the term "hand-carried ultrasound" or "HCU" for these devices. Although initially used to describe small ultrasound devices with basic two-dimensional and color Doppler imaging capabilities, the term HCU has deviated from this definition. The defining features of HCU platforms are their small size, ability to be battery powered, and being relatively low in price. Using these criteria, it is clear that HCU should not be used to describe devices that are essentially small full-featured echocardiograph platforms. Although a single person can carry these devices, they are not reasonably light for a physician to carry from bedside to bedside on rounds. In addition, their extensive functionality (including packages for contrast echocardiography, stress, and transesophageal echocardiography) makes them quite expensive and therefore not true HCU devices, even though they are less expensive than traditional platforms. The role of cardiac HCU in clinical practice is in evolution and is explored in this chapter.

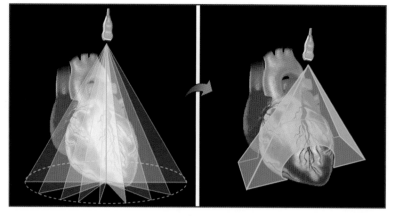

Figure 18-1. Earlier, three-dimensional echocardiography was performed from a sequential multiplane acquisition approach, gated to electrocardiography and respiration (*left panel*). This approach was tedious, time consuming, and prone to radial artifacts. This approach was recently replaced by real-time volumetric imaging that allows acquisition of a pyramid of data (*right panel*) using matrix array transducers.

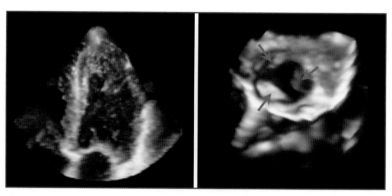

Figure 18-2. Transthoracic real-time three-dimensional images of the heart extracted from the pyramidal datasets show an apical four-chamber cross-sectional view obtained from a full volume acquisition (*left panel*) and zoomed acquisition of the aortic valve in early systole, shown from the LV perspective, depicting the three aortic valve leaflets (*right panel, arrows*).

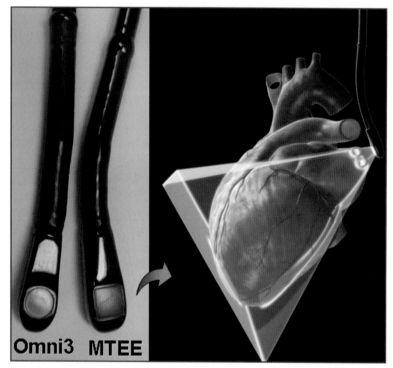

Figure 18-3. Multiplane Omni3 (Philips Medical Systems, Andover, MA) and matrix array transesophageal (MTEE) transducers, shown side by side (*left panel*). Although the dimensions of both transducers are similar, the MTEE probe that uses miniaturized beam forming technology allows fitting of nearly 3000 piezoelectric elements into the head of the probe, providing real-time volumetric imaging of the heart (*right panel*).

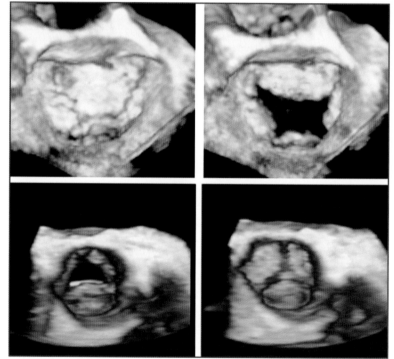

Figure 18-4. Examples of systolic (*left panels*) and diastolic (*right panels*) still frames, obtained from a zoomed real-time matrix transesophageal echocardiography dataset showing the mitral valve from the left atrial perspective (*top panels*) and the aortic valves (*bottom panels*) from the ascending aorta. (*From* Sugeng *et al.* [4]; with permission.)

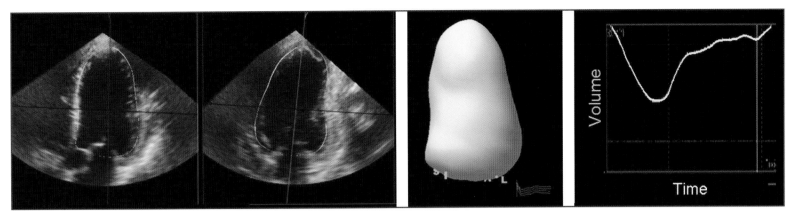

Figure 18-5. Semiautomated analysis of LV volume from a real-time three-dimensional dataset shows examples of apical four- and two-chamber cut planes (*left-hand panels*) obtained from a pyramidal dataset with the endocardial contours. Optimization of the boundaries in multiple planes results in a cast of the LV cavity (*middle panel*), which can be repeated frame by frame throughout the cardiac cycle to calculate LV volume over time (*right panel*).

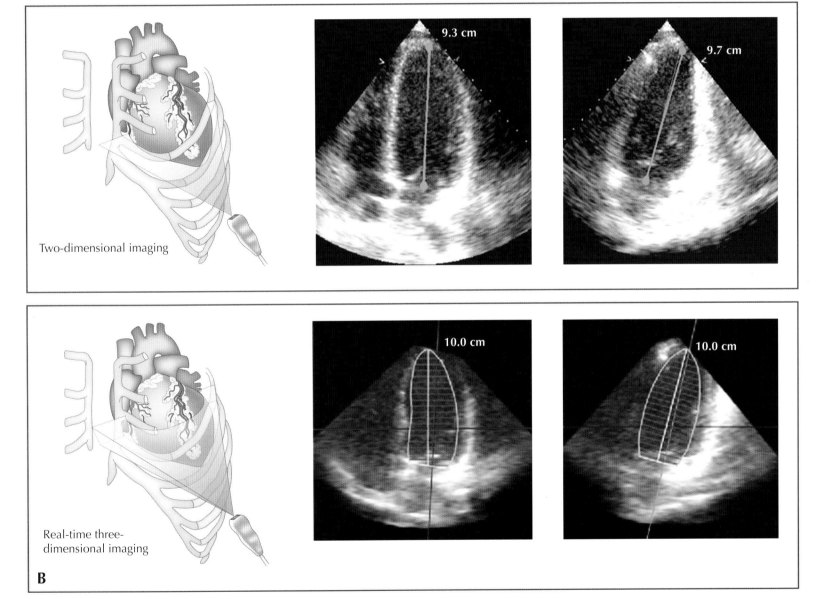

Figure 18-6. Imaging the LV from an apical window frequently results in foreshortened views. This is because the imaging plane, obtained through the intercostal space nearest to the LV apex (**A**, *left image*), may not necessarily contain the true LV apex. Tilting the transducer in order to improve endocardial visualization can result in even more anatomically oblique views, in which the long-axis dimension of the LV is foreshortened (**A**, *right images*). With real-time three-dimensional imaging from the same transducer position (**B**, *left image*), the entire LV is included in the full volume scan, which allows for the use of cropping identification of the anatomically correct nonforeshortened views for analysis (**B**, *right images*). In this example, the long-axis dimension was longer in both apical views when measured from the three-dimensional dataset.

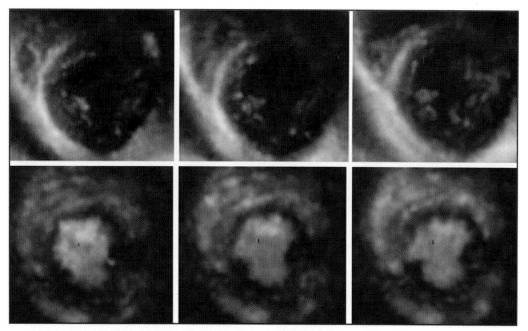

Figure 18-7. Three-dimensional endocardial visualization can be improved by contrast enhancement, as seen in these three LV short-axis cut planes extracted from a pyramidal dataset obtained in a patient with poor image quality. Note the poor endocardial definition in the non-enhanced images (*top panels*) and the improvement with contrast enhancement (*bottom panels*).

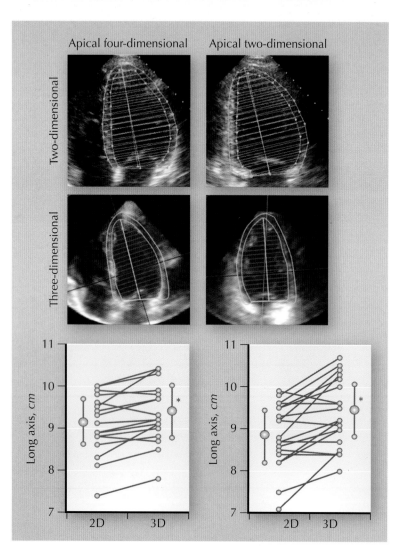

Figure 18-8. End-diastolic apical two- and four-chamber views of the LV obtained in a patient using conventional two-dimensional imaging (*top panels*) and anatomically correct apical four- and two-chamber cut planes selected from a real-time three-dimensional (*bottom panels*) dataset obtained in the same subject (*middle panels*). Manually traced endocardial and epicardial boundaries used to calculate LV mass are shown on the images. Note the increase in the length of the LV long axis in both apical views, as assessed by the three-dimensional–guided technique. Mean ± SD, $P < 0.05$, is represented (*large circles* and *error bars*). (*From* Mor-Avi *et al.* [27]; with permission.)

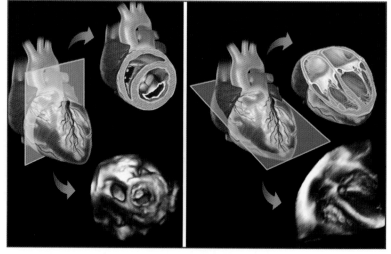

Figure 18-9. Schematic representation of how different cut planes of the heart can be extracted from a pyramidal three-dimensional dataset. The basal short-axis view of the LV depicts the mitral and tricuspid valves (*left panel, yellow cut plane*). The apical four-chamber view depicts the inferoseptal, inferior, and inferolateral walls (*right panel, green plane*). (*From* Nanda *et al.* [28]; with permission.)

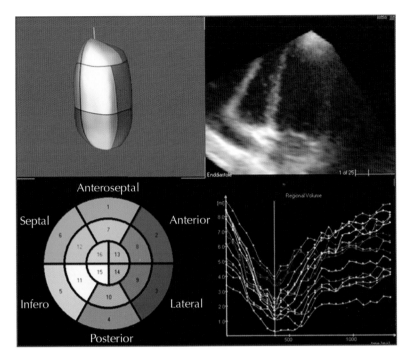

Figure 18-10. An apical four-chamber view extracted from the real-time three-dimensional dataset (*top right panel*) and the detected endocardial surface (*top left panel*) are used for three-dimensional analysis of regional LV wall motion. Schematic "bull's eye" represents the three-dimensional segmentation (*bottom left panel*), with the color notation used for the different segments in both the endocardial surface (*top left panel*) and the regional LV-volume–time curves (*bottom right panel*).

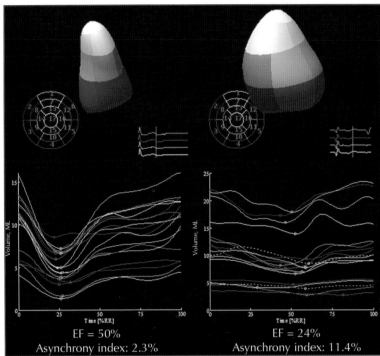

Figure 18-11. Two LV casts were obtained in a normal subject (*top left panel*) and in a patient with dilated cardiomyopathy (*top right panel*). The individual regional ejection fraction (EF) time intervals are used to calculate the asynchrony index, which is calculated as the standard deviation of the mean of these time intervals. In this example, the asynchrony index is considerably shorter in the synchronized normal ventricle (*bottom left panel*), compared with the disorganized contraction pattern in the patient with the dilated ventricle (*bottom right panel*).

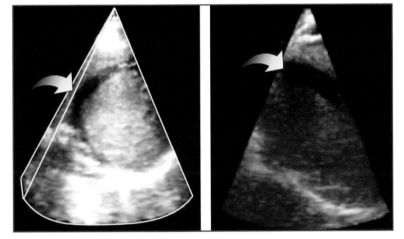

Figure 18-12. Narrow-angled end-systolic pyramidal dataset obtained in a patient with severe proximal left anterior descending stenosis (*left panel*) during steady state contrast infusion shows a lack of contrast enhancement in a section of the interventricular septum, indicating a perfusion defect (*left panel, arrow*). This defect was visible in multiple cross-sections (*right panel, arrow*). Therefore, this technique is likely to allow more accurate estimation of the extent of the hypoperfused area. (*From* Toledo *et al.* [15]; with permission.)

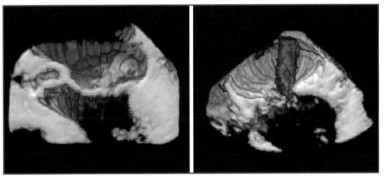

Figure 18-13. This three-dimensional rendering of a mitral valve, reconstructed from a gated sequential multiplane transesophageal acquisition (*left panel*), depicts a flail P2 leaflet scallop (*arrow*). The three-dimensional color Doppler image was obtained in a patient after unsuccessful mitral valve repair (*right panel*), demonstrating a central jet of mitral regurgitation.

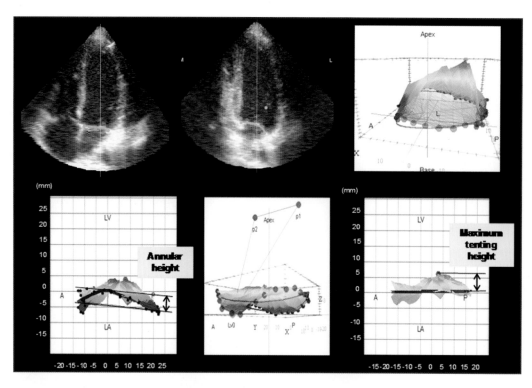

Figure 18-14. Quantification of mitral valve geometry from volumetric real-time three-dimensional datasets can be achieved by using specialized analysis software, which can be used to calculate annular height (*bottom left panel*), papillary muscle position in three-dimensional space (*bottom middle panel*), and tenting height and volume (*right panels*).

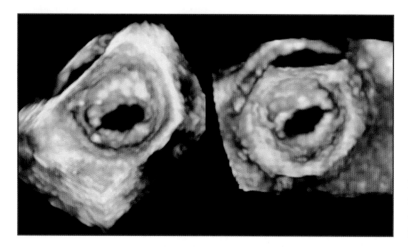

Figure 18-15. Real-time three-dimensional zoomed transesophageal views of a mitral valve from left atrial (*left panel*) and LV (*right panel*) perspectives obtained in a patient with severe rheumatic mitral stenosis are shown. Note the thickened mitral valve leaflets and fused medial and lateral commissures.

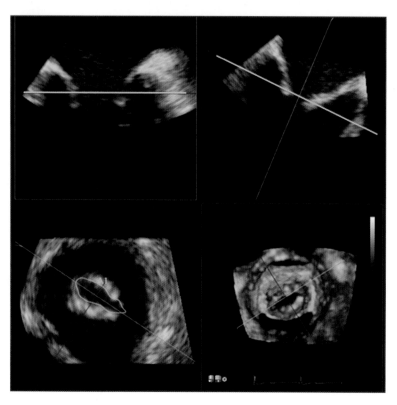

Figure 18-16. Mitral valve planimetry in a patient with mitral stenosis performed on a zoomed real-time three-dimensional transesophageal echocardiography dataset (*bottom right panel*). The advantage of three-dimensional echocardiography in the quantification of mitral valve orifice area is that it provides an en face display of the mitral apparatus, thus allowing planimetry to be performed at the tips of the mitral leaflets (*top panels, blue lines*).

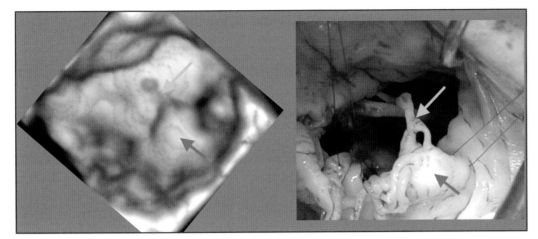

Figure 18-17. Real-time transthoracic zoomed acquisition of the mitral valve, as visualized from the left atrial perspective in a patient with P2 flail scallop (*green arrows in both panels*). Note the ruptured cord attached to the flail scallop (*blue arrows in both panels*). The surgical findings obtained in this patient (*right panel*) confirmed the three-dimensional diagnosis (*From* Sugeng *et al.* [18]; with permission.)

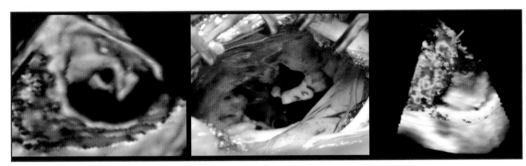

Figure 18-18. Real-time transthoracic zoomed acquisition of the mitral valve, as visualized from the left atrial perspective in a patient with a perforated anterior leaflet (*left panel*), secondary to bacterial endocarditis, is shown. The surgical findings obtained in this patient (*middle panel*) confirmed the three-dimensional diagnosis. The use of real-time three-dimensional color Doppler depicted the presence of a flow convergence jet through the perforation (*right panel, arrow*) (*From* Sugeng *et al.* [18]; with permission.)

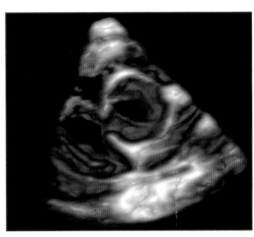

Figure 18-19. Real-time transthoracic zoomed acquisition of a bicuspid aortic valve as visualized from the aortic perspective.

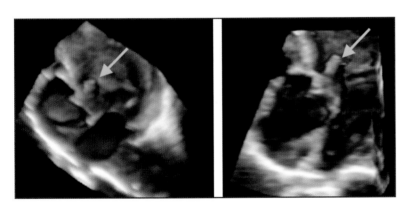

Figure 18-20. Real-time transthoracic zoomed acquisition of the aortic valve in a patient with aortic vegetations (*arrows*).

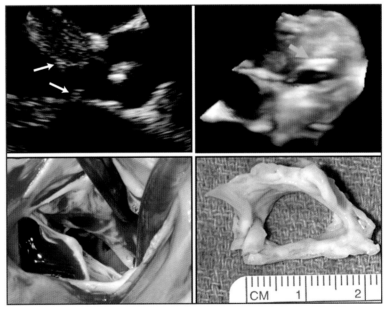

Figure 18-21. Parasternal transthoracic echocardiogram showing concentric LV hypertrophy and a subaortic membrane (*top left, arrows*). Narrowly angled three-dimensional acquisition, in which the LV outflow track has been cropped in order to visualize the rigid membrane with a single, slit-like opening, is shown (*top right, arrow*). Note the similarities between the morphology of the subaortic membrane and the orifice compared with the surgical findings (*bottom left*) and the view of the excised membrane (*bottom right*). (*From* Carr *et al.* [29]; with permission.)

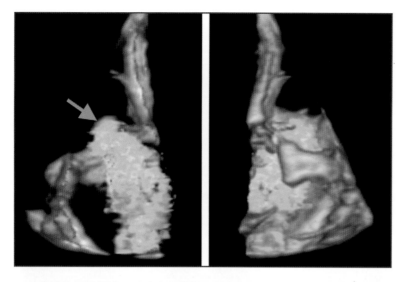

Figure 18-22. Real-time three-dimensional views of color flow, superimposed on a gray-scale image, in a patient with severe tricuspid regurgitation is shown. Note the area of flow convergence (*arrow*).

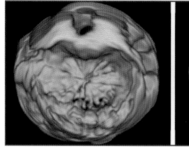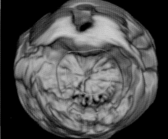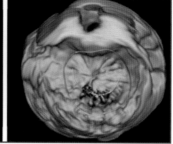

Figure 18-23. Gated sequential multiplane transesophageal acquisition of the mitral valve with mild regurgitation is visualized from the left atrial perspective (*left panel*). The mitral annulus as well as the area of leaflet coaptation is depicted (*middle panel, green line*). The three-dimensional color Doppler jet aids in the determination of the jet origin (*right panel*).

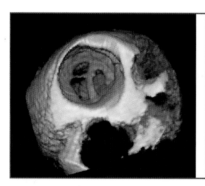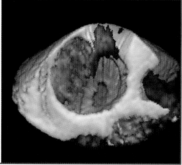

Figure 18-24. Sequential multiplane transesophageal acquisition of a dehisced mitral valve ring, as viewed from the left atrial perspective (*left panel*) with severe paravalvular mitral regurgitation is depicted by three-dimensional color Doppler (*right panel*).

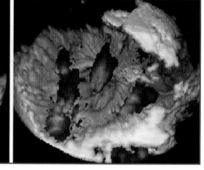

Figure 18-25. Gated sequential multiplane transesophageal acquisition of a bioprosthetic mitral valve with regurgitation is visualized, with the left atrial perspective in diastole (*left panel*) and midsystole (*right panel*). Note the multiple jets originating in the para-ring area [24].

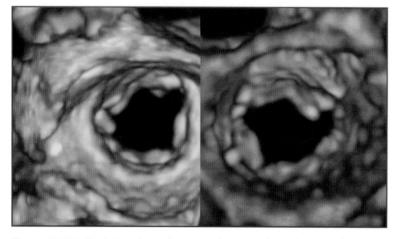

Figure 18-26. Real-time three-dimensional tranesophageal echocardiography views of the mitral valve from the left atrial (*left panel*) and LV (*right panel*) perspectives obtained during diastole.

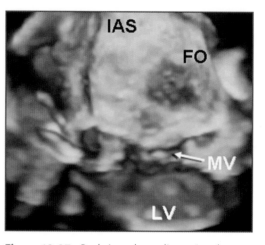

Figure 18-27. Real-time three-dimensional transesophageal echocardiography zoomed acquisition of the interatrial septum (IAS) depicting the foramen ovale (FO) from the left atrial perspective. (*From* Sugeng *et al.* [4]; with permission.) MV—mitral valve.

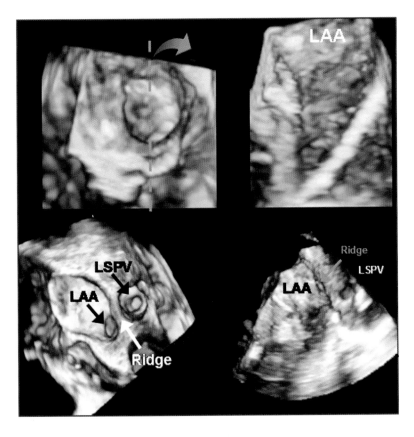

Figure 18-28. Examples of the left atrial appendage (LAA) visualized en face (*top left panel*) and in the long-axis view (*top right panel*). The ridge separating the LAA from the left upper pulmonary vein (LSPV) is depicted (*bottom panels*).

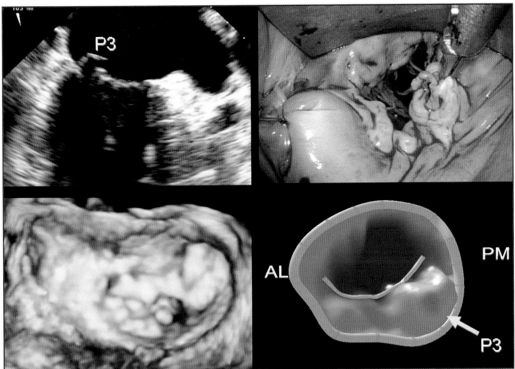

Figure 18-29. Example of a patient with a flail mitral valve (P3 scallop), as visualized with two-dimensional echocardiography (*top left panel*), real-time three-dimensional transesophageal echocardiography volume rendering (*bottom left panel*), as well a surgical view (*top right panel*) and a three-dimensional rendering obtained using software designed for quantitative analysis of the mitral apparatus (*bottom right panel*). The portion of the posterior mitral leaflet shaded in yellow (*arrow*) indicates the flail P3 scallop. AL—antero-lateral; PM—posteromedial. (*From* Sugeng *et al.* [4]; with permission.)

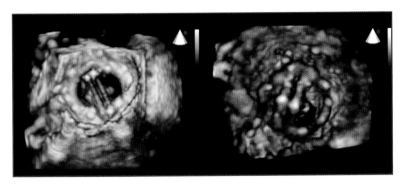

Figure 18-30. Real-time three-dimensional transesophageal echocardiography views of a mechanical bileaflet prosthetic mitral valve as visualized from the left atrial (*left panel*) and LV (*right panel*) perspectives.

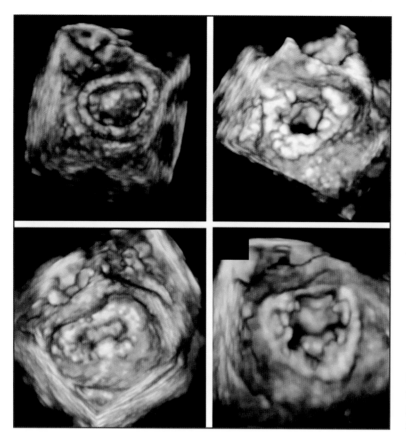

Figure 18-31. Real-time three-dimensional transesophageal echocardiography views of mitral valve rings, including a rigid ring (*top left panel*), flexible ring (*top right panel*), Geoform ring (Geoform, Inc., Inglewood, CA) (*bottom left panel*), and Simplicity (Medtronic, Minneapolis, MN) ring (*bottom right panel*).

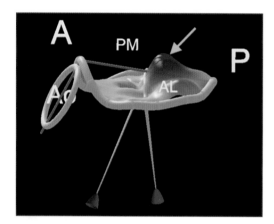

Figure 18-32. Quantitative analysis of the mitral valve geometry can be performed using specialized software capable of quantifying multiple parameters, including annular area, dimensions, height, leaflet surface area and length, prolapse volume (*arrow*), aortic mitral angle (*green lines*), and papillary muscle positions in three-dimensional space (*red carrots*). A—anterior; Ao—aorta; AL—anterolateral; P—posterior; PM—posteromedial.

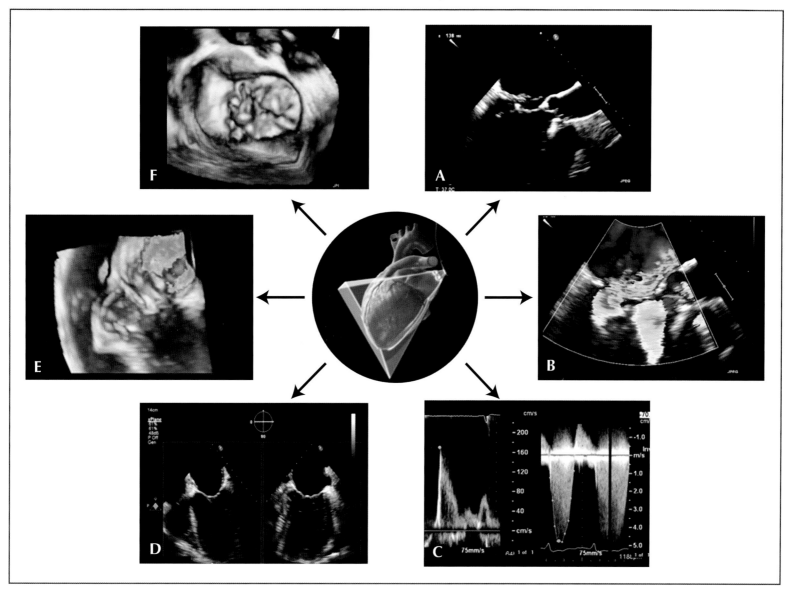

Figure 18-33. The three-dimensional matrix array transducer is capable of performing traditional two-dimensional and Doppler imaging (**A**, **B**, and **C**), as well as simultaneous biplane imaging, three-dimensional color flow, and real-time three-dimensional imaging (**D**, **E**, and **F**). (*From* Sugeng *et al.* [30]; with permission.)

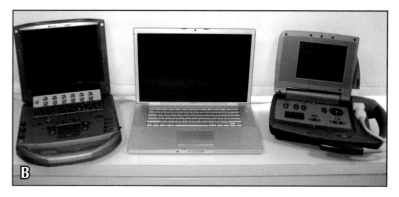

A Essential Features of a Hand-carried Ultrasound Device		
	Traditional Echocardiography Platform	**HCU**
Controls	Complex	Simple
Power supply	A/C	Battery
Weight	+++++	+
Price	+++++	++

Figure 18-34. Although devices of 10 to 20 lb can be "carried" (**A**), most would only consider using HCU device instruments that can be easily carried from patient room to patient room; this would typically mean platforms of less than 6 to 7 lb. More recent devices weighing less than 3 lb are currently available. The other key features are battery power, simplicity of operation, and relatively low cost. Typical hand-carried devices (**B**, *left and right*) are shown with a laptop computer (**B**, *middle*) for scale.

Comparison of Traditional and Hand-carried Ultrasound Platforms

	Traditional Echo Platform	HCU
Two-dimensional	+	+
Harmonics	+	+ / -
Color Doppler	+	+ / -
Spectral Doppler	+	+ / -
Tissue Doppler imaging	+	+ / -
Three-dimensional imaging	+	-
Image storage	Tape/hard drive/DVD	None or limited
Image analysis	Advanced	Limited

Figure 18-35. The small sizes of these hand-carried ultrasound (HCU) devices require a compromise in functionality. All have two-dimensional imaging, but tools used to enhance images in difficult patients, such as harmonics, lateral gain compensation, compression, persistence, colorization, and focus are not routinely available with HCU. Basic units lack the capabilities for assessing valve hemodynamic, diastolic function, or filling pressures, but are smaller and simpler to use, as well as being less expensive. Others are more full featured, but the additional functionality significantly increases their cost, which in turn limits their use in several of the proposed use models of HCU. In addition, more features greatly increase the training requirements, which also limit the use of these platforms for many of their proposed applications. There is a dual movement in device development—on one hand, providing more features; on the other, further miniaturization.

Comparison of Traditional and Hand-carried Ultrasound Echocardiography Examinations

	Traditional Echo Platform	HCU
Personnel	Sonographer/cardiologist	Health care provider
Examination	Complete	Focused, user defined
Examination duration	45–60 min	2–10 min
Examination location	Echocardiography laboratory	Bedside
Images	Archived	± Archived
Documentation	Formal report	?
Training	ASE/ACC guidelines	?

ACC—American College of Cardiology; ASE—American Society of Echocardiography.

Figure 18-36. In addition to differences in the platforms themselves, hand-carried ultrasound (HCU) examinations are inherently different from studies performed on a full featured platform. These devices are most often used at the bedside outside the echocardiographic laboratory in environments not optimal for imaging. With an HCU examination, the examiner decides which image acquisitions constitute a targeted study to address the relevant clinical question, yet remains within the scope of their training. One could envision a complex set of "limited examination" protocols that would differ depending on examiner expertise and clinical scenario. Acceptance of HCU beyond cardiology will depend on the willingness of users to accept responsibility for image acquisition, documentation, and interpretation, as well as how the information provided by HCU is used in patient care.

Uses of Hand-carried Ultrasound in Cardiovascular Medicine

Extension of the physical examination

Bedside evaluation of a patient by a cardiologist

Bedside evaluation of a patient by a noncardiologist

Screening for cardiovascular disease

Education

Figure 18-37. Although the role of hand-carried ultrasound (HCU) devices in cardiovascular medicine is still evolving, several use models have shown promise. These uses all leverage HCU's strengths of portability and ease of use compared with full platform ultrasound. The use of these devices to replace a standard examination with an inexpensive device is not appropriate because the image quality and diagnostic capabilities are inferior, and patient evaluation would be compromised.

Issues Affecting the Diagnostic Accuracy of Hand-carried Ultrasound

Device imaging quality

Harmonics

Image display size

Experience/training of personnel acquiring images

Experience/training of personnel interpreting images

Location/setting of imaging

Patient factors

Clinical question

Figure 18-38. The small size of these devices involves compromises related to image quality and display size. These concessions lead to the need to address whether the images are clinically useful. Additionally, hand-carried ultrasound (HCU) images may be acquired by personnel with substantially less experience than fully trained sonographers or level 2 trained echocardiographers. Not only acquisition experience, but also the experience of the persons interpreting the images will greatly affect the diagnostic accuracy of these devices. Patient factors, such as body size, play a role in the accuracy of HCU imaging, which is no different than traditional echocardiography. Some of the settings where rapid bedside HCU imaging would be useful, such as the intensive care settings, unfortunately involve patients and conditions that are most hostile to good echocardiographic images. It stands to reason that the devices with the most limited capabilities would perform more poorly in these settings [31].

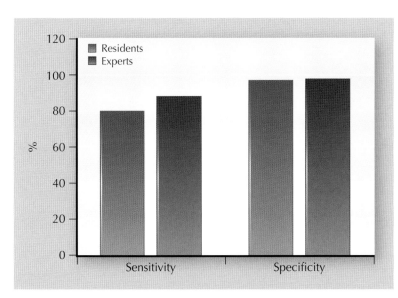

Figure 18-39. The accuracy of hand-carried ultrasound (HCU) devices is depicted. It is clear that when trained sonographers or physicians with level 2 or 3 echocardiographic training use HCU devices, their accuracy for the detection of two-dimensional and color Doppler findings is excellent [32–36]. Most of the studies comparing HCU and traditional ultrasound platforms are limited by only evaluating the agreement or sensitivity between the two modalities. This approach is limited by the significant intraobserver variability of standard echocardiography. Rugolotto *et al.* [34] demonstrated that major differences between HCU and standard echocardiography are no more common than the intraobserver differences of standard echocardiography. However, even in expert hands, HCU devices do show differences with full featured echocardiography for minor findings, especially in mild degrees of valvular regurgitation and the extent of regional wall motion abnormalities. When HCU devices are used by users less trained, their accuracy declines. The ability of inexperienced users to accurately diagnose echocardiographic abnormalities is partially dependent on what abnormality they are looking for and how much training they have received. After receiving 20 hours of didactic instruction and performing 20 supervised transthoracic studies, medical residents demonstrated the ability to detect clinically important abnormalities with lower sensitivity (88% vs 80%) and similar specificity (98% vs 97%) to that of level 3 trained echocardiographers [37]. Inexperienced imagers have more difficulty interpreting RV function and LV regional wall motion abnormalities.

Cardiac Pathology Detected by Physical Examination and Hand-carried Ultrasound

	HCU Superior to Physical Examination
Aortic regurgitation	Y
Aortic stenosis	N
Mitral regurgitation	Y
Tricuspid regurgitation	Y
RV dysfunction	Y
LV systolic dysfunction	Y
Pericardial effusion	Y
Elevated JVP	Y

JVP—jugular venous pressure

Figure 18-40. Although physical examination is essential when evaluating patients with suspected cardiac disease, studies assessing the accuracy of physical examination have shown significant error and omission rates for physicians at all levels of training. As echocardiography can diagnose cardiovascular conditions with excellent sensitivity and specificity, hand-carried ultrasound (HCU) has been evaluated as a tool for extending the physical examination. It is clear that when used by physicians with a broad range of echocardiographic and physical examination experience, HCU improves the detection of many cardiac findings [38–42]. Even when compared with those most experienced in cardiac physical examination, HCU improves the identification of cardiovascular pathology [41,42]. On the other hand, HCU will never replace the physical examination. For example, the detection of a cardiomyopathy does not tell a physician if the patient is in heart failure, and the presence of a pericardial rub certainly changes the evaluation of an echocardiographically detected pericardial effusion. HCU is best used in combination with a comprehensive cardiac physical examination.

Bedside Uses of Hand-carried Ultrasound Devices by a Cardiovascular Specialist

Patient Group	HCU Impact
Evaluation of patients presenting to outpatient cardiology clinic	Confirmed or rejected clinical diagnosis 78%, definite diagnosis 31%
Evaluation of hospitalized patients with cardiology consultation request	Immediate change in clinical management 48%, influenced treatment decision 63%
Evaluation of ED patients with CP	Negative predictive value for ACS, 100%
Inpatients on cardiology service	Expedited triage 25%, unanticipated clinically useful finding 21%

ACS—acute coronary syndrome; CP—chest pain; ED—emergency department

Figure 18-41. One of the early uses of hand-carried ultrasound (HCU) was by cardiovascular specialists with level 3 expertise in echocardiography at the bedside or in clinic. This use model is attractive because these physicians were already well trained in the performance and interpretation of echocardiography. On the other hand, patients with cardiovascular symptoms or signs probably merit complete evaluation with a full platform ultrasound device performed by an experienced sonographer. This HCU use model is best reserved for limited situations when a rapid bedside decision is required and an experienced echocardiographer is present. In this setting, the initial diagnostic impression and treatment plan formulated at the bedside may be confirmed or more importantly altered by the result of the bedside HCU [43–49].

Bedside Uses of Hand-carried Ultrasound Devices by Noncardiologists

Personnel	Patients
Emergency department physicians	All patients (like stethoscope)
Cardiology fellows	High-risk patients
Intensivists	Patients with cardiac symptoms
Internists/hospitalists	Bedside (when full echocardiography
Medical residents	is not available)
Medical students	Bedside targeted echocardiography
Nurses	

Figure 18-42. A growing use of cardiac hand-carried ultrasound (HCU) is the performance of directed bedside evaluation by noncardiologists [37,50–58]. There are a number of reasons why this use model is attractive. For example, there are many situations in which rapid answers are needed, and cardiologists are not immediately available, such as the emergency department and medical intensive care unit. In other settings, such as remote or underserved clinics, access to echocardiography is limited or unavailable [59,60]. For many patients, the internist or hospitalist is their contact with medical care. In these situations, increasing the detection of cardiovascular abnormalities might allow earlier treatment and referral to a cardiovascular specialist. Some disorders might benefit from daily bedside echocardiography, which is impractical for anyone but for the treating physician. Congestive heart failure is such a disorder, and daily bedside HCU of the inferior vena cava has shown promise in identifying patients who remain volume overloaded and are at high risk for hospital readmission. For medical residents and students, HCU use may be most useful because these are the groups in which physical examination is more likely to miss findings. For these trainees, the HCU serves to ensure that findings are not missed, as well as serving as a training tool to improve their physical examination skills [61]. Lastly, HCU by nurses could be used before the physician encounter in order to provide information additional to the vital signs [62]. As the positive predictive value in nonexperienced users is lower, it is clear that all abnormal findings should be confirmed with a traditional echocardiographic examination. Likewise, a "negative" HCU examination in a patient with a cardiovascular symptom or sign should prompt a complete echocardiographic evaluation because of the lower sensitivity of less experienced HCU users and the more limited diagnostic capabilities of these devices.

Cardiovascular Abnormalities That Can Be Detected by Screening with Hand-carried Ultrasound Devices

Abdominal aortic aneurysm

Left atrial enlargement

LV hypertrophy

LV dysfunction

Pericardial effusion

Regional wall motion abnormalities

RV dysfunction

Valvular heart disease

Figure 18-43. One of the greatest potential uses for hand-carried ultrasound (HCU) devices is in screening for cardiovascular disease, such as performing HCU examinations on subjects who do not have an indication for echocardiography. A number of approaches have been used. The first is simply to perform an abbreviated echocardiographic examination, screening for valvular heart disease, ventricular dysfunction, regional wall motion abnormalities, and pericardial effusion. The rate of abnormal findings depends on the population screened. When patients on an inpatient medical service are screened, 39% are found to have a clinically important finding [40]. When outpatients at an underserved clinic are screened, the abnormal finding incidence is 12.4% [60]. A second approach is to perform focused screening examinations for a specific finding. HCU has proven to be a valuable tool in screening for abdominal aortic aneurysms, left atrial enlargement, and LV hypertrophy [63–65].

Advantages of Using Hand-Carried Ultrasound to Screen for LV Systolic Dysfunction

Relatively inexpensive compared with traditional echocardiography

Portable, allowing screening outside hospital setting

Excellent accuracy for detecting LVSD

Superior to physical examination for detecting LVSD

Negative predictive value of HCU is excellent

Positive predictive value of HCU higher than BNP screening

More cost effective than traditional echocardiography screening

Can be performed by personnel with limited training

BNP—brain natriuretic factor

Figure 18-44. Left ventricular systolic dysfunction (LVSD) is probably the most important cardiovascular condition that hand-carried ultrasound (HCU) can be used to screen for. LVSD is an ideal target for screening for several reasons. It is prevalent (2%–8%, depending on age), it may be asymptomatic, it is often undetected on physical examination, it is associated with significant morbidity and mortality, and very effective therapies can be implemented once it is detected. It is clear that HCU (when performed by experienced imagers) can assess LVSD with accuracies of 96% to 98% compared with traditional echocardiography [36,66]. In comparison with several other screening techniques, HCU screening for LVSD appears to be cost effective, particularly when performed in high-risk subgroups. However, in order to be effective as a screening technique, the use of less experienced personnel is critical; not only does this lower cost, but it opens screening to a much broader group of patients. Several studies have evaluated using physicians with limited echocardiographic training to screen for LVSD. When outpatients without cardiac symptoms were screened with HCU, LVSD was detected in 3.3% [60]. This is similar to the rate of asymptomatic LVSD reported in the community using full platform devices (1.8% to 4.0%) [67]. When more significantly ill patients, such as hospitalized patients, are screened with HCU, the rate of LVSD rises to 10% [40]. Early experience suggests that nurses can be trained to use HCU to perform LVSD screening in high-risk patients [40,62].

A Unresolved Issues in HCU

Training

Who should be trained

What is adequate training duration

Should training be specific to type of examination

Assessment of competency

Recertification

Reimbursment for HCU

Documentation

Image documentation

Documentation of findings/report generation

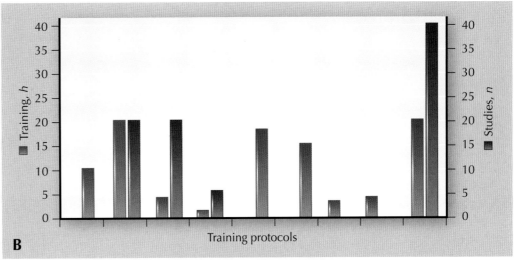

Figure 18-45. Unresolved issues in cardiac hand-carried ultrasound (HCU) are shown. There are a number of issues that merit more research and sub-specialty professional society recommendations regarding HCU (**A**). Should only level 2 and 3 echocardiographers perform these studies? These devices have proven to be useful in less experienced hands, but what should the training requirements be? The training variation in the published literature is significant (**B**). Some propose 1 to 4 hour hands-on sessions, whereas others recommend 20 hours of didactic training together with 20 to 40 supervised HCU examinations. Contrast this with the American College of Cardiology/American Society of Echocardiography requirements for level 1 and 2 training in echocardiography, which include 480/960 hours of training and performing 75/150 examinations with interpretation of an additional 75/150 studies. Hellmann *et al.* [68] studied the rate at which medical residents learned to perform a limited HCU examination, which included acquiring two-dimen-sional images (parasternal short, long, and apical four), color flow Doppler (mitral and aortic), as well as measurement of LV size, LV wall thickness, aortic root size, and left atrial dimension. Their data suggested that an acceptable level of skill might be obtained with 20 to 40 one-on-one supervised studies. In many respects, the required training will depend on what the examiner is going to look for. No one would argue that the skill required to assess LV systolic function from one view is easier to learn than the assessment of regional wall motion, which requires a multiview approach. Newer devices allow continuous and pulsed-wave Doppler and Doppler tissue imaging to be recorded, but the knowledge to perform and interpret these images is substantial. Equally controversial is the documentation of HCU examinations. Should cardiac HCU be considered part of the physical examination, meaning that findings are recorded, but no images stored for review or should there be image documentation?

References

1. Matsumoto M, Inoue M, Tamura S, *et al.*: Three-dimensional echocardiography for spatial visualization and volume calculation of cardiac structures. *J Clin Ultrasound* 1981, 9:157–165.

2. Stickels KR, Wann LS: An analysis of three-dimensional reconstructive echocardiography. *Ultrasound Med Biol* 1984, 10:575–580.

3. von Ramm OT, Smith SW: Real time volumetric ultrasound imaging system. *J Digit Imaging* 1990, 3:261–266.

4. Sugeng L, Shernan SK, Salgo IS, *et al.*: Live three-dimensional transesophageal echocardiography: initial experience using the fully-sampled matrix array probe. *J Am Coll Cardiol* 2008, In press.

5. King DL, Harrison MR, King DL Jr, *et al.*: Improved reproducibility of left atrial and left ventricular measurements by guided three-dimensional echocardiography. *J Am Coll Cardiol* 1992, 20:1238–1245.

6. Buck T, Hunold P, Wentz KU, *et al.*: Tomographic three-dimensional echocardiographic determination of chamber size and systolic function in patients with left ventricular aneurysm: comparison to magnetic resonance imaging, cineventriculography, and two-dimensional echocardiography. *Circulation* 1997, 96:4286–4297.

7. Jenkins C, Bricknell K, Hanekom L, Marwick TH, *et al.*: Reproducibility and accuracy of echocardiographic measurements of left ventricular parameters using real-time three-dimensional echocardiography. *J Am Coll Cardiol* 2004, 44:878–886.

8. Jacobs LD, Salgo IS, Goonewardena S, *et al.*: Rapid online quantification of left ventricular volume from real-time three-dimensional echocardiographic data. *Eur Heart J* 2006, 27:460–468.

9. Caiani EG, Coon P, Corsi C, *et al.*: Dual triggering improves the accuracy of left ventricular volume measurements by contrast-enhanced real-time 3-dimensional echocardiography. *J Am Soc Echocardiogr* 2005, 18:1292–1298.

10. Frielingsdorf J, Franke A, Kuhl HP, *et al.*: Evaluation of regional systolic function in hypertrophic cardiomyopathy and hypertensive heart disease: a three-dimensional echocardiographic study. *J Am Soc Echocardiogr* 1998, 11:778–786.

11. Corsi C, Lang RM, Veronesi F, *et al.*: Volumetric quantification of global and regional left ventricular function from real-time three-dimensional echocardiographic images. *Circulation* 2005, 112:1161–1170.

12. Krenning BJ, Szili-Torok T, Voormolen MM, *et al.*: Guiding and optimization of resynchronization therapy with dynamic three-dimensional echocardiography and segmental volume–time curves: a feasibility study. *Eur J Heart Fail* 2004, 6:619–625.

13. van der Heide JA, Mannaerts HF, Spruijt HJ, *et al.*: Noninvasive mapping of left ventricular electromechanical asynchrony by three-dimensional echocardiography and semi-automatic contour detection. *Am J Cardiol* 2004, 94:1449–1453.

14. Kapetanakis S, Kearney MT, Siva A, *et al.*: Real-time three-dimensional echocardiography: a novel technique to quantify global left ventricular mechanical dyssynchrony. *Circulation* 2005, 112:992–1000.

15. Toledo E, Lang RM, Collins KA, *et al.*: Imaging and quantification of myocardial perfusion using real-time three-dimensional echocardiography. *J Am Coll Cardiol* 2006, 47:146–154.

16. Iwakura K, Ito H, Okamura A, *et al.*: Comparison of two- versus three-dimensional myocardial contrast echocardiography for assessing subendocardial perfusion abnormality after percutaneous coronary intervention in patients with acute myocardial infarction. *Am J Cardiol* 2007, 100:1502–1510.

17. Levine RA, Handschumacher MD, Sanfilippo AJ, *et al.*: Three-dimensional echocardiographic reconstruction of the mitral valve, with implications for the diagnosis of mitral valve prolapse. *Circulation* 1989, 80:589–598.

18. Sugeng L, Coon P, Weinert L, *et al.*: Use of real-time three-dimensional transthoracic echocardiography in the evaluation of mitral valve disease. *J Am Soc Echocardiogr* 2006, 19:413–421.

19. Binder TM, Rosenhek R, Porenta G, *et al.*: Improved assessment of mitral valve stenosis by volumetric real-time three-dimensional echocardiography. *J Am Coll Cardiol* 2000, 36:1355–1361.

20. Chen Q, Nosir YF, Vletter WB, *et al.*: Accurate assessment of mitral valve area in patients with mitral stenosis by three-dimensional echocardiography. *J Am Soc Echocardiogr* 1997, 10:133–140.

21. Zamorano J, Cordeiro P, Sugeng L, *et al.*: Real-time three-dimensional echocardiography for rheumatic mitral valve stenosis evaluation: an accurate and novel approach. *J Am Coll Cardiol* 2004, 43:2091–2096.

22. Ge S, Warner JG Jr, Abraham TP, *et al.*: Three-dimensional surface area of the aortic valve orifice by three-dimensional echocardiography: clinical validation of a novel index for assessment of aortic stenosis. *Am Heart J* 1998, 136:1042–1050.

23. Breburda CS, Griffin BP, Pu M, *et al.*: Three-dimensional echocardiographic planimetry of maximal regurgitant orifice area in myxomatous mitral regurgitation: intraoperative comparison with proximal flow convergence. *J Am Coll Cardiol* 1998, 32:432–437.

24. Sugeng L, Spencer KT, Mor-Avi V, *et al.*: Dynamic three-dimensional color flow Doppler: an improved technique for the assessment of mitral regurgitation. *Echocardiography* 2003, 20:265–273.

25. Lang RM, Mor-Avi V, Sugeng L, *et al.*: Three-dimensional echocardiography: the benefits of the additional dimension. *J Am Coll Cardiol* 2006, 48:2053–2069.

26. Roelandt J, Wladimiroff JW, Baars AM: Ultrasonic real time imaging with a hand-held-scanner. Part II: initial clinical experience. *Ultrasound Med Biol* 1978, 4:93–97.

27. Mor-Avi V, Sugeng L, Weinert L, *et al.*: Fast measurement of left ventricular mass with real-time three-dimensional echocardiography: comparison with magnetic resonance imaging. *Circulation* 2004, 110:1814–1818.

28. Nanda NC, Kisslo J, Lang R, *et al.*: Examination protocol for three-dimensional echocardiography. *Echocardiography* 2004, 21:763–768.

29. Carr JA, Sugeng L, Weinert L, *et al.*: Images in cardiovascular medicine. Subaortic membrane in the adult. *Circulation* 2005, 112:e347.

30. Sugeng L, Mor-Avi V, Lang RM: Three-dimensional echocardiography: coming of age (Editorial). *Heart* 2008, In press.

31. Goodkin GM, Spevack DM, Tunick PA, Kronzon I: How useful is hand-carried bedside echocardiography in critically ill patients? *J Am Coll Cardiol* 2001, 37:2019–2022.

32. Coletta C, De Marchis E, Lenoli M, *et al.*: Reliability of cardiac dimensions and valvular regurgitation assessment by sonographers using hand-carried ultrasound devices. *Eur J Echocardiogr* 2006, 7:275–283.

33. Kobal SL, Tolstrup K, Luo H, *et al.*: Usefulness of a hand-carried cardiac ultrasound device to detect clinically significant valvular regurgitation in hospitalized patients. *Am J Cardiol* 2004, 93:1069–1072.

34. Rugolotto M, Hu BS, Liang DH, Schnittger I: Rapid assessment of cardiac anatomy and function with a new hand-carried ultrasound device (OptiGo): a comparison with standard echocardiography. *Eur J Echocardiogr* 2001, 2:262–269.

35. Scholten C, Rosenhek R, Binder T, *et al.*: Hand-held miniaturized cardiac ultrasound instruments for rapid and effective bedside diagnosis and patient screening. *J Eval Clin Pract* 2005, 11:67–72.

36. Vourvouri EC, Schinkel AF, Roelandt JR, *et al.*: Screening for left ventricular dysfunction using a hand-carried cardiac ultrasound device. *Eur J Heart Fail* 2003, 5:767–774.

37. DeCara JM, Lang RM, Koch R, *et al.*: The use of small personal ultrasound devices by internists without formal training in echocardiography. *Eur J Echocardiogr* 2003, 4:141–147.

38. Brennan JM, Blair JE, Goonewardena S, *et al.*: A comparison by medicine residents of physical examination versus hand-carried ultrasound for estimation of right atrial pressure. *Am J Cardiol* 2007, 99:1614–1616.

39. DeCara JM, Lang RM, Spencer KT: The hand-carried echocardiographic device as an aid to the physical examination. *Echocardiography* 2003, 20:477–485.

40. Fedson S, Neithardt G, Thomas P, *et al.*: Unsuspected clinically important findings detected with a small portable ultrasound device in patients admitted to a general medicine service. *J Am Soc Echocardiogr* 2003, 16:901–905.

41. Spencer KT, Anderson AS, Bhargava A, *et al.*: Physician-performed point-of-care echocardiography using a laptop platform compared with physical examination in the cardiovascular patient. *J Am Coll Cardiol* 2001, 37:2013–2018.

42. Xie T, Chamoun AJ, McCulloch M, *et al.*: Rapid screening of cardiac patients with a miniaturized hand-held ultrasound imager: comparisons with physical examination and conventional two-dimensional echocardiography. *Clin Cardiol* 2004, 27:241–245.

43. Atar S, Feldman A, Darawshe A, *et al.*: Utility and diagnostic accuracy of hand-carried ultrasound for emergency room evaluation of chest pain. *Am J Cardiol* 2004, 94:408–409.

44. Bruce CJ, Montgomery SC, Bailey KR, *et al.*: Utility of hand-carried ultrasound devices used by cardiologists with and without significant echocardiographic experience in the cardiology inpatient and outpatient settings. *Am J Cardiol* 2002, 90:1273–1275.

45. de Groot-de Laat LE, ten Cate FJ, Vourvouri EC, *et al.*: Impact of hand-carried cardiac ultrasound on diagnosis and management during cardiac consultation rounds. *Eur J Echocardiogr* 2005, 6:196–201.

46. Giannotti G, Mondillo S, Galderisi M, *et al.*: Hand-held echocardiography: added value in clinical cardiological assessment. *Cardiovasc Ultrasound* 2005, 3:7.

47. Gorcsan J 3rd, Pandey P, Sade LE: Influence of hand-carried ultrasound on bedside patient treatment decisions for consultative cardiology. *J Am Soc Echocardiogr* 2004, 17:50–55.

48. Trambaiolo P, Papetti F, Posteraro A, *et al.*: A hand-carried cardiac ultrasound device in the outpatient cardiology clinic reduces the need for standard echocardiography. *Heart* 2007, 93:470–475.

49. Vourvouri EC, Poldermans D, Deckers JW, *et al.*: Evaluation of a hand carried cardiac ultrasound device in an outpatient cardiology clinic. *Heart* 2005, 91:171–176.

50. Alexander JH, Peterson ED, Chen AY, *et al.*: Feasibility of point-of-care echocardiography by internal medicine house staff. *Am Heart J* 2004, 147:476–481.

51. Croft LB, Duvall WL, Goldman ME: A pilot study of the clinical impact of hand-carried cardiac ultrasound in the medical clinic. *Echocardiography* 2006, 23:439–446.

52. Lapostolle F, Petrovic T, Lenoir G, *et al.*: Usefulness of hand-held ultrasound devices in out-of-hospital diagnosis performed by emergency physicians. *Am J Emerg Med* 2006, 24:237–242.

53. Lemola K, Yamada E, Jagasia D, Kerber RE: A hand-carried personal ultrasound device for rapid evaluation of left ventricular function: use after limited echo training. *Echocardiography* 2003, 20:309–312.

54. Manasia AR, Nagaraj HM, Kodali RB, *et al.*: Feasibility and potential clinical utility of goal-directed transthoracic echocardiography performed by noncardiologist intensivists using a small hand-carried device (SonoHeart) in critically ill patients. *J Cardiothorac Vasc Anesth* 2005, 19:155–159.

55. Rugolotto M, Chang CP, Hu B, *et al.*: Clinical use of cardiac ultrasound performed with a hand-carried device in patients admitted for acute cardiac care. *Am J Cardiol* 2002, 90:1040–1042.

56. Vignon P, Chastagner C, Francois B, *et al.*: Diagnostic ability of hand-held echocardiography in ventilated critically ill patients. *Crit Care* 2003, 7:R84–R91.

57. Weston P, Alexander JH, Patel MR, *et al.*: Hand-held echocardiographic examination of patients with symptoms of acute coronary syndromes in the emergency department: the 30-day outcome associated with normal left ventricular wall motion. *Am Heart J* 2004, 148:1096–1101.

58. Brennan JM, Ronan A, Goonewardena S, *et al.*: Handcarried ultrasound measurement of the inferior vena cava for assessment of intravascular volume status in the outpatient hemodialysis clinic. *Clin J Am Soc Nephrol* 2006, 1:749–753.

59. Kobal SL, Lee SS, Willner R, *et al.*: Hand-carried cardiac ultrasound enhances healthcare delivery in developing countries. *Am J Cardiol* 2004, 94:539–541.

60. Kirkpatrick JN, Davis A, DeCara JM, *et al.*: Hand-carried cardiac ultrasound as a tool to screen for important cardiovascular disease in an underserved minority health care clinic. *J Am Soc Echocardiogr* 2004, 17:399–403.

61. DeCara JM, Kirkpatrick JN, Spencer KT, *et al.:* Use of hand-carried ultrasound devices to augment the accuracy of medical student bedside cardiac diagnoses. *J Am Soc Echocardiogr* 2005, 18:257–263.

62. Kirkpatrick JN, Belka V, Furlong K, *et al.:* Effectiveness of echocardiographic imaging by nurses to identify left ventricular systolic dysfunction in high-risk patients. *Am J Cardiol* 2005, 95:1271–1272.

63. Bruce CJ, Spittell PC, Montgomery SC, *et al.:* Personal ultrasound imager: abdominal aortic aneurysm screening. *J Am Soc Echocardiogr* 2000, 13:674–679.

64. Kimura BJ, Fowler SJ, Fergus TS, *et al.:* Detection of left atrial enlargement using hand-carried ultrasound devices to screen for cardiac abnormalities. *Am J Med* 2005, 118:912–916.

65. Vourvouri EC, Poldermans D, Schinkel AF, *et al.:* Left ventricular hypertrophy screening using a hand-held ultrasound device. *Eur Heart J* 2002, 23:1516–1521.

66. Galasko GI, Lahiri A, Senior R: Portable echocardiography: an innovative tool in screening for cardiac abnormalities in the community. *Eur J Echocardiogr* 2003, 4:119–127.

67. Wang TJ, Levy D, Benjamin EJ, Vasan RS: The epidemiology of "asymptomatic" left ventricular systolic dysfunction: implications for screening. *Ann Intern Med* 2003, 138:907–916.

68. Hellmann DB, Whiting-O'Keefe Q, Shapiro EP, *et al.:* The rate at which residents learn to use hand-held echocardiography at the bedside. *Am J Med* 2005, 118:1010–1018.

Myocardial Strain Echocardiography

Veronica Lea J. Dimaano and Theodore P. Abraham

Strain is a measure of tissue deformation, and it is defined as the change in length normalized to the original length (*see* Fig. 19-1). The rate at which this change occurs is strain rate (SR). Deformation in a one-dimensional object is limited to lengthening or shortening [1]. Strain measures the extent of shortening or lengthening relative to its original length, whereas SR is the speed at which this change occurs. SR and strain are analogous to shortening velocity and shortening fraction, respectively. Peak systolic SR closely reflects local contractility. It is relatively volume independent and less pressure independent than strain.

Strain and strain rate can be derived by tissue Doppler echocardiography (TDE) or by speckle tracking (ST) using ultrasound. With TDE, SR is the difference in velocity between two points along the myocardial wall (velocity gradient) normalized to the distance between the two points [2]. A similar velocity gradient exists between the endocardium, which moves faster than the epicardium, a concept used to derive myocardial velocity gradient (radial SR) [3]. SR measures the rate at which the two points of interest move towards or away from each other. Integration of SR yields strain, which is the normalized change in length between these two points.

The use of strain (deformation) to examine the properties of the heart is not a new concept. Mirsky and Parmley [4] used strain to study the elastic properties of the myocardium. Although myocardial strain is a three-dimensional tensor, it has traditionally been simplified to focus on three primary directions of strain in the heart. The heart shortens and lengthens in the longitudinal direction, it thickens and thins in the radial direction, and it shortens and lengthens in the circumferential direction (*see* Fig. 19-2). There is also a torsion, or wringing motion, between the base and apex. When viewed from the apex, the apex rotates counterclockwise, and the base rotates clockwise in systole (twisting) with the opposite motion (untwisting) in diastole (*see* Fig. 19-2). SR and strain are theoretically less susceptible to translational motion and tethering artifacts and thus may be superior to tissue velocity in depicting regional or global myocardial function.

Tissue-Doppler—derived strain variables have been extensively validated in experimental and clinical models [5–9]. Strain and strain rate are more sensitive than current measures of cardiac function. Preclinical and clinical studies suggest that these novel quantitative measures of cardiac function may have a potential role in the clinical assessment of several cardiac pathologies, such as coronary artery disease, heart failure, and cardiomyopathies. Additionally, strain and SR may allow better assessment of cardiac structures that are challenging to evaluate with conventional echocardiography and are therefore traditionally ignored, such as the right ventricle and the left atrium [10].

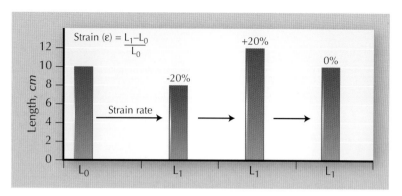

Figure 19-1. Strain measures tissue deformation, and it is defined as the change in dimension or length ($L_1 - L_0$) normalized to the initial length (L_0) of the region of interest. For example, if the initial length of a myocardial segment is 10 cm, then shortening by 2 cm to 8 cm indicates a strain or -20%. Likewise, a lengthening of the segment to 12 cm indicates a strain of +20%. No change in length would suggest 0% strain. The rate at which any of these length (dimension) changes occur is strain rate [10]. ε—strain.

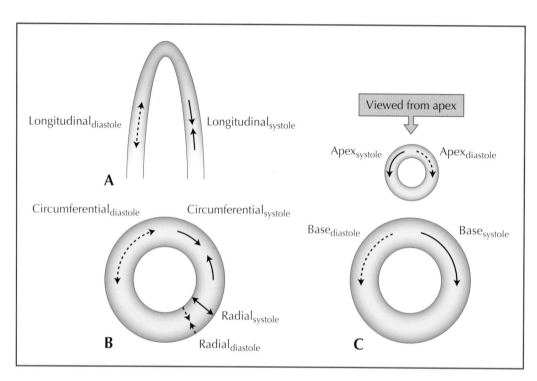

Figure 19-2. Graphic representation of the principal myocardial deformations—longitudinal (**A**), radial and circumferential (**B**), and torsion (**C**). The direction of deformation in systole is shown in *solid lines* and that in diastole shown in *dashed lines* [10].

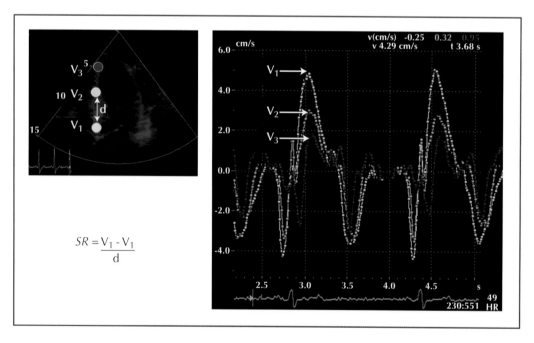

Figure 19-3. In the longitudinal orientation, normal heart motion is such that the base moves towards the apex, which moves very little or not at all. Thus, tissue velocity is maximal at the base (V_1), lower in the middle (V_2), and least at the apex (V_3). This gradient in velocities is used to calculate strain rates (SR). SR is calculated (using tissue Doppler) as the difference between two tissue velocities along the ultrasound beam ($V_2 - V_1$) normalized to the intervening distance (d) between these two velocities. *Colored circles* indicate the positions of the region of interest in the myocardium (*left panel*) for the corresponding tissue velocity traces (*right panel*). (*From* Abraham *et al.* [10]; with permission.)

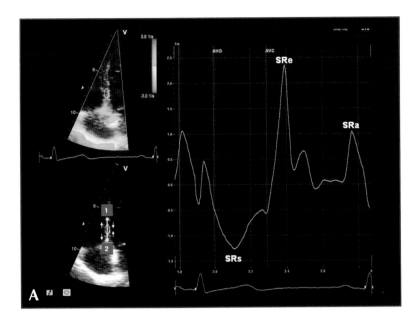

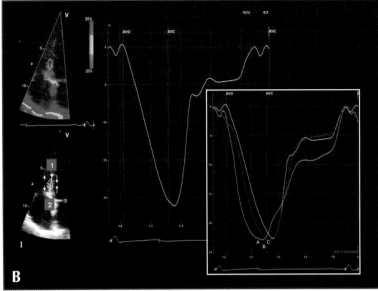

Figure 19-4. Myocardial strain rate (SR) in the longitudinal direction. This is a Doppler-derived SR curve with sample volume placed at the base of the LV septum using a strain length of 18 mm (distance between points 1 and 2). **A,** SR is the spatial derivation of tissue velocity. The rate by which two reference points (1 and 2) in the myocardium move closer to each other during systole (myocardial contraction) is the systolic strain rate (SRs). Because the distance between these two reference points becomes progressively shorter, the resulting SRs curve takes on a negative magnitude. SRs normally peak at early- to mid-systole. The rate at which the reference points in the myocardium move away from each other during relaxation is termed diastolic SR. Because the distance between these reference points becomes longer, the resulting early diastolic SR (SRe) and late diastolic SR (SRa) curves have positive polarity. **B,** Representative normal longitudinal strain tracing obtained from the basal septum. Using tissue Doppler imaging, strain is the integration of SR. In the longitudinal direction, strain has a negative polarity. It normally peaks during late systole (*A in inset*), end systole at aortic valve closure (*B in inset*), or just after the aortic valve closure (*C in inset*). AVO—aortic valve opening; AVC—aortic valve closure.

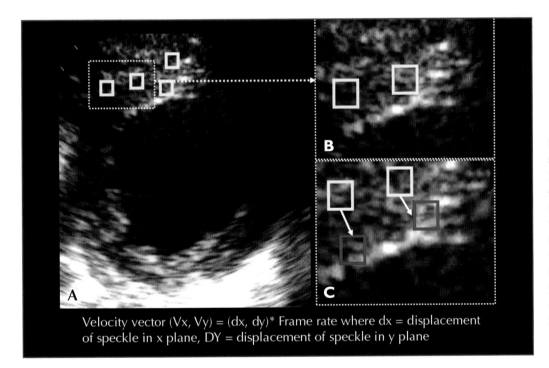

Velocity vector (Vx, Vy) = (dx, dy)* Frame rate where dx = displacement of speckle in x plane, DY = displacement of speckle in y plane

Figure 19-5. Two-dimensional speckle tracking strain measurement. In this technique, displacement is measured by tracking a speckle over the cardiac cycle. Speckles are unique acoustic patterns that are detected automatically by the software (**A**). Original speckle locations (*yellow boxes*) are recorded at end diastole (**B**) and tracked over time to their new location (*blue boxes*) in end systole (**C**). Displacement is integrated in order to yield strain. The derivative of strain yields SR. The advantage of two-dimensional speckle tracking strain is that it is not angle dependent, and it can potentially be measured in multiple planes, unlike tissue Doppler imaging–derived strain.

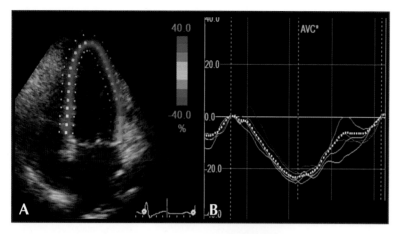

Figure 19-6. A representative figure of two-dimensional speckle tracking strain measurement of longitudinal strain. The color overlay indicates peak systolic strain along the longitudinal direction per the color scale in the right upper corner (**A**). Absolute values of strain per segment (*individual traces in solid line*) and global strain (*dotted white line*) are shown (**B**). AVC—aortic valve closure.

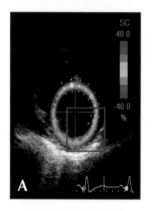
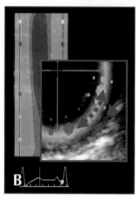
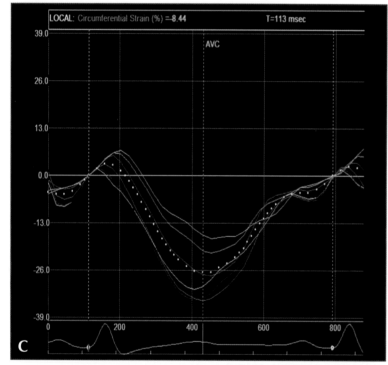

Figure 19-7. Example of circumferential strain, measured along or parallel to the direction of the ventricular wall in the short axis. Automated tracking on the midventricular region in the short-axis view with color-coded identification of the 6-segment LV model is shown (**A**). Inset (**B**) shows the direction of deformation in systole (*solid arrows*) and diastole (*dotted arrow*). Representative circumferential strain traces are presented (**C**).

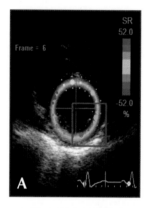
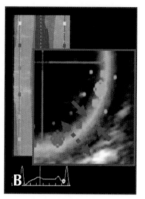
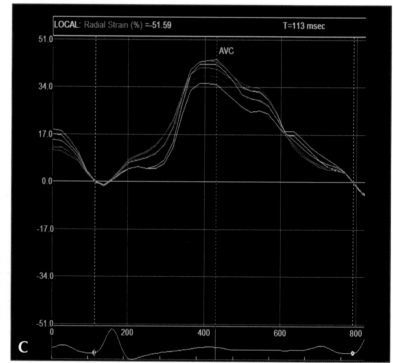

Figure 19-8. Example of radial strain, measured perpendicular to the direction of the ventricular wall in the short axis. Automated tracking performed on the midventricular region in the short-axis view with color-coded identification of the 6-segment LV model is shown (**A**). Inset (**B**) shows the direction of deformation in systole (*solid arrows*) and diastole (*dotted arrow*). Representative radial strain traces are presented (**C**).

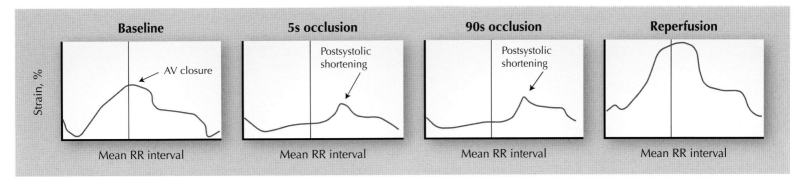

Figure 19-9. Acute and chronic ischemia results in reduced strain rate (SR) and strain. Acute occlusion of a coronary artery, as occurs during inflation of an angioplasty balloon, results in rapid decrease in systolic strain with the appearance of postsystolic strain. Postsystolic strain lasts throughout this transient ischemia and subsides immediately after restoration of myocardial perfusion with balloon deflation along with restoration of normal systolic strain. (*Adapted from* Jamal *et al.* [11]; with permission.)

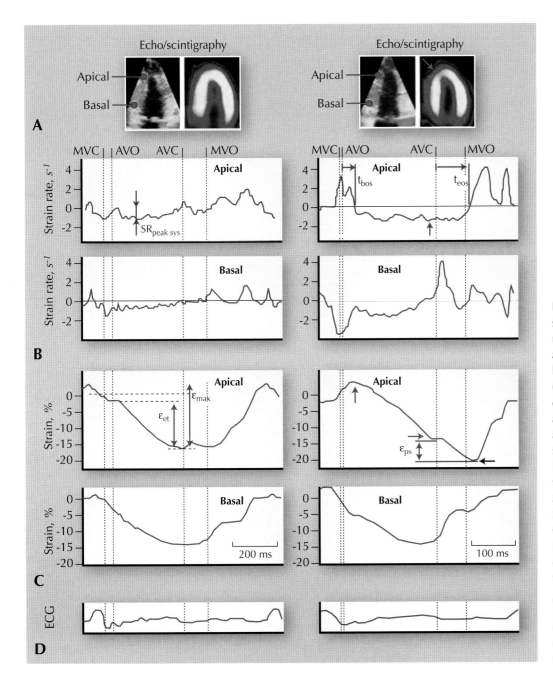

Figure 19-10. Inducible ischemia occurring with stress, such as dobutamine stimulation, results in reduction of systolic strain. In this example, there are no changes in strain at the basal segment between rest (**C**, *lower left panel*) and stress images (**C**, *lower right panel*), whereas there is a significant decrease in systolic strain (*blue arrow*) and the appearance of postsystolic strain (*black arrow*) at the apex. These strain changes coincided with stress-induced decrements in myocardial perfusion by thallium scintigraphy. (*From* Voigt *et al.* [12]; with permission.) **A**, Echo and scintigraphy images at rest and during dobutamine stress stimulation. **B**, Strain rate (SR) curves at apical and basal segments. **C**, Strain curves at apical and basal segments. **D**, ECG tracing; event-timings. AVC—aortic valve closure; AVO—aortic valve opening; MVC—mitral valve closure; MVO—mitral valve opening; $SR_{peak\ sys}$—peak systolic SR; t_{bos}—time to beginning of myocardial shortening; t_{eos}—time to end of myocardial shortening; ε_{max}—maximum length change during the entire cardiac cycle; ε_{et}—strain during ejection time; ε_{ps}—postsystolic strain.

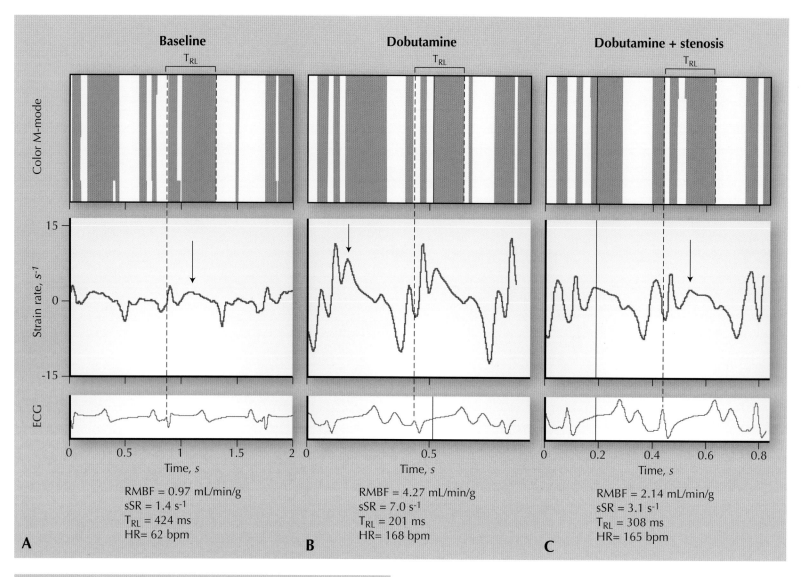

Baseline

T_{RL}

Color M-mode

Strain rate, s^{-1}

15

0

-15

ECG

| 0 | 0.5 | 1 | 1.5 | 2 |

Time, s

RMBF = 0.97 mL/min/g
sSR = 1.4 s^{-1}
T_{RL} = 424 ms
HR= 62 bpm

A

Dobutamine

T_{RL}

0   0.5

Time, s

RMBF = 4.27 mL/min/g
sSR = 7.0 s^{-1}
T_{RL} = 201 ms
HR= 168 bpm

B

Dobutamine + stenosis

T_{RL}

0   0.2   0.4   0.6   0.8

Time, s

RMBF = 2.14 mL/min/g
sSR = 3.1 s^{-1}
T_{RL} = 308 ms
HR= 165 bpm

C

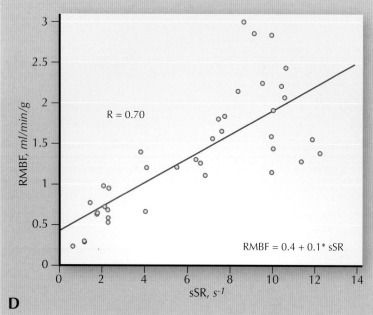

R = 0.70

RMBF = 0.4 + 0.1* sSR

RMBF, ml/min/g

sSR, s^{-1}

D

Figure 19-11. In an experimental, closed-chest model, systolic strain rate (SRs) increases severalfold with dobutamine stimulation in the absence of any coronary stenosis (**B**) compared with baseline (**A**). Introduction of a nonocclusive coronary stenosis (**C**) results in a significant blunting of this increase in SRs at peak dobutamine stress. Absolute SRs closely correlates with regional myocardial perfusion as measured by microspheres (**D**). RMBF—regional myocardial blood flow; sSR—peak systolic SR; T_{RL}—time to regional lengthening; HR—heart rate. (*From* Yip *et al.* [13]; with permission.)

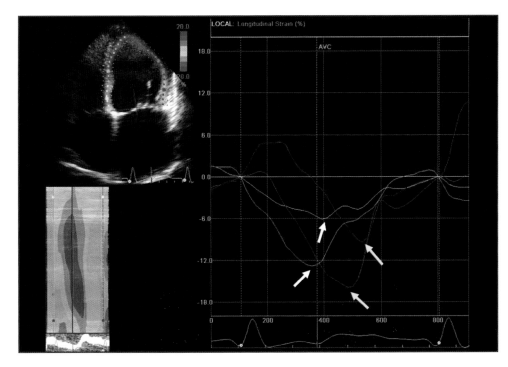

Figure 19-12. Intraventricular dyssynchrony using longitudinal two-dimensional strain analysis by speckle tracking in a heart failure patient. Automated tracking was performed on all segments of the septum and the lateral wall of the LV using an apical four-chamber view. Tracings from the basal (*yellow line*), midseptum (*aqua line*), basal (*red line*), and midlateral (*blue line*) wall are shown. Septal peak strains (*white arrows*) occurred near the AV closure and those of the lateral wall (*yellow arrows*) were noted in diastole.

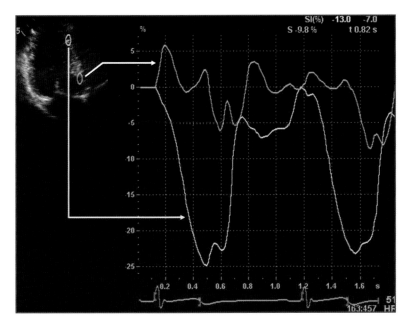

Figure 19-13. In hypertrophic cardiomyopathy, regional systolic strain is significantly reduced in the basal hypertrophied anterior septum (*white arrow*) relative to normal systolic strain at the apex (*yellow arrow*). A regional systolic strain greater than 10% is thought to support a diagnosis of hypertrophic cardiomyopathy, separating it from hypertension-related hypertrophy wherein regional strain is preserved [14].

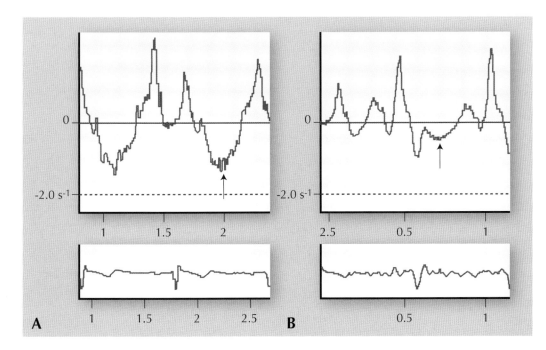

Figure 19-14. Systolic strain rate is significantly reduced in a patient with primary amyloidosis (**B**, *arrow*) with normal wall thickness, normal wall motion, and normal ejection fraction compared with a healthy, age-matched control (**A**, *arrow*). The *solid line* is 0 and the *dashed line* is -2.0 s⁻¹. Echocardiographic tracing is shown at the bottom for time reference.

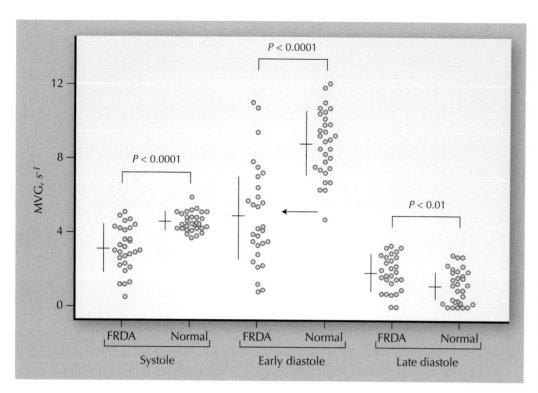

Figure 19-15. Early diastolic strain rate (*black arrow*) is significantly lower in asymptomatic subjects who are gene positive for Friedreich's ataxia compared with normal controls. Thus, strain rate may help in screening subjects with family history of inherited myopathies to screen for cardiac involvement [15]. FRDA—Friedreich's ataxia; MVG—myocardial velocity gradient.

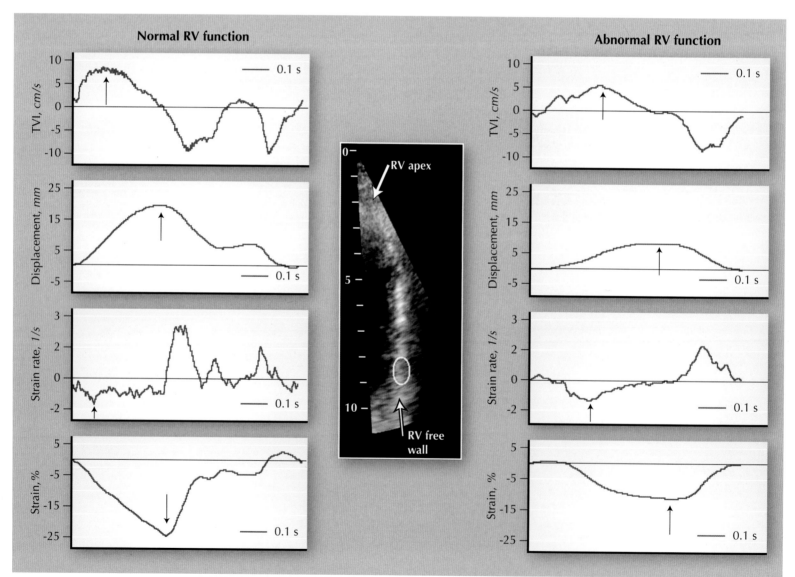

Figure 19-16. Systolic strain derived from the RV free wall closely correlates with RV stroke volume as determined by thermodilution or Fick method. Strain appears superior to other Doppler-based indices, such as the index of myocardial performance and tissue Doppler-based isovolumic acceleration. Representative traces from the basal RV free wall illustrate tissue velocity (TVI), tissue displacement, strain rate, and strain from a normal subject (*left*) as well as a subject with primary pulmonary hypertension (*right*) [16].

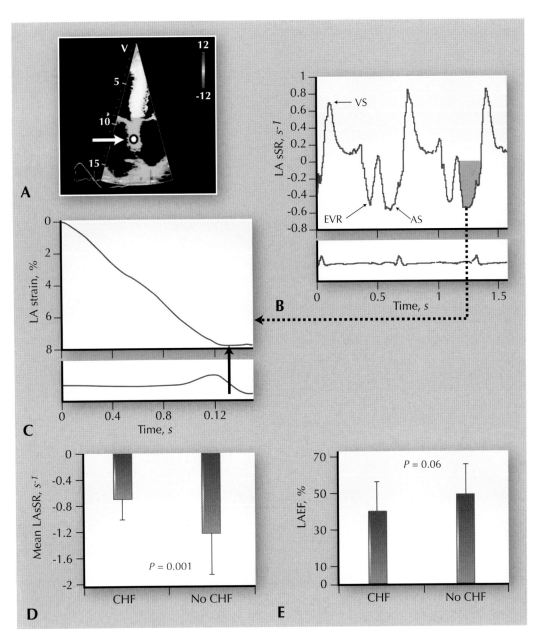

Figure 19-17. Measurement of left atrial strain from the interatrial septum is illustrated (**A**, *arrow*). Representative left atrial strain rate (SR) traces (**B**) illustrate the various phases of atrial mechanical activity, consisting of ventricular systole (VS), early ventricular relaxation (EVR), and atrial systole (AS). Integration of atrial systole strain rate (SR) yields atrial strain (**C**). Left atrial SR was significantly lower in patients with amyloidosis who had heart failure symptoms compared to those without symptoms (**D**). In contrast, left atrial ejection fraction was similar in both groups (**E**) [17]. CHF—congestive heart failure; LAsSR—left atrial systolic SR; LAEF—left atrial ejection fraction; sSR—systolic SR.

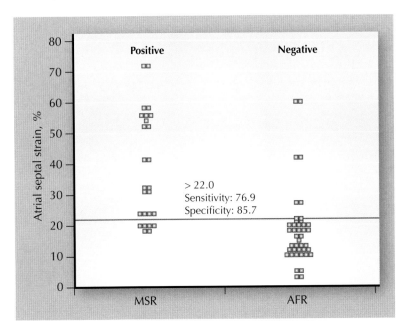

Figure 19-18. Left atrial strain rate predicted maintenance of sinus rhythm in patients with atrial fibrillation undergoing electrical cardioversion. A cutoff value of 1.8 s^{-1} for atrial inferior wall peak systolic strain rate was associated with a sensitivity of 92%, specificity of 79%, positive predictive value of 77%, and negative predictive value of 86% (area under the receiving operating characteristics [ROC] curve, 0.878; SE, 0.047; 95% CI, 0.77–0.94). For atrial septal peak systolic strain, a cutoff value of 22% was associated with a sensitivity of 77%, specificity of 86%, positive predictive value of 73%, and negative predictive value of 94% (area under the ROC curve, 0.852; SE, 0.05; 95% CI, 0.76–0.93). MSR—maintenance of sinus rhythm; AFR—atrial fibrillation recurrence [18].

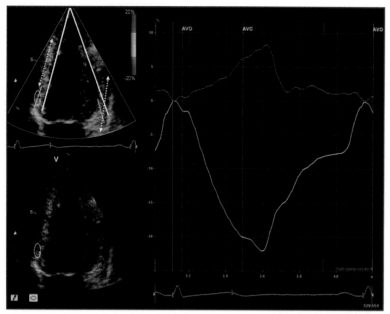

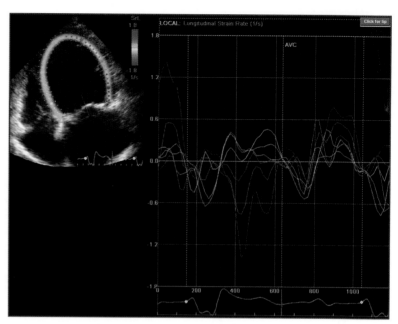

Figure 19-19. Angle-related issues could significantly affect strain measurements with tissue-Doppler—derived strain. In this example, the direction of motion of the basal segment of the septal wall (*upper left panel, yellow dashed line*) is almost parallel to the ultrasound beam (*upper left panel, white solid line*). In contrast, there is a substantial angle between the direction of motion of the basal segment of the lateral wall (*upper left panel, white dashed line*) and the ultrasound beam (*upper left panel, white solid line*). Subsequently, the septal strain tracing (*right panel, yellow*) appears normal, whereas the lateral strain tracing (*right panel, red*) demonstrates stretching (pseudodyskinesis) in this healthy, normal volunteer.

Figure 19-20. Strain tracings can be very noisy. In such circumstances, the strain data are unreliable and highly variable. In this example from a heart failure patient, there are multiple peaks in systole (*right panel*) precluding reliable analysis of regional function or assessment of dyssynchrony.

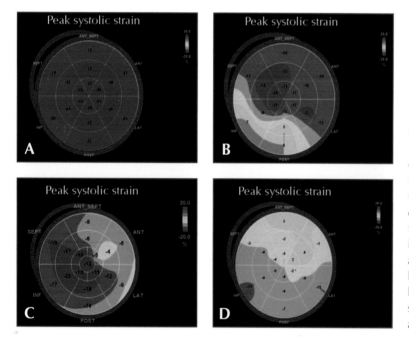

Figure 19-21. Bull's eye plots generated by a semiautomated strain analysis program using a two-dimensional speckle tracking technique in order to calculate strain. Plots are color coded based on longitudinal strain derived from the three standard apical views. The strain color code is depicted in the right upper corner of each figure. **A**, Normal volunteer with normal strain (*shades of red*) in all segments. **B**, A patient with inferior-posterior myocardial infarction who demonstrated reduced and abnormal (*shades of blue*) systolic strain in the inferior and posterior and preserved strain elsewhere. **C**, Patient with a myocardial infarction related to proximal left-anterior descending artery lesion demonstrating reduced strain in the anterior septum and anterior and lateral LV free walls. **D**, Patient with nonischemic cardiomyopathy demonstrating reduced strain in all segments and abnormal systolic strains in the anterior septum and anterior LV free wall (*shade of blue*).

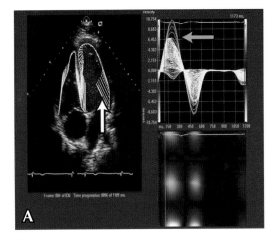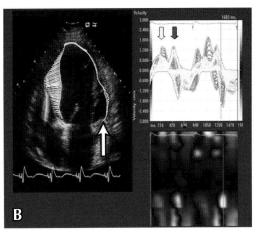

Figure 19-22. Representative images from a semiautomated technique that uses two-dimensional speckle tracking, along with mitral annulus and endocardial border tracking, to calculate tissue velocity and strain. The arrow direction indicates the direction of motion, and the length of the arrow indicates the amplitude of motion. In a normal volunteer (**A**), there is normal motion in all segments including the lateral wall (*left panel, white arrow*); there is only one systolic peak (*upper right panel, blue arrow*), and the color M-mode image shows a synchronous contraction (*lower right panel*). In a heart failure patient with low ejection fraction (**B**), there is little motion (*left panel, white arrow*), there are two systolic peaks (*upper right panel*), with the septum peaking early (*yellow arrow*) and a delayed lateral wall peak (*red arrow*). Color M-mode image (*lower right panel*) shows dyssynchronous mechanical activity. In color M-mode images, *red shades* are systole (motion towards the transducer) and *blue shades* are diastole (motion away from the transducer). (*From* Abraham *et al.* [10]; with permission.)

Acknowledgments

Dr. Abraham receives honoraria (modest) and research support (modest) from GE Ultrasound. This work was partially supported by grants from the National Institutes of Health (AG22554-01 and HL076513-01).

References

1. D'hooge J, Heimdal A, Jamal F, *et al.*: Regional strain and strain rate measurements by cardiac ultrasound: principles, implementation and limitations. *Eur J Echocardiogr* 2000, 1:154–170. [Published erratum appears in *Eur J Echocardiogr* 2000, 1:295–299.

2. Heimdal A, Stoylen A, Torp H, Skjaerpe T: Real-time strain rate imaging of the left ventricle by ultrasound. *J Am Soc Echocardiogr* 1998, 11:1013–1019.

3. Uematsu M, Miyatake K, Tanaka N, *et al.*: Myocardial velocity gradient as a new indicator of regional left ventricular contraction: detection by a two-dimensional tissue Doppler imaging technique. *J Am Coll Cardiol* 1995, 26:217–223.

4. Mirsky I, Parmley WW: Assessment of passive elastic stiffness for isolated heart muscle and the intact heart. *Circ Res* 1973, 33:233–243.

5. Belohlavek M, Bartleson VB, Zobitz ME: Real-time strain rate imaging: validation of peak compression and expansion rates by a tissue-mimicking phantom. *Echocardiography* 2001, 18:565–571.

6. Abraham T, Laskowski C, Zhan W, *et al.*: Myocardial contractility by strain echocardiography: comparison with physiological measurements in an in vitro model. *Am J Physiol Heart Circ Physiol* 2003, 285:H2599–H2604.

7. Urheim S, Edvardsen T, Torp H, *et al.*: Myocardial strain by Doppler echocardiography: validation of a new method to quantify regional myocardial function. *Circulation* 2000, 102:1158–1164.

8. Edvardsen T, Gerber BL, Garot J, *et al.*: Quantitative assessment of intrinsic regional myocardial deformation by Doppler strain rate echocardiography in humans: validation against three-dimensional tagged magnetic resonance imaging. *Circulation* 2002, 106:50–56.

9. Kowalski M, Kukulski T, Jamal F, *et al.*: Can natural strain and strain rate quantify regional myocardial deformation? A study in healthy subjects. *Ultrasound Med Biol* 2001, 27:1087–1097.

10. Abraham TP, Dimaano VL, Liang HY: Role of tissue Doppler and strain echocardiography in current clinical practice. *Circulation* 2007, 116:2597–2609.

11. Jamal F, Kukulski T, D'hooge J, *et al.*: Abnormal post-systolic thickening in acutely ischemic myocardium during coronary angioplasty: a velocity, strain, and strain rate Doppler myocardial imaging study. *J Am Soc Echocardiogr* 1999, 12:994–996.

12. Voigt JU, Exner B, Schmiedehausen K, *et al.*: Strain-rate imaging during dobutamine stress echocardiography provides objective evidence of inducible ischemia. *Circulation* 2003, 107:2120–2126.

13. Yip G, Khandheria B, Belohlavek M, *et al.*: Strain echocardiography tracks dobutamine-induced decrease in regional myocardial perfusion in nonocclusive coronary stenosis. *J Am Coll Cardiol* 2004, 44:1664–1671.

14. Kato TS, Noda A, Izawa H, *et al.*: Discrimination of nonobstructive hypertrophic cardiomyopathy from hypertensive left ventricular hypertrophy on the basis of strain rate imaging by tissue Doppler ultrasonography. *Circulation* 2004, 110:3808–3814.

15. Dutka DP, Donnelly JE, Palka P, *et al.*: Echocardiographic characterization of cardiomyopathy in Friedreich's ataxia with tissue Doppler echocardiographically derived myocardial velocity gradients. *Circulation* 2000, 102:1276–1282.

16. Urheim S, Cauduro S, Frantz R, *et al.*: Relation of tissue displacement and strain to invasively determined right ventricular stroke volume. *Am J Cardiol* 2005, 96:1173–1178.

17. Modesto KM, Dispenzieri A, Cauduro SA, *et al.*: Left atrial myopathy in cardiac amyloidosis: implications of novel echocardiographic techniques. *Eur Heart J* 2005, 26:173–179.

18. Di Salvo G, Caso P, Lo Piccolo R, *et al.*: Atrial myocardial deformation properties predict maintenance of sinus rhythm after external cardioversion of recent-onset lone atrial fibrillation: a color Doppler myocardial imaging and transthoracic and transesophageal echocardiographic study. *Circulation* 2005, 112:387–395.

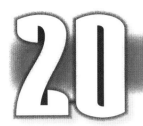

Echocardiographic Assessment of Cardiac Dyssynchrony

Gabe B. Bleeker, Cheuk-Man Yu, and Jeroen J. Bax

There has been increasing interest in accurately diagnosing cardiac dyssynchrony. This has been primarily due to the recent promising clinical results of novel therapeutic modalities, such as cardiac resynchronization therapy (CRT), which aims to reduce cardiac dyssynchrony [1–3]. Several large randomized trials, such as MIRACLE and COMPANION, have demonstrated that CRT can result in an impressive improvement in clinical symptoms and LV function in selected patients with moderate to severe heart failure, depressed LV function, and wide QRS complex. Moreover, the recent CARE-HF trial demonstrated that these beneficial effects are also associated with a reduction in patient mortality [1–7].

Smaller trials have suggested that CRT may be beneficial if cardiac dyssynchrony is present [8]. A dyssynchronous activation of the heart is a relatively common problem in patients with heart failure and can be divided into three types: 1) atrioventricular dyssynchrony (ie, prolonged AV conduction), 2) interventricular dyssynchrony (ie, dyssynchrony between the RV and the LV, and 3) LV dyssynchrony (ie, dyssynchrony within the LV). Few studies have suggested that interventricular dyssynchrony is valuable for response to CRT; instead, the vast majority of studies indicate that the key mechanism of benefit from CRT is related to the presence and subsequent reduction of LV dyssynchrony [8,9]. Adequate diagnosis of baseline LV dyssynchrony is therefore of utmost importance in order to select patients with the highest likelihood of response following CRT. Traditionally, the duration of the QRS complex has been used as a marker of LV dyssynchrony. However, QRS duration has proved to be a poor predictor of response following CRT [10–13]. This may be explained by the fact that QRS duration is closely related to interventricular dyssynchrony but not to LV dyssynchrony (*see* Fig. 20-1) [11–13]. Since this observation was made, a wide variety of echocardiographic techniques have been introduced for the direct assessment of LV dyssynchrony [8]. This chapter will provide an overview of the relative merits of the most important echocardiographic techniques that are currently available for the assessment of LV dyssynchrony, as well as other forms of cardiac dyssynchrony.

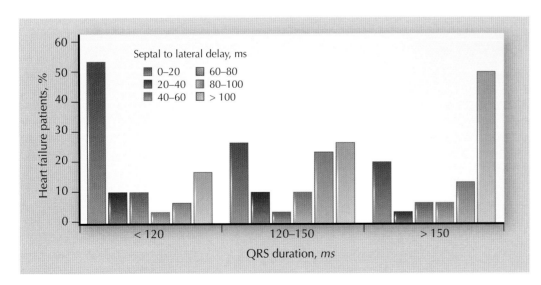

Figure 20-1. Distribution of septal to lateral delay as a marker of LV dyssynchrony (*see* Fig. 20-6) and QRS duration in patients with heart failure is shown. Thirty percent to 40% of heart failure patients with a QRS duration of 120 ms or greater do not have substantial LV dyssynchrony (septal to lateral delay > 60 ms). In addition, 27% of heart failure patients with a narrow QRS complex (< 120 ms) had substantial LV dyssynchrony. (*From* Bleeker *et al.* [12]; with permission.)

Diagnosis of Cardiac Dyssynchrony

Conventional Echocardiographic Methods

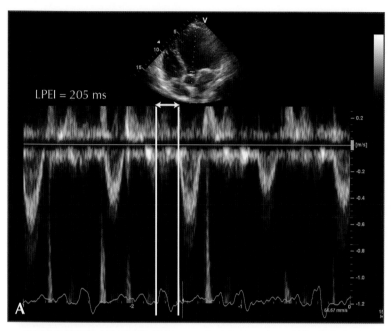

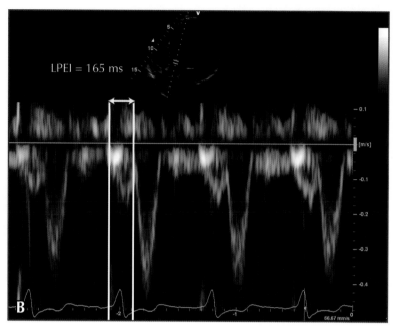

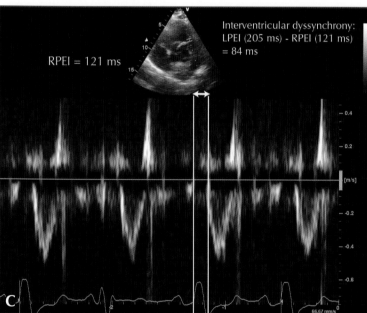

Figure 20-2. Measurement of interventricular dyssynchrony is shown. The aortic preejection time (LPEI) is measured as the time interval between the beginning of the QRS complex and the onset of aortic flow [14] (measured from the pulsed-wave Doppler signal through the LV outflow tract). An LPEI of more than 140 ms has been proposed as a marker of interventricular dyssynchrony, with an early activated RV and late activation of the LV [14]. A heart failure patient with LPEI of 205 ms is shown (**A**), indicating severe interventricular dyssynchrony, which is reduced to 165 ms after implantation of a cardiac resynchronization device (**B**).

A second marker proposed for the measurement of interventricular dyssynchrony is the delay between the preejection times of the LV and RV [14]. A difference in ejection time exceeding 40 ms is thought to represent substantial interventricular dyssynchrony. The measurement of a pulmonic preejection time (with RPEI equaling the time from the beginning of the QRS complex to the onset of pulmonic flow as measured with pulsed-wave Doppler in the RV outflow tract) of 121 ms in the same patient displayed previous (**A**), results in a substantial interventricular dyssynchrony of 84 ms (**C**). However, recent studies have now suggested that the presence of baseline interventricular dyssynchrony is a poor predictor of response to CRT [6,7].

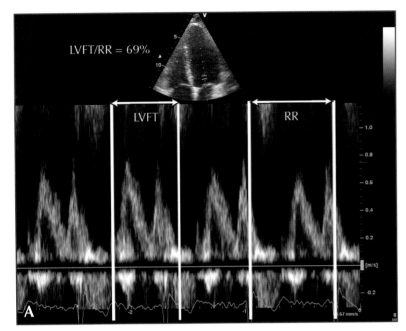

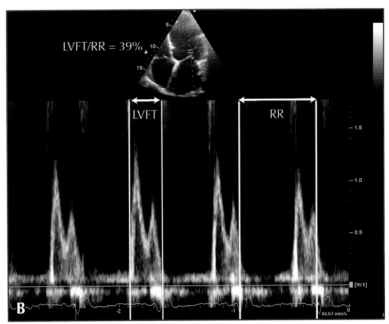

Figure 20-3. Measurement of the duration of LV filling time (LVFT) as a marker of atrioventricular (AV) dyssynchrony is shown. The measurement of LVFT in relation to the duration of the cardiac cycle (RR interval) has been proposed as a marker of AV dyssynchrony. The LVFT is similar to the duration of mitral inflow as measured by pulsed-wave Doppler, and the RR interval can be measured from the ECG. An arbitrary cut-off value of an LVFT of less than 40% of the cardiac cycle has been proposed in order to identify patients who were likely to benefit from cardiac resynchronization therapy (CRT). AV dyssynchrony in patients with heart failure leads to a shortening of the LVFT with subsequent suboptimal diastolic LV filling. By definition, CRT reduces the AV conduction interval (in patients with intact AV conduction) because the ventricles have to be preexcited in order to achieve biventricular stimulation. **A,** An example of a normal individual with an LVFT/RR of 69%. **B,** An example of a heart failure patient with an LVFT/RR of 39%, which is below the proposed cut-off value of 40%, indicating impaired diastolic filling of the heart [15,16].

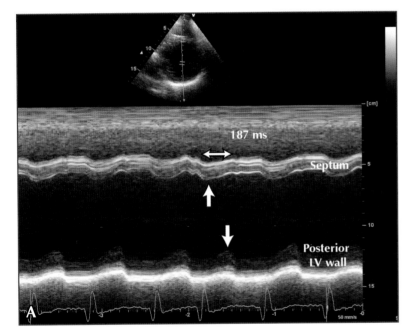

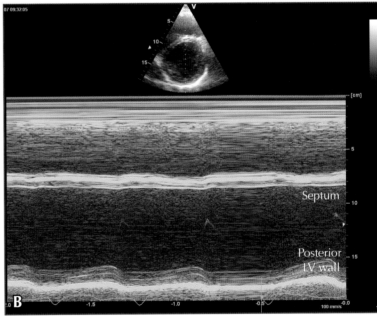

Figure 20-4. Septal to posterior wall motion delay (SPWMD) as a measure of LV dyssynchrony is shown. An M-mode recording is obtained through the septum and posterior LV wall in the parasternal short-axis view. LV dyssynchrony is defined as the shortest interval between the maximum systolic displacement of the septum and posterior wall. Using a cut-off value of 130 ms, Pitzalis *et al.* [15,16] were able to predict response after cardiac resynchronization therapy (CRT) with an accuracy of 85% (sensitivity of 100% and specificity of 63%). An example of the SPWMD measurement in a heart failure patient is shown (**A**). The SPWMD is 187 ms, which is above the cut-off value of 130 ms, indicating the presence of substantial LV dyssynchrony. Septal and posterior systolic displacement is indicated (*arrows*). Recently, however, Marcus *et al.* [17] reported (in a retrospective analysis of patients included in the CONTAK-CD trial) a sensitivity of 24% with a specificity of 66% to predict a response to CRT; the SPWMD could not be assessed in 50% of patients. Reduced interpretability of the SPWMD can be the result of akinesia of the interventricular septum after infarction (**B**), the posterior wall (or both), or a poor acoustic window in the parasternal view [17,18].

Methods Based on Tissue Doppler Imaging

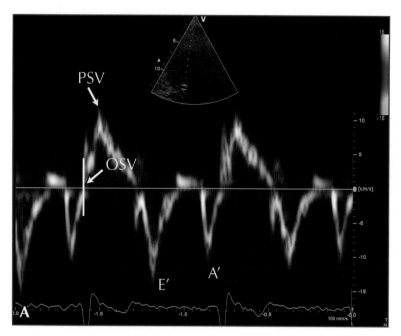

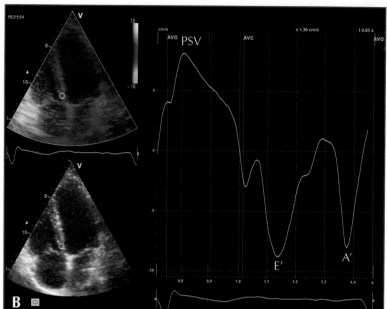

Figure 20-5. Tissue Doppler imaging (TDI) is one of the most widely studied techniques for the assessment of LV dyssynchrony [5–7,19–22]. TDI allows measurement of the (peak systolic) velocities of different regions of the myocardium and detection of the timing of these velocities throughout the cardiac cycle among different myocardial regions. The myocardial velocity curves can be constructed on-line using pulsed-wave TDI (**A**) and off-line using color-coded TDI (**B**) by placing a sample in the region of interest (in this example, in the basal septum on the four-chamber view). The sample area has the same color as the corresponding myocardial velocity curve. The

main advantage of color-coded TDI is the possibility for off-line analysis and the ability to evaluate multiple myocardial segments within one single heart beat, thereby avoiding potential errors from differences in cardiac frequency. The differences in time-to-peak systolic velocities (PSV) among different myocardial segments are used as a marker of LV dyssynchrony. Using pulsed-wave TDI, the PSV is often difficult to define, and therefore the onset of systolic velocity (OSV) is often used when pulsed wave Doppler is applied (**A**). E′ and A′ represent diastolic parameters. AVO—aortic valve opening; AVC—aortic valve closure.

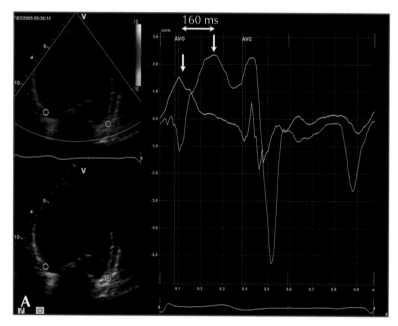

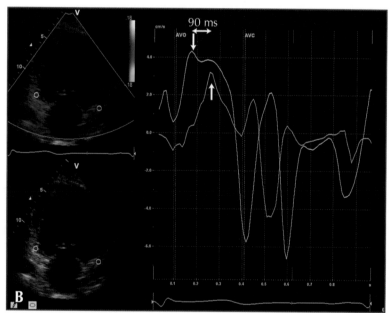

Figure 20-6. Two- and four-segmental color-coded tissue Doppler imaging (TDI) models for measurement of LV dyssynchrony [6,23] are shown. The two-segmental model measures the difference in time-to-peak systolic velocity between the basal septum and lateral wall on the four-chamber color-coded image and is referred to as the septal-to-lateral delay. This technique has been validated in 25 heart failure patients and an optimal cut-off value of 60 ms for substantial LV dyssynchrony has been proposed [23]. The four-segmental model is a further refinement of this approach and is defined as the largest time difference among the four basal LV segments on the four- and two-chamber

views (*ie*, septum, lateral, anterior, and inferior) [6]. In a group of patients undergoing cardiac resynchronization therapy (CRT), the largest delay was observed between the septum and the lateral wall in 89% of patients. Using receiver operating characteristic curve analysis, an optimal cut-off value of 65 ms was derived in 85 patients undergoing CRT with a sensitivity and specificity of 80% to predict clinical response and 92% to predict echocardiographic response. Four-chamber (**A**) and two-chamber (**B**) views of a heart failure patient with dyssynchrony of 160 ms between the septum and the lateral wall (**A**) and dyssynchrony of 90 ms between the anterior and posterior wall (**B**) are shown.

Continued on the next page

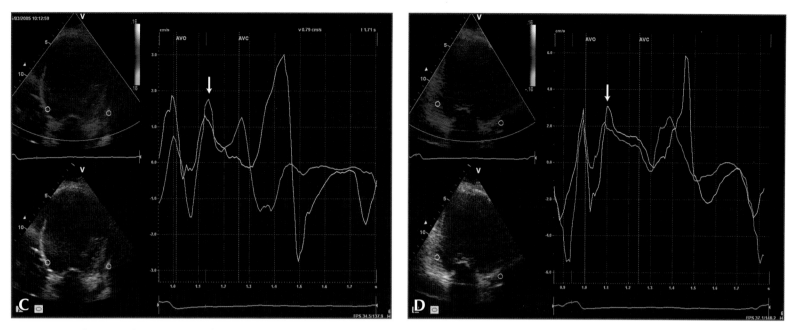

Figure 20-6. *(Continued)* Immediately after CRT implantation, LV dyssynchrony has disappeared (**C** and **D**). Peak systolic velocities are shown (*arrows*). AVO—aortic valve opening; AVC—aortic valve closure.

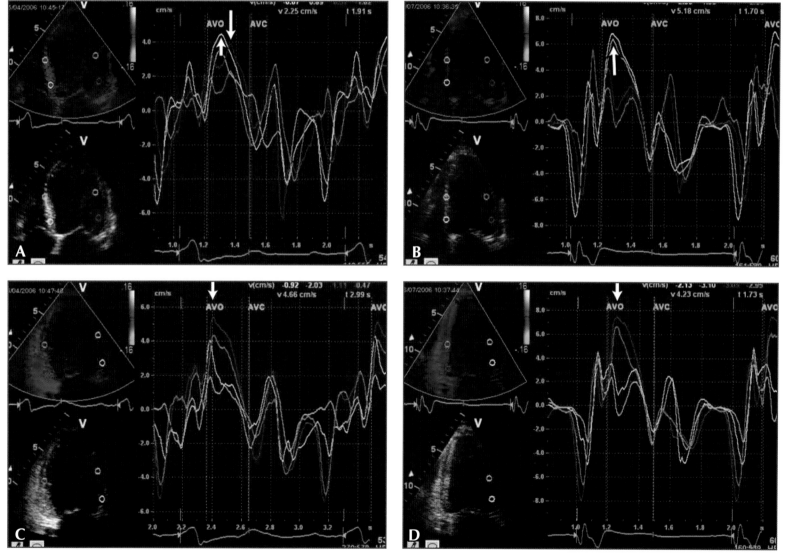

Figure 20-7. Twelve-segmental color-coded tissue Doppler imaging (TDI) models for measurement of LV dyssynchrony is shown. Yu *et al.* [5] proposed measuring the standard deviation of the time-to-peak systolic velocity among 12 LV segments (six basal and six mid) on the apical two-, three-, and four-chamber images in order to calculate the dyssynchrony index (Ts-SD). Examples of color-coded TDI at apical four-chamber (**A** and **B**), apical two-chamber (**C** and **D**), and apical three-chamber (**E** and **F**) views before (**A**, **C**, and **E**) and after (**B**, **D**, and **F**) CRT are shown.

Continued on the next page

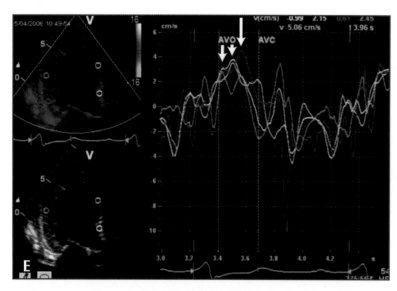

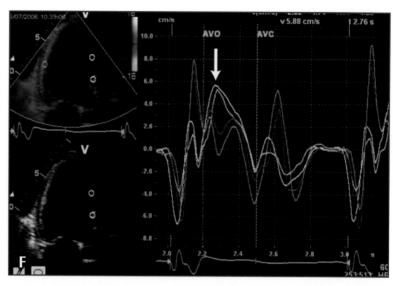

Figure 20-7. *(Continued)* The use of three apical views can establish the six-basal and six-midsegmental LV model for assessing LV dyssynchrony. Delay in the time-to-peak systolic velocity is evident in the lateral (**A**) and posterior walls (**C**) at baseline. Peak systolic velocities are shown (**A** and **C**, *arrows*). After cardiac resynchronization therapy (CRT), there is a realignment of the systolic velocities, in particular in the ejection phase where the peak systolic velocities occur almost at the same time. Peak systolic velocities are shown (*all panels, arrows*) The Ts-SD can be calculated from the standard deviation of time-to-peak systolic velocity in the ejection phase of the 12 LV segments, which is decreased from 51 ms before CRT to 20 ms after the therapy. The cut-off value of Ts-SD for substantial LV dyssynchrony is 33 ms [5]. AVC—aortic valve closure; AVO—aortic valve opening.

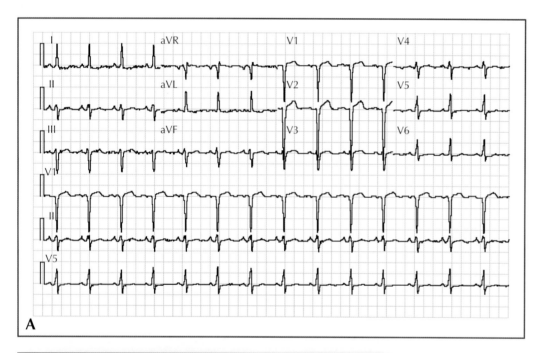

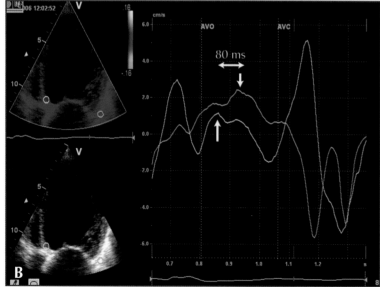

Figure 20-8. Tissue Doppler imaging (TDI) in a patient with a narrow QRS complex is shown. In patients with a QRS complex of less than 120 ms, evidence of substantial LV dyssynchrony can be demonstrated in 25% to 50% of patients, suggesting that these patients may benefit from cardiac resynchronization therapy (CRT) [11–13]. Recent small studies have indicated that CRT has similar effects in heart failure patients with narrow QRS complex as long as substantial baseline LV dyssynchrony is present [24,25]. However, the recent RethinQ study suggested a limited effect of CRT in patients with narrow QRS complex [26]. An example of a heart failure patient (New York Heart Association class III and LV ejection fraction < 35%) with a narrow QRS complex (90 ms) and substantial LV dyssynchrony (80 ms) is shown (**A** and **B**). Peak systolic velocity is indicated (*arrows*). AVC—aortic valve closure; AVO—aortic valve opening.

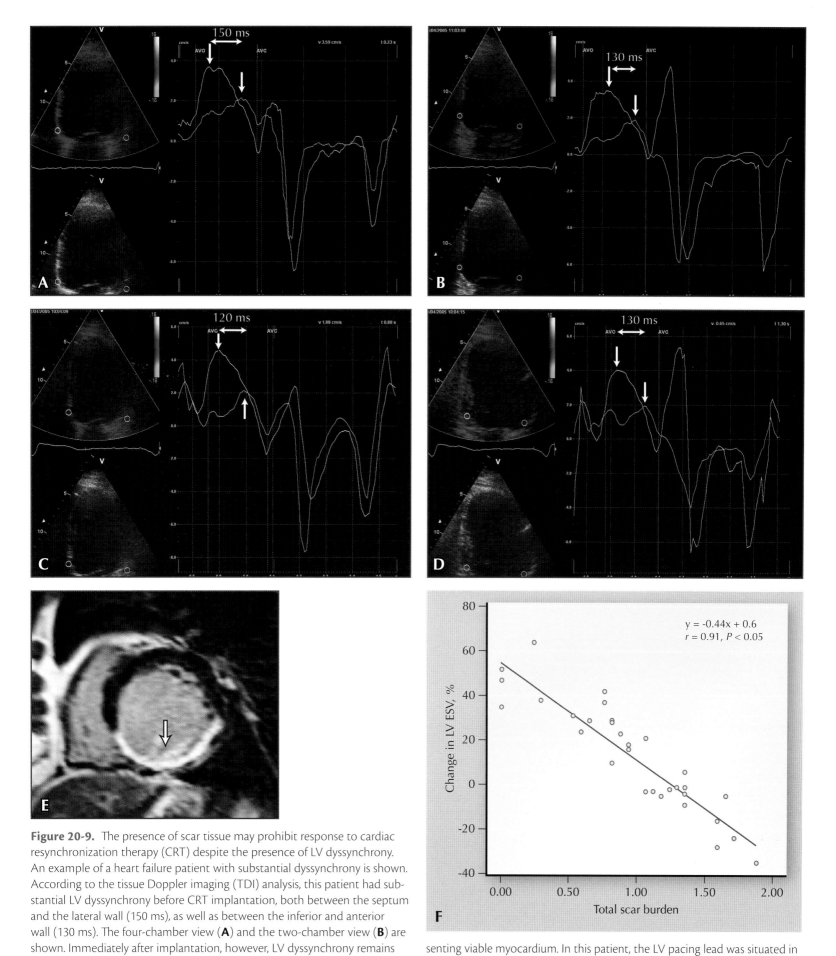

Figure 20-9. The presence of scar tissue may prohibit response to cardiac resynchronization therapy (CRT) despite the presence of LV dyssynchrony. An example of a heart failure patient with substantial dyssynchrony is shown. According to the tissue Doppler imaging (TDI) analysis, this patient had substantial LV dyssynchrony before CRT implantation, both between the septum and the lateral wall (150 ms), as well as between the inferior and anterior wall (130 ms). The four-chamber view (**A**) and the two-chamber view (**B**) are shown. Immediately after implantation, however, LV dyssynchrony remains largely unchanged (**C** and **D**). Peak systolic velocity is shown (**A–D**, *arrows*). At 6 months follow-up, this patient did not improve in clinical symptoms or LV function. A preimplantation contrast-enhanced MRI revealed the presence of scar tissue in the inferolateral region. The short-axis view (**E**) shows an area (*white*) representing scar tissue (*arrow*) and another area (*black*) repre-

senting viable myocardium. In this patient, the LV pacing lead was situated in a posterolateral branch of the venous system, which resulted in ineffective LV stimulation as a result of the scar tissue in the area of the LV pacing lead. A recent study has demonstrated that patients with scar tissue in the posterolateral LV segments have a low likelihood of response to CRT [27]. In addition, the extent of scar tissue in the entire LV is also important.

Continued on the next page

Figure 20-9. *(Continued)* Ypenburg *et al.* [28] recently demonstrated (using contrast-enhanced MRI) that patients with extensive scar formation did not respond to CRT. In 34 patients undergoing CRT, a close correlation was observed between the total scar burden (defined as the mean scar score among 17 LV segments) and the change in LV end-systolic volume at 6 months follow-up (**F**). (*From* Ypenburg *et al.* [28]; with permission.) AVC—aortic valve closure; AVO—aortic valve opening; ESV—end-systolic volume.

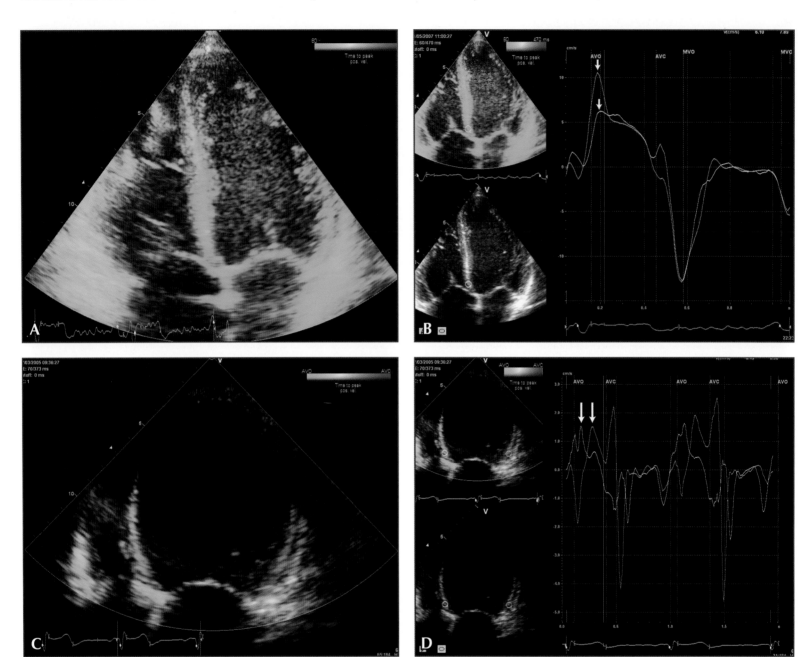

Figure 20-10. Semiautomatic measurement of LV dyssynchrony using tissue synchronization imaging (TSI) is shown. The TSI approach is a novel derivation of color-coded tissue Doppler imaging (TDI), which allows a quick and qualitative visualization of segments with an early peak systolic velocity (indicated in *green in all panels*) and segments with a late peak systolic velocity (indicated in *orange/red in all panels*) without the need for the myocardial velocity curves. If needed, quantitative assessment of LV dyssynchrony is still possible through construction of the myocardial velocity curves (similar to color-coded TDI). Yu *et al.* [22] studied this qualitative approach in 56 heart failure patients and reported a sensitivity of 82% with a specificity of 87% in order to predict response to cardiac resynchronization therapy. An example of a normal individual without LV dyssynchrony (with all segments colored green, indicating an early peak systolic velocity through the LV) is shown (**A**). An example of a heart failure patient with late mechanical activation of the lateral wall (**C**, *orange*) is shown. The myocardial velocity curves are displayed (**B** and **D**) (derived by postprocessing of the TSI images) illustrating complete synchrony in the normal individual (**A**) and the presence of LV dyssynchrony between the basal septum and lateral wall in the patient (**C**). Peak systolic velocity is shown (**B** and **D**, *arrows*). AVC—aortic valve closure; AVO—aortic valve opening.

Methods Based on Strain Imaging

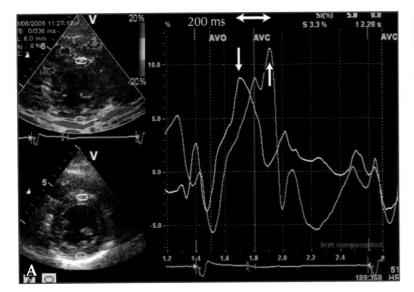

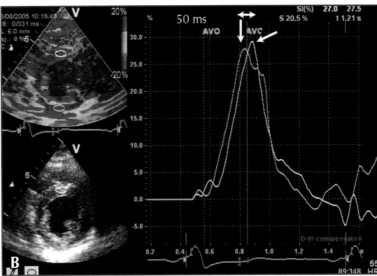

Figure 20-11. Strain imaging is able to measure deformation of the myocardium in contrast to tissue Doppler imaging (TDI), which measures myocardial velocities. A potential advantage of strain imaging over TDI therefore is its ability to distinguish active deformation from passive myocardial motion. Examples of radial strain derived from short-axis views at the midventricular level are shown (**A** and **B**). Normal systolic radial strain derived from short-axis views yields positive deflections, with the largest cumulated value occurring during the end of systole. In this patient, systolic dyssynchrony at baseline (**A**) before cardiac resynchronization therapy (CRT) is illustrated by the difference in time to maximal positive strain (*arrows*) between the midanteroseptal and posterior segments (in this case, 200 ms). This mechanical delay is reduced to 50 ms after CRT (**B**). A recent study by Dohi *et al.* [29] proposed an optimal cut-off value of 130 ms in dyssynchrony based on radial strain for prediction of response to CRT. AVC—aortic valve closure; AVO—aortic valve opening.

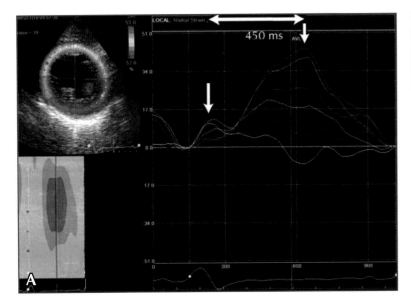

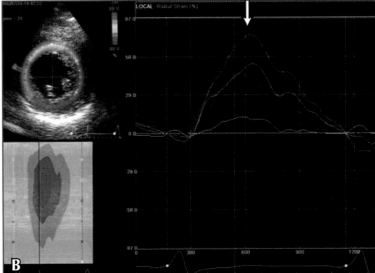

Figure 20-12. Two-dimensional speckle tracking to assess strain from a short-axis image at the level of the papillary muscles is shown. Images before (**A**) and after (**B**) cardiac resynchronization therapy (CRT) are shown; normal radial strain yields positive deflections during systole. LV dyssynchrony at baseline is reflected by the difference of time to maximal radial strain (*arrows*) between the midanteroseptal (*yellow curve*) and midposterior segments (*purple curve*) of 450 ms, which was reduced to 30 ms after CRT. Suffoletto *et al.* [30] proposed an optimal cut-off value of 130 ms for two-dimensional radial strain derived by speckle tracking to predict response to CRT.

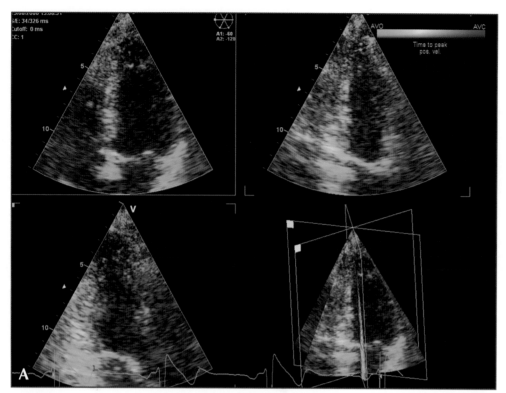

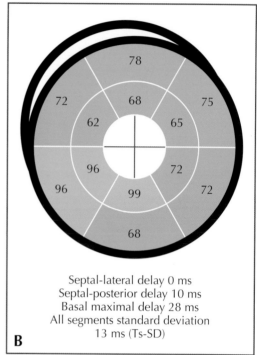

Septal-lateral delay 0 ms
Septal-posterior delay 10 ms
Basal maximal delay 28 ms
All segments standard deviation
13 ms (Ts-SD)

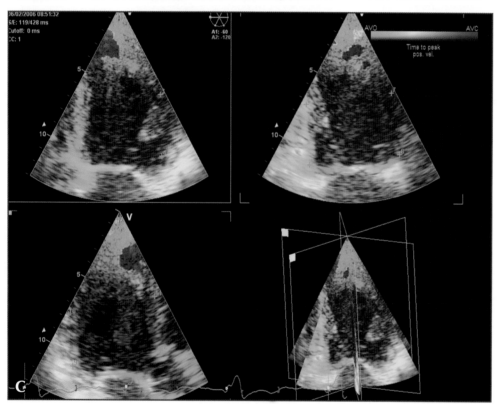

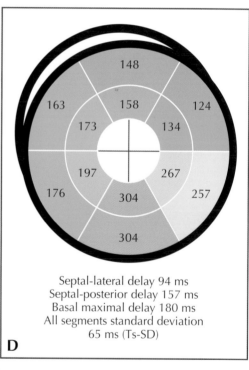

Septal-lateral delay 94 ms
Septal-posterior delay 157 ms
Basal maximal delay 180 ms
All segments standard deviation
65 ms (Ts-SD)

Figure 20-13. Triplane tissue synchronization imaging (TSI) is shown. This approach permits the recording of the two-, three-, and four-chamber TSI images in one single heart beat and provides a three-dimensional reconstruction of the LV dyssynchrony. Similar to single-plane TSI (*see* Fig. 20-10), this technique displays LV dyssynchrony qualitatively. Early (indicated in *green*) and late (indicated in *orange/red*) peak systolic velocities are shown, which allows immediate visualization of the area of latest activation. The program is also able to automatically deliver quantitative information on LV dyssynchrony (eg, the two-, four, or 12-segmental tissue Doppler imaging [TDI] dyssynchrony models), and a bull's eye plot with information on time-to-peak systolic velocity for each individual LV segment. An example of a normal individual (**A**) with a synchronous contraction of the LV is shown. The two-,

three-, and four-chamber views do not display significant dyssynchrony. A bull's eye plot (**B**) of the same patient (**A**) is depicted. The numbers represent the automatically calculated time-to-peak systolic velocities for 12 myocardial segments (six basal and six mid segments). In this patient, the time-to-peak systolic velocities are comparable between the 12 segments, indicating a synchronous activation. In addition, the calculations of the different LV dyssynchrony models are displayed automatically (eg, the two-, four-, or 12-segmental TDI dyssynchrony models). An example of a heart failure patient (**C**) with a clear dyssynchrony in the basal and mid inferior/posterior LV segments (*orange/red*) is shown . A bull's eye plot (**D**) of the same patient (**C**) is depicted. The time-to-peak systolic velocity in the posterolateral segments is clearly prolonged compared with the anterior and septal LV regions.

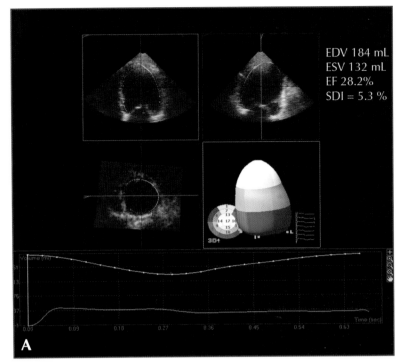

EDV 184 mL
ESV 132 mL
EF 28.2%
SDI = 5.3 %

A

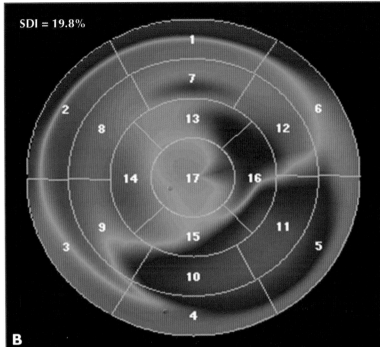

SDI = 19.8%

B

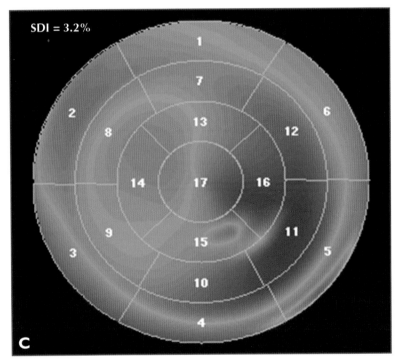

SDI = 3.2%

C

Figure 20-14. LV dyssynchrony measurement using real time three-dimensional echocardiography is shown. First LV volumes can be calculated (**A**). The time to minimal regional volume is then calculated for each segment (16-segment model), and the systolic dyssynchrony index (SDI) is calculated as a marker of LV dyssynchrony, which is defined as the standard deviation of the time taken to reach minimal regional volume for each LV segment. Kapetanakis *et al.* [31] defined an arbitrary SDI cut-off value of more than 3SD above the mean for normal subjects (*ie*, 8.3%). Similar to tissue synchronization imaging (TSI), real-time three-dimensional echocardiography is also able to provide a semiautomatic bull's eye plot representing the area of latest activation (referred to as parametric imaging). An example of a heart failure patient with LV dyssynchrony (**B**) located in the inferolateral LV regions is shown; the SDI is 19.8%. Early activated segments (*green*) and the area of last mechanical activation (*red*) are displayed. After implantation of the cardiac resynchronization therapy (CRT) device, resynchronization of the LV is obtained, and the SDI is reduced to 3.2% (**C**). EDV—end-diastolic volume; EF—ejection fraction; ESV—end-systolic volume.

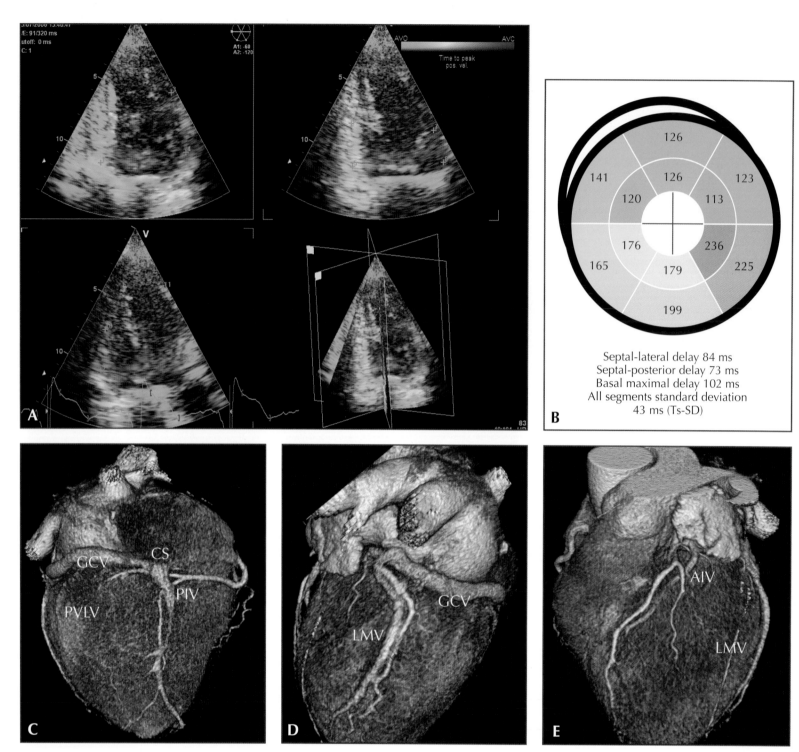

Figure 20-15. Integration of imaging modalities in cardiac resynchronization therapy (CRT) is shown. Recent data have suggested that the LV pacing lead should ideally be positioned in the area of latest mechanical activation. Murphy *et al.* [32] demonstrated that patients with the LV lead positioned in the area of latest mechanical activation have a superior improvement in LV function compared with patients with the LV lead positioned in an adjacent LV segment. Moreover, patients with the LV lead positioned in a remote LV segment showed no improvement in LV function after CRT. Novel techniques, such as triplane tissue synchronization imaging (TSI) and real-time three-dimensional echocardiography, allow identification of the area of latest mechanical activation, which should be targeted for optimal LV lead placement. Multislice CT can then be used in order to visualize the anatomy of the coronary sinus and its tributes in order to verify the presence of a suitable branch of the venous system draining the area of latest mechanical activation. In the absence of a suitable vein, a minimally invasive surgical approach may be preferred to position the LV pacing lead in the area of latest mechanical activation.

This figure provides an illustration of this integrated imaging approach for optimal LV lead placement using triplane TSI in combination with multislice CT in a patient with nonischemic cardiomyopathy considered for CRT implantation. The preimplantation triplane TSI image is displayed (**A**). The bull's eye plot (**B**) illustrates that the area of latest mechanical activation was located in the lateral LV segments; the LV dyssynchrony according to the 12-segment model was 43 ms (cut-off value 33 ms; *see* Fig. 20-7). A preimplantation three-dimensional volume-rendered multislice CT reconstruction [33] demonstrates the various cardiac veins in posterior view (**C**), lateral view (**D**), and anterior view (**E**). The multislice CT image indicates that the area of latest activation is located in the area of the left marginal vein (LMV); this branch of the coronary sinus would therefore be a perfect target for the LV pacing lead.

Continued on the next page

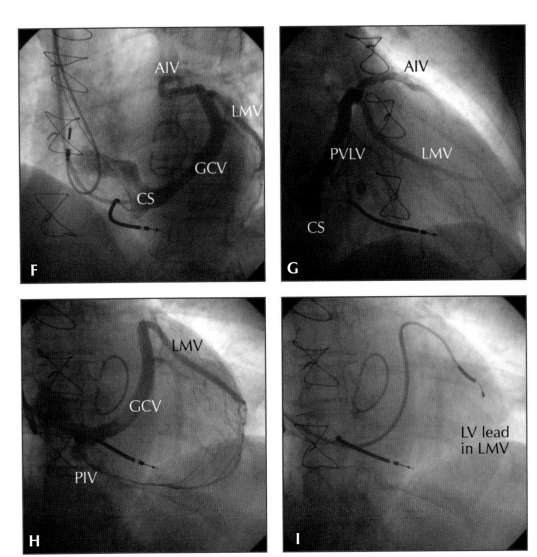

Figure 20-15. (Continued) Next, invasive venography confirms that multislice CT has provided an excellent representation of the venous anatomy (F, G, and H). AIV—anterior interventricular vein; CS—coronary sinus; GCV—great cardiac vein; PVLV—posterior vein of the LV.

The LV pacing lead was positioned in the LMV (I). Immediately after CRT implantation, triplane TSI demonstrated a significant reduction in dyssysnchrony (using the 12-segment model) to 25 ms (not shown).

At 6 month's follow-up, the patient had improved in clinical symptoms (New York Heart Association class from III to II) and LV function (LV end-diastolic volume from 193 to 185 mL, LV end-systolic volume from 160 to 134 mL, and LV ejection fraction from 14% to 27%).

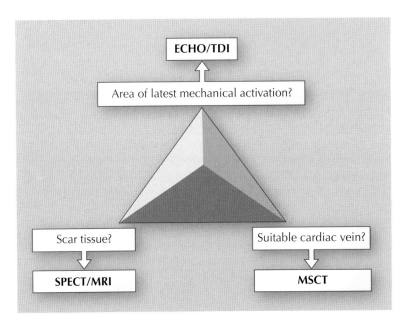

Figure 20-16. Potential approach to the use of cardiac imaging for optimal selection of patients for cardiac resynchronization therapy (CRT) is shown [34]. At present, no consensus exists on which technique is optimal for the prediction of response following CRT. A large number of different techniques measuring different myocardial segments and applying differ-

ent cut-off values have been tested in a large number of relatively small single-center studies. To date, no study has directly compared the relative merits of the different echocardiographic techniques in large multicenter studies. It has been demonstrated that patients with LV dyssynchrony appear to benefit more from CRT [8]; however, not all patients with LV dyssynchrony respond well to CRT, and it has recently been demonstrated that the correction of LV dyssynchrony was mandatory in order to result in good response to CRT [9]. Recent studies have suggested various reasons for this failure to correct LV dyssynchrony by CRT. Two major issues are important: the presence of scar tissue and the LV lead position. Patients with extensive transmural scar formation in the region where the LV lead is positioned do not benefit from CRT [27]. Moreover, the total extent of scar tissue in the LV may also be important for response to CRT, and it has been shown that patients with too extensive scar formation may not respond to CRT [28]. In addition, data are emerging that the LV lead needs to be positioned in the area of latest mechanical activation. In that respect, it may be may preferred in some patients to have information before CRT on the venous anatomy. This information can be obtained noninvasively with multislice CT (see Fig. 20-15). Accordingly, in selected patients, optimal LV lead positioning could be guided by these different imaging modalities, taking into consideration the presence and extent of scar tissue, the location of LV dyssynchrony, and the venous anatomy. MSCT—multislice CT; SPECT—single photon emission CT. TDI—tissue Doppler imaging. From Van de Veire et al. [33]; with permission.)

References

1. Abraham WT, Fisher WG, Smith AL, *et al.*: Cardiac resynchronization in chronic heart failure. *N Engl J Med* 2002, 346:1845–1853.

2. Bristow MR, Saxon LA, Boehmer J, *et al.*: Cardiac-resynchronization therapy with or without an implantable defibrillator in advanced chronic heart failure. *N Engl J Med* 2004, 350:2140–2150.

3. Cleland JG, Daubert JC, Erdmann E, *et al.*: The effect of cardiac resynchronization on morbidity and mortality in heart failure. *N Engl J Med* 2005, 352:1539–1549.

4. St John Sutton MG, Plappert T, Abraham WT, *et al.*: Effect of cardiac resynchronization therapy on left ventricular size and function in chronic heart failure. *Circulation* 2003, 107:1985–1990.

5. Yu CM, Chau E, Sanderson JE, *et al.*: Tissue Doppler echocardiographic evidence of reverse remodeling and improved synchronicity by simultaneously delaying regional contraction after biventricular pacing therapy in heart failure. *Circulation* 2002, 105:438–445.

6. Bax JJ, Bleeker GB, Marwick TH, *et al.*: Left ventricular dyssynchrony predicts response and prognosis after cardiac resynchronization therapy. *J Am Coll Cardiol* 2004, 44:1834–1840.

7. Bordachar P, Lafitte S, Reuter S, *et al.*: Echocardiographic parameters of ventricular dyssynchrony validation in patients with heart failure using sequential biventricular pacing. *J Am Coll Cardiol* 2004, 44:2154–2165.

8. Bax JJ, Abraham T, Barold SS, *et al.*: Cardiac resynchronization therapy: part 1—issues before implantation. *J Am Coll Cardiol* 2005, 46:2153–2167.

9. Bleeker GB, Mollema SA, Holman ER, *et al.*: Left ventricular resynchronization is mandatory for response to cardiac resynchronization therapy: analysis in patients with echocardiographic evidence of left ventricular dyssynchrony at baseline. *Circulation* 2007, 116:1440–1448.

10. Yu CM, Fung WH, Lin H, *et al.*: Predictors of left ventricular reverse remodeling after cardiac resynchronization therapy for heart failure secondary to idiopathic dilated or ischemic cardiomyopathy. *Am J Cardiol* 2003, 91:684–688.

11. Yu CM, Lin H, Zhang Q, Sanderson JE: High prevalence of left ventricular systolic and diastolic asynchrony in patients with congestive heart failure and normal QRS duration. *Heart* 2003, 89:54–60.

12. Bleeker GB, Schalij MJ, Molhoek SG, *et al.*: Relationship between QRS duration and left ventricular dyssynchrony in patients with end-stage heart failure. *J Cardiovasc Electrophysiol* 2004, 15:544–549.

13. Ghio S, Constantin C, Klersy C, *et al.*: Interventricular and intraventricular dyssynchrony are common in heart failure patients, regardless of QRS duration. *Eur Heart J* 2004, 35:571–578.

14. Cazeau S, Bordachar P, Jauvert G, *et al.*: Echocardiographic modeling of cardiac dyssynchrony before and during multisite stimulation: a prospective study. *PACE* 2003, 26(1 Pt 2):137–143.

15. Pitzalis MV, Iacoviello M, Romito R, *et al.*: Cardiac resynchronization therapy tailored by echocardiographic evaluation of ventricular asynchrony. *J Am Coll Cardiol* 2002, 40:1615–1622.

16. Pitzalis MV, Iacoviello M, Romito R, *et al.*: Ventricular asynchrony predicts a better outcome in patients with chronic heart failure receiving cardiac resynchronization therapy. *J Am Coll Cardiol* 2005, 45:65–69.

17. Marcus GM, Rose E, Viloria EM, *et al.*: Septal to posterior wall motion delay fails to predict reverse remodeling or clinical improvement in patients undergoing cardiac resynchronization therapy. *J Am Coll Cardiol* 2005, 46:2208–2214.

18. Bleeker GB, Schalij MJ, Boersma E, *et al.*: Relative merits of M-mode echocardiography and tissue Doppler imaging for prediction of response to cardiac resynchronization therapy in patients with heart failure secondary to ischemic or idiopathic dilated cardiomyopathy. *Am J Cardiol* 2007, 99:68–74.

19. Notabartolo D, Merlino JD, Smith AL, *et al.*: Usefulness of the peak velocity difference by tissue Doppler imaging technique as an effective predictor of response to cardiac resynchronization therapy. *Am J Cardiol* 2004, 94:817–820.

20. Yu CM, Fung JW, Zhang Q, *et al.*: Tissue Doppler imaging is superior to strain rate imaging and postsystolic shortening on the prediction of reverse remodeling in both ischemic and nonischemic heart failure after cardiac resynchronization therapy. *Circulation* 2004, 110:66–73.

21. Penicka M, Bartunek J, de Bruyne B, *et al.*: Improvement of left ventricular function after cardiac resynchronization therapy is predicted by tissue Doppler imaging echocardiography. *Circulation* 2004, 109:978–983.

22. Yu CM, Zhang Q, Fung JW, *et al.*: A novel tool to assess systolic asynchrony and identify responders of cardiac resynchronization therapy by tissue synchronization imaging. *J Am Coll Cardiol* 2005, 45:677–684.

23. Bax JJ, Marwick TH, Molhoek SG, *et al.*: Left ventricular dyssynchrony predicts benefit of cardiac resynchronization therapy in patients with end-stage heart failure before pacemaker implantation. *Am J Cardiol* 2003, 92:1238–1240.

24. Bleeker GB, Holman ER, Steendijk P, *et al.*: Cardiac resynchronization therapy in patients with a narrow QRS complex. *J Am Coll Cardiol* 2006, 48:2243–2250.

25. Yu CM, Chan YS, Zhang Q, *et al.*: Benefits of cardiac resynchronization therapy for heart failure patients with narrow QRS complexes and coexisting systolic asynchrony by echocardiography. *J Am Coll Cardiol* 2006, 48:2251–2257

26. Beshai JF, Grimm RA, Nagueh SF, *et al.*: Cardiac-resynchronization therapy in heart failure with narrow QRS complexes. *N Engl J Med* 2007, 357:2461–2471.

27. Bleeker GB, Kaandorp TA, Lamb HJ, *et al.*: Effect of posterolateral scar tissue on clinical and echocardiographic improvement after cardiac resynchronization therapy. *Circulation* 2006, 113:969–967.

28. Ypenburg C, Roes SD, Bleeker GB, *et al.*: Effect of total scar burden on contrast-enhanced magnetic resonance imaging on response to cardiac resynchronization therapy. *Am J Cardiol* 2007, 99:657–660.

29. Dohi K, Suffoletto MS, Schwartzman D, *et al.*: Utility of echocardiographic radial strain imaging to quantify left ventricular dyssynchrony and predict acute response to cardiac resynchronization therapy. *Am J Cardiol* 2005, 96:112–116.

30. Suffoletto MS, Dohi K, Cannesson M, *et al.*: Novel speckle-tracking radial strain from routine black-and-white echocardiographic images to quantify dyssynchrony and predict response to cardiac resynchronization therapy. *Circulation* 2006, 113:960–968.

31. Kapetanakis S, Kearney MT, Siva A, *et al.*: Real-time three-dimensional echocardiography: a novel technique to quantify global left ventricular mechanical dyssynchrony. *Circulation* 2005, 112:992–1000.

32. Murphy RT, Sigurdsson G, Mulamalla S, *et al.*: Tissue synchronization imaging and optimal left ventricular pacing site in cardiac resynchronization therapy. *Am J Cardiol* 2006, 97:1615–1621.

33. Van de Veire NR, Schuijf JD, De Sutter J, *et al.*: Non-invasive visualization of the cardiac venous system in coronary artery disease patients using 64-slice computed tomography. *J Am Coll Cardiol* 2006, 48:1832–1838.

34. Bleeker GB, Yu CM, Nihoyannopoulos P, *et al.*: Optimal use of echocardiography in cardiac resynchronization therapy. *Heart* 2007, 93:1339–1350.

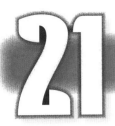

Contrast Echocardiography

Roxy Senior and Brijesh Anantharam

Ultrasound contrast agents have been used clinically for nearly 40 years; however, the past decade has seen great refinements in agents, as well as echocardiographic technologies, which have resulted in a new range of clinical applications. The development of ultrasound contrast agents has undergone significant advances. Initially, contrast agents were air-filled microbubbles, which were relatively unstable in the blood and could not pass the pulmonary capillary bed, rendering them unsuitable for the assessment of the left side of the heart during intravenous injection. Second-generation contrast agents contain a gas with low solubility and diffusibility as well as a shell of lipids, albumin, or galactose to prolong their life span. The microbubbles are a diameter less than that of a red blood cell, they resist arterial pressure, and they remain intravascular in the intact circulation. These properties allow passage of the pulmonary vasculature, opacification of the LV cavity, and imaging of myocardial perfusion. Currently, the most frequently used second-generation contrast agents are sulphur hexafluoride (SonoVue; Bracco Research SA, Geneva, Switzerland), perflutren protein-type A microspheres (Optison; GE Healthcare Inc., Princeton, NJ), and perflutren lipid microspheres (Definity; Bristol-Myers Squibb, Billerica, MA), which differ in terms of their shell constituents and gas content.

The first part of the chapter details the common clinical applications of LV opacification with contrast agents, which are explained with echocardiographic images. The second part of the chapter details the usefulness of contrast in the assessment of myocardial perfusion.

Contrast-Enhanced Endocardial Definition

In spite of substantial improvement in endocardial definition through the use of tissue harmonic imaging, there is still a significant number of patients in whom endocardial definition remains inadequate for proper assessment of LV function. LV opacification can be achieved using microbubbles. These microbubbles increase back scatter in an ultrasound field, opacifying LV cavity, and at the same time making the myocardium dark, enhancing the interface that is the endocardium. This also allows for more accurate assessment of LV volumes and ejection fraction [1,2]. The LV endocardial walls are not smooth borders, but instead are irregularly trabeculated. With contrast, the small spaces between the trabeculations are filled, and the contour for border tracing will include a larger area than observed with unenhanced echocardiography where the inner border of the trabeculated area is traced. Accurate assessment of regional and global LV function and structure is pivotal in the clinical management of patients with suspected cardiovascular disease.

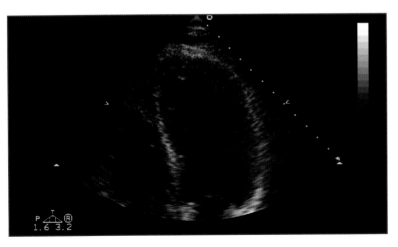

Figure 21-1. Image in apical four-chamber view. This image, along with Fig. 21-2, is taken during tissue harmonic imaging, showing poor delineation of the endocardium, particularly in the distal septum, apex, and lateral wall. This makes it difficult to assess regional wall motion and LV function.

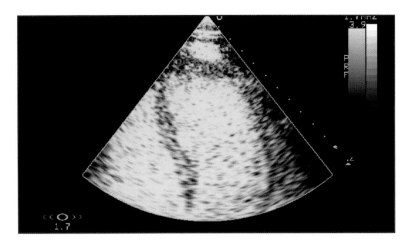

Figure 21-2. Image in apical four-chamber view. Following contrast injection, there is marked improvement of the endocardial border visualization of the LV and the ability to fully identify the distal septum, apex, and lateral wall. Normal wall motion and LV function was observed.

Thrombus in the LV

Transthoracic echocardiography is currently the standard diagnostic procedure for the diagnosis of LV thrombus. Transthoracic imaging suffers from near-field artifacts where apical LV thrombi are usually located. LV opacification with contrast agents in patients with suboptimal acoustic windows enhances the identification of thrombus in LV. Contrast is also useful in the differential diagnosis of masses. A thrombus typically shows up as a nonopacified structure. This can be important in rare conditions when the mass is found in a ventricle with normal contractility and a tumor is suspected. Tumor opacification is usually related to the degree of vascularization.

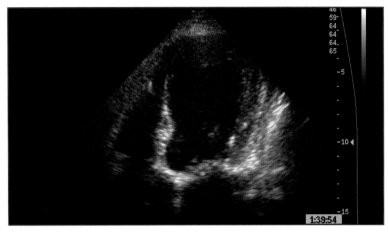

Figure 21-3. Tissue harmonic imaging in a patient with dilated cardiomyopathy and a vague echo density in the LV apex is suggestive of an apical LV thrombus.

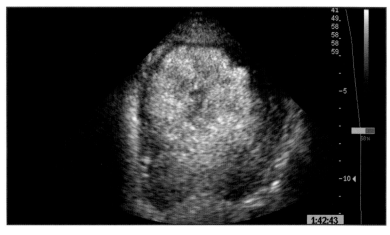

Figure 21-4. Apical four-chamber view. Image enhancement with intravenous contrast demonstrates LV opacification and outlines the normal smooth endocardial border. The apical image artifact is eliminated, thus excluding an LV thrombus.

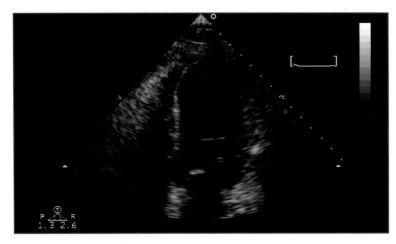

Figure 21-5. Apical four-chamber view. Tissue harmonic imaging in a patient with recent anteroseptal acute myocardial infarction demonstrates suboptimal endocardial borders. A vague echo density at the apex suggests an apical thrombus.

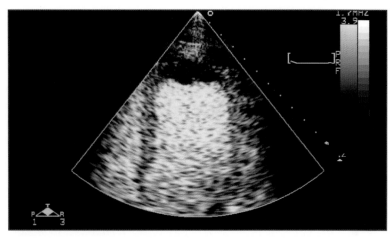

Figure 21-6. Apical four-chamber view. After contrast enhancement, a distinct filling defect is noted in the apex consistent with LV apical thrombus.

Apical Hypertrophic Cardiomyopathy

Apical hypertrophic cardiomyopathy is characterized by LV hypertrophy localized to the apex and is a rare form of hypertrophic cardiomyopathy. The typical features consist of "giant" T-wave negativity in the electrocardiogram and a spade-like configuration of the LV cavity at end diastole on left ventriculography, mild symptoms, and a more benign course compared with other forms of hypertrophic cardiomyopathy. Atrial fibrillation is the most common complication.

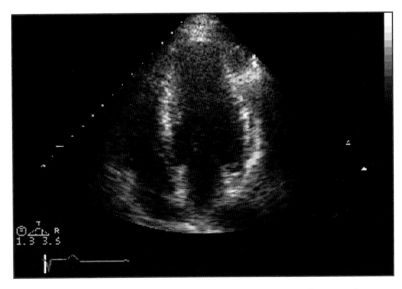

Figure 21-7. Apical four-chamber view. The apex appears akinetic, whereas the rest of the LV contracts normally.

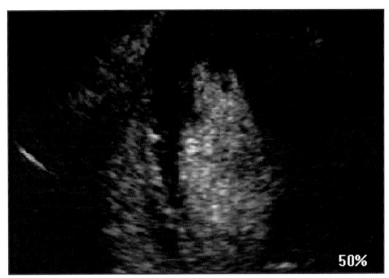

Figure 21-8. Apical four-chamber view. The classical spade-like appearance of the LV cavity is seen with an intravenous injection of contrast agent, confirming the diagnosis of apical hypertrophic cardiomyopathy. The unenhanced echocardiography missed the diagnosis, as the harmonics of the myocardium in the apex is poor and therefore myocardium is not well visualized.

Noncompaction of the Ventricular Myocardium

These morphological abnormalities predominantly involve the distal (apical) portion of the LV. RV noncompaction is seen in up to 40% of patients. The noncompact trabeculated myocardium becomes thicker, and the compact layer gets thinner. It is easy to misdiagnose this disease because the compacted layer often resembles a thickened myocardium, especially if the acoustic windows are not optimal, and fine trabeculations are missed. With contrast echocardiography, the two myocardial layers can be clearly displayed. Quantitative evaluation for the diagnosis has been proposed by determining the ratio of maximal thickness of the noncompacted to compacted layers (at end systole in a parasternal short-axis view), with a ratio greater than 2 diagnostic of isolated noncompaction. This disorder is considered to be the result of an arrest of the normal process of intrauterine endomyocardial morphogenesis.

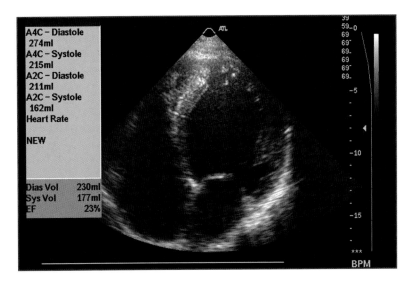

Figure 21-9. Apical four-chamber view. The unenhanced image shows dilated LV with no other pathology. A2C—apical two-chamber; A4C—apical four-chamber; BPM—beats per minute

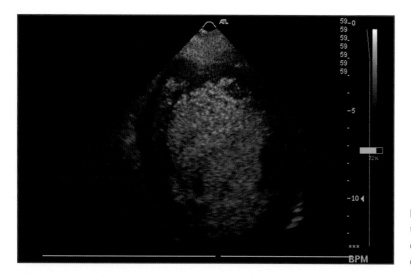

Figure 21-10. Apical four-chamber view. The figure demonstrates hypertrophied LV with multiple trabeculations and deep intertrabecular recesses communicating with the ventricular cavity, suggestive of noncompaction of ventricular myocardium. BPM—beats per minute.

Stress Echocardiography

Stress echocardiography is shown to have a high sensitivity and specificity for the detection of coronary heart disease, but is limited by the quality of the images. Contrast echocardiography enhances endocardial definition and improves the quality of the images, resulting in improved interpretation.

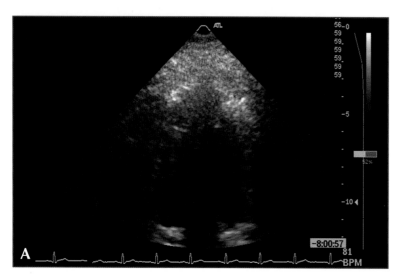
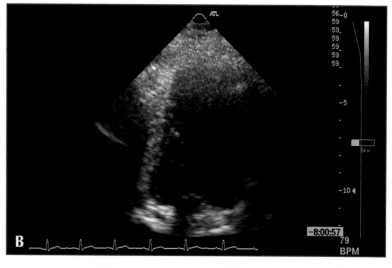

Figure 21-11. Rest images in apical four- (**A**) and two-chamber (**B**) views of a patient presenting with chest pain and nondiagnostic exercise ECG. These views show poor delineation of the endocardial border, thus precluding assessment of wall motion at rest. BPM—beats per minute.

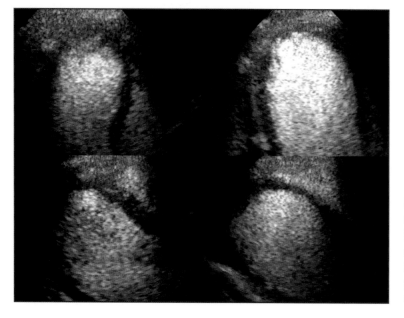

Figure 21-12. The same patient (*see* Fig. 21-11) underwent stress echocardiography after injection of contrast, which shows rest and exercise stress images in apical and parasternal long-axis views. There is clear definition of endocardial borders. The images also demonstrate dilated LV after exercise (treadmill) with akinesia involving apex and anterior septum, suggestive of proximal left anterior descending (LAD) stenosis. The patient underwent coronary angioplasty and stent to proximal LAD.

Myocardial Contrast Echocardiography

Myocardial contrast echocardiography can assess myocardial perfusion because the microbubbles remain entirely intravascular and possess a rheology similar to that of red blood cells.

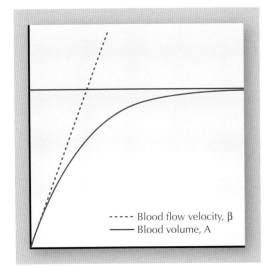

Figure 21-13. Microbubbles are administered as a constant infusion through a peripheral intravenous route and when a steady state is signal intensity from the myocardium, it represents the myocardial blood volume (A). At steady state, the microbubbles within the myocardium may be cleared with high-energy ultrasound pulse, and when imaging is performed, one can measure the rate of microbubble reappearance, which reflects red blood cell velocity (β). The product of the A x β represents myocardial blood flow (MBF) [3]. It has been shown that MBF (as assessed above) has an excellent correlation with that assessed by positron emission tomography [4].

Normal Microbubble Destruction and Replenishment

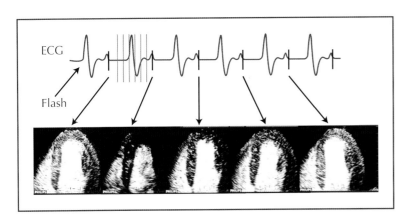

Figure 21-14. Triggered replenishment imaging. Myocardial contrast echocardiographic (MCE) images demonstrate normal replenishment after microbubble destruction at rest using high-energy ultrasound pulses (*red stripes*). These MCE images demonstrate myocardial perfusion at rest. Following stress, the microbubble velocity increases 3 to 4 times in the regions of myocardium not subtended by coronary stenosis. However, microbubble velocity is reduced in the myocardium with greater than 50% diameter stenosis. Furthermore, capillary derecruitment occurs in these regions resulting in diminished contrast signal intensity, which is seen as a perfusion defect.

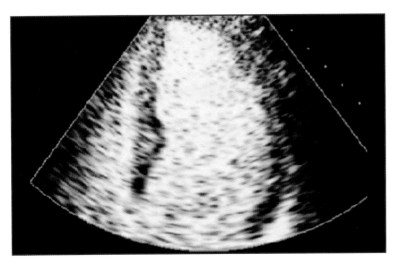

Figure 21-15. Image in apical four-chamber view. Myocardial contrast echocardiography during rest. After a steady state of contrast is achieved in the myocardium, complete destruction of myocardial contrast is achieved by high-mechanical index. There is replenishment of myocardial contrast within five cardiac cycles at rest, which is suggestive of normal myocardial blood flow.

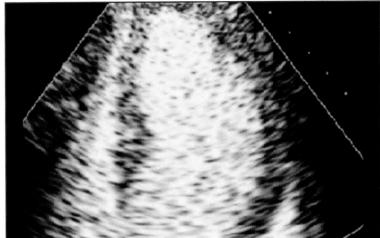

Figure 21-16. Image in apical four-chamber view. Myocardial contrast echocardiography during hyperemia using dipyridamole. After myocardial contrast destruction using high-mechanical index, there is immediate myocardial contrast replenishment within two cardiac cycles, suggestive of normal coronary flow reserve. Normal myocardial perfusion at rest and stress, respectively, is shown (*see* Fig. 21-15).

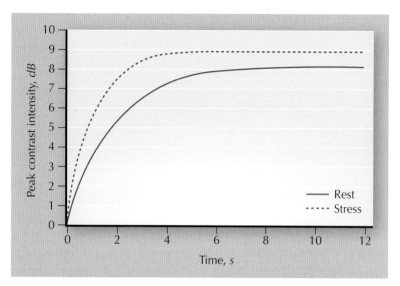

Figure 21-17. Figure shows an increase in microbubble velocity during stress, with a slight increase in capillary blood volume. The coronary blood volume is comprised of the coronary arteries, arterioles, capillaries, venules, veins, and coronary sinus; the myocardial blood volume is made up of vessels, which are less than 300 μm in diameter, most of which (> 90%) lie within the capillaries. In order to quantify myocardial blood flow (MBF), the use of specialist software is required to determine regions of interest, at rest and stress.

The software can automatically construct background subtracted plots of peak myocardial contrast intensity (*see* Figs. 21-15 and 21-16) versus pulsing intervals, from which the slope of the replenishment curve depicting mean microbubble velocity, β reserve, and MBF, can be derived. Coronary flow reserve (*ie*, stress MBF/rest MBF) can then be calculated.

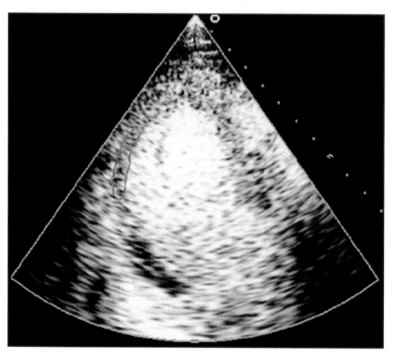

Figure 21-18. Image in apical three-chamber view. Myocardial contrast during rest demonstrates normal perfusion at rest.

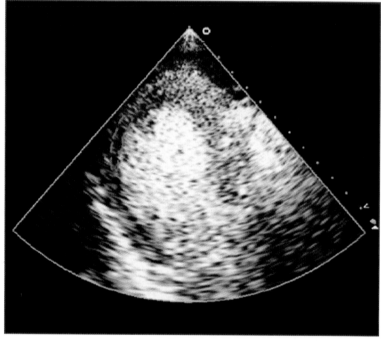

Figure 21-19. Image in apical three-chamber view. Myocardial contrast echocardiography during hyperemia using dipyridamole demonstrates slow replenishment of the posterior wall compared with septum with a persistent perfusion defect in the posterior wall. Coronary angiography subsequently demonstrated flow, limiting stenosis of the left circumflex artery.

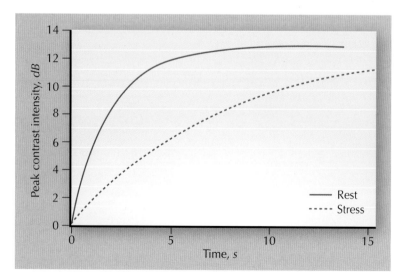

Figure 21-20. The quantification software shows reduced microbubble velocity and capillary volume during rest compared with stress in the posterior wall. Coronary flow reserve is thus markedly reduced.

Qualitative Assessment of Myocardial Perfusion

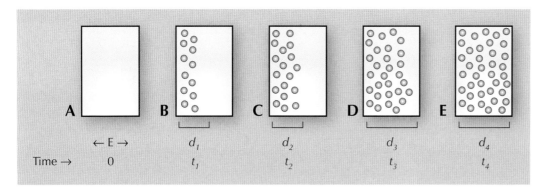

Figure 21-21. Destruction/replenishment imaging. The elevation of the ultrasound beam is 5 mm, represented as E (A). If all the microbubbles in the elevation are destroyed by a single pulse of ultrasound at t0, then replenishment of the beam elevation (d1 through d4, B through E) will depend on the velocity of the microbubbles and the ultrasound. At rest, the capillary blood flow is 1 mm/s, and microbubble replenishes by 5 seconds (t in seconds). Because coronary flow reserve in normal myocardium increases by 5 times during stress, however, the ultrasound beam replenishes in 1 second. In the myocardium (subtended by > 50% of coronary stenosis), coronary flow reserve is less than 5 times; therefore, the ultrasound beam replenishment takes longer than 1 second. The lengths of the replenishment time and perfusion defect, which can be assessed qualitatively, form the basis of detection of coronary artery stenosis. (*Adapted from* Wei *et al* [5].) d—distance traveled by the microbubble.

Sensitivity and Specificity of MCE, SPECT, and DSE

	Patients, *n*	Definition Stenosis, %	Imaging Mode	MCE Sensitivity, %	MCE Specificity, %	SPECT/DSE Sensitivity, %	SPECT/DSE Sensitivity, %
Shimoni *et al.* [6]	44	> 50	All	75	100	75	81
Olszowska *et al.* [7]	44	> 60	RTHI	97	93	83	84
Rocchi *et al.* [8]	25	> 70	HPD	89	100	100	88
Elhendy *et al.** [9]	169	> 50	RTPI	91	51	70	74
Senior *et al.* [10]	55	> 50	IPI	83	58	49	92
Peltier *et al.* [11]	35	> 70	PM	86	69	82	85
Tsutsui *et al.* [12]	16	> 50	RTI	64	92	68	61
Xie *et al.* [13]	27	> 50	PPI	66	65	33	72
Jeetley *et al.* [14]	123	> 50	TRI	84	56	82	52
Korosoglou *et al.* [15]	89	> 75	PPI	84	93	77	52
Karavidas *et al.* [16]	47	> 50	TPD	91	92	73	72
Pooled estimate				85 (81.5–88.5)	74 (67.7–80.3)	71 (66–76)	71 (64–78)

*Compared with DSE.
DSE—dobutamine stress echocardiography; MCE—myocardial contrast echocardiography; SPECT—single-photon emission CT

Figure 21-22. Sensitivity and specificity of myocardial contrast echocardiography (MCE), single-photon emission CT (SPECT), and dobutamine stress echocardiography (DSE) to detect stable coronary artery stenosis compared with coronary arteriography. The pooled estimate is a percentage (95% CI). There are a number of studies that have compared perfusion abnormalities by MCE to coronary angiography as a gold standard, suggesting MCE is a reliable and accurate technique for the identification of coronary artery stenosis. (*Adapted from* Dijkmans *et al.* [17]; with permission.) All—accelerated intermittent imaging; HPD—harmonic power Doppler; IPI—intermittent pulse inversion; PM—power modulation; PPI—power pulse inversion; RTHI—real-time harmonic imaging; RTI—real-time imaging; RTPI—real-time perfusion imaging; THI—triggered harmonic imaging; TPD—triggered power Doppler; TRI—triggered replenishment imaging.

Myocardial Contrast Echocardiography in Acute Heart Failure

Myocardial contrast echocardiography (MCE) can be used early in patients presenting with acute heart failure (AHF) in order to rapidly assess LV function (regional and global) and perfusion (rest and stress). Demonstration of normal resting myocardial perfusion in patients with AHF indicates viable myocardium. The presence of significant reversible myocardial perfusion defects in these patients establishes the diagnosis of flow-limiting coronary artery disease, and it should prompt the attending physician to plan for urgent coronary arteriography and revascularization. Coronary arteriography may not be warranted in patients with no demonstrable myocardial perfusion defects; however, even in the absence of obvious myocardial perfusion defects, determination of myocardial blood flow reserve may help to predict the outcome in patients with heart failure.

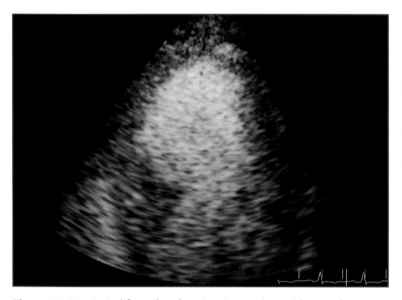

Figure 21-23. Apical four-chamber view in a patient with acute heart failure (AHF) and LV dysfunction (LV ejection fraction, 42%), demonstrating normal myocardial perfusion at rest (5 seconds after myocardial contrast destruction).

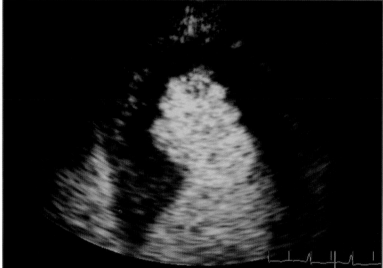

Figure 21-24. Apical four-chamber view, after dipyridamole stress, displayed 3 seconds after myocardial contrast destruction. Note the perfusion defect in the septum, apex, and lateral wall. This suggests left anterior descending (LAD) and left circumflex (LCx) flow-limiting stenosis, which was confirmed by coronary arteriography.

Postmyocardial Infarction

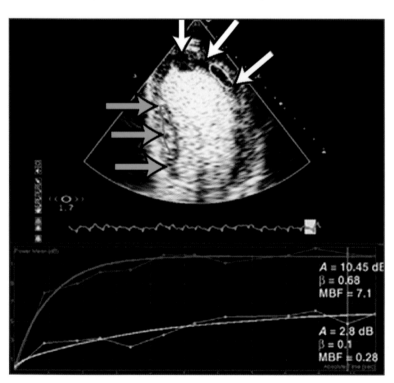

Figure 21-25. Myocardial contrast echocardiography in a patient who sustained an anterior myocardial infarction. **Top**, Apical two-chamber view on myocardial contrast echocardiography demonstrates absence of contrast opacification (*white arrows*) at the apex and anterior wall, which were akinetic. The normally contracting remote segments (*blue arrows*) show normal contrast intensity. **Bottom**, Replenishment curves in the akinetic segment (*yellow*) demonstrate very low peak contrast intensity (A), microbubble velocity (β), and myocardial blood flow (MBF), in comparison with remote normal segment (*red*).

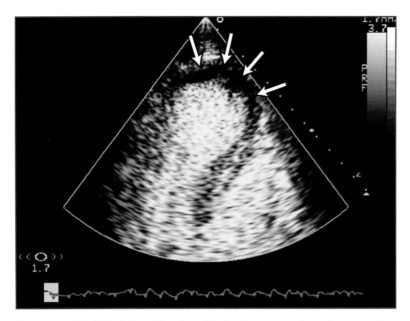

Figure 21-26. Apical three-chamber view in the same patient, demonstrating absence of contrast opacification (*arrows*) in apex.

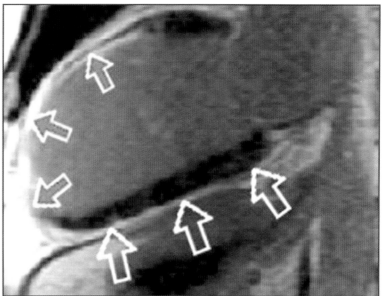

Figure 21-27. The corresponding image on contrast magnetic resonance demonstrates greater than 75% transmural extent of infarction (delayed hyperenhancement) in the akinetic segments (*orange arrows*) and no infarction in the remote normal segments (*white arrows*). Myocardial contrast echocardiography accurately reflects transmurality of myocardial necrosis and predicts contractile reserve after acute myocardial infarction.

Acute Chest Pain

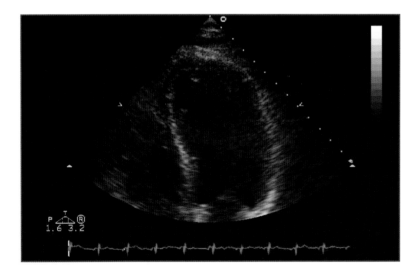

Figure 21-28. Echocardiographic image in apical four-chamber view in a patient with acute chest pain. The image shows tissue harmonic imaging demonstrating akinetic septum and apex, which suggest acute coronary syndrome.

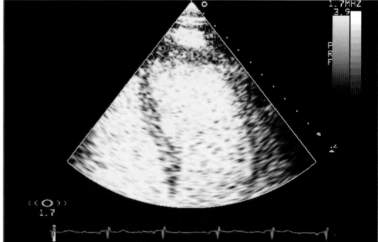

Figure 21-29. Apical four-chamber view shows myocardial contrast echocardiography (MCE) of the same patient (*see* Fig. 21-28). The image shows normal perfusion of the septum, but reduced perfusion of the apex, which suggests stunned septal myocardium and partially necrotic apex. MCE provides improved diagnostic and prognostic information over and above clinical, echodardiogram, and cardiac troponin data in patients presenting to emergency department with chest pain [18].

References

1. Malm S, Frigstad S, Sagberg E, et al.: Accurate and reproducible measurement of left ventricular volume and ejection fraction by contrast echocardiography: a comparison with magnetic resonance imaging. *J Am Coll Cardiol* 2004, 44:1030–1035.

2. Lim TK, Burden L, Janardhanan R, et al.: Improved accuracy of low-power contrast echocardiography for the assessment of left ventricular remodeling compared with unenhanced harmonic echocardiography after acute myocardial infarction: comparison with cardiovascular magnetic resonance imaging. *J Am Soc Echocardiogr* 2005, 18:1203–1207.

3. Wei K, Jayaweera AR, Firoozan S, et al.: Quantification of MBF flow with ultrasound-induced destruction of micro bubbles administered as a constant venous infusion. *Circulation* 1998, 97:473–483.

4. Vogel R, Indermühle A, Reinhardt J, et al.: The quantification of absolute myocardial perfusion in humans by contrast echocardiography: algorithm and validation. *J Am Coll Cardiol* 2005, 45:754–762.

5. Wei K, Jayaweera AR, Firoozan S, et al.: Quantification of MBF flow with ultrasound-induced destruction of micro bubbles administered as a constant venous infusion. *Circulation* 1998, 97:473–483.

6. Shimoni S, Zoghbi WA, Xie F, et al.: Real-time assessment of myocardial perfusion and wall motion during bicycle and treadmill exercise echocardiography: comparison with single photon emission computed tomography. *J Am Coll Cardiol* 2001, 37:741–747.

7. Olszowska M, Kostkiewicz M, Tracz W, Przewlocki T: Assessment of myocardial perfusion in patients with coronary artery disease. Comparison of myocardial contrast echocardiography and 99mTc MIBI single photon emission computed tomography. *Int J Cardiol* 2002, 90:49 –55.

8. Rocchi G, Fallani F, Bracchetti G, et al.: Non-invasive detection of coronary artery stenosis: a comparison among power-Doppler contrast echo, 99Tc-sestamibi SPECT and echo wall-motion analysis. *Coron Artery Dis* 2003, 14:239–245.

9. Elhendy A, O'Leary EL, Xie F, et al.: Comparative accuracy of real-time myocardial contrast perfusion imaging and wall motion analysis during dobutamine stress echocardiography for the diagnosis of coronary artery disease. *J Am Coll Cardiol* 2004, 44:2185–2191.

10. Senior R, Lepper W, Pasquet A, et al.: Myocardial perfusion assessment in patients with medium probability of coronary artery disease and no prior myocardial infarction: comparison of myocardial contrast echocardiography with 99mTc single-photon emission computed tomography. *Am Heart J* 2004, 147:1100–1105.

11. Peltier M, Vancraeynest D, Pasquet A, et al.: Assessment of the physiologic significance of coronary disease with dipyridamole realtime myocardial contrast echocardiography. Comparison with technetium-99m sestamibi single-photon emission computed tomography and quantitative coronary angiography. *J Am Coll Cardiol* 2004, 43:257–264.

12. Tsutsui JM, Xie F, McGrain AC, et al.: Comparison of low–mechanical index pulse sequence schemes for detecting myocardial perfusion abnormalities during vasodilator stress echocardiography. *Am J Cardiol* 2005, 95:565–570.

13. Xie F, Tsutsui JM, McGrain AC, et al.: Comparison of dobutamine stress echocardiography with and without real-time perfusion imaging for detection of coronary artery disease. *Am J Cardiol* 2005, 96:506–511.

14. Jeetley P, Hickman M, Kamp O, et al.: Myocardial contrast echocardiography for the detection of coronary artery stenosis: a prospective multicenter study in comparison with single-photon emission computed tomography. *J Am Coll Cardiol* 2006, 47:141–145.

15. Korosoglou G, Dubart AE, DaSilva KG, et al.: Real-time myocardial perfusion imaging for pharmacologic stress testing: added value to single photon emission computed tomography. *Am Heart J* 2006, 151:131–138.

16. Karavidas AI, Matsakas EP, Lazaros GA, et al.: Comparison of myocardial contrast echocardiography with SPECT in the evaluation of coronary artery disease in asymptomatic patients with LBBB. *Int J Cardiol* 2006, 112:334–340.

17. Dijkmans PA, Senior R, Becher H, et al.: Myocardial contrast echocardiography evolving as a clinically feasible technique for accurate, rapid, and safe assessment of myocardial perfusion: the evidence so far. *J Am Coll Cardiol* 2006, 48:2168–2177.

18. Tong KL, Kaul S, Wang XQ, et al.: Myocardial contrast echocardiography versus thrombolysis in myocardial infarction score in patients presenting to the emergency department with chest pain and a nondiagnostic electrocardiogram. *J Am Coll Cardiol* 2005, 46:920–927.

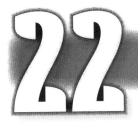

Echocardiographic Emergencies

Judy R. Mangion

Echocardiography is often the first line imaging modality for diagnosing life threatening cardiac disease because of its portability and ability to provide instantaneous real time information regarding cardiovascular structure and function. For this reason, echocardiography laboratories must be prepared at all times for "stat" requests from every area of the hospital, and the echocardiographer must be prepared to make immediate decisions at the bedside that rapidly affect patient management. Therefore, it is paramount for practicing echocardiographers to be aware of common echocardiographic emergencies and the diverse ways in which they may present themselves.

This chapter will cover common scenarios, in which echocardiography is used in the emergency setting, including cardiac tamponade. The multiple ways that tamponade may present itself will be emphasized, including pericardial effusions, loculated postoperative pericardial hematomas, pacer perforations, and coronary perforations, as well as unusual causes of tamponade, including large pleural effusions and tense ascites. The chapter will also cover the role of echocardiography in patients with pulmonary embolism with emphasis on the echocardiographic features, both on transthoracic as well as transesophageal echocardiography. Various presentations of acute aortic pathology, including aortic dissection, aneurysm, intramural hematoma, and transection are also demonstrated. Other uses of echocardiography in the emergency setting, including acute coronary syndromes, penetrating trauma, and various complications of myocardial infarction (eg, LV free wall rupture, ventricular septal defect, papillary muscle rupture, and ventricular pseudoaneurysm) will also be presented.

Cardiac Tamponade

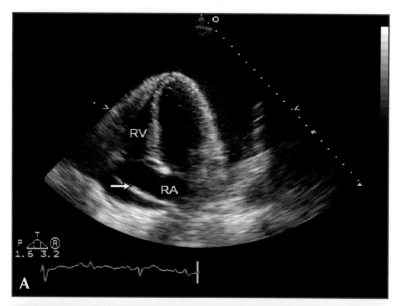

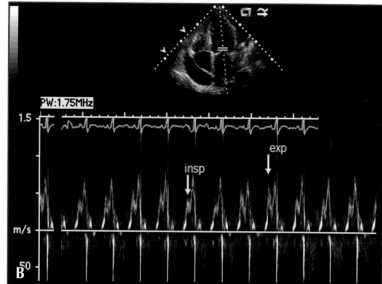

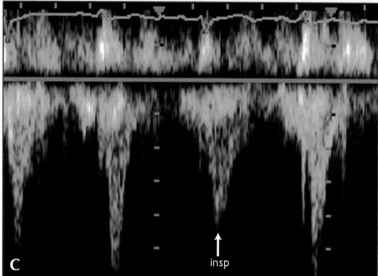

Figure 22-1. A, Physiology of cardiac tamponade, right atrial inversion. The urgent need to use echocardiography in assessing pericardial effusions always involves determining the presence or absence of tamponade physiology. Cardiac tamponade physiology occurs when the pressure in the pericardium exceeds the pressure in the cardiac chambers, resulting in impaired cardiac filling. The compressive effect of the pericardium is seen most clearly in the phase of the cardiac cycle when the pressure is lowest in that chamber. Hence, one of the earliest manifestations of tamponade is late diastolic early systolic collapse of the right atrium (RA), as is present in this apical four-chamber image (*arrow*) of a patient with massive circumferential pericardial effusion.

B, Respiratory variation in transmitral E wave with pulsed Doppler, apical four-chamber view. This image demonstrates an inspiratory decrease in transmitral E wave velocities of greater than 25% (*arrows*), which is highly suggestive of cardiac tamponade. Intrapericardial and intrathoracic pressures normally decrease to the same degree with inspiration. In tamponade, intrapericardial pressures fall substantially with inspiration as opposed to intrathoracic pressures, and as a consequence there is decreased left atrial filling pressure, which results in a decrease in E wave peak velocity. The diagnosis of pericardial tamponade always includes both clinical hemodynamic parameters and the echocardiographic findings. insp—inspiration; exp—expiration.

C, Respiratory variation in transaortic spectral Doppler, apical five-chamber view. This image demonstrates an inspiratory decrease in transaortic spectral Doppler velocities of greater than 25%, which is highly suggestive of cardiac tamponade (*arrow*). In cardiac tamponade, the increased venous return to the RV with inspiration causes a shift of septal motion towards the LV, which in turn leads to decreased LV filling and resultant pulsus paradoxus or inspiratory decrease in transaortic spectral Doppler velocities. Insp—inspiration.

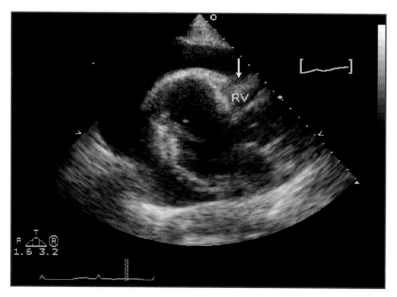

Figure 22-2. Physiology of cardiac tamponade, RV diastolic collapse (*arrow*), parasternal long-axis view. When intrapericardial pressure exceeds RV diastolic pressure, collapse of the free wall of the RV occurs. This is a less sensitive, but more specific finding, consistent with cardiac tamponade.

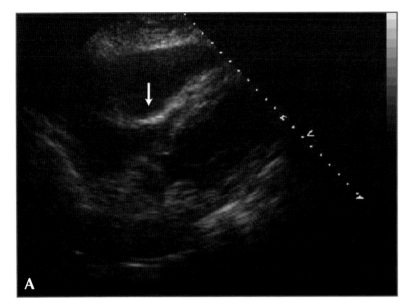

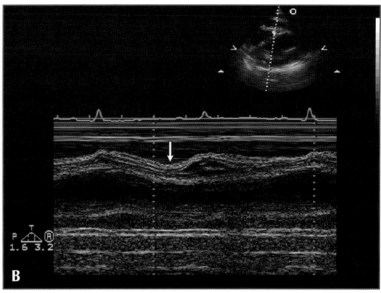

Figure 22-3. **A**, Physiology of cardiac tamponade, RV diastolic collapse (*arrow*), subcostal view. In addition to the parasternal long-axis view, the subcostal four-chamber view is often the best view for visualizing RV diastolic collapse due to pericardial tamponade. **B**, M-Mode examination, subcostal view, demonstrating diastolic collapse of the RV (*arrow*). Because of its greater spatial and temporal resolution, M-mode echocardiography can be very helpful in establishing the presence of tamponade physiology.

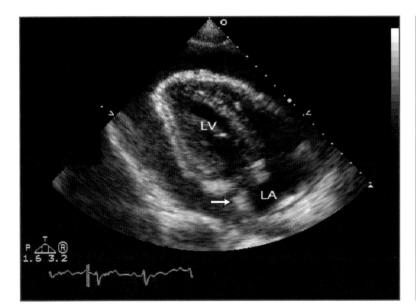

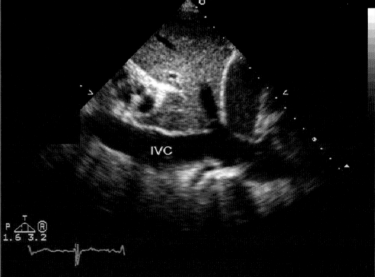

Figure 22-4. Physiology of cardiac tamponade, parasternal long-axis view, demonstrating left atrial compression (*arrow*). In fully developed cardiac tamponade, intrapericardial pressures exceed intracardiac pressures in all four chambers of the heart. Diastolic pressures in all four cardiac chambers are then elevated and equalized. LA—left atrium.

Figure 22-5. Physiology of cardiac tamponade, subcostal view, demonstrating inferior vena cava (IVC) plethora. Plethora of the inferior vena cava refers to dilatation (usually > 2 cm) with less than 50% inspiratory collapse (on sniff or deep inspiration) in diameter near the inferior vena cava, right atrial junction. This is a highly sensitive (97%), although nonspecific (40%) finding, simply reflecting high right atrial pressures.

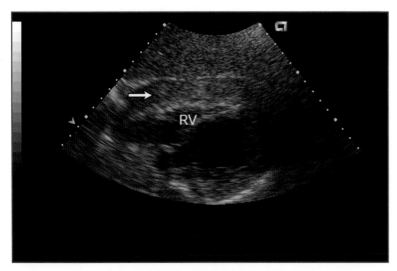

Figure 22-6. Loculated pericardial hematoma from right coronary artery perforation during cardiac catheterization, causing tamponade. In this subcostal four-chamber view, there is a small layered hematoma identified along the diaphragmatic surface of the RV (*arrow*). Loculated hematomas are particularly important to recognize because hemodynamic compromise can occur even with a small but strategically located collection. Although this loculated hematoma is clearly identified with transthoracic scanning, it is important to recognize that transesophageal echocardiography is frequently required in order to identify loculated effusions, which cause tamponade.

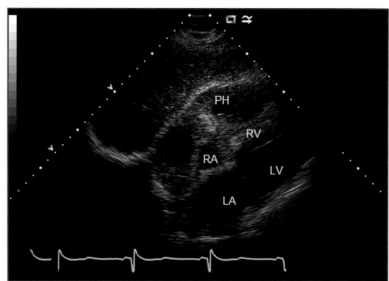

Figure 22-7. Loculated pericardial hematoma in postoperative coronary artery bypass graft patient causing tamponade, subcostal four-chamber view. The large pericardial hematoma is identified along the diaphragmatic surface of the RV. Loculated pericardial effusions often occur in postoperative patients or patients with recurrent pericardial disease. The effusion is localized by adhesions to a small area of the pericardial space. In this scenario, the clinical history is of paramount importance in assessing the likelihood of tamponade (*ie*, low cardiac output symptoms, hypotension, large output from chest tubes). Traditional markers of tamponade, such as respiratory variation in Doppler spectral profiles and right atrial or RV diastolic collapse, are often missing in postoperative patients. LA—left atrium; PH—pericardial hematoma; RA—right atrium.

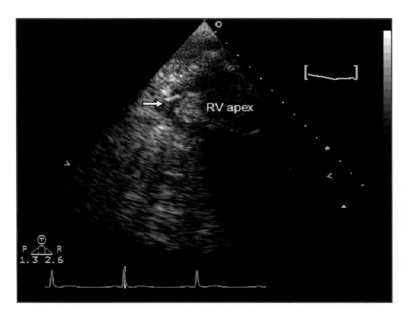

Figure 22-8. Cardiac tamponade secondary to permanent pacer perforation (*arrow*) of the RV apex, RV inflow view. A patient presented to the emergency department with chest pain, two days following pacer implantation. Serial echocardiograms demonstrated an enlarging pericardial effusion associated with decreasing blood pressure. In this setting, visualizing the true RV apex is critical in establishing the diagnosis.

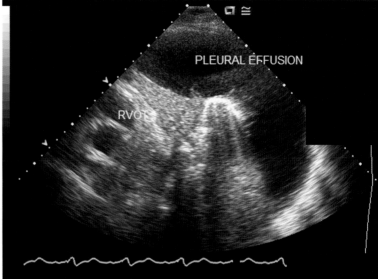

Figure 22-9. Cardiac tamponade secondary to massive left pleural effusion, parasternal short-axis view. It is important to recognize that cardiac tamponade may be caused by large pleural effusions. In this situation, the large left pleural effusion is causing compression of the RV outflow tract (RVOT). Emergency treatment required a left-sided thoracentesis with resolution of symptoms.

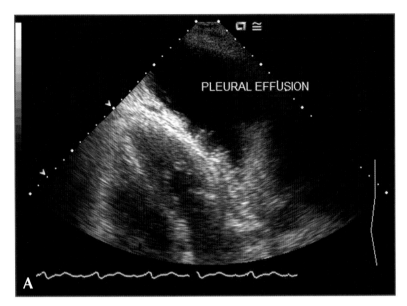

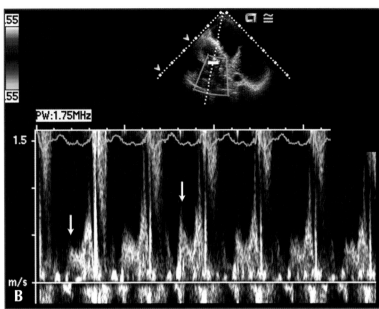

Figure 22-10. **A**, Cardiac tamponade secondary to massive left pleural effusion, apical four-chamber view. When distinguishing pleural from pericardial effusions, a left pleural effusion will extend posterolateral to the descending aorta, whereas a pericardial effusion will track anterior to the descending aorta. Once there is 1 cm of pericardial fluid posteriorly, the fluid will begin to accumulate anteriorly. A large 3-cm posterior echo free space with no anterior accumulation is therefore more likely to be pleural than pericardial. **B**, Pulsed wave Doppler of the mitral valve of the same patient with a large left pleural effusion, apical four-chamber view, demonstrating significant inspiratory decrease in the transmitral E wave velocities of greater than 25%, (*arrows*) consistent with tamponade physiology.

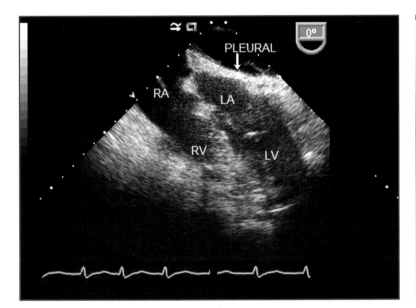

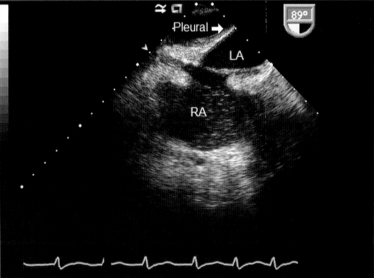

Figure 22-11. Cardiac tamponade secondary to pleural effusion and pleural hematoma, identified on transesophageal echocardiogram, midesophageal four-chamber view. In this example, the pleural collection is causing significant compression of the left atrium (LA) (*arrow*). RA—right atrium.

Figure 22-12. Cardiac tamponade secondary to pleural effusion and pleural hematoma, same patient as in Figure 22-11 from the transesophageal bicaval view. This figure also shows compression of the left atrium (LA) (*arrow*) by the effusion/hematoma. RA—right atrium.

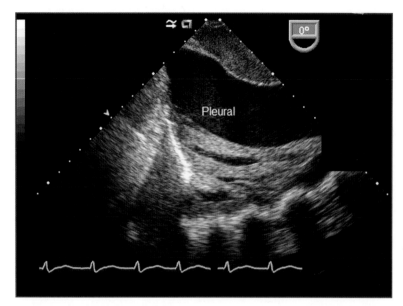

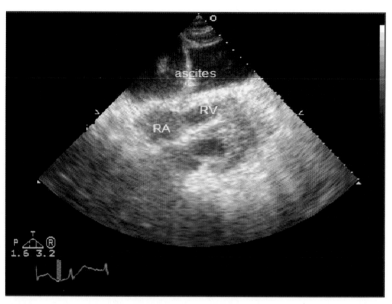

Figure 22-13. Cardiac tamponade secondary to pleural effusion with pleural hematoma identified on transesophageal image of the left pleural space. This image illustrates how pleural effusions can present in combination with hematoma in order to create loculated collections, which may cause focal compression of the cardiac chambers, resulting in tamponade. Transesophageal echocardiography is often required to confirm the diagnosis.

Figure 22-14. Cardiac tamponade from tense ascites, identified on the subcostal view in an acutely hypotensive patient with cirrhosis of the liver. The massive ascites are causing compression of the right side of the heart. This patient clinically improved following paracentesis. RA—right atrium.

Acute Pulmonary Embolism

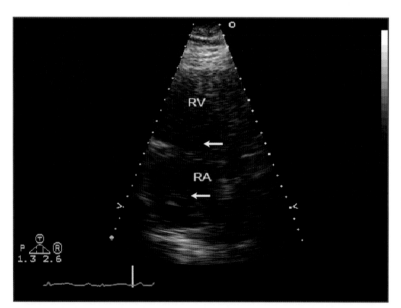

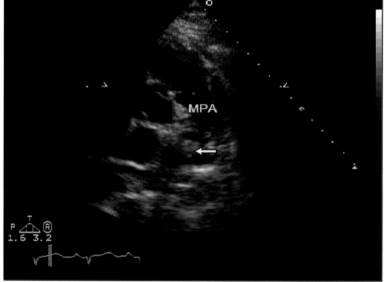

Figure 22-15. Apical four-chamber view demonstrating massive thrombus in transit within the right atrium (RA) and RV (*arrows*). The appearance of thrombus in transit is diagnostic, although not highly sensitive in patients with pulmonary embolism. Echocardiography is used more and more often in the setting of pulmonary embolism. However, echocardiography is not recommended as a routine imaging test for the diagnosis of pulmonary embolism, as many patients with pulmonary embolism will have a normal echo. However, echocardiography is recommended for patients with known pulmonary emboli, as it can help direct therapy towards thrombolysis versus catheter-based or surgical embolectomy.

Figure 22-16. Main pulmonary artery (MPA) and bifurcation view showing thrombus within the right pulmonary artery (*arrow*). This view should be obtained in all patients with suspected pulmonary embolism. Direct visualization of pulmonary emboli usually occurs only when the thrombus is large and centrally located.

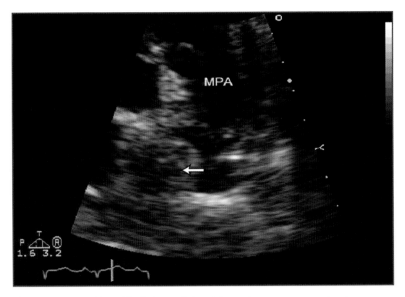

Figure 22-17. Magnified view of the right pulmonary artery in the same patient as Figure 22-16, again showing large thrombus (*arrow*). MPA—main pulmonary artery.

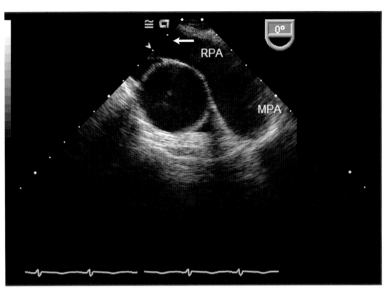

Figure 22-18. Main pulmonary artery (MPA) and bifurcation view, transesophageal image illustrating right pulmonary artery (RPA) thrombus (*arrow*).

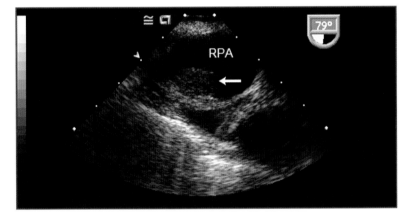

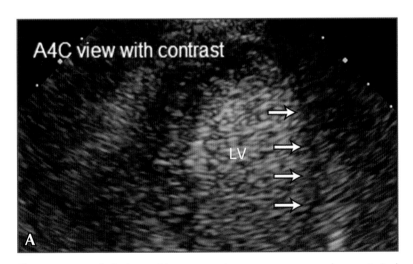

Figure 22-19. Thrombus (*arrow*) in right pulmonary artery (RPA) in transverse plane transesophageal image.

Acute Coronary Syndromes

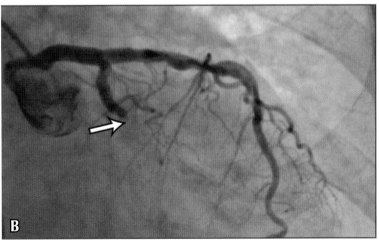

Figure 22-20. A, Patient with suspected acute coronary syndrome. Apical four-chamber (A4C) view obtained with an ultrasound contrast agent to enhance endocardial border definition. This demonstrates regional LV wall motion abnormality involving the lateral wall (*arrows*). **B**, Coronary angiography, demonstrating an occluded left circumflex coronary artery (*arrow*), which correlates with the wall motion abnormality observed above. Echocardiographic assessment of segmental and global wall motion can be extremely helpful in clinical decision making. Presence of a segmental wall motion abnormality indicates coronary artery disease, but does not necessarily differentiate between an acute infarction, ischemia, or an old infarction. Echocardiography has great value in assessing left circumflex-related ischemia and infarction (lateral and posterior wall myocardial infarction), as this type of acute coronary syndrome is often electrocardiographically silent.

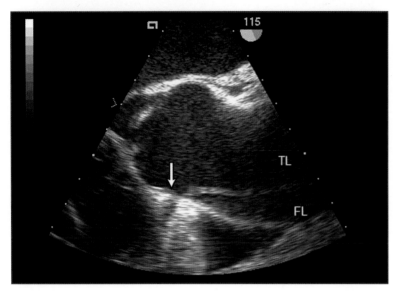

Figure 22-21. Transesophageal echocardiogram, longitudinal view of the aorta, demonstrating a Debakey type I aortic dissection. A mobile linear dissection flap originates just distal to the right coronary artery (*arrow*). According to the Debakey classification, type I dissection starts in the ascending aorta and extends to the arch and often beyond. These are surgical emergencies. FL—false lumen; TL—true lumen.

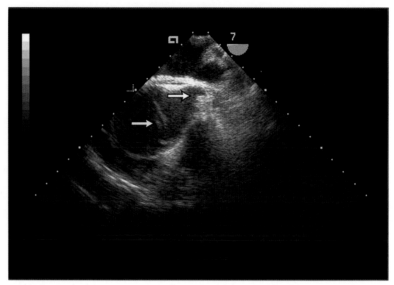

Figure 22-22. Type I aortic dissection, same patient as in Figure 22-21. Transesophageal transverse view of the aortic root and ascending aorta, demonstrating no left coronary artery involvement (*white arrow*) by the dissection flap (*yellow arrow*). It is important to carefully examine the left and right coronary artery ostia in all patients with dissection involving the ascending aorta, as flaps can often dissect into the coronary artery, causing myocardial infarction. The identification of coronary artery involvement would warrant coronary artery bypass grafting at the time of surgical repair.

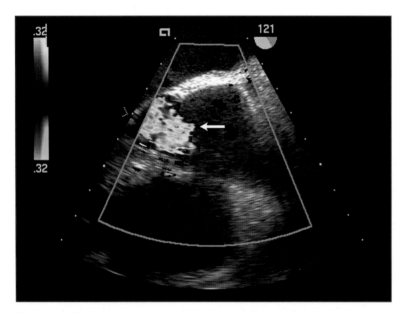

Figure 22-23. Type I aortic dissection, transesophageal echocardiogram, longitudinal view with color Doppler, demonstrating severe aortic insufficiency (*arrow*). The dissection flap can extend to the aortic leaflets, causing aortic leaflet prolapse and aortic insufficiency, or the flap can cause aortic root dilatation, leading to aortic insufficiency. Acute severe aortic insufficiency can be a life threatening complication of aortic dissection and warrants either surgical resuspension of the native valve or surgical valve replacement.

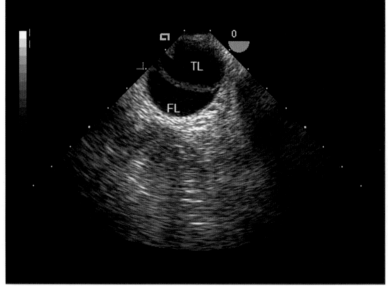

Figure 22-24. Type I aortic dissection, transesophageal echocardiogram, transverse view of descending aorta, demonstrating mobile linear dissection flap. The intimal flap moves towards the false lumen in systole. FL—false lumen; TL—true lumen.

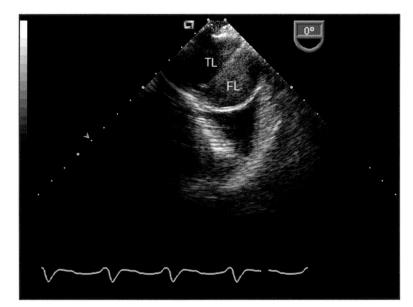

Figure 22-25. Type I aortic dissection, transesophageal echocardiogram, transverse view of descending aorta, demonstrating partial thrombosis of false lumen (FL). Spontaneous echo contrast or partial thrombosis of the false lumen is indicative of stasis of blood within the false lumen. This is usually a good prognostic sign and represents healing of the dissection. TL—true lumen.

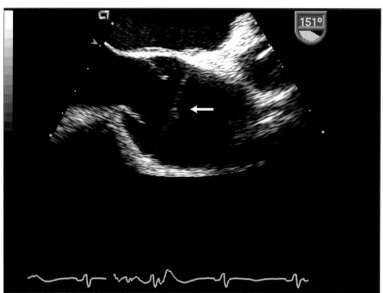

Figure 22-26. Transesophageal echocardiogram, longitudinal view of the ascending aorta, demonstrating a Debakey type II aortic dissection. In this case, the cause of the dissection was believed to be iatrogenic and occurred during coronary angiography. There is a discrete mobile linear flap (*arrow*). The Debakey type II aortic dissection is confined entirely to the ascending aorta with no involvement of the descending thoracic aorta.

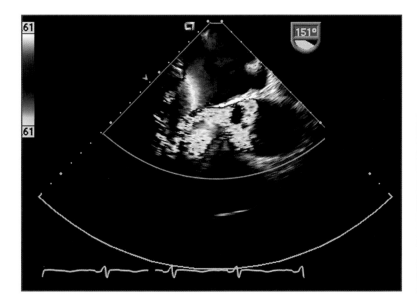

Figure 22-27. Type II aortic dissection, same patient as in Figure 22-26. This transesophageal longitudinal view of ascending aorta with color Doppler interrogation reveals severe aortic insufficiency. Severe acute aortic insufficiency can be a life threatening complication of aortic dissection.

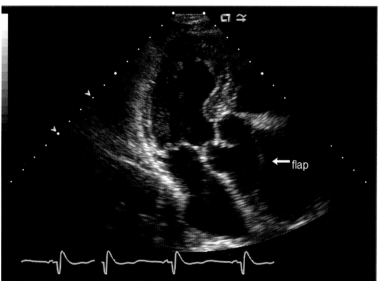

Figure 22-28. Type II aortic dissection, apical three-chamber view, showing linear mobile flap (*arrow*). Transthoracic echocardiography is less sensitive and less specific than transesophageal echocardiography for diagnosing aortic dissection (59%–85% sensitive, 63%–96% specific). Nevertheless, transthoracic echocardiography can provide valuable information that can be clinically useful, particularly when awaiting transesophageal echocardiography.

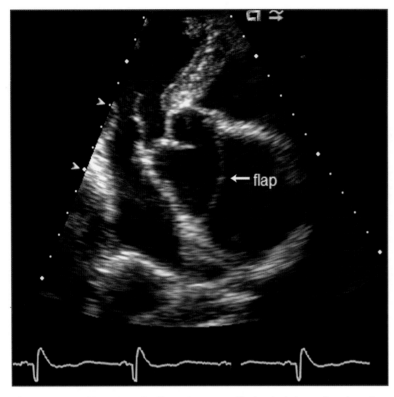

Figure 22-29. Type II aortic dissection, magnified apical three-chamber view, showing mobile linear flap (*arrow*). The parasternal long and apical three-chamber views allow visualization of the aortic root and a segment of the proximal ascending aorta.

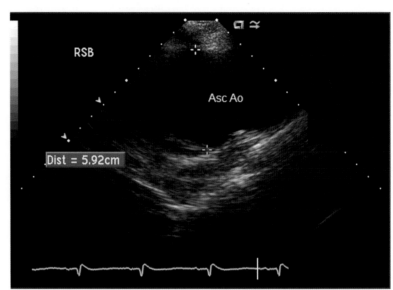

Figure 22-30. Same patient as in Figures 22-28 and 22-29. Right parasternal view, demonstrating an associated ascending aortic aneurysm measuring 5.9 cm in caliber. The right parasternal window is obtained by having the patient lie in the right lateral decubitus position. The transducer is placed between the third and fourth intercostal space with the transducer notch pointed towards 1 o'clock. This view is most valuable for the visualization of the ascending aorta (AscAo) and identifying ascending aortic aneurysms, which can be missed if special efforts are not made to obtain this view.

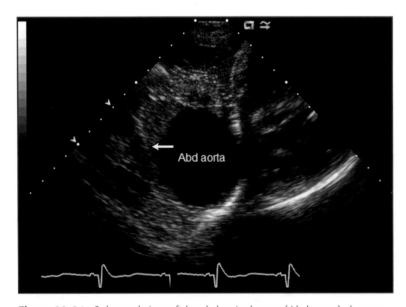

Figure 22-31. Subcostal view of the abdominal aorta (Abd aorta), demonstrating aortic aneurysm and associated aortic dissection with thrombosed false lumen (*arrow*). With the subcostal window, the distal thoracic and proximal abdominal aorta can be evaluated.

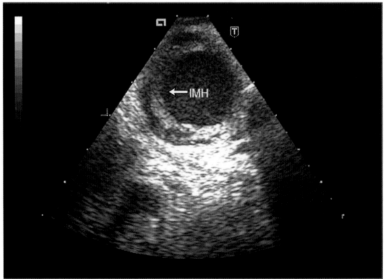

Figure 22-32. Intramural hematoma (IMH) (*arrow*) involving the descending thoracic aorta identified with transesophageal echocardiography. Intramural hematomas are often pathologically different from aortic dissections, and they are usually caused by the rupture of the vasa vasorum without tearing of the intima of the aorta. Therefore, with intramural hematomas, there is no communication with the lumen of the aorta. Often, it is not possible to distinguish between a spontaneous intramural hematoma and a focal aortic dissection with completely thrombosed false lumen; however, the clinical presentation and natural history of these patients are usually the same.

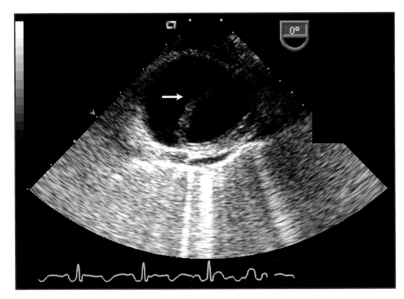

Figure 22-33. Transesophageal echocardiogram demonstrating a thick vertical mobile and linear dissection flap (*arrow*) involving the descending thoracic aorta in a patient with aortic trauma secondary to a motor vehicle accident. Aortic transections often have extremely thick flaps, which unlike dissections are directed vertically instead of horizontally.

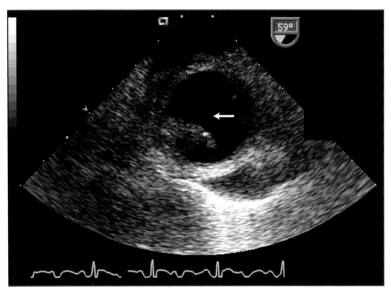

Figure 22-34. Transesophageal echocardiogram in the same patient as Figure 22-33. Another hallmark of aortic transection is the presence of extensive aortic luminal thrombus (*arrow*), as is visualized in the descending thoracic aorta in this patient.

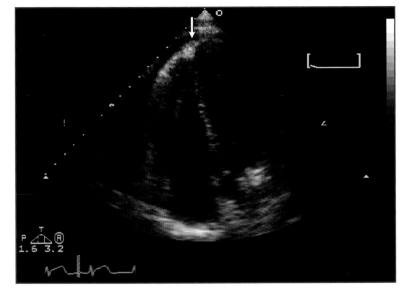

Figure 22-35. Apical four-chamber view in a patient presenting to the emergency department with a history of a gunshot wound to the chest. A highly reflective metal object is identified at the RV apex, consistent with a bullet (*arrow*). There is also a trace of pericardial effusion. The patient has remained stable for many years with the bullet remaining at the RV. The patient often presents to the hospital with recurrent chest pain consistent with pericarditis.

Complications of Myocardial Infarction

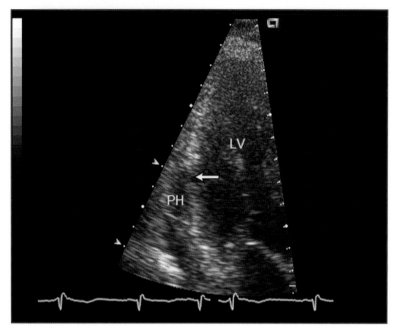

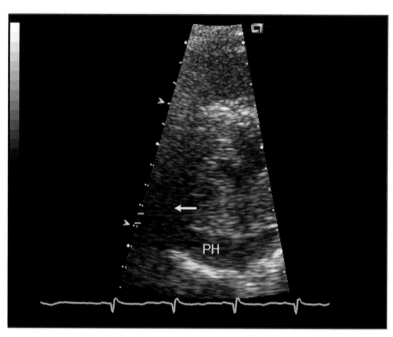

Figure 22-36. After myocardial infarction, subacute LV posterior lateral free wall rupture (*arrow*). Apical three-chamber view. Patient had had a myocardial infarction and complained of chest pain, nausea, and vomiting and was hypotensive. LV free wall rupture is a cause of in-hospital mortality among patients with acute myocardial infarction. Because free wall rupture does not always present as a catastrophic event that results in immediate death, if it is recognized early and diagnosed accurately, emergency surgery can allow for successful treatment. PH—pericardial hematoma.

Figure 22-37. After myocardial infarction, subacute LV posterior lateral free wall rupture (*arrow*), parasternal short-axis view. This is the same patient as Figure 22-36. PH—pericardial hematoma.

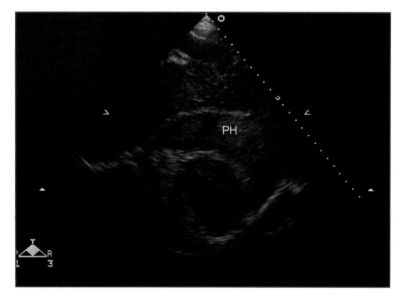

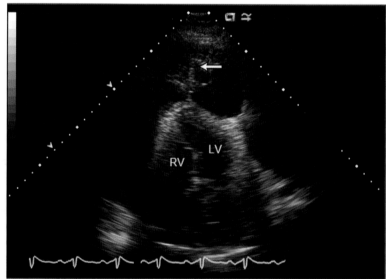

Figure 22-38. After myocardial infarction, acute LV free wall rupture. Emergency echocardiography performed during code blue with chest compressions. Subcostal view. There is massive pericardial hematoma (PH).

Figure 22-39. After myocardial infarction, acute LV free wall rupture, apical four-chamber view, performed during code blue. There is massive pericardial hematoma (*arrow*). The presence of pericardial hematoma in a patient after myocardial infarction should always warrant careful echocardiographic assessment for the presence of possible subacute free wall rupture.

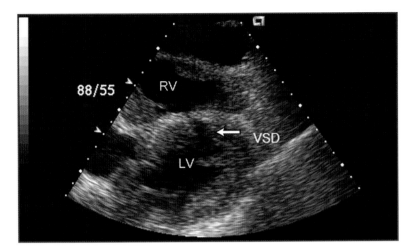

Figure 22-40. After myocardial infarction ventricular septal defect (VSD), subcostal view. The patient became acutely hypotensive with new systolic murmur. The ventricular septal defect is located at the midinterventricular septum and appears as an abrupt interruption in the septal musculature (*arrow*). Ventricular septal rupture is associated with a grave prognosis, although survival is improved with early diagnosis and prompt surgical repair.

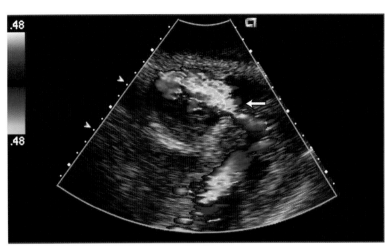

Figure 22-41. After myocardial infarction, ventricular septal defect (same patient as in Figure 22-40), subcostal view with color Doppler interrogation of the interventricular septum, demonstrating significant left to right shunting across the defect (*arrow*).

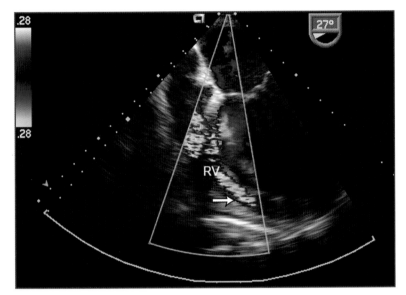

Figure 22-42. After myocardial infarction, ventricular septal defect, transesophageal echocardiogram, midesophageal four-chamber view with color Doppler demonstrating significant left to right shunting at the apical level, as illustrated by turbulent color flow signal within the RV (*arrow*). Transeophageal echocardiography can establish the diagnosis of mechanical complications of myocardial infarction in cases in which the transthoracic images are suboptimal.

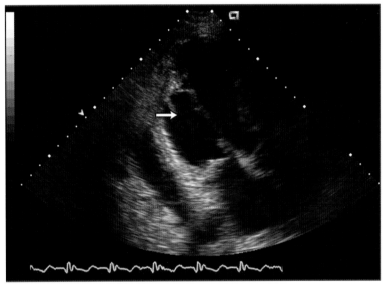

Figure 22-43. After myocardial infarction, rupture of the head of the posteromedial papillary muscle represented by a highly mobile structure within the LV cavity (*arrow*) in this apical three-chamber view. The patient became acutely hypotensive. Papillary muscle rupture, like ventricular septal rupture, has a high likelihood of death. Prompt diagnosis and early surgical intervention may improve prognosis.

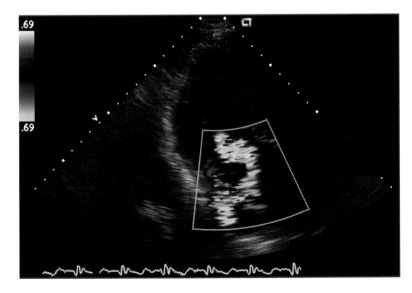

Figure 22-44. After myocardial infarction, rupture of the head of the posteromedial papillary muscle. The same patient as Figure 22-43. Apical three-chamber view with color Doppler interrogation of the mitral valve demonstrates resultant severe mitral insufficiency.

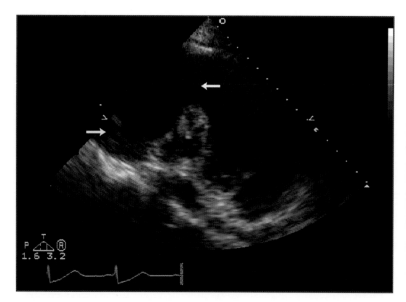

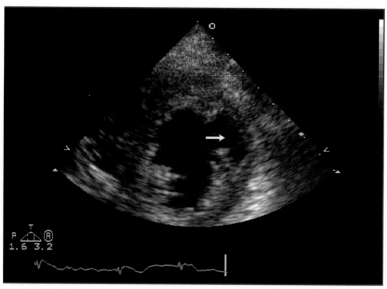

Figure 22-45. Apical two-chamber view, demonstrating large inferior apical LV pseudoaneurysm (*white arrow*), with layered thrombus (*yellow arrow*). Pseudoaneurysms result from myocardial rupture with the extravasated blood being contained by adherent parietal pericardium. Pseudoaneurysms are pathologically described as having a narrow neck (less than 40% of the diameter of the aneurysm) that connects the LV to a large aneurysmal sac, which is lined by fibrous pericardial tissue. They are associated with high mortality unless recognized early and promptly treated surgically.

Figure 22-46. Parasternal short-axis view, demonstrating anterior-lateral LV pseudo-aneurysm (*arrow*). Because of the high incidence of late myocardial rupture and death, this patient was referred for prompt cardiac surgery.

Suggested Reading

Goldhaber S: Echocardiography in the management of pulmonary embolism. *Ann Intern Med* 2002, 136:691–700.

Romano S, Dagianti A, Penco M, *et al.*: Usefulness of echocardiography in the prognostic evaluation of non-Q—wave myocardial infarction. *Am J Cardiol* 2000, 86:43G–45G.

Solomon SD, ed: *Essential Echocardiography*. Totowa, NJ: Humana Press; 2007.

Weyman A, ed: *Principles and Practice of Echocardiography*, edn 2. Philadelphia: Lea & Febiger; 1994.

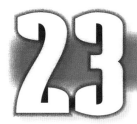

Echocardiography in Adult Congenital Heart Disease

Meryl S. Cohen, Theodore Plappert, Rita Novello, and Martin St. John Sutton

The prevalence of congenital heart disease (CHD) is 0.8% of all live births. The abnormalities in intracardiac anatomy vary in severity and complexity from simple bicuspid aortic valve to complex anomalies, such as transposition of the great arteries with univentricular connection. Hemodynamic measurements and noninvasive imaging have clarified the structural and functional changes in CHD and spawned advances in palliative and corrective surgical techniques, which have improved survival even in the most complicated lesions. Survival to adulthood is now the rule rather than the exception, occurring in 85% of patients. When CHD patients reach adulthood, they should ideally transition to an adult cardiologist with special expertise in CHD who assumes their cardiac care throughout life. The aim of this chapter is to provide a diagnostic framework for physicians caring for adults with CHD. This is achieved using two-dimensional echocardiographic imaging for sequential chamber analysis and assessment of the cardiac structural and functional abnormalities that drive clinical decision making. The initial step is to establish atrial situs by determining the spatial relationships of the abdominal aorta, the inferior vena cava, and the spine. Once atrial situs is known, sequential chamber analysis is performed, wherein the two atria are distinguished by their internal landmarks, atrial appendages, defects of atrial septation, and anomalies of pulmonary venous and systemic venous drainage. The atrioventricular connections are described next, and the morphology of the ventricular chambers is identified. The presence and location of ventricular septal defects are noted. Next, the RV and LV outflow tracts and ventriculoarterial connections are determined. Lastly, the spatial orientation of the two great arteries—their relative sizes and the presence of anomalous origins or stenoses of the primary branch arteries—must be established.

We have selected a portfolio of still images in the sequential chamber analysis format described for most cardiac lesions that are likely to be encountered in an established adult CHD service, including patients who have undergone palliative or corrective cardiothoracic surgery.

Situs

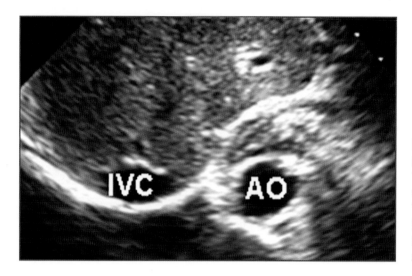

Figure 23-1. The first image to be obtained in a congenital heart disease study in order to determine situs is the transaxial or coronal subcostal view. This view helps to determine the position of the aorta (AO) and the inferior vena cava (IVC) and whether the IVC connects directly to the right atrium. The transaxial image shows that the liver is on the right, the spine in the far field, the IVC is anterior to the right of the abdominal AO, and the stomach (not shown) is to the left. This anatomic arrangement is known as normal situs or situs solitus.

Venous Anomalies

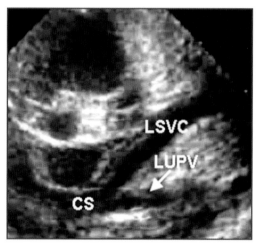

Figure 23-2. Complete assessment of the segmental anatomy of the heart includes demonstration of systemic venous anatomy. Left superior vena cava (LSVC) to the coronary sinus (CS) is a common abnormality in both structurally abnormal and normal hearts. An LSVC has implications regarding cardiopulmonary bypass; important abnormal systemic venous anatomy must be identified in those with univentricular hearts that are staged to the Fontan palliation. In this high parasternal view, angled posteriorly, the LSVC is seen entering the CS just superior to the entrance of the left upper pulmonary vein (LUPV). The LSVC passes anterior to the left pulmonary artery in order to reach the heart. The CS is typically dilated from increased flow. Further imaging is required when an LSVC is identified to determine if a bridging vein (from LSVC to right SVC) is present.

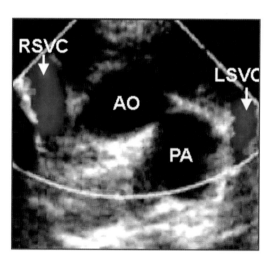

Figure 23-3. If a bridging vein is not present in patients with univentricular hearts, then bilateral bidirectional Glenn shunts are necessary so that the blood flow from the left superior vena cava (LSVC) can reach the left pulmonary artery. This suprasternal frontal view demonstrates bilateral LSVC, with the right superior vena cava (RSVC) to the right of the aorta (AO) directed toward the right atrium and the LSVC, crossing anterior to the left pulmonary artery to the left of the main pulmonary artery (PA) and headed toward the coronary sinus. Rarely does the LSVC enter the left atrium directly (this typically only happens in heterotaxy [isomerism] syndrome).

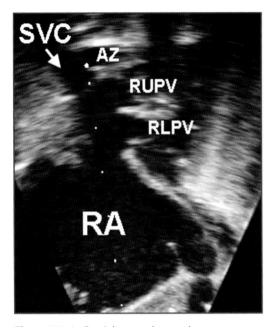

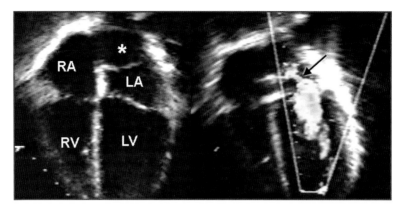

Figure 23-4. Partial anomalous pulmonary venous return can be difficult to diagnose by transthoracic echocardiography, but it is particularly important to assess in the patient with a sinus venosus atrial septal defect. The right pulmonary veins often connect anomalously, usually to the right superior vena cava (SVC). This subcostal sagittal view shows the right upper and right lower pulmonary veins (RUPV, RLPV) connecting directly to the right SVC posteriorly, with the azygos vein (AZ) draining superior to the pulmonary veins. The right atrium (RA) becomes dilated from increased flow.

Figure 23-5. When the common pulmonary vein is not absorbed in early embryologic development, cor triatriatum is the resulting cardiac abnormality. These membranous structures are typically funnel-like and separate the left atrium into two chambers—the pulmonary venous chamber (posteriorly) and the true left atrium (LA) including the left atrial appendage (anteriorly). There is usually a narrow opening between the two chambers. This diminutive orifice results in increased pressure in the pulmonary veins, and in some cases, pulmonary arterial hypertension. In milder forms, the diagnosis may occur late, and the common presenting symptom is exercise intolerance. This apical four-chamber view in two-dimensional echo (*left panel*) and color flow (*right panel*) shows cor triatriatum. The membrane is seen between the pulmonary venous chamber (*asterisk*) and the true LA. When the probe sweeps anteriorly, color Doppler demonstrates the very narrow orifice (*black arrow*) with accelerated flow, which causes pulmonary venous chamber hypertension. RA—right atrium.

Atrial Septal Anomalies

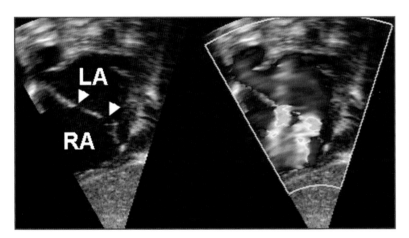

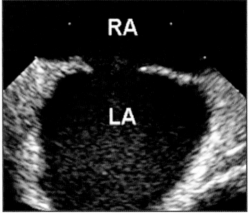

Figure 23-6. Ostium secundum-type atrial septal defects can occur in several regions of the atrial septum and can be multiple or fenestrated. This subcostal left anterior oblique view highlights most of the atrial septum and shows the right atrium (RA) and left atrium (LA) with draining pulmonary veins (*left panel*). The atrial septum, which divides the RA from the LA, has two small defects (*arrows*) with blood flow predominantly from left to right. This is shown by the aliased flow acceleration (*right panel, two pale blue regions*).

Figure 23-7. An intracardiac echocardiogram shows an ostium secundum-type atrial septal defect with the right atrium (RA) above the septum and the left atrium (LA) below.

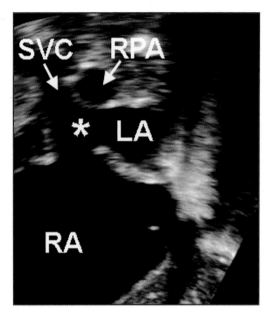

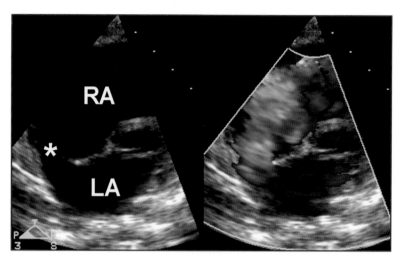

Figure 23-8. Atrial septal defects of the sinus venosus type are more challenging to diagnose than secundum defects. They can be missed in traditional views, such as subcostal frontal and parasternal short axis. In those with good subcostal windows, subcostal sagittal view is ideal in demonstrating a sinus venosus atrial septal defect of the superior vena cava (SVC) type. In other cases, a high right parasternal view may be used. In some cases, transesophageal echocardiography is required to locate the abnormality. This subcostal sagittal image demonstrates the defect. The sinus venosus defect (*asterisk*) is seen just inferior to the entry of the SVC into the right atrium (RA). The right pulmonary artery (RPA), which is slightly dilated from the left to right shunt, is seen in cross-section as it passes posterior to the SVC. LA—left atrium.

Figure 23-9. Sinus venosus atrial septal defects of the inferior vena cava type are even more challenging and can be difficult to distinguish from an inferior secundum-type atrial septal defect. This distinction is important because sinus venosus defects cannot be closed with occluder devices. This parasternal short-axis view, angled inferiorly, demonstrates a sinus venosus atrial septal defect (*left panel, asterisk*) at the mouth of the inferior vena cava. The right atrium (RA) is markedly dilated from the left to right shunting, which is demonstrated with color Doppler (*right panel*). LA—left atrium.

Atrioventricular Junction

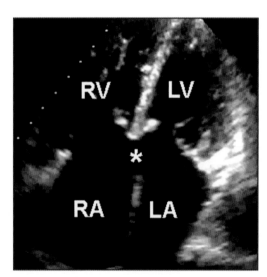

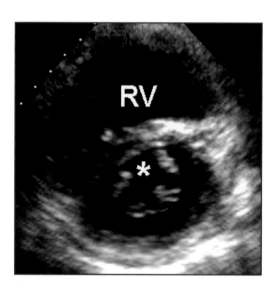

Figure 23-10. Partial (incomplete) atrioventricular canal (septal) defects have an atrial septal defect component (ostium primum atrial septal defect), but are considered abnormalities of the endocardial cushion and therefore fall into the category of anomalies of the atrioventricular junction. The apical four-chamber view of a partial atrioventricular canal defect shows the ostium primum atrial septal defect (*asterisk*) just superior to the common atrioventricular inlet. This defect results in a left to right shunt at atrial level. Note the enlarged right atrium (RA) and enlarged RV that forms the apex. The atrioventricular valves are at the same level because they share a common annulus. In the normal heart, the septal leaflet of the tricuspid takes its origin from the septum more apically than does the anterior mitral valve leaflet. LA—left atrium.

Figure 23-11. In the partial (incomplete) form of common atrioventricular canal (septal) defect (ostium primum atrial septal defect with no shunting at ventricular level), the atrioventricular valve is adherent to the ventricular septum and allows no ventricular level shunting. Although there are two atrioventricular valve orifices, there is only one annulus. The so-called mitral valve "cleft" seen in association with this lesion is in fact the approximation of the superior and inferior bridging leaflets at the ventricular septum. The parasternal short-axis view demonstrates this cleft (*asterisk*) that is directed toward the ventricular septum. The left atrioventricular valve is not a true mitral valve in this abnormality. The RV is usually dilated as a result of the typically large atrial-level left to right shunt.

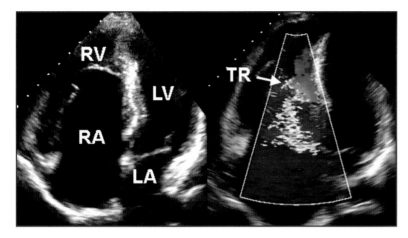

Figure 23-12. Ebstein's anomaly (particularly the milder form) often goes undiagnosed until adulthood. This apical four-chamber view of Ebstein's anomaly of the tricuspid valve (TV) shows the diagnostic features, which include apical displacement and restricted movement of the septal leaflet of the TV, the atrialized portion of the RV, and the markedly enlarged right atrium (RA) (*left panel*). The apical four-chamber view in Ebstein's anomaly with color flow Doppler shows that the tricuspid regurgitation (TR) begins at the TV leaflets coaptation point close to the RV apex, indicating that the functional part of the RV is small (*right panel*). LA—left atrium.

Ventricular Septal Anomalies

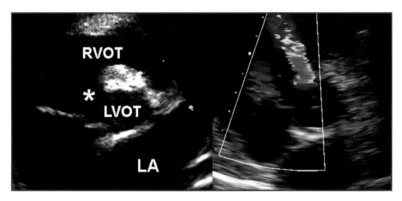

Figure 23-13. The most common type of ventricular septal defect is the perimembranous defect, which is located under the septal leaflet of the tricuspid valve and under the aortic valve. The proximity of this defect to the aortic valve can typically result in prolapse of the right coronary cusp into the defect. Perimembranous defects can become more restrictive and may even close because of the formation of aneurysmal tissue from the septal leaflet of the tricuspid valve. This parasternal short-axis view of the aorta shows a perimembranous ventricular septal defect (*asterisk*) under the septal leaflet of the tricuspid valve (*left panel*) with RV outflow tract (RVOT) hypertrophy. The infundibular septum is prominently displayed between the RVOT and the LV outflow tract (LVOT). Left to right flow across the perimembranous defect in the parasternal short-axis view into the RVOT (*right panel*) is shown. The color jet is seen at approximately eleven o'clock. If the defect was subpulmonary or doubly committed (also called conoseptal hypoplasia type) the color jet would be directed closer to one o'clock. LA—left atrium.

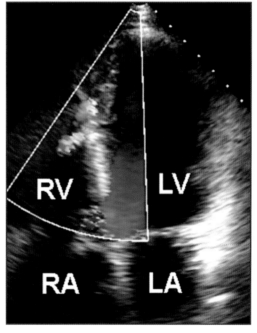

Figure 23-14. Muscular ventricular septal defects can occur anywhere within the ventricular septum and can vary in size. There are often multiple defects in the same patient. This apical four-chamber view demonstrates the location of two restrictive midseptal muscular defects by color flow Doppler. These defects are often so small that they cannot be seen without color flow Doppler. LA—left atrium; RA—right atrium.

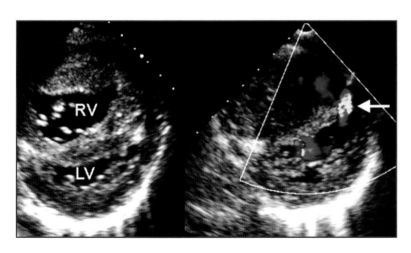

Figure 23-15. Eisenmenger syndrome occurs when pulmonary vascular obstructive disease becomes so severe that the pulmonary vascular resistance is higher than the systemic vascular resistance. Reversal of shunting patterns ensues when there is a communication, such as an atrial septal defect, ventricular septal defect, patent ductus arteriosus, or aortopulmonary window. Shunting occurs from the pulmonary vasculature to the systemic vasculature, resulting in cyanosis. Eisenmenger syndrome can occur when a hemodynamically significant cardiac lesion is left unrepaired for a protracted period of time. Once it develops, repair of the cardiac defect is usually not possible. In Eisenmenger syndrome, the parasternal short-axis view (*left panel*) demonstrates the abnormal position of the ventricular septum, which is bowing into the LV as a result of severe RV hypertension. Marked RV hypertrophy is also seen. Color flow Doppler is seen across an anterior muscular ventricular septal defect, which is shunting right to left (*right panel, arrow*).

Outflow Tract Abnormalities

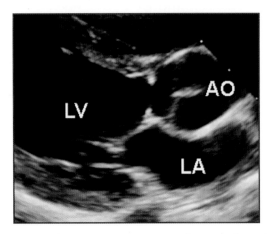

Figure 23-16. Left ventricular outflow tract (LVOT) obstruction can occur at multiple levels. Discrete subaortic membranes are usually fibrous and can be associated with significant obstruction and aortic insufficiency. Surgical intervention is usually successful, but there is a recurrence risk of up to 10% to 20%. The parasternal long-axis view demonstrates a discrete fibrous membrane just proximal to the aortic valve, which impinges on the LVOT. The membrane is seen on the anterior leaflet of the mitral valve as well. AO—aorta; LA—left atrium.

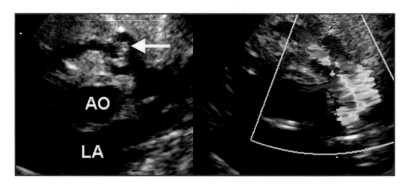

Figure 23-17. Right ventricular outflow tract obstruction can also occur at multiple levels, and is often amenable to catheter-directed intervention. A parasternal short-axis view (*left panel*) demonstrates severe valvar pulmonary stenosis. The pulmonary valve leaflets are dysplastic and are thickened with limited excursion (*arrow*). Marked infundibular hypertrophy is also seen. This hypertrophy often resolves slowly after intervention. Poststenotic dilation of the main pulmonary artery is also seen. Color flow Doppler demonstrates a narrowed high-velocity jet (aliased color) through the pulmonary valve in systole (*right panel*). It is important to interrogate velocity within this narrow jet in order to obtain an accurate measure of the severity of obstruction. AO—aorta; LA—left atrium.

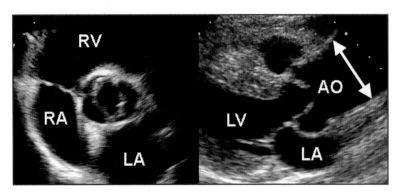

Figure 23-18. The most common congenital anomaly by far is the bicuspid aortic valve (BAV). These valves can develop progressive stenosis, regurgitation, or both. The ascending aorta (AO) is often dilated in this disorder. This parasternal short-axis view shows a BAV in systole with a mildly reduced valve orifice and equivalent cusp sizes within an enlarged AO root (*left panel*). In this example, fusion of the right and noncoronary cusps is seen. Parasternal long-axis view shows the associated dilated ascending AO or aortopathy, in which the aneurysmal AO dilatation is out of proportion to the severity of the hydraulics across the AO valve (*right panel*). An enlarged ascending aorta, which is associated with bicuspid aortic valve (diameter = 4.9 cm) is shown (*arrows*). LA—left atrium; RA—right atrium.

Conotruncal Anomalies

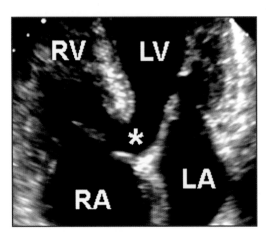

Figure 23-19. Tetralogy of Fallot is the most common conotruncal defect seen in the adult population with congenital heart disease. An apical four-chamber view of a patient with tetralogy of Fallot shows a normal LV, a non-restrictive perimembranous malalignment ventricular septal defect (*asterisk*), RV hypertrophy and an enlarged aorta (not shown) overriding the ventricular septum. LA—left atrium; RA—right atrium..

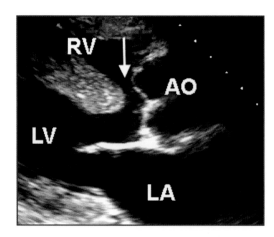

Figure 23-20. Parasternal long-axis view of tetralogy of Fallot shows a large unrestrictive malalignment-type ventricular septal defect (*arrow*) and an enlarged aorta (AO) overriding the outlet septum. The anterior RV is hypertrophied. LA—left atrium.

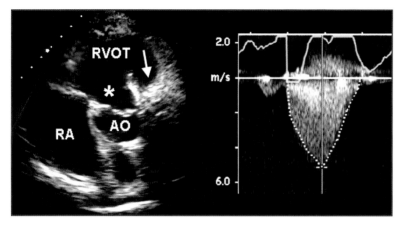

Figure 23-21. Parasternal short-axis view of the aorta (AO) in tetralogy of Fallot shows the ventricular septal defect (*asterisk*). The RV outflow tract (RVOT) is narrowed as a result of anterior malalignment of the infundibular septum (the muscle is between the *asterisk* and *arrow*), which impinges upon the RVOT and causes obstruction (*left panel*). The malaligned infundibular septum is the cause of all of the components in tetralogy of Fallot, including the ventricular septal defect, the overriding AO, the infundibular stenosis, and the RV hypertrophy (from the systemic RV pressure). Continuous wave Doppler estimate of the RVOT systolic gradient is shown demonstrating severe RVOT obstruction with peak velocity of 5 m/s (*right panel*). RA—right atrium.

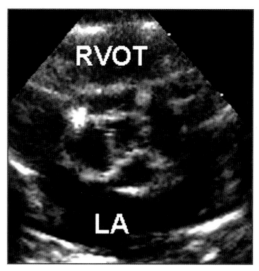

Figure 23-22. Truncus arteriosus is a diagnosis where a common trunk gives rise to the aorta and the pulmonary arteries. It is almost exclusively diagnosed in the newborn period. However, the long-term consequences usually involve the truncal valve, which can be stenotic, regurgitant, or both. The number of valve leaflets ranges from 2 to 5, with 3 being the most common. This parasternal short-axis view demonstrates a quadracuspid truncal valve with thickened leaflets that do not coapt normally. The truncal valve is also larger than a normal aortic valve. RVOT—RV outflow tract; LA—left atrium.

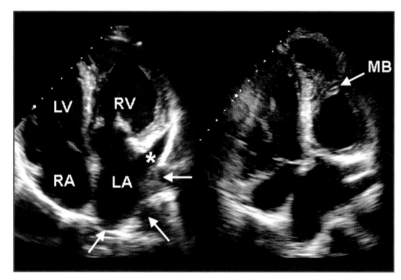

Figure 23-23. Congenitally corrected transposition of the great arteries (L-TGA) presents many complex management problems. Patients who have L-TGA use their RV as the systemic pumping chamber. This can be associated with the development of RV failure and tricuspid regurgitation. Ebstein's anomaly can also be seen with L-TGA. Some patients have a ventricular septal defect with obstruction of one of the outflow tracts (most commonly the pulmonary), but some have intact ventricular septum with no outflow tract obstruction. Because the blood flows in series like a normal heart, it is difficult to know when and if to intervene. A double switch, including both an atrial and arterial switch, has recently been advocated to designate the LV as the systemic pumping chamber. In this example of an unrepaired L-TGA, the apical four-chamber view in diastole (*left panel*) and in systole (*right panel*) is shown. The left atrium (LA) is identified by the draining pulmonary veins (*arrows*) and the morphology of the left atrial appendage (*asterisk*). The LA empties into the morphologic RV with the septal leaflet of the left-sided tricuspid valve taking origin from the interventricular septum more apically than the septal leaflet of the right-sided mitral valve (*left panel*). The moderator band (MB) is also a useful landmark in recognizing the RV. RA—right atrium.

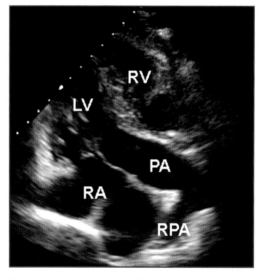

Figure 23-24. Parasternal long-axis view of congenitally corrected transposition of the great arteries shows that blood passes from the right atrium (RA) to the LV and then to the main pulmonary artery (PA). The PA is seen bifurcating into the right (RPA) and left pulmonary primary branch arteries. The aorta sits anterior to the pulmonary artery and typically to the left.

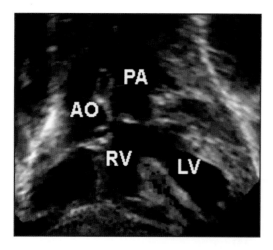

Figure 23-25. The double-outlet RV is a heterogeneous group of defects that describes when both great arteries are assigned to the RV. The Taussig-Bing anomaly is a particular form of double-outlet RV where the ventricular septal defect is subpulmonary (*ie*, underneath the pulmonary valve), and the great vessels are side by side, with the aorta (AO) to the right of the pulmonary artery (PA). The blood flow from the LV ejects almost exclusively into the PA, resulting in physiology similar to transposition of the great arteries. In the subcostal frontal view at the anterior aspect of the sweep, both great vessels are seen side by side, with the AO rightward of the PA. The PA is overriding the ventricular septal defect.

Coronary Anomalies

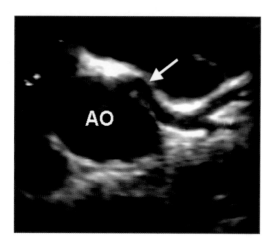

Figure 23-26. The origin of the coronary artery may be abnormal, coming from the wrong cusp. This can have serious implications, particularly if the coronary artery passes between the aorta (AO) and the pulmonary artery and/or if it takes an intramural course in the wall of the AO. Sudden death has occurred in children and adults with anomalous origin of the coronary artery, but prophylactic surgical intervention is controversial. In the parasternal short-axis view, the left coronary artery is demonstrated as originating from the anterior right coronary cusp. It is seen branching into the left anterior descending and circumflex artery. As a result of the anomalous origin, the left coronary artery courses between the AO and pulmonary artery. In some cases of anomalous origin of the coronary artery, the opening is narrowed and slit-like, which may contribute to the risk of ischemia and sudden death. The anomolous origin of the left coronary artery from the right coronary sinus of Valsalva is shown (*arrow*).

Aortic Arch and Tributaries

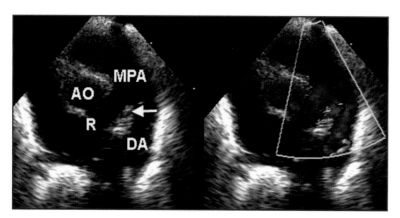

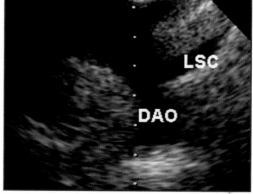

Figure 23-27. Patent ductus arteriosus (DA) is common in premature infants and newborns, but it can be seen in adults as well. Often it is too small to cause a significant hemodynamic burden. The risk of the development of endarteritis is small but present. A high parasternal view best images the DA when normally related great arteries are present. A large DA is demonstrated (*left panel*). This classic three-finger view shows the right pulmonary artery (R), the takeoff of the left pulmonary artery (*arrow*), and the DA. The connection of the DA from the main pulmonary artery (MPA) to the descending aorta (AO) is seen. Color flow Doppler shows low velocity left to right flow from the AO to the pulmonary artery, indicating that the pressures in both great vessels is similar (*right panel*).

Figure 23-28. Coarctation of the aorta can sometimes present in adolescence and adulthood. The most common findings presented are upper extremity systemic hypertension, blood pressure gradient from upper to lower extremities, and diminished femoral pulses. Claudication, frequent headaches, and nosebleeds can also occur with late presentation. Imaging the entire aortic arch when there is severe narrowing at the isthmus can be difficult. The suprasternal sagittal view shows that the descending aorta (DAO) tapers down just distal to the left subclavian artery (LSC).

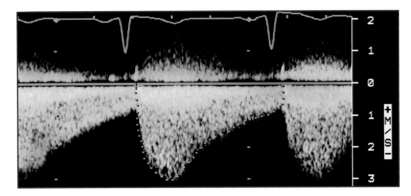

Figure 23-29. Continuous wave Doppler through the isthmus in a patient with coarctation of the aorta demonstrates accelerated flow to a peak velocity of 3 m/s with the diastolic runoff pattern classically associated with this lesion. The diastolic runoff occurs because the aortic pressure is always lower distally to the isthmus narrowing, and therefore forward flow continues throughout the cardiac cycle.

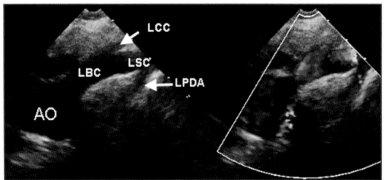

Figure 23-30. Arch anomalies can occur in isolation or in association with other congenital heart defects. Right aortic arch with mirror image branching is typically seen in association with conotruncal lesions, such as tetralogy of Fallot and truncus arteriosus, or with complex heart disease in heterotaxy syndrome. In these disorders, 20% to 30% of patients have a right aortic arch. If identified, it should raise concern that deletion of chromosome 22q11.2 may be present. Suprasternal frontal view is used to determine arch sidedness. In this anterior sweep (*left panel*), the first branch seen arising from the aorta (AO) is the left brachiocephalic artery (LBC), which then branches into the left common carotid artery (LCC) and the left subclavian artery (LSC), indicating a right aortic arch with mirror image branching. In this example, a left ductus arteriosus (LPDA) is seen coming off the LBC. Doppler indicating direction of flow in the aortic arch and the LPDA is shown (*right panel*).

Univentricular Hearts

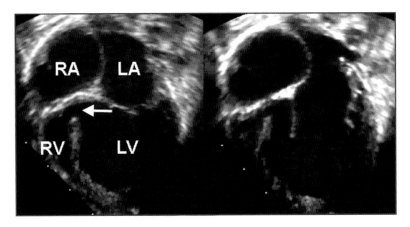

Figure 23-31. There are a range of abnormalities that result in a univentricular heart as shown in systole (*left panel*) and diastole (*right panel*). In most forms, there is either a common atrioventricular valve or two atrioventricular valves entering a single ventricular chamber. Although tricuspid atresia and hypoplastic left-sided heart syndrome also result in a single functioning ventricular chamber, they are not considered true univentricular hearts. Tricuspid atresia is associated with severe RV hypertrophy and usually has a ventricular septal defect as well. The great vessels can be normally or abnormally related (*ie*, transposition of the great arteries or double outlet RV). Outflow tract obstruction is variable. This apical four-chamber view shows muscular tricuspid atresia with severe RV hypoplasia. A ventricular septal defect is seen (*arrow*), which allows the only inflow into the RV. The atrial septum bows right to left as a result of the obligatory right to left shunt. LA—left atrium; RA—right atrium.

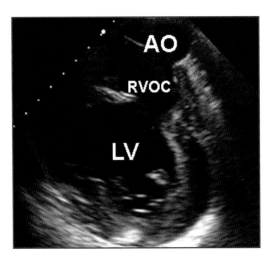

Figure 23-32. In the double inlet LV, the RV outflow tract typically provides blood flow to the aorta (AO). If the ventricular septal defect decreases in size, the patient develops subaortic obstruction unless an aortopulmonary anastomosis (Damus-Kaye-Stansel) is constructed. The apical five-chamber view, angled toward the outflow tracts, demonstrates the RV outflow chamber (RVOC) with the ventricular septal defect seen just inferiorly. The AO arises from the RVOC.

Postoperative Imaging

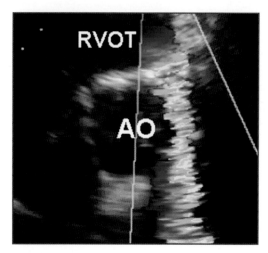

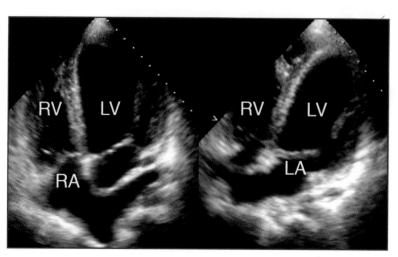

Figure 23-33. Conduits from the RV to the pulmonary artery are commonly used in patients with conotruncal abnormalities, such as tetralogy of Fallot with pulmonary atresia and truncus arteriosus. They are also used in the Ross procedure to replace the RV outflow tract (RVOT). Conduit stenosis is common because of the development of calcification over time. In addition, although some conduits are valved, these valves invariably fail, and severe pulmonary regurgitation is the norm. This parasternal short-axis view with color flow Doppler shows a diffusely narrowed conduit with acceleration that begins at the takeoff of the conduit from the RVOT. AO—aorta.

Figure 23-34. The atrial switch operation (either the Mustard or the Senning procedure) performed for D-transposition of the great arteries baffles the systemic and pulmonary venous channels to the contralateral ventricle with the RV as the systemic-pumping chamber. The pulmonary and systemic venous pathways are at risk for obstruction and baffle leaks can occur. These apical four-chamber images of D-transposition of the great arteries demonstrate the atrial level pathways in the atrial switch operation (Mustard). A baffle to direct the oxygenated blood from the pulmonary veins to the aorta via the RV is demonstrated (pulmonary venous channel) (*left panel*). The systemic venous blood flow is directed to the pulmonary artery via the LV (systemic venous channel) (*right panel*). LA—left atrium; RA—right atrium..

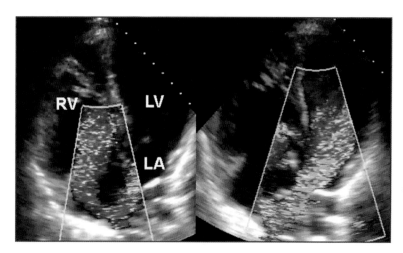

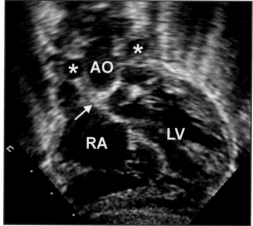

Figure 23-35. An apical four-chamber image of D-transposition of the great arteries with Doppler velocity color flow mapping of the pulmonary venous blood baffled into the RV and then to the aorta is shown (*left panel*). Doppler color flow velocity mapping of systemic venous blood baffled into the LV and subsequently into the pulmonary artery (*right panel*). LA—left atrium.

Figure 23-36. The arterial switch operation has recently been performed for patients with D-transposition of the great arteries. The advantage of this operation compared with the atrial switch operation is that the LV becomes the systemic pumping chamber. In the arterial switch operation, both great vessels are transected and switched, and the coronary arteries are also moved to the neoaorta. The LeCompte maneuver is performed in order to bring the aorta (AO) posteriorly. The result of this maneuver is that the branch pulmonary arteries both cross anterior to the AO. In this subcostal frontal view, the suture line of the neoaorta is seen (*arrow*). On either side of the AO are the branch pulmonary arteries (*asterisks*), which are clearly visible because of the LeCompte maneuver. RA—right atrium.

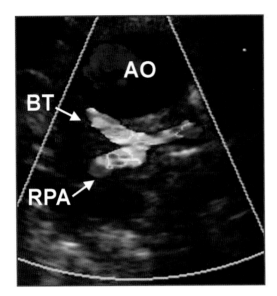

Figure 23-37. The Blalock-Taussig (BT) shunt, first introduced in the 1940s, is used in patients with pulmonary atresia or severe pulmonary valvar stenosis. It is also performed in patients with hypoplastic left-sided heart syndrome because the pulmonary valve becomes the designated neoaortic valve. The modified BT shunt is a Gore-Tex tube graft from the brachiocephalic artery to the pulmonary artery. Although many patients with tetralogy of Fallot now undergo primary closure in infancy, the BT shunt is still used frequently in the population of patients with univentricular hearts. This suprasternal frontal view with color flow Doppler demonstrates a right modified BT shunt from the right brachiocephalic artery to the right pulmonary artery (RPA). In some cases, distortion of the branch pulmonary arteries can occur. AO—aorta.

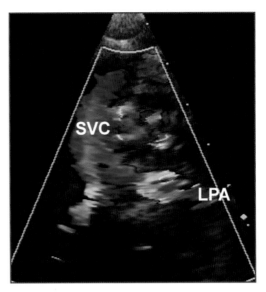

Figure 23-38. The Glenn shunt (or superior cavopulmonary anastomosis), which was originally performed as a connection of the superior vena cava (SVC) to the right pulmonary artery, has been modified in recent years and is now a shunt from the SVC directed to both branch pulmonary arteries (bidirectional). This shunt is performed in the surgical reconstructive staging that culminates in the Fontan operation. This suprasternal image demonstrates the connection of the SVC to the pulmonary arteries with low velocity (venous pattern) flow. LPA—left pulmonary artery.

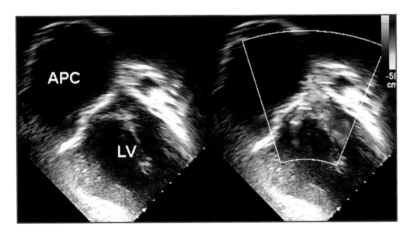

Figure 23-39. The Fontan operation (total cavopulmonary anastomosis) was first successfully performed in the 1970s and has been modified over time. The goal of the Fontan is to shunt all of the systemic venous blood flow directly to the pulmonary arteries. This operation is generally performed in patients with univentricular hearts or biventricular hearts that cannot be septated. The oldest patients who have undergone this procedure have atrio-pulmonary connections (APC), whereby the atrium is connected directly to the pulmonary artery. The long-term consequences of this type of Fontan are shown in the figure. The atrium dilates significantly with sluggish blood flow into the pulmonary arteries and there is significant risk for the development of thrombus. Many patients with APC develop atrial arrhythmias, which are likely secondary to the atrial dilatation. This apical four-chamber view demonstrates a massively dilated right atrium connected to the pulmonary arteries (APC) in a patient with a single LV. The color flow Doppler (*left panel*) shows that right pulmonary veins and atrial septal defect flow can become obstructed because of the Fontan baffle mass. The color flow Doppler indicates location and direction of blood flow (*right panel*).

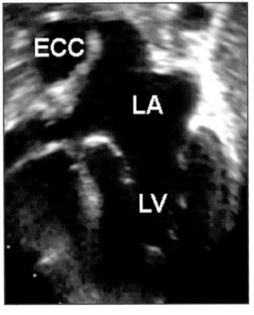

Figure 23-40. The most recent modification of the Fontan operation is the extra cardiac conduit (ECC), which is a tube graft connecting the inferior vena cava directly to the pulmonary arteries. The ECC has potential advantages over other Fontan types. The heart is not entered in order to perform the procedure, and thus these patients may have a lower risk for the development of atrial arrhythmias. In addition, the pathway does not dilate, and the flow dynamics may be improved. This apical four-chamber view demonstrates an ECC along the free wall of the right atrium in a patient with tricuspid atresia. The wall surrounding the Fontan baffle often appears thickened, and in rare cases atrial septal defect restriction can occur. LA—left atrium.

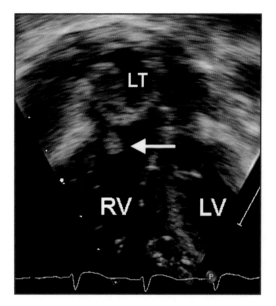

Figure 23-41. Another modification of the Fontan operation is the lateral tunnel (LT) Fontan, whereby a baffle wall is placed from the inferior vena cava to the superior vena cava, which is connected to the pulmonary arteries. Although the flow profile is better than in the atriopulmonary connection, the risk of thrombus formation is still present because of the low-flow state of the Fontan baffle. This apical four-chamber view in a patient with double outlet RV demonstrates a pedunculated thrombus on the pulmonary venous side (*arrow*) of the LT Fontan baffle. There is also a wedge of thrombus seen within the baffle (next to LT).

Suggested Reading

Ammash NM, Seward JB, Warnes CA, *et al.*: Partial anomalous pulmonary venous connection: diagnosis by transesophageal echocardiography. *J Am Coll Cardiol* 1997, 29:1351–1358.

Bharati S, Lev M: The spectrum of common atrioventricular orifice (canal). *Am Heart J* 1973, 86:553-561.

Blalock A, Taussig HB: The surgical treatment of malformations of the heart in which there is pulmonary stenosis or pulmonary atresia. *JAMA* 1945, 128:189–202.

Fontan F, Baudet E: Surgical repair of tricuspid atresia. *Thorax* 1971, 26:240–248.

Gatzoulis MA, Li J, Ho SY: The echocardiographic anatomy of ventricular septal defects. *Cardiol Young* 1997, 7:471–484.

Glenn WW: Circulatory bypass of the right side of the heart. IV. Shunt between the superior vena cava and distal right pulmonary artery: report of clinical application. *N Engl J Med* 1958, 259:117–120.

Hausmann D, Daniels WG, Mugge A, *et al.*: Value of transesophageal color Doppler echocardiography for detection of different types of atrial septal defects in adults. *J Am Soc Echocardiogr* 1992, 5:481–489.

Hoffman JI, Kaplan S: The incidence of congenital heart disease. *J Am Coll Cardiol* 2002, 39:1890–1900.

Huhta JC, Seward JB, Tajik AJ, *et al.*: Two-dimensional echocardiographic spectrum of univentricular atrioventricular connection. *J Am Coll Cardiol* 1985, 5:149–157.

Jatene AD, Fontes VF, Souza LC, et al.: Anatomic correction of transposition of the great arteries. *J Thorac Cardiovasc Surg* 1982, 83:20–26.

Keane MG, Wiegers SE, Plappert T, *et al.*: Bicuspid aortic valve is associated with aortic dilatation out of proportion to coexisting valvular lesions. *Circulation* 2000, 102(19 Suppl 3):III35–III39.

LeCompte Y, Zannini L, Hazan E, *et al.*: Anatomic correction of transposition of the great arteries. *J Thorac Cardiovasc Surg* 1981, 82:629–631.

Marino BS, Wernovsky G, Dieuwertje LK, *et al.*: Neo-aortic valvular function after the arterial switch. *Cardiol Young* 2006, 16:481–489.

Murphy JG, Gersh BJ, Mair DD, *et al.*: Long-term outcome of patients undergoing surgical repair of tetralogy of Fallot. *N Engl J Med* 1993, 329:539–599.

Mustard WT, Chute AL, Keith JD, *et al.*: The surgical approach to transposition of the great vessels with extracorporeal circuit. *Surgery* 1954, 36:39–51.

Senning A: Surgical correction of transposition of the great vessels. *Surgery* 1959, 45:966–980.

Shiina A, Seward JB, Edwards WD, *et al.*: Two-dimensional echocardiographic spectrum of Ebstein's anomaly: detailed anatomic assessment. *J Am Coll Cardiol* 1984, 3:356–370.

Shinebourne EA, Macartney FJ, Anderson RH: Sequential chamber localization: logical approach to diagnosis in congenital heart disease. *Br Heart J* 1976, 38:327–340.

Smallhorn JF, Tommasini G, Anderson RH, Macartney FJ: Assessment of atrioventricular defects by two-dimensional echocardiography. *Br Heart J* 1982, 47:109–121.

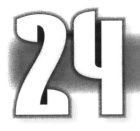

24 Perioperative Echocardiography

Stanton K. Shernan

Intraoperative echocardiography was first introduced into clinical practice in the early 1970s in the form of epicardial echocardiographic evaluation during open mitral valve commissurotomy. The introduction of intraoperative transesophageal echocardiography (TEE) in the early 1980s provided a catalyst for subsequent innovative developments, including Doppler echocardiography, high-resolution two-dimensional, and most recently, three-dimensional echocardiographic imaging. Over the past 30 years, the use of perioperative echocardiography has become increasingly more evident as anesthesiologists, cardiologists, and surgeons continue to appreciate its potential application as an invaluable diagnostic tool and monitor of cardiac performance for the management of surgical patients. Currently, perioperative TEE has been shown to influence cardiac anesthesia and surgical management of patients in over 50% of cases according to various reports.

The essential information provided by perioperative TEE regarding hemodynamic management, cardiac valve function, congenital heart lesions, and great vessel pathology has contributed to its widespread popularity. Intraoperative epicardial echocardiography has also been used both as an adjunct to TEE and as a primary diagnostic tool in patients with contraindications to TEE, or in those in whom a TEE probe cannot be inserted. Furthermore, direct epivascular or epiaortic ultrasonographic imaging of the ascending aorta and aortic arch have also gained recent prominence as part of a multidimensional intraoperative strategy to reduce atherosclerotic emboli by facilitating the delineation of significant atheromatous disease of the ascending aorta, as well as serving as a guide in identifying aortic cross-clamp and cardioplegia delivery sites used during cardiopulmonary bypass for cardiac surgery.

The future of perioperative echocardiography remains exceptionally bright. Novel approaches directed toward repairing dysfunctional valves and congenital anomalies using complex percutaneous interventional techniques are becoming more dependent on echocardiographic imaging to assist in the positioning of devices. In addition, new technological developments in three-dimensional echocardiography will perhaps allow for the development of virtual surgical programs that can be used for preoperative planning, as well as more efficient and accurate acquisition of comprehensive intraoperative echocardiographic examinations, which should facilitate the communication of important diagnostic information to surgeons and interventional cardiologists. As the clinical profile of surgical patients continues to shift towards higher-risk populations with cardiovascular disease who are predisposed to increased perioperative morbidity and mortality, the value of perioperative echocardiography as an important primary imaging modality, diagnostic tool, and monitor of cardiac performance, will almost certainly increase substantially.

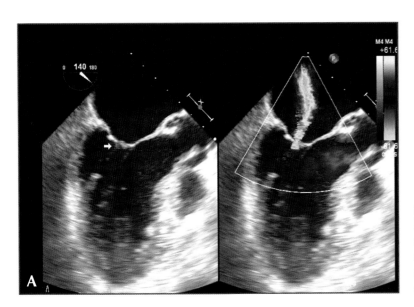

Figure 24-1. A transesophageal echocardiographic (TEE) midesophageal long-axis two-dimensional view (**A**, *left panel*) with color flow Doppler (**A**, *right panel*) demonstrates abnormal apical tethering (**A**, *arrow*) of both anterior and posterior mitral leaflets and a moderate central jet of mitral regurgitation in a patient who presented for coronary artery bypass grafting and mitral annuloplasty.

Continued on the next page

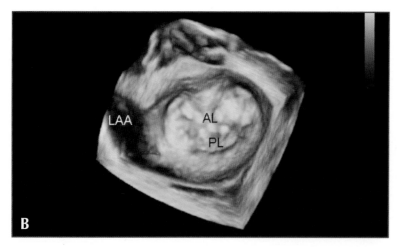

B

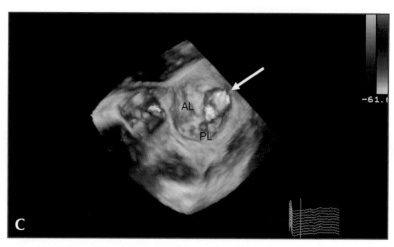

C

Figure 24-1. *(Continued)* A real time three-dimensional TEE enface view (*ie*, "surgeon's view") of the mitral valve (**B**) demonstrates an echolucent central zone of malcoaptation between the middle anterior (AL) and posterior leaf-

let (PL) scallops. A real time three-dimensional TEE enface view (*ie*, "surgeon's view") of the mitral valve (**C**) demonstrates central jet of mitral regurgitation (*arrow*). LAA—left atrial appendage.

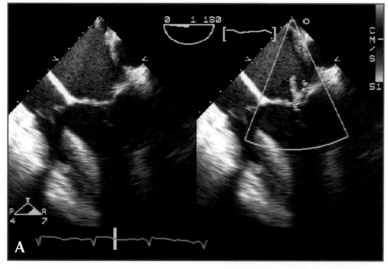

A

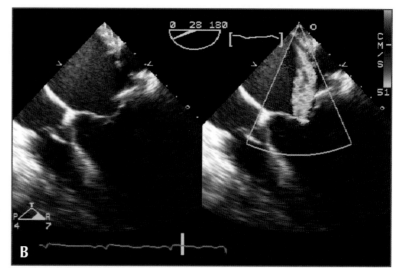

B

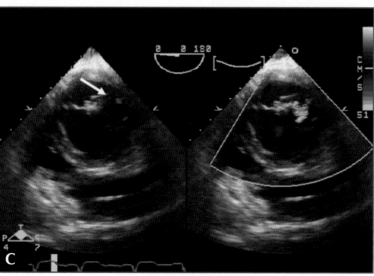

C

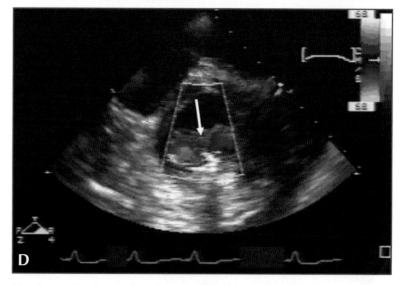

D

Figure 24-2. A transesophageal echocardiographic (TEE) midesophageal four-chamber view demonstrates the effects of general anesthesia induction on mitral regurgitation severity in a patient scheduled for coronary artery bypass grafting and mitral valve repair for moderate to severe functional mitral regurgitation (**A** and **B**). Two-dimensional (**A**, *left panel*) and color flow Doppler (**A**, *right panel*) images demonstrate the impact of a decrease in the patient's blood pressure from preoperative values following induction of general anesthesia, which is associated with an eccentric jet of only mild mitral regurgitation (**A**). After restoration of blood pressure to preoperative values with the intravenous administration of vasopressors, two-dimensional

(**B**, *left panel*) and color flow Doppler (**B**, *right panel*) images demonstrate a more moderate jet of central functional mitral regurgitation develops as shown. TEE midtransgastric short-axis two-dimensional (**C**, *left panel*) and color flow Doppler (**C**, *right panel*) views of the mitral valve in a patient with functional mitral regurgitation demonstrates primary posterior leaflet tethering (**C**, *arrow*) and an eccentric jet. An epicardial echocardiographic view demonstrates a short-axis view of the same mitral valve after an edge-to-edge mitral valve repair to optimize coaptation and create a double orifice (**D**, *arrow*) by suturing the central portion of the anterior and posterior leaflet middle scallops together.

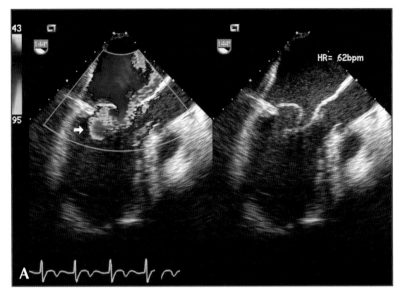

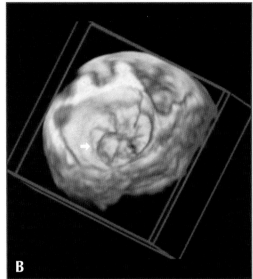

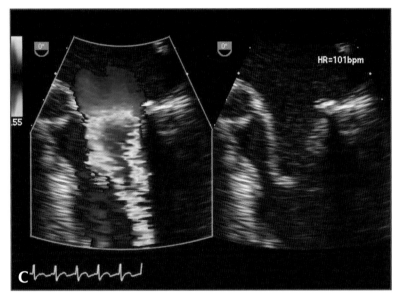

Figure 24-3. A transesophageal echocardiographic (TEE) midesophageal long-axis two-dimensional (**A**, *right panel*) view with color flow Doppler (**A**, *left panel*) demonstrates severe prolapse of the posterior mitral valve leaflet middle scallop. The color flow baseline has been shifted in the direction of the eccentric regurgitant jet to highlight the flow convergence (**A**, *arrow*) on the LV side. A three-dimensional TFE reconstruction shows severe prolapse of the posterior mitral valve leaflet middle scallop (**B**, *arrow*). A TEE midesophageal four-chamber two-dimensional (**C**, *right panel*) and color flow Doppler (**C**, *left panel*) view demonstrates a repaired mitral valve with resection of prolapsed posterior leaflet and ring annuloplasty.

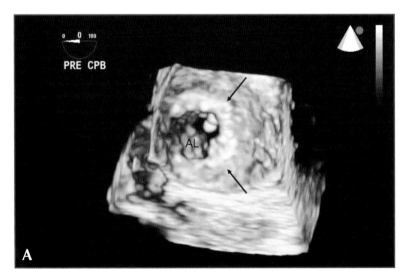

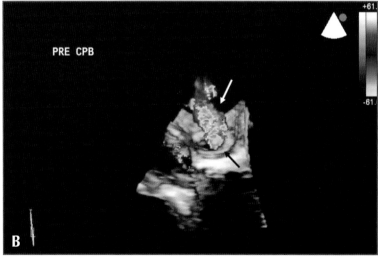

Figure 24-4. A real time three-dimensional transesophageal echocardiographic (TEE) enface view (*ie*, "surgeon's view") of mitral annuloplasty ring is shown (**A**, *black arrows*). A real time three-dimensional TEE enface view of the same mitral annuloplasty ring (**B**, *black arrow*) demonstrates a severe jet of mitral regurgitation (**B**, *white arrow*) between lateral scallops of the anterior and posterior leaflets.

Continued on the next page

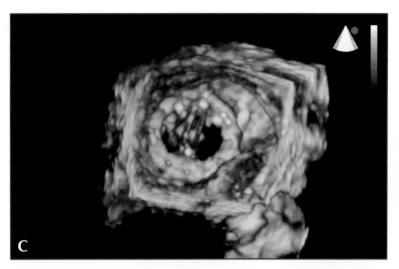

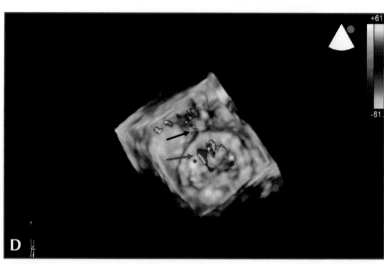

Figure 24-4. (*Continued*) Real time three-dimensional intraoperative TEE enface view with color flow Doppler demonstrates normal, bileaflet mechanical mitral valve prosthetic (**C** and **D**). Note the normal washing jets (**D**, *red arrow*) and small, insignificant perivalvular jet (**D**, *black arrow*). AL—middle anterior; CPB—cardiopulmonary bypass

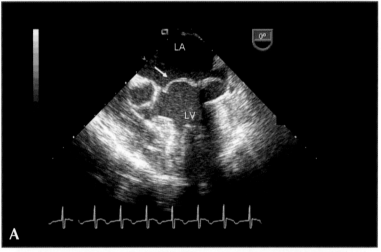

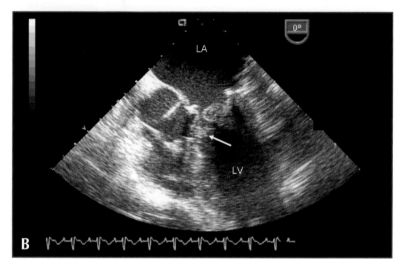

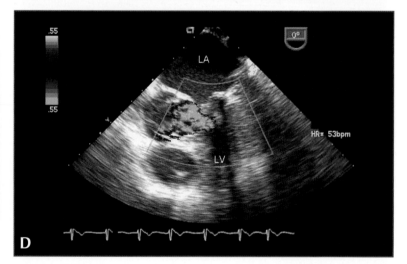

Figure 24-5. Transesophageal echocardiographic midesophageal four-chamber views show the development of systolic anterior motion and mitral regurgitation following mitral annuloplasty. The preoperative view of the mitral valve highlights bileaflet prolapse (**A**, *white arrow*) due to myxomatous degeneration (Barlow's Valve). Initial postcardiopulmonary bypass images show systolic anterior motion of the subvalvular apparatus (**B**, *white arrow*) and associated mitral regurgitation due to leaflet malcoaptation (**B** and **C**). Resolution of the systolic anterior motion after optimizing hemodynamics intraoperatively by augmenting preload and afterload is shown (**D**). The patient remained stable throughout the postoperative course. LA—left atrium.

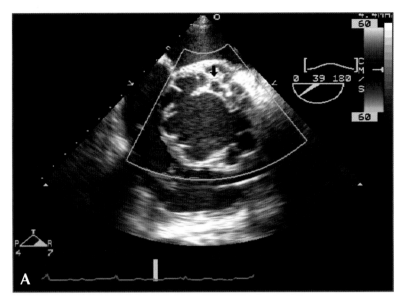

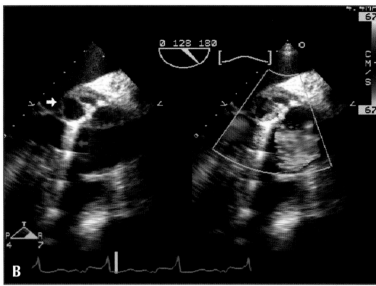

Figure 24-6. Transesophageal echocardiographic midesophageal aortic valve short-axis (**A**) and long-axis two-dimensional (**B**, *left panel*) views with color flow Doppler (**B**, *right panel*) in a patient with a bioprosthetic aortic valve who presented with large perivalvular abscess (**A**, *black arrow* and **B**, *white arrow*) and dehisced aortic valve prosthetic (**B**, *red arrow*) necessitating valve replacement are shown.

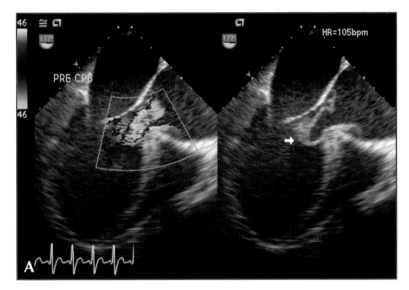

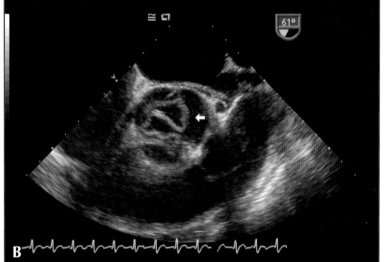

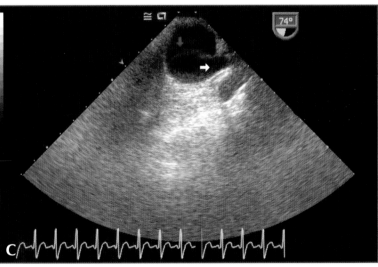

Figure 24-7. A transesophageal echocardiographic (TEE) midesophageal long-axis two-dimensional (**A**, *right panel*) view with color flow Doppler (**A**, *left panel*) demonstrating an acute ascending aortic dissection with a mobile flap is shown (**A**, *white arrow*) prolapsing across the aortic valve during diastole and moderate aortic insufficiency. A TEE midesophageal aortic valve short-axis view shows a dissection flap (**B**, *white arrow*). A TEE upper-esophageal ascending aortic short-axis view shows the dissection flap (**C**, *red arrow*) extending toward brachiocephalic artery (**C**, *white arrow*). CPB—cardiopulmonary bypass

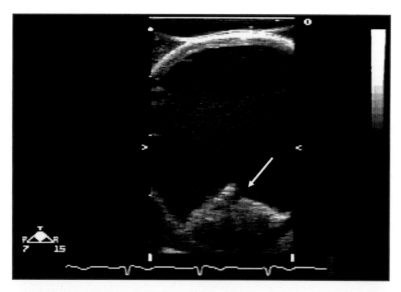

Figure 24-8. Intraoperative epiaortic ultrasonographic imaging using a linear array demonstrating a highly mobile, grade V atherosclerotic plaque (*arrow*) in the midascending aorta is shown. The patient was originally scheduled only for coronary artery bypass graft surgery, but as a result of the finding of atherosclerotic disease in the ascending aorta, hypothermic arrest was also performed during cardiopulmonary bypass in order to excise the aortic atheroma.

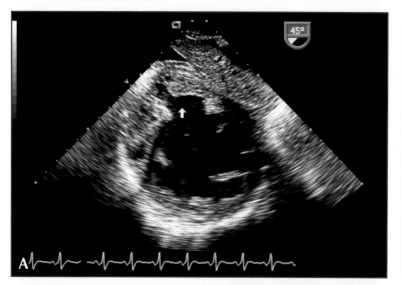

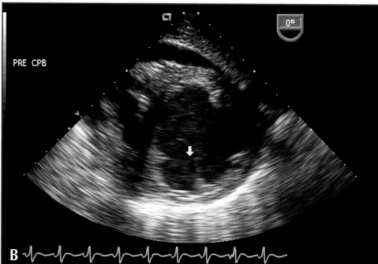

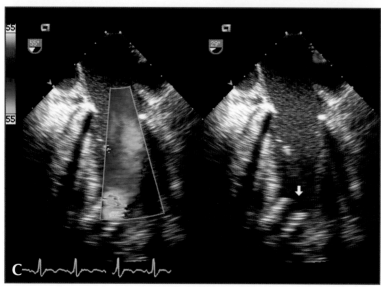

Figure 24-9. A transesophageal echocardiographic (TEE) transgastric short-axis view demonstrating an LV pseudoaneurysm in the vicinity of the inferior septum is shown (**A**, *white arrow*). A TEE transgastric short-axis view demonstrating an LV aneurysm in the vicinity of the anterior wall is also shown (**B**, *white arrow*). The patient had end-stage ischemic biventricular cardiomyopathy and presented for both LV and RV assist device placement. A TEE midesophageal four-chamber two-dimensional (**C**, *right panel*) and color flow Doppler (**C**, *left panel*) view shows the inflow cannula of the LV assist device (**C**, *white arrow*). TEE midesophageal ascending aortic long-axis (**D**, *right panel*) view with color flow Doppler (**D**, *left panel*) demonstrates the LV assist device outflow cannula (**D**, *white arrow*).

Continued on the next page

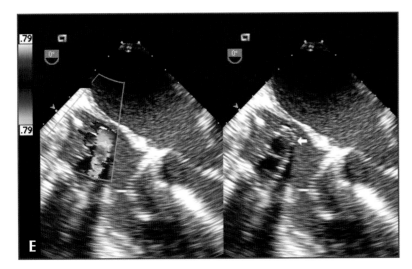

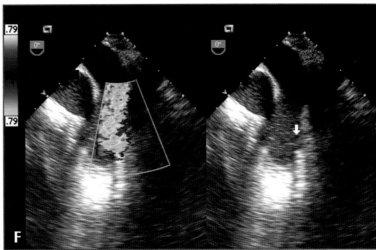

Figure 24-9. *(Continued)* TEE midesophageal four-chamber two-dimensional (**E**, *right panel*) and color flow Doppler (**E**, *left panel*) views show the inflow cannula of the RV assist device (**E**, *white arrow*). TEE midesophageal ascending aortic short-axis two-dimensional (**F**, *right panel*) view with color flow Doppler (**F**, *left panel*) demonstrates the RV assist device outflow cannula (**F**, *white arrow*) in the main pulmonary artery. CPB—cardiopulmonary bypass.

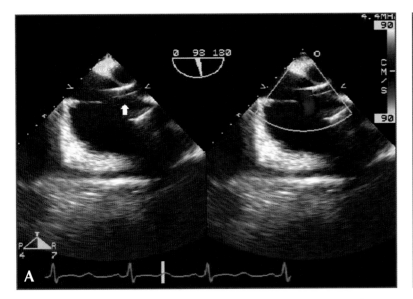

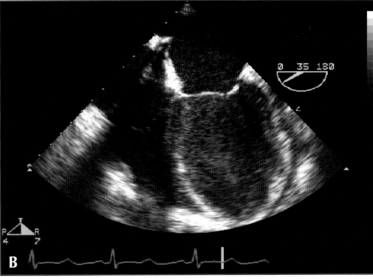

Figure 24-10. A percutaneously placed LV assist device inflow cannula (**A**, *white arrow*) is shown in the inferior cava and traversing the interatrial septum in transesophageal echocardiographic (TEE) midesophageal bicaval two-dimensional (**A**, *left panel*) and color flow Doppler (**A**, *right panel*) views. The intraoperative TEE midesophageal four-chamber view shows inflow cannula of LV assist device traversing the interatrial septum to its position in the left atrium (**B**).

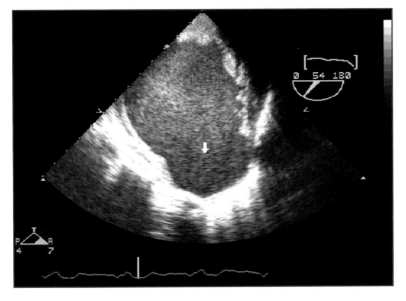

Figure 24-11. A transesophageal echocardiographic transgastric short-axis view demonstrates an LV aneurysm (*white arrow*) in the vicinity of the anterior wall. The patient underwent coronary artery bypass grafting, mitral valve repair, and resection of the ventricular aneurysm.

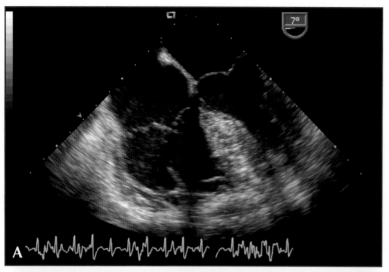

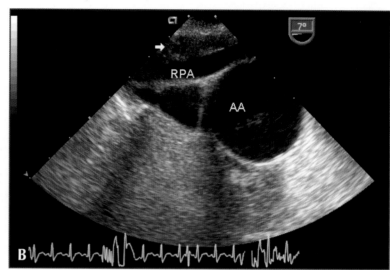

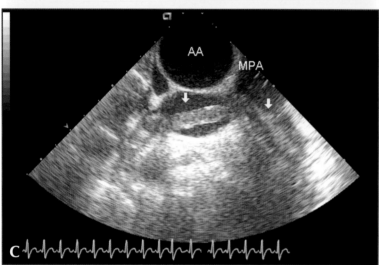

Figure 24-12. An intraoperative transesophageal echocardiographic midesophageal four-chamber view shows RV dilatation and hypokinesis in a patient with an acute pulmonary embolus (**A**). A midesophageal ascending aortic (AA) short-axis view shows thromboembolus (**B**, *white arrow*) in the right pulmonary artery (RPA). Epiaortic AA short-axis view shows pulmonary embolus (**C**, *white arrows*) in both right and left pulmonary arteries. MPA—main pulmonary artery.

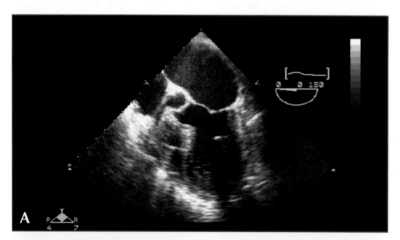

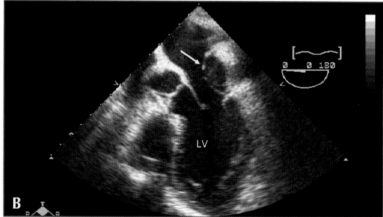

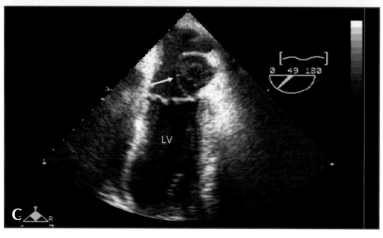

Figure 24-13. A transesophageal echocardiographic midesophageal four-chamber view shows initial normal anatomy before initiating cardiopulmonary bypass (**A**). Subsequent views in the same imaging plane (**B** and **C**) obtained after weaning from cardiopulmonary bypass show a coronary sinus dissection (**B**, *arrow*) with a progressively increasing lumen (**C**, *arrow*) due to traumatic cannulation following attempted retrograde cardioplegia catheter placement. The patient remained hemodynamically stable without further intervention and had a benign postoperative course.

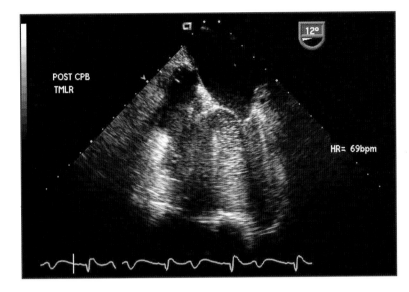

Figure 24-14. An intraoperative transesophageal echocardiographic midesophageal four-chamber view in a patient undergoing transmyocardial laser revascularization (TMLR) is shown. Visualization of bubbles within the LV cavity immediately after creation of the channel is necessary to confirm endocardial penetration by the laser. CPB—cardiopulmonary bypass.

Recommended Reading

Eltzschig HK, Rosenberger P, Löffler M, *et al.*: Impact of intraoperative transesophageal echocardiography on surgical decision-making in 12566 cardiac surgical patients. *Ann Thorac Surg* 2008, 85:845–852.

Fox J, Friedrich A, Formanek V, Shernan S: Intraoperative echocardiography. In: *Cardiac Surgery in the Adult*, edn 2. Edited by Cohn L, Edmunds LH. New York: McGraw-Hill; 2003:283–314.

Fox J, Glas K, Swaminathan M, Shernan S: Impact of intraoperative echocardiography during cardiac surgery. *Semin Cardiothorac Vasc Anesth* 2005, 9:25–40.

Hung J, Lang R, Flachskampf F, *et al.*: 3D echocardiography: a review of the current status and future directions. *J Am Soc Echocardiogr* 2007, 20:213–233.

Reeves S, Glas K, Eltzschig H, *et al.*: Guidelines for performing a comprehensive epicardial echocardiographic examination: recommendations of the American Society of Echocardiography and the Society of Cardiovascular Anesthesiologists. *J Am Soc Echocardiogr* 2007, 20:427–437.

Rosenberger P, Shernan SK, Löffler M, *et al.*: The influence of epiaortic ultrasonography on intraoperative decision making in 6051 cardiac surgical patients. *Ann Thorac Surg* 2008, 85:548–553.

Sugeng L, Shernan S, Salgo S, *et al.*: Real-time three-dimensional transesophageal echocardiography using fully-sampled matrix array probe. *J Am Coll Cardiol* 2008, In Press.

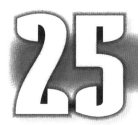

Echocardiographic Findings in Patients with Noncardiac Disease

Suma H. Konety and Elyse Foster

Various systemic illnesses lead to morphological and functional abnormalities of the heart. Among the cardiac manifestations of systemic diseases are various forms of cardiomyopathy (*eg*, dilated, hypertrophic, and infiltrative), valvular disease, pericardial disease (*eg*, pericardial thickening, constriction, and pericardial effusion), intracardiac masses, and endocarditis (nonbacterial thrombotic endocarditis). The majority of cardiac involvement can be readily detected by echocardiography. Two-dimensional echocardiography provides morphological and functional assessment, whereas Doppler and color-flow studies provide hemodynamic assessment of intracardiac pressures, valvular competencies, and diastolic function.

This chapter provides an overview of some of the common cardiac abnormalities noted in frequently encountered systemic illnesses and the key two-dimensional, Doppler, and color flow features that are helpful in diagnosing these clinical conditions.

Amyloidosis

Amyloidosis is due to deposition of the abnormal protein in various organs. Cardiac involvement occurs in up to 50% of patients with systemic primary (AL) [1] compared with less than 5% with secondary amyloidosis [2], and it can also occur in senile systemic amyloidosis because of pathologic deposition of wild-type transthyretin (TTR) molecules [3]. This disorder differs from the familial TTR-associated amyloidoses that generally occur in a younger population due to deposition of mutated forms of the amyloidogenic precursor protein. In the heart, the deposition of the amyloid protein typically leads to a restrictive cardiomyopathy. Other manifestations that can occur include syncope due to arrhythmia or heart block and angina or infarction due to amyloid accumulation in the coronary arteries. The hallmark of cardiac amyloidosis is a low QRS voltage on ECG with increased myocardial thickness and a characteristic "speckled" appearance on two-dimensional echocardiography [4]. Symptomatic heart involvement is associated with a median survival of 6 months [5]. Treatment of symptomatic cardiac amyloidosis is usually ineffective and generally consists of supportive measures. Cardiac transplantation is an option in select patients with AL amyloidosis; hepatocardiac transplantation is an option in patients with hereditary amyloidosis with advanced cardiomyopathy [6].

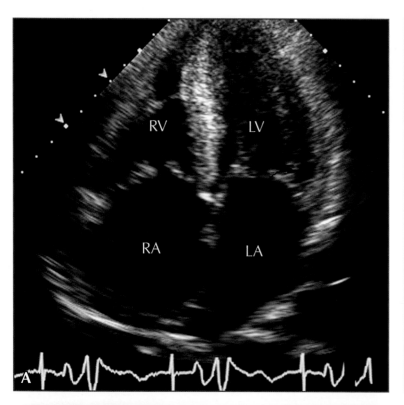

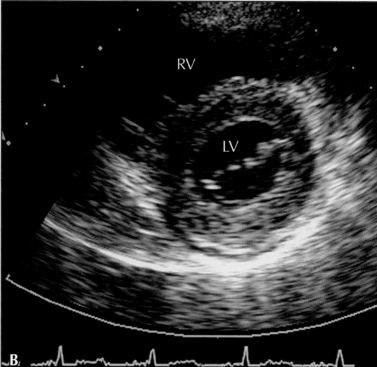

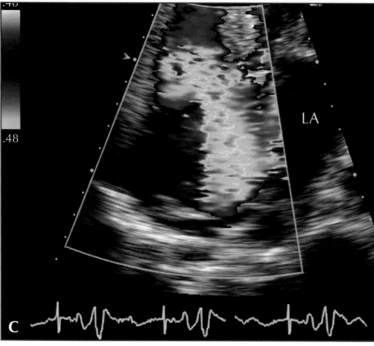

Figure 25-1. Two-dimensional echocardiography shows restrictive cardiomyopathy in a patient with cardiac amyloidosis. **A,** Apical four-chamber view shows LV hypertrophy, small LV size, and biatrial enlargement. LV ejection fraction was estimated to be 55% in this patient. LV systolic function is usually preserved initially without dilatation of the ventricular chamber, and as the disease progresses, the systolic function can gradually deteriorate. **B,** Short-axis view of the LV in the same patient shows concentric LV hypertrophy and thickening of the mitral valve. Amyloid deposits can also occur diffusely in the heart valves, resulting in thickening of the heart valves, which can lead to significant valvular insufficiency. **C,** Severe mitral insufficiency due to involvement of the mitral valve in cardiac amyloidosis is shown. LA—left atrium; RA—right atrium.

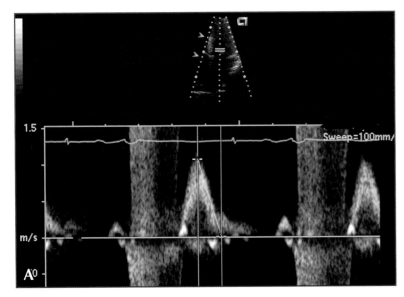

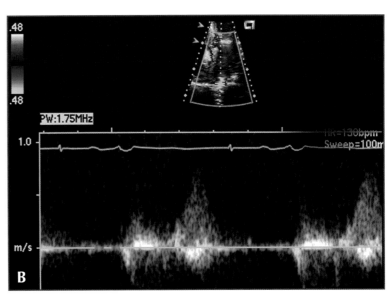

Figure 25-2. Cardiac amyloidosis is also associated with a spectrum of abnormal diastolic function, which can be evaluated with Doppler echocardiography. In early stages, abnormal relaxation (grade I diastolic dysfunction) due to increased ventricular wall thickness is seen, which later progresses to a restrictive pattern (grade IV diastolic dysfunction) when amyloidosis causes decreased LV compliance and increased left atrial pressure. The pulmonary vein flow signal should always be sought as an adjunct to the mitral inflow pattern. **A,** Mitral inflow shows an abnormal mitral inflow velocity with an E to A wave velocity ratio greater than 2 and a very short deceleration time of the E wave velocity, which is suggestive of severe diastolic dysfunction. **B,** Pulmonary vein Doppler shows a diastolic-dominant pattern consistent with elevated left-sided heart filling pressures.

Carcinoid Heart Disease

Carcinoid heart disease is caused by metastasis of a slow-growing tumor, which most commonly originates in the ileum, but can also originate in the bronchial tree. Patients can present with a constellation of symptoms, including flushing, diarrhea, bronchospasm, and hypotension, which is mediated by various vasoactive substances, including serotonin, histamine, bradykinin, and prostaglandins. Cardiac involvement occurs almost exclusively with hepatic involvement. The pathognomonic lesions of carcinoid heart disease include plaque-like deposits of fibrous tissue on the endocardium of valvular cusps, leaflets, and cardiac chambers, predominantly on the right side of the heart because the humoral substances are inactivated by the lungs [7]. Occasionally, the left-sided heart structures can be involved (< 10% of patients) [8,9]. This occurs in the presence of primary bronchial carcinoid, pulmonary metastasis, or atrial right-to-left shunt. The major therapeutic modality in such patients consists of symptom control, usually with a somatostatin analogue. Carcinoid heart disease remains a major cause of morbidity and mortality among patients with carcinoid syndrome. Cardiac valve replacement surgery prolongs survival and alleviates otherwise intractable symptoms [10].

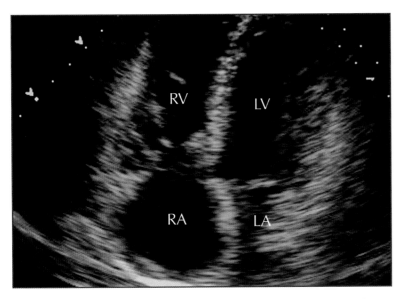

Figure 25-3. Two-dimensional echocardiography in a patient with cardiac carcinoid shows marked thickening and fibrosis of the tricuspid valve and the chordae tendinae, with restricted motion of the tricuspid valve. There is also enlargement of the right atrium (RA). LA—left atrium.

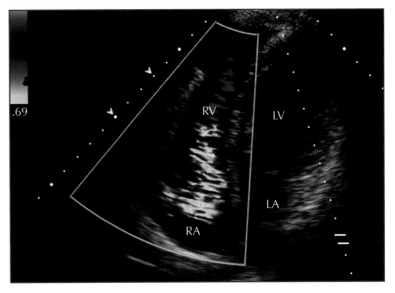

Figure 25-4. Color Doppler shows moderate to severe tricuspid regurgitation in a patient with cardiac carcinoid. LA—left atrium; RA—right atrium.

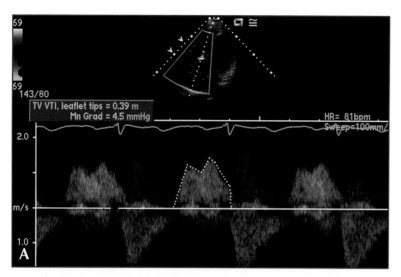

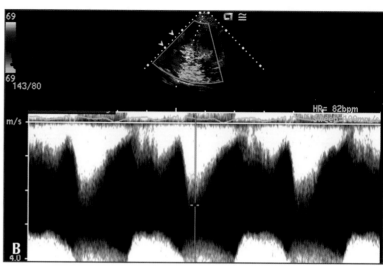

Figure 25-5. Valvular involvement could lead to varying degrees of stenosis and regurgitation in cardiac carcinoid. **A**, Continuous Doppler of the tricuspid valve (TV) shows mild to moderate tricuspid stenosis in the same patient. The calculated TV area was 2.5 cm² with a mean transvalvular gradient of 5 mm Hg. **B**, Saline-enhanced continuous Doppler across the TV estimates a pulmonary artery systolic pressure of 35 mm Hg, with an estimated right atrial pressure of 10 mm Hg in this patient. VTI—velocity time integral.

Hemochromatosis

Hemochromatosis occurs because of increased absorption of iron (*ie*, hereditary hemochromatosis) or because of secondary iron overload states (*ie*, increased oral intake of iron or secondary to multiple blood transfusions). There is deposition of iron stores in various organs, including the heart, liver, testes, and pancreas. Cardiac involvement is usually seen in advanced stages, but can present as the initial manifestation of the disease as well. Myocardial deposition of iron interferes with myocardial cellular function, and can initially present as a restrictive cardiomyopathy, which can then progress into a dilated cardiomyopathy. The typical echocardiographic findings of cardiac hemochromatosis include mild to moderate ventricle dila-

tion and LV systolic dysfunction, normal wall thickness, normal heart valves, and bilateral enlargement. Mitral and tricuspid regurgitation can result from annular dilatation. The LV diastolic filling pattern is restrictive when patients present with congestive heart failure. Given the nonspecific echocardiographic findings in hemochromatosis, cardiac MRI can be very helpful and diagnostic. Although mortality is high in untreated patients, chronic phlebotomy with control of iron levels can reverse LV dysfunction in hereditary hemochromatosis [11]. Iron chelation therapy, if initiated early, may prevent or reverse the cardiac abnormalities in iron overload states in thalassemia and sideroblastic anemia [12].

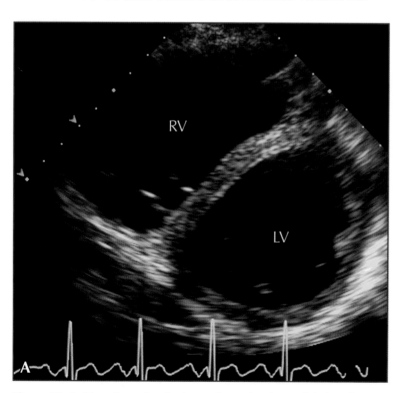

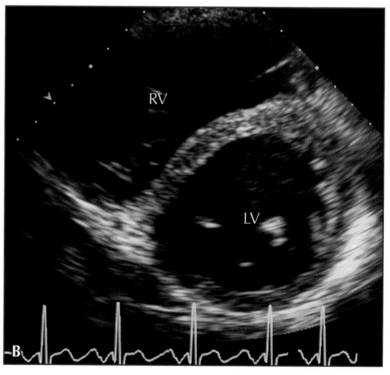

Figure 25-6. Two-dimensional echocardiography shows global LV dysfunction in a patient with hemochromatosis. **A**, Short-axis view of the LV in end-diastole shows a dilated LV. **B**, LV in end-systole shows global LV dysfunction. The estimated LV ejection fraction was 20%.

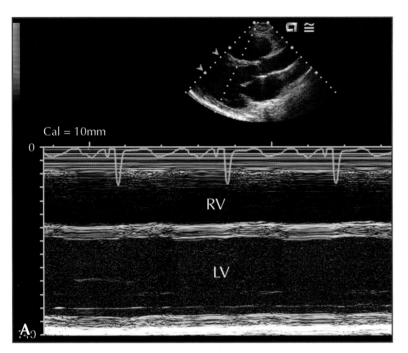
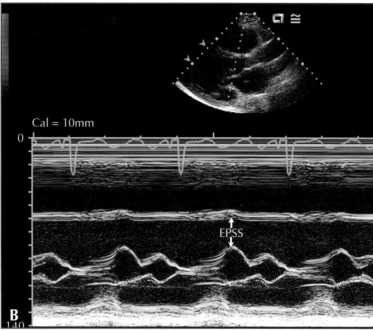

Figure 25-7. M-mode echocardiography recorded in a patient with hemochromatosis demonstrates several signs of LV dysfunction. **A**, M-mode recorded in the parasternal long-axis view shows dilated LV with an LV internal dimension of 5.8 cm in end-systole. **B**, M-mode recorded in the same patient shows an increased mitral E-point septal separation (EPSS) of 2.1 cm (normal < 6 mm). Cal—calibration.

Endomyocardial Fibrosis

Endomyocardial fibrosis is an idiopathic condition that is characterized by fibrosis of the apical RV, LV, or both. Both ventricles are affected in about half of the cases, with isolated LV involvement in 40% and pure RV involvement in the remaining 10% of cases [13]. The clinical manifestations are largely related to the consequences of impaired ventricular filling, including left- and right-sided heart failure. As a result, ventricles do not dilate, but the atria enlarge. In addition, atrioventricular valvular insufficiency can result from distortion of the subvalvular apparatus. Only in advanced cases RV failure develops with evidence of peripheral edema, hepatomegaly, and ascites. Pulmonary congestion and pulmonary hypertension are usually features of LV involvement. Medical management is often difficult. In early stages, diuretics can be used for management of volume status. Endocardial resection with atrioventricular valve replacement can result in appreciable improvement and 10-year survival of approximately 70% [14].

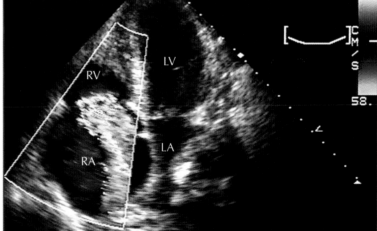

Figure 25-8. Two-dimensional echocardiography shows dense fibrous thickening of the apex and inflow tract of the RV with obliteration of the apex, which is consistent with RV endomyocardial fibrosis. Systolic function is preserved. There is massive enlargement of the right atrium (RA). LA—left atrium.

Figure 25-9. Color Doppler shows moderate to severe tricuspid regurgitation in RV endomyocardial fibrosis. The cause for tricuspid regurgitation is the tethering of the septal tricuspid papillary muscle and chordae tendinae from the fibrous process. LA—left atrium; RA—right atrium.

Hyperparathyroidism

Cardiovascular disease usually occurs in hyperparathyroidism as part of multiple endocrine neoplasia with pheochromocytoma or hyperaldosteronism. In primary hyperparathyroidism, hypertension occurs in as many as 50% of patients, with LV hypertrophy in 80% and aortic or mitral calcifications in 40% [15]. Long-standing hypercalcemia can lead to the deposition of calcium in heart valves, coronary arteries, and myocardial fibers. Dense valvular and annular calcifications can lead to varying degree of functional valvular stenosis, requiring valve replacement therapy for definitive treatment.

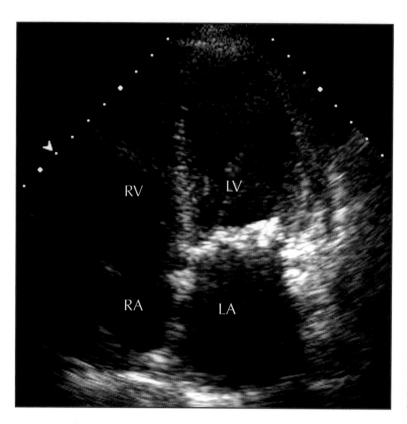

Figure 25-10. Two-dimensional echocardiography in a patient with primary hyperparathyroidism shows significant thickening and calcification of the anterior mitral valve leaflets and the annulus. The left atrium (LA) is severely enlarged. RA—right atrium.

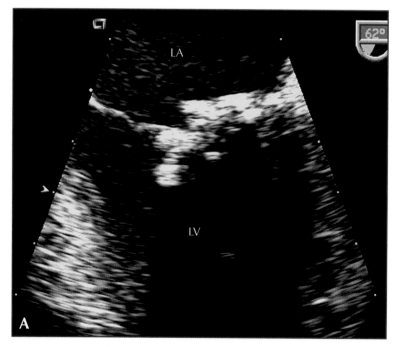

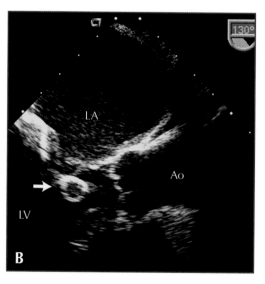

Figure 25-11. Transesophageal echocardiography in a patient with primary hyperparathyroidism identifies the mitral valve abnormalities clearly. Calcific deposits in the heart valves and in the annuli can present as mobile echobright densities with differential diagnoses that include benign cardiac tumors, metastatic tumors, or healed vegetations. **A**, Four-chamber view shows marked thickening calcification and restricted motion of the anterior mitral leaflet in real time imaging. **B**, LV outflow view demonstrates a spherical mobile mass with a calcific ring (*arrow*) attached to the ventricular side of the mitral valve. Ao—aorta; LA—left atrium.

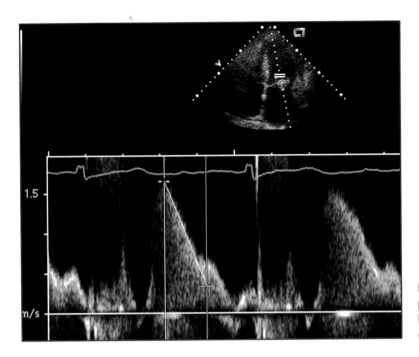

Figure 25-12. Continuous wave Doppler across the mitral valve in the same patient indicates moderate mitral stenosis with a mitral valve area of 2.7 cm² by the pressure half-time method and transmitral valvular gradients 7 mm Hg (mean) and 11 mm Hg (peak).

Systemic Lupus Erythematosus

Systemic lupus erythematosus is an autoimmune disorder with immune complexes and antinuclear antibodies with a multiorgan involvement that includes the heart. Cardiac manifestations occur in up to 50% of patients with lupus and can include pericardial disease, coronary artery disease, valvular involvement, or myocarditis [16]. Valvular thickening is a common finding in lupus and can occur in over 50% of patients. Mitral valve is commonly involved. Noninfectious vegetations (Libman-Sacks endocarditis) are usually located near the edge of the valve and consist of accumulations of immune complexes, mononuclear cells, fibrin, and platelet thrombi. Some studies suggest an association of significantly elevated levels of antiphospholipid antibodies and valvular disease [17]. These vegetations can fragment and produce systemic emboli; additionally, infective endocarditis can develop on previously damaged valves. Sequential echocardiographic studies may be necessary to document decline in LV function because the changes can be subtle. Treatment strategies are similar to treatment for systolic dysfunction and valvular dysfunction from other causes.

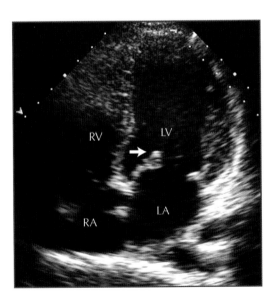

Figure 25-13. Two-dimensional echocardiography shows thickening of the mitral leaflet (*arrow*) and a verrucous nonmobile mass on the anterior mitral valve leaflet in a patient with lupus. LA—left atrium; RA—right atrium.

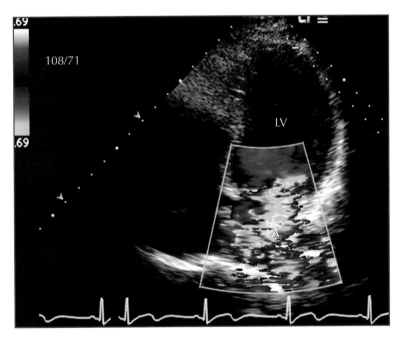

Figure 25-14. Color Doppler shows severe mitral insufficiency due to involvement of mitral valve in lupus. Valvular insufficiency occurs due to fibrosis and retraction of the valves. Less commonly, valvular stenosis can occur due to occlusion of the valvular orifice by the vegetations on the valve. LA—left atrium.

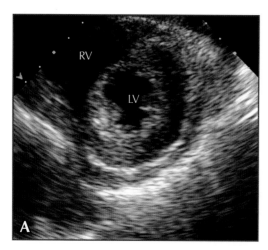

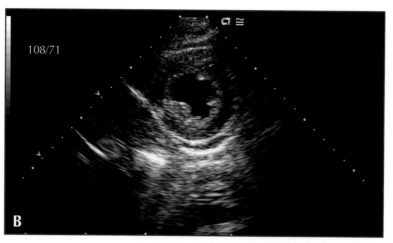

Figure 25-15. Two-dimensional echocardiography shows a decline in systolic function over a 2-year time period in the same patient with lupus. This patient had no evidence of underlying coronary artery disease. **A**, Short-axis view of the LV in end-systole demonstrates preserved LV systolic func- tion. The estimated LV ejection fraction was 70%. **B**, Short-axis view of the LV in end-systole 2 years later in the same patient shows a decline in systolic function. Estimated ejection fraction was 55%, and elevated end-systolic volume index was 40 mL/m².

Sarcoidosis

Sarcoidosis is a granulomatous disease involving multiple organs. The common manifestation is pulmonary involvement with pulmo- nary fibrosis, hilar lymphadenopathy, right-sided heart failure, and pulmonary hypertension. Cardiac involvement can be benign or life-threatening, and it is present in approximately 5% of patients with sarcoidosis; however, autopsy reports indicate presence of subclinical cardiac involvement in 20% to 30% of cases [18]. Both systolic and diastolic dysfunction can occur. Involvement of the conduction sys- tem is common, and can include heart block, ventricular arrhythmias, and sudden death [19]. Diagnosis is suspected in patients with hilar lymphadenopathy and pulmonary findings with concomitant cardiac abnormalities. Endomyocardial biopsy may be of low yield given the nonuniform involvement of the heart by sarcoidosis. Management of cardiac sarcoidosis is difficult. Pacemaker implantation may be neces- sary for advanced heart block, and implantable cardioverter defibril- lators may be needed in order to prevent sudden death. Severity of heart failure is one of the most significant independent predictors of mortality for cardiac sarcoidosis. Initiating corticosteroids prior to the onset of systolic dysfunction has shown excellent clinical out- come [20]. Heart transplantation should be considered in patients with intractable heart failure symptoms because there is significant improvement in survival of transplant recipients [21].

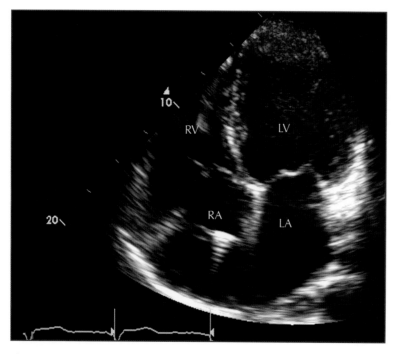

Figure 25-16. Two-dimensional echocardiography in a patient with sarcoid- osis shows a dilated and spherically remodeled LV, with significant wall thin- ning. The myocardium can sometimes be more echogenic. LA—left atrium; RA—right atrium.

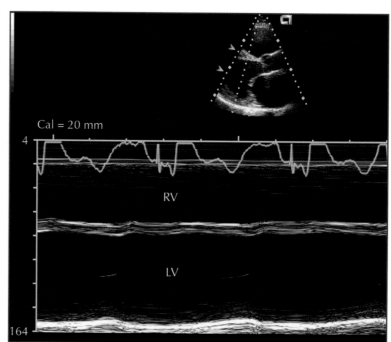

Figure 25-17. M-mode echocardiography recorded in cardiac sarcoidosis dem- onstrates that the LV is significantly dilated and is severely hypokinetic. The myo- cardium can be involved by noncaseating granulomas in sarcoidosis, resulting in myocardial fibrosis and regional wall motion abnormalities. Cal—calibration.

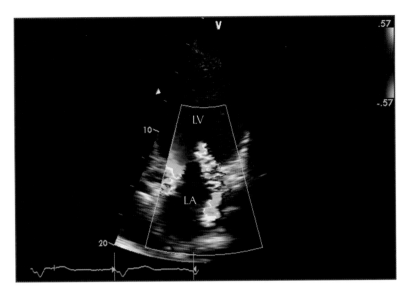

Figure 25-18. Color Doppler of the mitral valve in the same patient shows moderate to severe mitral regurgitation. Mitral insufficiency is a common finding in patients with cardiac sarcoidosis because of annular dilatation. LA—left atrium.

Sickle Cell Disease

Cardiac involvement in sickle cell disease is an important but poorly characterized entity. The presence of pulmonary hypertension is a poor prognostic factor, with a higher mortality rate in patients with pulmonary hypertension compared with those without [22]. Right ventricular dysfunction from pulmonary hypertension occurs in as many as 9% of patients [23]. Management options are very limited and include use of exchange transfusion and supplemental oxygen as required.

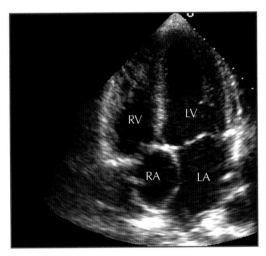

Figure 25-19. Two-dimensional echocardiography shows characteristic findings of pulmonary hypertension in a patient with sickle cell disease. There is evidence of RV hypertrophy and right atrial enlargement with bowing of the interatrial septum to the left, suggestive of elevated right atrial pressure exceeding left atrial pressure. LA—left atrium; RA—right atrium.

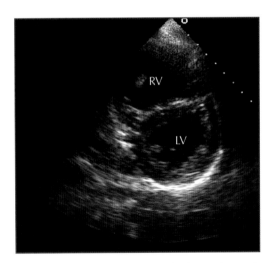

Figure 25-20. Two-dimensional echocardiography shows RV pressure overload in a patient with sickle cell disease. There is flattening of the interventricular septum during systole with a D-shaped configuration, suggestive of elevated RV pressure.

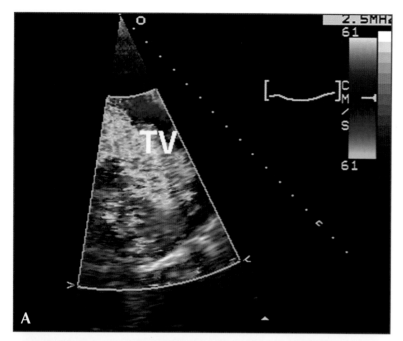

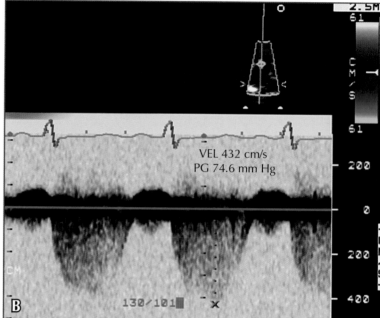

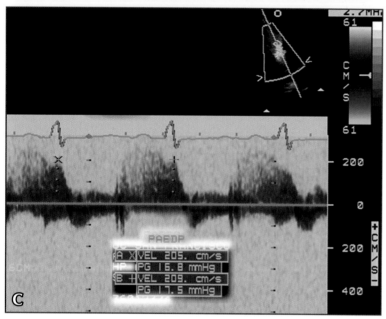

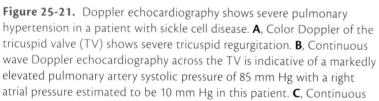

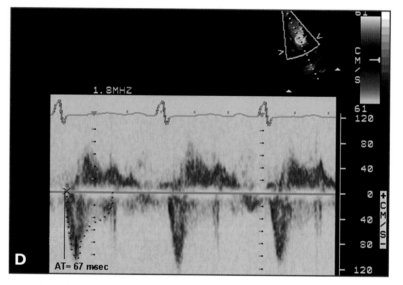

Figure 25-21. Doppler echocardiography shows severe pulmonary hypertension in a patient with sickle cell disease. **A,** Color Doppler of the tricuspid valve (TV) shows severe tricuspid regurgitation. **B,** Continuous wave Doppler echocardiography across the TV is indicative of a markedly elevated pulmonary artery systolic pressure of 85 mm Hg with a right atrial pressure estimated to be 10 mm Hg in this patient. **C,** Continuous wave Doppler suggests a significantly elevated pulmonary artery end-diastolic pressure of 27 mm Hg in the same patient. **D,** Pulsed wave Doppler of the RV outflow tract flow shows an abnormal flow pattern with a shortened acceleration time (time interval between onset of the flow to its peak velocity), suggestive of severe pulmonary hypertension. PG—peak gradient.

References

1. Dubrey SW, Cha K, Anderson J, *et al.*: The clinical features of immunoglobulin light-chain (AL) amyloidosis with heart involvement. *QJM* 1998, 91:141–157.

2. Dubrey SW, Cha K, Simms RW, *et al.*: Electrocardiography and Doppler echocardiography in secondary (AA) amyloidosis. *Am J Cardiol* 1996, 77:313–315.

3. Klein AL, Hatle LK, Taliercio CP, *et al.*: Serial Doppler echocardiographic follow-up of left ventricular diastolic function in cardiac amyloidosis. *J Am Coll Cardiol* 1990, 16:1135–1141.

4. Rahman JE, Helou EF, Gelzer-Bell R, *et al.*: Noninvasive diagnosis of biopsy-proven cardiac amyloidosis. *J Am Coll Cardiol* 2004, 43:410–415.

5. Falk RH, Comenzo RL, Skinner M: The systemic amyloidoses. *N Engl J Med* 1997, 337:898–909.

6. Sack FU, Kristen A, Goldschmidt H, *et al.*: Treatment options for severe cardiac amyloidosis: heart transplantation combined with chemotherapy and stem cell transplantation for patients with AL-amyloidosis and heart and liver transplantation for patients with ATTR-amyloidosis. *Eur J Cardiothorac Surg* 2008, 33:257–262.

7. Modlin IM, Kidd M, Latich I, *et al.*: Current status of gastrointestinal carcinoids. *Gastroenterology* 2005, 128:1717–1751.

8. Pellikka PA, Tajik AJ, Khandheria BK, *et al.*: Carcinoid heart disease. Clinical and echocardiographic spectrum in 74 patients. *Circulation* 1993, 87:1188–1196.

9. Lundin L, Norheim I, Landelius J, *et al.*: Carcinoid heart disease: relationship of circulating vasoactive substances to ultrasound-detectable cardiac abnormalities. *Circulation* 1988, 77:264–269.

10. Connolly HM, Nishimura RA, Smith HC, *et al.*: Outcome of cardiac surgery for carcinoid heart disease. *J Am Coll Cardiol* 1995, 25:410–416.

11. Rahko PS, Salerni R, Uretsky BF: Successful reversal by chelation therapy of congestive cardiomyopathy due to iron overload. *J Am Coll Cardiol* 1986, 8:436–440.

12. Glickstein H, El RB, Link G, *et al.*: Action of chelators in iron-loaded cardiac cells: accessibility to intracellular labile iron and functional consequences. *Blood* 2006, 108:3195–3203.

13. Schneider U, Jenni R, Turina J, *et al.*: Long-term follow up of patients with endomyocardial fibrosis: effects of surgery. *Heart* 1998, 79:362–367.

14. Wynne J, Braunwald E: The cardiomyopathies. In: *Braunwald's Heart Disease.* Edited by Zipes DP, Libby P, Bonow RO, Braunwald E. Philadelphia: Elsevier Saunders; 2005:1659–1696.

15. Stefenelli T, Abela C, Frank H, *et al.*: Cardiac abnormalities in patients with primary hyperparathyroidism: implications for follow-up. *J Clin Endocrinol Metab* 1997, 82:106–112.

16. Moder KG, Miller TD, Tazelaar HD: Cardiac involvement in systemic lupus erythematosus. *Mayo Clin Proc* 1999, 74:275–284.

17. Hojnik M, George J, Ziporen L, Shoenfeld Y: Heart valve involvement (Libman-Sacks endocarditis) in the antiphospholipid syndrome. *Circulation* 1996, 93:1579–1587.

18. Chapelon-Abric C, de Zuttere D, Duhaut P, *et al.*: Cardiac sarcoidosis: a retrospective study of 41 cases. *Medicine (Baltimore)* 2004, 83:315–334.

19. Roberts WC, McAllister HA, Ferrans VJ: Sarcoidosis of the heart. A clinicopathologic study of 35 necropsy patients (group 1)and review of 78 previously described necropsy patients (group 11). *Am J Med* 1977, 63:86–108.

20. Yazaki Y, Isobe M, Hiroe M, *et al.*: Prognostic determinants of long-term survival in Japanese patients with cardiac sarcoidosis treated with prednisone. *Am J Cardiol* 2001, 88:1006–1010.

21. Zaidi AR, Zaidi A, Vaitkus PT: Outcome of heart transplantation in patients with sarcoid cardiomyopathy. *J Heart Lung Transplant* 2007, 26:714–717.

22. Gladwin MT, Sachdev V, Jison ML, *et al.*: Pulmonary hypertension as a risk factor for death in patients with sickle cell disease. *N Engl J Med* 2004, 350:886–895.

23. Rich S, McLaughlin VV: Pulmonary hypertension. In *Braunwald's Heart Disease.* Edited by Zipes DP, Libby P, Bonow RO, Braunwald E. Philadelphia: Elsevier Saunders; 2005:1807–1842.

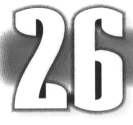

26

Clinicopathologic Correlates

Justina C. Wu and Robert F. Padera

The ultrasound examination of the heart displays structural and functional characteristics in real time. However, the final diagnosis is ultimately revealed by the pathology found at the time of biopsy, surgery, or autopsy. Follow-up with the surgeon and the pathologist is essential to refining the art of echocardiography. In many instances, diagnoses that are made by echocardiography are confirmed, and in other cases, unsuspected diagnoses or sequelae, such as microthrombi, intracardiac shunts, preexisting conditions, and tissue degeneration, are uncovered. In all cases, the astute cardiologist and sonographer should integrate the information into his or her knowledge base in hopes of improving the accuracy and clinical use of future studies.

In this chapter, we present the gross and microscopic pathology underlying both classic and unusual cases. The premise for this collection grew from a longstanding collaboration between the cardiac non-invasive and pathology laboratories at Brigham and Women's Hospital,

where pre- and postmortem data from inpatients are reviewed regularly at cardiology morbidity and mortality conferences. Furthermore, the actual gross heart specimens from explant or autopsy are reviewed with the corresponding imaging at specialized echocardiography-pathology correlation conferences. These cases were selected in order to illustrate diverse etiologies (*ie*, acquired infectious, inflammatory, oncologic, infiltrative, and vascular diseases, in addition to congenital or developmental states), which affect the different cardiovascular tissues in pathognomonic patterns. One or two examples highlight the increasing use of intracardiac and prosthetic devices with the ensuing potential for associated complications due to infection, thrombosis, or foreign body degradation. Although this chapter represents only a small sample of our growing archives, it is illustrative of the increased knowledge of cardiovascular anatomy and disease that can be gained through detailed corroboration between echocardiography and pathology studies.

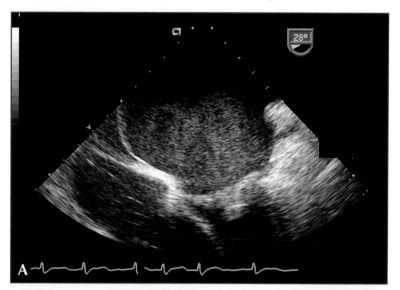

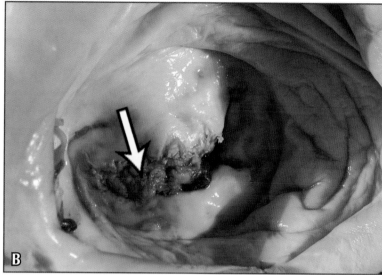

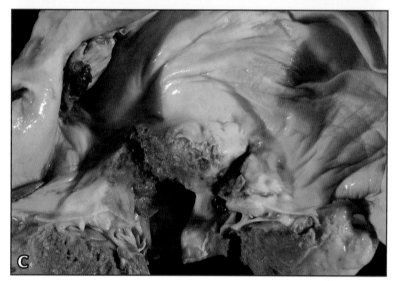

Figure 26-1. Rheumatic mitral stenosis complicated by bacterial endo-carditis. **A,** Transesophageal echocardiogram, four-chamber view of a 75-year-old woman who presented with septic shock, showing the thickened and restricted mitral valve leaflets doming in systole. There is spontaneous echocardiographic contrast, representing blood stasis in a prominently distended left atrium. The electrocardiogram shows atrial fibrillation, which is an additional risk factor for thrombus formation in the left atrial appendage. An organized thrombus was found in the left atrial appendage by transesophageal echocardiography and pathology. **B,** The mitral valve, seen from the left atrial viewpoint, demonstrates the diffuse fibrous thickening, distortion, and calcification of the valve leaflets and commissural fusion, which are characteristic of rheumatic mitral stenosis. Bacterial endocarditis is superimposed on this chronic pathology, manifest as large friable vegetation (*arrow*), causing destruction of the lateral aspect of the anterior and posterior valve leaflets. **C,** With the left side of the heart opened along the lateral wall, the massively enlarged left atrium and thickened, fused, and shortened chordae tendinea can be appreciated along with the vegetation.

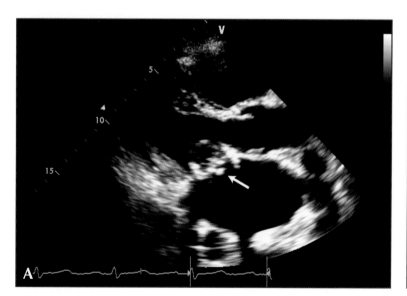

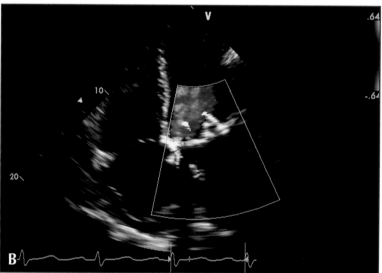

Figure 26-2. Bacterial endocarditis of a bioprosthetic mitral valve compli-cated by paravalvular leak. The patient was a 41-year-old former intravenous drug abuser who presented with an embolic stroke several months after a dental procedure. **A,** Transthoracic echocardiogram, parasternal long-axis window, showing a Carpentier-Edwards porcine bioprosthesis with thickened and degenerated leaflets. The independently mobile echogenic structure (*arrow*) on the left atrial side of the leaflet represents discrete vegetation. **B,** Apical four-chamber view with color Doppler showing a small paravalvular leak at the anteromedial aspect of the sewing ring, causing mitral regurgitation into a dilated left atrium.

Continued on the next page

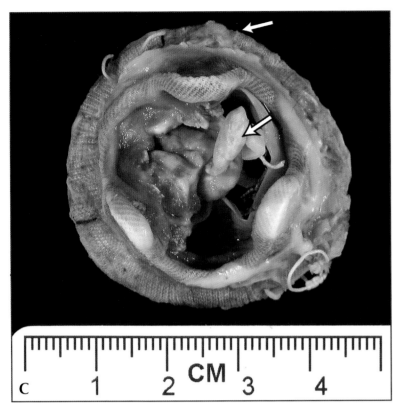

Figure 26-2. *(Continued)* **C**, The explanted valve viewed retrograde from the LV viewpoint contained large and bulky vegetation (*bottom arrow*) that traverses the axial length of the valve. The vegetation was likely caused by both stenosis, by virtue of its size and location within the orifice, and by regurgitation, by preventing adequate closure of the bioprosthetic valve cusps. The infection also involved the sewing ring (*top arrow*) and adjacent myocardium, accounting for the paravalvular leak. Microscopically, the vegetation consisted of fibrin, acute inflammatory cells and innumerable bacterial colonies, consistent with prosthetic valve bacterial endocarditis.

Oncologic Correlates

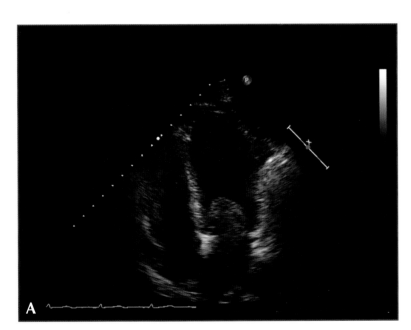

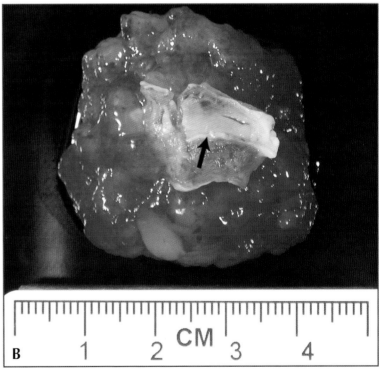

Figure 26-3. Cardiac myxoma in the left atrium. Cardiac myxoma is the most common primary tumor of the heart, and it is part of the constellation of findings in the autosomal dominant condition of Carney complex (cardiac and cutaneous myxomas with endocrinopathy) [1]. **A**, Apical four-chamber view of the heart of a 30-year-old woman with Carney complex. Classic echocardiographic features include an echogenic ovoid solid lobulated mass attached via narrow peduncle to the interatrial septum with prolapse of the mass through the mitral valve into the LV in diastole. **B**, The surgically excised specimen consisted of a myxoid, gelatinous mass with an irregular surface and attached fragment of atrial myocardium (*arrow*).

Continued on the next page

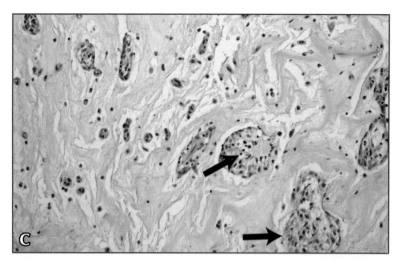

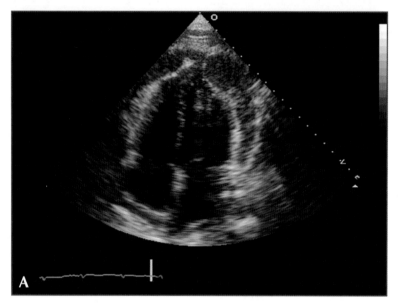

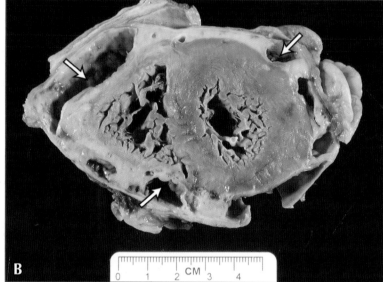

Figure 26-3. *(Continued)* **C**, Histologically, the mass is largely composed of a proteoglycan-rich extracellular matrix with relatively low cellularity. The diagnostic polygonal or stellate syncytial cells of the tumor, literally called "myxoma cells," are arranged in cords and small nests, which often form rings around small blood vessels (*arrows*), particularly near the surface of the mass.

Figure 26-4. Pericardial metastasis as well as constriction and effusion. **A**, Apical four-chamber transthoracic window of a 41-year-old man with a history of lung adenocarcinoma who presented with acute respiratory decompensation and hypotension. There are heterogenous solid thick echodensities as well as cystic spaces seen in the pericardial space circumferentially around the heart. The septum deviates leftwards with inspiration due to interventricular interdependence, and there is focal diastolic inversion at the LV apex where a small pericardial effusion is localized laterally. Spectral Doppler recordings at the mitral valve inflow and LV outflow tract confirmed significant respiratory variation consistent with effusive constrictive physiology. **B**, A transverse cross-section of the heart demonstrates metastatic tumor involving the pericardial space. There is significant degeneration and necrosis of the tumor, accounting for the cystic spaces (*arrows*) seen on the echocardiogram within the otherwise tan-white solid tumor.

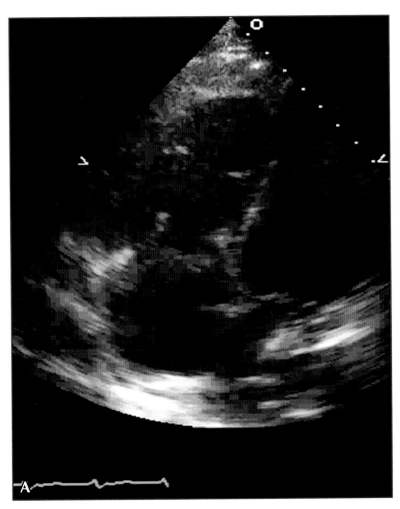

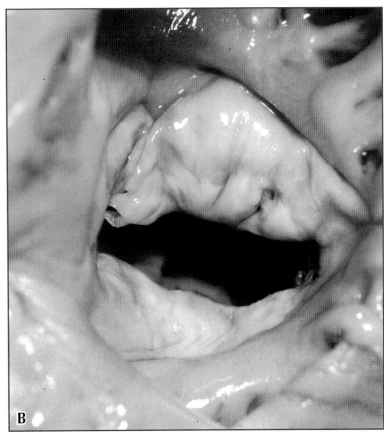

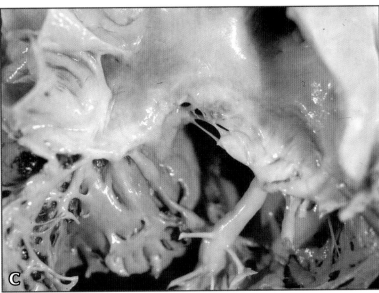

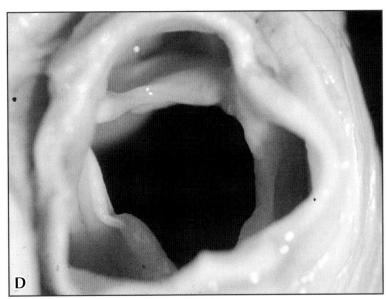

Figure 26-5. Carcinoid heart. This 64-year-old woman presented with ascites and was found to have widespread carcinoid tumor involving the gastrointestinal tract and peritoneum. She died from secondary progressive right-sided heart failure. **A**, Apical four-chamber view of the thickened and retracted tricuspid valve, which is tethered open even during systole, and the accompanying right atrial and RV enlargement, which is due to severe tricuspid regurgitation. **B**, The tricuspid valve is shown from the right atrial viewpoint, demonstrating thickened fibrotic leaflets, which essentially fix the valve in a half opened, half closed configuration leading to both tricuspid stenosis and regurgitation. **C**, The tricuspid valve is shown after opening the right side of the heart, demonstrating densely fibrotic and shortened chordae, which contribute to the regurgitation by preventing the valve leaflets from completely coapting during systole. **D**, The pulmonic valve is shown from the distal pulmonary artery viewpoint, demonstrating dense stiff cuspal fibrosis resulting in both stenosis and regurgitation. Similar pathology is seen in patients taking fenfluramine and phentermine for weight loss or ergot derivatives, such as methysergide, for migraine headaches.

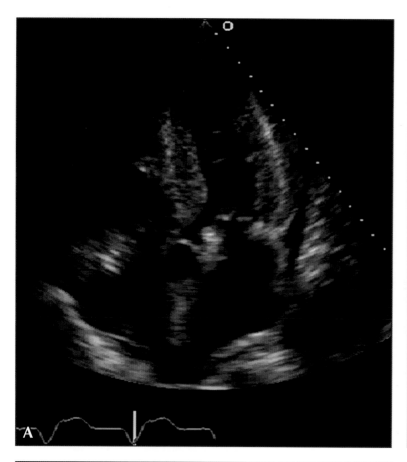

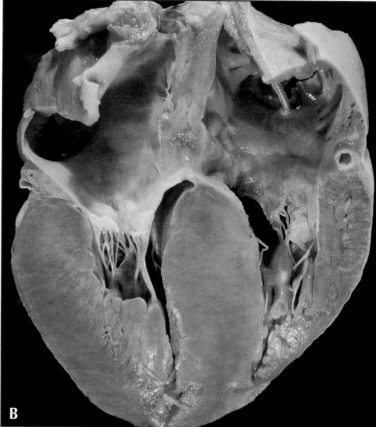

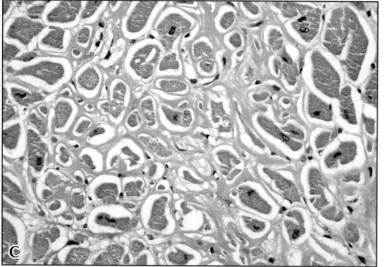

Figure 26-6. Amyloid heart. This is the heart of an 82-year-old man with refractory biventricular congestive heart failure and chronic renal insufficiency. **A**, Apical five-chamber echocardiogram revealing severe biventricular hypertrophy with a characteristic homogeneous echogenic myocardial texture. Note the biatrial enlargement, valvular thickening, pericardial effusion, and intraventricular conduction delay typically seen in this restrictive cardiomyopathy. **B**, The heart is stiff, the ventricular walls are dramatically thickened, and both atria are markedly enlarged; these are all common findings in amyloid heart specimens. The cut surface of the myocardium has a waxy appearance, and the left atrial endocardial surface is textured, giving the appearance of wax droppings. **C**, Microscopically, amyloid is found in the interstitium, encircling the cardiac myocytes in a "bricks-and-mortar" pattern and can be found in vessel walls as well (20x objective). With the routine hematoxylin and eosin staining shown here, the amyloid is light pink. A Congo-red stain will be positive in amyloid and will show apple-green birefringence under polarized light. A sulfated Alcian-blue stain would highlight amyloid in green, whereas the collagen of interstitial fibrosis would stain deep magenta.

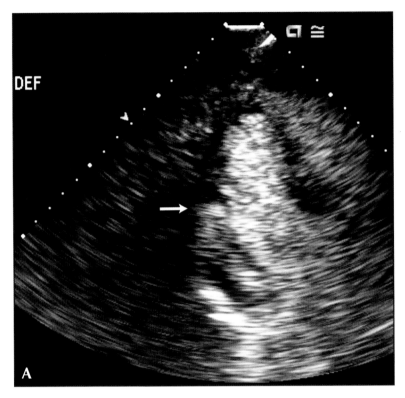

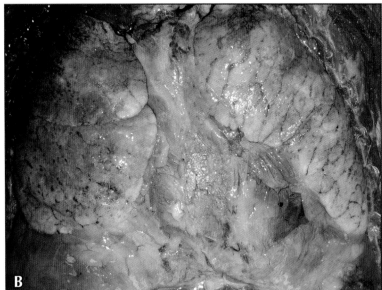

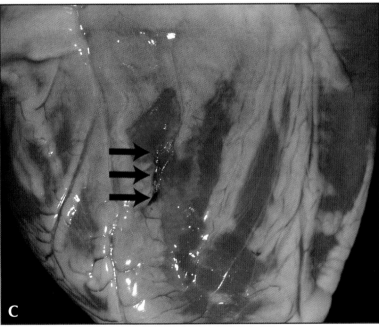

Figure 26-7. Cardiac rupture after myocardial infarction. This elderly woman died 5 days after delayed diagnosis of a large posterior myocardial infarction. **A**, Transthoracic apical three-chamber view of the heart in systole, (*arrow*) showing tracking of intravenous echocardiographic contrast from the LV cavity through the rupture site in a thinned and akinetic LV posterior wall, entering the pericardial sac (*courtesy of* Judy Mangion, Brigham and Women's Hospital, Boston, MA). **B**, The pericardium and lungs are seen after removal of the chest plate at the time of autopsy. The pericardium is distended, bulging, and filled with blood from the myocardial rupture, accounting for the abnormal blueish discoloration. **C**, A linear myocardial rupture (*arrows*) is seen in the posterolateral LV in this posterior view of the heart.

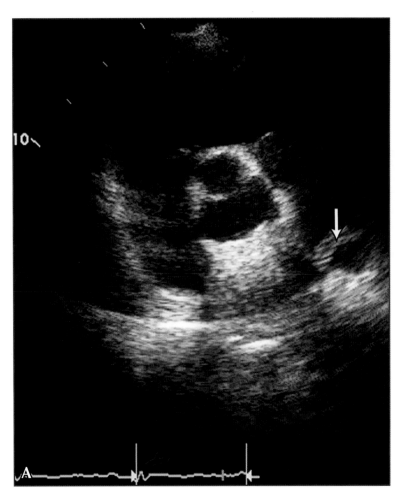

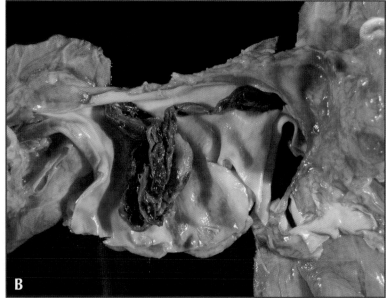

Figure 26-8. Saddle pulmonary embolus. The patient had a history of lung cancer and a known occlusive deep venous thrombus and presented with increasing dyspnea and new pleuritic chest pain. Following this echocardiogram, he was treated with alteplase, but inevitably died. **A**, Transthoracic short-axis views of the pulmonary artery bifurcation, demonstrating a long cylindrical thrombus (*arrow*) straddling the pulmonary artery bifurcation. Other views, which are not shown, demonstrate a concomitantly dilated RV with free wall hypokinesis and "strain" pattern [2]. **B**, The thromboemboli are lodged in the main pulmonary artery and extend into both the left and right main pulmonary arteries in the saddle region.

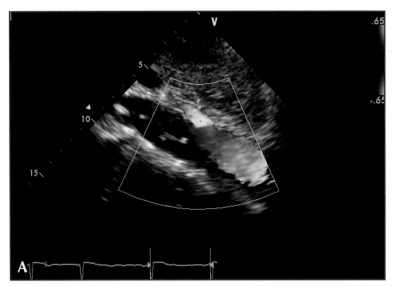

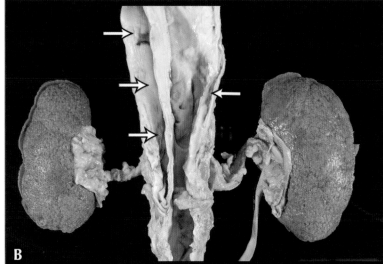

Figure 26-9. Chronic aortic dissection extending into the abdominal aorta. The patient had a history of a remote type I aortic dissection, which had been repaired with aortic valve and root replacement to the level of the arch. **A**, Subcostal echocardiographic view of the abdominal aorta. A dissection flap is seen in the lower (anatomically posterior) section of the abdominal aorta with the intima running parallel to the aortic long axis.

The false lumen is thrombosed. Systolic flow by color Doppler is seen in the true lumen and continues into the superior mesenteric artery. **B**, The dissection extended from the distal anastomosis of the graft in the thorax to the iliac bifurcation in the pelvis. The aorta has been opened posteriorly to demonstrate the false lumen (*arrows*) extending past the ostia of the renal arteries.

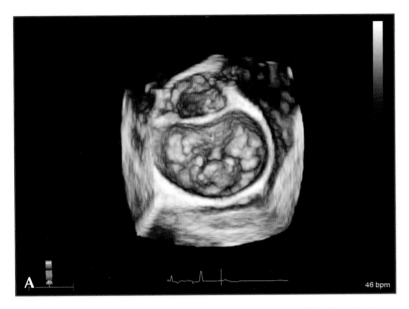

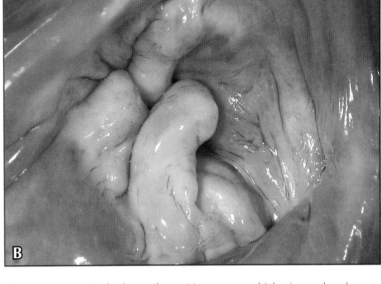

Figure 26-10. Mitral valve prolapse. Myxomatous thickening and prolapse of the mitral valve can occur in isolation in 2% to 3% of the general population [3], or may be associated with heritable collagen vascular disorders and aortic root dilatation, such as Marfan syndrome [4]. Myxomatous degeneration of the valve predisposes to severe regurgitation and chordal rupture and is a frequent indication for mitral valve repair or replacement [5]. Prolapse can affect only one or both leaflets to varying degrees. **A**, Three-dimensional transesophageal echocardiogram showing a myxomatous mitral valve from the left atrial *en face* aspect. There is billowing and prolapse of the entire middle scallop of the posterior leaflet (*courtesy of* Douglas C. Shook, Brigham and Women's Hospital, Boston, MA). **B**, The posterior leaflet of the mitral valve demonstrates marked prolapse and hooding in all segments and severe redundancy in this photograph taken from the vantage point of the left atrium. **C**, Opening the left side of the heart reveals prominent mitral leaflet hooding (*arrows*). The chordae are focally thickened but are not fused, which would be the case in rheumatic valve disease.

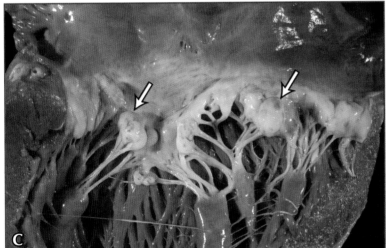

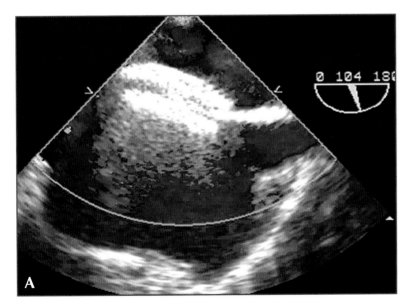

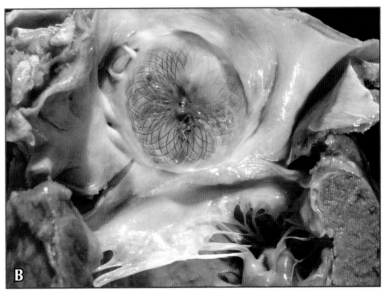

Figure 26-11. Amplatzer Nitinol (Nitinol Devices and Components, Fremont, CA) device, a self-expanding double disk made of Nitinol mesh and polyester, used for percutaneous closure of secundum atrial septal defects. Ultrasound is used to guide implantation and assess the degree of interatrial shunting. **A**, Long-axis 120°, or bicaval transesophageal view showing an Amplatzer device in cross-section, which is sandwiched securely across the interatrial septum, with no residual shunting seen by color Doppler. **B**, The left atrial aspect of the device is seen with patchy white fibrous tissue overgrowth (pannus) and focal entrapped thrombus. This device was in place for 20 months; the patient died from complications of lung transplantation for cystic fibrosis.

References

1. Reynen K: Cardiac myxomas. *N Engl J Med* 1995, 333:1610–1617.

2. McConnell MV, Solomon SD, Rayan ME, *et al.*: Regional right ventricular dysfunction detected by echocardiography in acute pulmonary embolism. *Am J Cardiol* 1996, 78:469–473.

3. Freed LA, Levy D, Levine RA, *et al.*: Prevalence and clinical outcome of mitral-valve prolapse. *N Engl J Med* 1999, 341:1–7.

4. Weyman AE, Scherrer-Crosbie M: Marfan syndrome and mitral valve prolapse. *J Clin Invest* 2004, 114:1543–1546.

5. Wilcken DE, Hickey AJ: Lifetime risk for patients with mitral valve prolapse of developing severe valve regurgitation requiring surgery. *Circulation* 1988, 78:10–14.

Index

Diastolic indices, 51
Dilated cardiomyopathy, 204–209
  mitral valve in, 29–30
Display monitor, 1
Dobutamine stress echocardiography, 81–86, 275–276
Doppler echocardiography
  Bernoulli equation in, 36, 41–44
  cardiac hemodynamics assessed by, 7–8, 35–51
  color flow, 12–14, 35
  comparison of imaging modes in, 14
  continuous wave, 12, 35
  Doppler effect in, 8
  Doppler equation in, 9, 35, 37
  in myocardial strain assessment, 271–274
  pressure-velocity relationship assessed by, 36, 41–44
  of prosthetic valves, 146–160
  pulsed wave, 9–12, 35
  quantitation and continuity of flow assessed by, 36, 38–41
  in systolic function assessment, 59–61
  tissue. See Tissue Doppler echocardiography
  valvular regurgitation assessed by, 36, 44–50
  ventricular function assessed by, 37, 50–51
Doppler equation, 9, 35, 37
Doppler velocity index
  in prosthetic valve function, 147
Dyssynchrony
  cardiac, 283–295. See also Cardiac dyssynchrony

E

Ebstein's anomaly, 31, 169, 325
Echocardiography
  artifact in, 5–6
  B-mode, 1
  clinicopathologic correlates with, 355–363
  contrast, 4, 297–305
  Doppler principles in, 7–14. See also Doppler echocardiography
  emergency, 307–320
  harmonic imaging in, 3
  image resolution in, 3
  M-mode, 25–34. See also M-mode echocardiography
  myocardial strain, 34, 271–281
  in noncardiac disease, 343–352
  perioperative, 333–341
  phased array transducers in, 2
  principles and modalities of, 1–14
  stress, 81–88
  three-dimensional, 251–253. See also Three-dimensional echocardiography
  tomographic anatomy in, 15–23
  transesophageal, 91–111. See also Transesophageal echocardiography
  transthoracic, 15–23, 141, 143–144, 162
  ultrasound waves in, 1–2
Effective orifice area
  in prosthetic valves, 148
Eisenmenger syndrome, 221–222, 325
Ejection fraction
  in dilated cardiomyopathy, 204–205
  in systolic function assessment, 57–58, 63
Electrocardiography, 186
Embolism
  evaluation of cardiac sources of, 100, 241, 244–246, 248
  pulmonary, 215–217. See also Pulmonary embolism
Emergency echocardiography, 307–320
  in acute coronary syndromes, 313
  in aortic dissection, 314–316
  in cardiac tamponade, 308–312

in cardiac trauma, 317
  overview of, 307
  postinfarction, 318–320
  in pulmonary embolism, 312–313
Emotional trauma
  cardiomyopathy from, 180, 209
Endocarditis. See also Infective endocarditis
  stroke in nonbacterial, 246
Endomyocardial fibrosis, 347
European Society of Cardiology
  cardiomyopathy classification of, 201–203
Exercise stress echocardiography, 81–85, 87–88

F

Fabry's disease, 74
Fibroelastoma
  aortic valve, 101, 126, 239
Fibrosis
  endomyocardial, 347
Filling pressures
  in diastolic function assessment, 71
Fontan operation, 331–332
Four-chamber scan planes, 15, 21
Freestyle Medtronic stentless bioprosthetic valve, 142
Friedreich's ataxia, 278

G

Gated sequential multiplane echocardiography
  real-time imaging versus, 254, 260
Genetic disorders, 195
Genetic mutations
  in hypertrophic cardiomyopathy, 183, 192–195
Glenn shunt, 331

H

Hancock porcine stented bioprosthetic valve, 142
Hand-carried cardiac ultrasound, 253, 263–267
  accuracy of, 264–265
  bedside uses for, 265–266
  equipment for, 263–264
  overview of, 253
  training for, 267
Harmonic imaging
  principles of, 3
Heart failure, 304
Hemangiosarcoma, 238
Hemochromatosis, 346–347
Hemodynamics. See Cardiac hemodynamics
Hiatal hernia
  tumor versus, 238
Hyperparathyroidism, 348–349
Hypertension
  diastolic dysfunction in, 77
  pulmonary. See Pulmonary hypertension
Hypertrophic cardiomyopathy, 183–199
  alcohol septal ablation for, 197–199
  athlete's heart versus, 194–195
  contrast imaging of, 299
  genetic mutations in, 183, 192–195
  myocardial strain echocardiography in, 277
  other genetic disorders versus, 195
  overview of, 183
  preclinical, 194
  remodeling of phenotype of, 192–194
  sudden death risk assessment in, 199
  surgical myectomy for, 196–197

I

Infective endocarditis
  aortic valve in, 127

embolization in, 245
  mitral valve in, 29, 356–357
  prosthetic valves in, 156–158
  pulmonic valve in, 170
  transesophageal imaging of, 102–105
  tricuspid valve in, 168
Inferior vena cava
  in cor pulmonale, 220
  in elevated right atrial pressure, 32, 43
Interatrial shunt, 247
Intraoperative echocardiography, 333–342
Intraventricular pressure gradient, 78
Ischemia
  myocardial strain echocardiography in, 275–276
  stress echocardiography in, 82–86

L

Lambl's excrescence
  aortic valve, 126, 249
Left atrial appendage
  normal, 99
  reduced peak emptying velocity in, 99
  spontaneous echocontrast in, 99
  three-dimensional imaging of, 261
  thrombotic, 98, 244
Left atrial pressure, 43, 69
Left atrial thrombus, 237
Left atrium, 241–249
  color M-mode imaging of, 33
  overview of, 241
  stroke and, 241, 245–249
  volumetric calculations in, 242
Left bundle branch block, 30
Left superior vena cava, 322
Left ventricle
  color M-mode imaging of, 33
  in cor pulmonale, 31
  in left bundle branch block, 30
  morphology in hypertrophic cardiomyopathy of, 184–186
  normal, 26
  normal systolic function of, 54. See also Systolic function assessment
  septal bounce in, 30
  strain imaging in, 34, 60–62
  three-dimensional imaging of, 255–257, 259
Left ventricular foreshortening, 58
Left ventricular function
  Doppler assessment of, 37, 50–51
  three-dimensional assessment of, 252
Left ventricular mass calculation, 57
Left ventricular noncompaction, 208, 299–300
Left ventricular outflow obstruction, 187–191, 326
Left ventricular scan planes, 23
Left ventricular segmentation schema, 173
Left ventricular thrombus, 236–237
Lipoma, 239–240
Lipomatous interatrial septum hypertrophy, 239
Long-axis scan planes, 15–17
Lung cancer
  pericardial metastases in, 358
  pulmonary embolism in, 362

M

Marfan's syndrome, 133–134
Masses
  cardiac, 237–240
Matrix array transesophageal transducer, 254, 263
Medtronic Hall prosthetic valve, 142
Microbubble imaging, 301–302

Rheumatic heart disease
  aortic valve in, 129
  mitral valve in, 29, 115–116, 356–357
  tricuspid valve in, 167
Right atrial pressure estimates, 43
Right atrial thrombus, 237
Right ventricular dysfunction
  in cor pulmonale, 218–219
  postinfarction, 65
  in pulmonary hypertension, 218–221
Right ventricular dysplasia, 225
Right ventricular enlargement, 222
Right ventricular infarction, 179, 223–224
Right ventricular shortening, 65
Right ventricular stroke volume calculation, 65
Right-ventricle
  double-outlet, 328
Ring down artifacts, 6

S

Sarcoidosis, 350–351
Scan converter, 1
Septal bounce, 30
Short-axis scan planes, 15, 18–20
Sickle cell disease, 351–352
Side lobe artifacts, 6
Simpson's rule method, 57
Situs solitus, 322
Speckle tracking imaging
  of myocardial strain, 273–274, 281
  of systolic function, 62–63
St. Jude's prosthetic valve, 32
Strain imaging. See Myocardial strain
  echocardiography
Strain rate
  defined, 271
  in systolic function assessment, 60–62
Stress echocardiography, 81–88
  in cardiomyopathy, 86
  contrast-enhanced, 300
  in coronary artery disease, 81–83, 85–86
  in diastolic function assessment, 79
  dobutamine, 81–86
  exercise, 81–85, 87–88
  ischemic responses to, 82–86
  normal responses to, 82
  overview of, 81
  postinfarction, 86
  in preoperative risk stratification, 85
  prognostic value of, 81, 83–84
  in valvular disease, 86–88
Stress-induced cardiomyopathy, 180, 209
Stroke, 98, 241, 244–249
  myxoma-induced, 245
Stroke volume
  Doppler assessment of, 38–40, 48
  in systolic function assessment, 58, 65
Subaortic membrane
  discrete, 129
Suprasternal notch scan plane, 15, 22
Surgery
  echocardiography during, 333–341

Systemic lupus erythematosus, 349–350
Systolic anterior motion, 187–191
Systolic function assessment, 53–65
  Doppler, 50, 59–61
  M-mode, 56
  myocardial strain rate in, 60–62
  normal physiology in, 54, 61
  overview of, 53
  postinfarction, 63–64
  right ventricular, 64–65
  three-dimensional, 55, 58
  wall motion abnormalities in, 55–56

T

Tako-tsubo cardiomyopathy, 180, 209
Tei index
  in systolic function assessment, 59
Teichholz method
  in systolic function assessment, 56
Tetralogy of Fallot, 326–327
Three-dimensional echocardiography
  in cardiac dyssynchrony, 292–295
  in myocardial infarction, 181
  overview of, 251–253
  in prosthetic valve assessment, 162
  real-time, 251–263. See also Real-time
    three-dimensional echocardiography
  in systolic function assessment, 55, 58
Thrombi
  in dilated cardiomyopathy, 208
  left atrial, 98, 237, 244
  left ventricular, 236–237, 298
  postinfarction, 175
  in pulmonary embolism, 216–217
  right atrial, 237
Thrombosis
  prosthetic mitral valve, 158–160
Time velocity integral
  in aortic valve disease, 131–132, 136
Tissue Doppler echocardiography
  in cardiac dyssynchrony, 284–285
  in diastolic function assessment, 69
  strain variables derived from, 271
  in systolic function assessment, 60
Tomographic anatomy, 15–23
Torsion
  in myocardial strain echocardiography, 272
  systolic and diastolic, 63, 77–78
Transducers, 1–2
  for three-dimensional imaging, 254, 263
Transesophageal echocardiography, 91–111
  in acute aortic syndromes, 107
  anatomy and nomenclature in, 93
  in aortic dissection, 88
  in atrial fibrillation, 98–99
  embolic event evaluation in, 100–101
  equipment for, 93
  indications for, 91
  in infective endocarditis, 102–105
  overview of, 91
  in pericardial disease, 227

preparation for, 92
  of prosthetic valves, 106, 141, 144–146, 158–160, 162
  real-time three-dimensional, 108–110
  risks and contraindications to, 92
  stages of standard examination in, 93–97
  three-dimensional, 252–253
  in valvular dysfunction, 105–106
Transient ischemic attack, 243
Transmyocardial laser revascularization, 341
Transposition of the great arteries, 327, 330
Transthoracic echocardiography
  imaging planes in, 15–23
  of prosthetic valves, 141, 143–144, 162
Trauma
  cardiac, 317
Tricuspid atresia, 169
Tricuspid regurgitation, 46, 167–168, 260
Tricuspid stenosis
  prosthetic, 154
Tricuspid valve, 165–168
  in cor pulmonale, 218–219
  in Ebstein's anomaly, 31, 169
  in endocarditis, 168
  flail leaflet in, 168
  normal, 26, 165–166
  prosthetic, 145–146, 154, 162
  in pulmonary hypertension, 218
Truncus arteriosus, 327
Tumors
  cardiac, 237–240

U

Ultrasound waves
  in echocardiographic image generation, 1–2
Unicuspid aortic valve, 124
Univentricular heart, 329

V

Valvular disease. See also specific disorders
  in infective endocarditis, 102–104
  M-mode imaging of, 27–31
  three-dimensional imaging of, 252
  transesophageal imaging of, 105–106
Valvular regurgitation. See also specific disorders
  Doppler assessment of, 36, 38–41, 44–50
Ventricular compliance assessment, 70
Ventricular relaxation assessment, 68–69
Ventricular septal defect, 319, 325
  pulmonary hypertension in, 221–222
Ventricular septal rupture
  postinfarction, 176
Ventricular tachycardia, 225
Volumetric assessment
  of systolic function, 55, 57–58
  three-dimensional imaging in, 255, 258

W

Wall motion abnormalities
  in myocardial infarction, 172–173
  pseudodyskinesis as, 181
  in stress echocardiography, 84–85
  in systolic function assessment, 55–56